D0856395

Control of
Communicable
Diseases Manual

James Chin, MD, MPH, Editor

Seventeenth Edition   2000

An official report of the American Public Health Association

American Public Health Association
800 I Street, NW
Washington, DC 20001-3710

American Public Health Association
800 I Street, NW
Washington, DC 20001-3710

Mohammad N. Akhter, MD, MPH
Executive Vice President

Ellen T. Meyer
Director of Publications

Judith B. Castagna
Production Manager

Printed and bound in the United States of America

Cover Design: Yianni Papadopoulos,
Chevy Chase, MD
Typesetting: The Mack Printing Group, Science Press Division,
Ephrata, Pa
Set in: Garamond
Printing and Binding: United Book Press, Inc., Baltimore, Md

Note on the cover design: The cover illustrates four basic
aspects of communicable disease control. Grain—proper nutrition; flask—research; syringe—prevention and treatment; hand
and soap—sanitation.

ISBN 0-87553-242-X soft cover
ISBN 0-87753-182-2 hardcover
100M 11/99

EDITORS

James Chin, MD, MPH
Editor
Clinical Professor of Epidemiology
School of Public Health
University of California, Berkeley
Mailing Address:
4578 Pine Valley Circle
Stockton, CA 95219
jchin@socrates.berkeley.edu

Michael S. Ascher, MD
Associate Editor
Chief, Viral and Rickettsial Disease Laboratory
2151 Berkeley Way
Berkeley CA 94704
Mascher@dhs.ca.gov

EDITORIAL BOARD MEMBERS

John E. Bennett, MD
Head, Clinical Mycology Section, LCI
NIAID, NIH
Clinical Center Room 11C304
National Institutes of Health
9000 Rockville Pike
Bethesda MD 20892
JBENNETT@atlas.niaid.nih.gov

John H. Cross, PhD
Professor, Tropical Public Health
Department of Preventive Medicine and Biometrics
Uniformed Services University of the Health Sciences
4301 Jones Bridge Road
Bethesda MD 20814-4799
CROSS@USUHSB.USUHS.MIL

Roger A. Feldman, MD
Emeritus Professor of Clinical Epidemiology
St Bartholemew's and the
Royal London School of Medicine and Dentistry
Whitechapel Road, London E1 1BB
r.a.feldman@qmw.ac.uk

James L. Hadler, MD, MPH
    State Epidemiologist
    State of Connecticut Department of Public Health
    410 Capitol Avenue, PO Box 340308
    Hartford CT 06134-0308
    james.hadler@po.state.ct.us

Neal A. Halsey, MD
    Professor and Director, Division of Disease Control
    Johns Hopkins University School of Hygiene and Public Health
    615 North Wolfe Street
    Baltimore MD 21205
    nhalsey@jhsph.edu

Scott B. Halstead, MD
    Adjunct Professor
    Department of Preventive Medicine and Biostatistics
    Uniformed Services University of Health Sciences
    5824 Edson Lane
    N. Bethesda MD 20852
    halsteads@erols.com

Richard B. Hornick, MD
    Vice President, Medical Education Administration
    Orlando Regional Healthcare System
    1414 Kuhl Avenue
    Orlando FL 32806-2093
    dickh@orhs.org

COL Patrick W. Kelley, MD, DrPH
    Director, DoD Global Emerging Infections System
        and the Division of Preventive Medicine
    Walter Reed Army Institute of Research
    Washington DC 20307-5100
    patrick.kelley@ana.amedd.army.mil

Ann Marie Kimball, MD, MPH
    Director, MPH Program and Community Medicine
    Associate Professor of Epidemiology and Health Services
    School of Public Health and Community Medicine, Box 357660
    University of Washington
    Seattle, Washington 98195
    akimball@u.washington.edu

John R. LaMontagne, PhD
Deputy Director, NIAID
National Institutes of Health
31 Center Drive
Building 31, Room 7A03
Bethesda, MD 20892
jlamontagn@niaid.nih.gov

Myron M. Levine, MD, DTPH
Professor and Director
University of Maryland School of Medicine
Center for Vaccine Development
685 W. Baltimore Street-HSF 480
Baltimore MD 21201
mlevine@medicine.umaryland.edu

Yvonne A. Maldonado, MD
Associate Professor
Department of Pediatrics, Room G312
Stanford University School of Medicine
300 Pasteur Drive
Stanford CA 94305
mn.yam@forsythe.stanford.edu

Stanley A. Plotkin, MD
Medical and Scientific Advisor
Pasteur Mérieux Connaught
Emeritus Professor, University of Pennsylvania
Emeritus Professor, Wistar Institute
4650 Wismer Road
Doylestown, PA 18901
splotkin@us.pmc-vacc.com

Robert E. Shope, MD
Professor of Pathology
University of Texas Medical Branch
11th and Texas Avenue
Galveston TX 77555
rshope@utmb.edu

James H. Steele, DVM, MPH
Professor Emeritus
Center for Infectious Diseases
School of Public Health
University of Texas Health Science Center
1200 Herman Pressler
Houston TX 77225
[c/o] pcoleman@utsph.sph.uth.tmc.edu

Karl A. Western, MD, DTPH
   Assistant Director for International Research
   NIAID, Office of Tropical Medicine and International Research
   Room 3155
   6700-B Rockledge Drive
   Bethesda, MD 20892-7610
   kwestern@niaid.nih.gov

LIAISON REPRESENTATIVES

George W. Beran, DVM, PhD, LHD
   Conference of Public Health Veterinarians

Stephen Corber, MD
   Pan American Health Organization

Jacques A. Drucker, MD, MSc
   Réseau National de Santé Publique, France

David Goldberg, MB, ChB
   Scottish Centre for Infection and Environmental Health, Scotland

Neal Halsey, MD
   American Academy of Pediatrics

David L. Heymann, MD
   World Health Organization

J. Z. Losos, MD, DECH, FRCP(C) FACPM
   Department of National Health and Welfare, Canada

Edward D. O'Brien, BAppSc BMed MAppEpid MIEEE FAFPHM
   National Centre for Disease Control, Department of Health
   and Aged Care, Australia

Alison Roberts
   Ministry of Health, New Zealand

Eileen Rubery, MD
   Department of Health, England

Dixie E. Snider, Jr., MD, MPH
   Centers for Disease Control and Prevention

F. E. Thompson, Jr., MD, MPH
   Association of State and Territorial Health Officers

CAPT David H. Trump, MD, MPH
   U.S. Department of Defense

TABLE OF CONTENTS

EDITORIAL BOARD iii
LIAISON REPRESENTATIVES vi
FOREWORD xv
PREFACE xvii
ORGANIZATION AND CONTENTS OF CCDM xxi
SURVEILLANCE AND REPORTING OF COMMUNICABLE DISEASES. xxv
ACQUIRED IMMUNODEFICIENCY SYNDROME 1
ACTINOMYCOSIS 9
AMOEBIASIS 11
ANGIOSTRONGYLIASIS 15
   ABDOMINAL 17
   INTESTINAL 17
ANISAKIASIS 18
ANTHRAX 20
ARENAVIRAL HEMORRHAGIC FEVERS IN SOUTH AMERICA 26
ARTHROPOD-BORNE VIRAL DISEASES 28
   INTRODUCTION 28
   TABLE: DISEASES IN HUMANS CAUSED BY ARTHROPOD-
     BORNE VIRUSES 30
ARTHROPOD-BORNE VIRAL ARTHRITIS AND RASH 37
ARTHROPOD-BORNE VIRAL ENCEPHALITIDES 39
   I. MOSQUITO-BORNE VIRAL ENCEPHALITIDES 39
   II. TICKBORNE VIRAL ENCEPHALITIDES 43
ARTHROPOD-BORNE VIRAL FEVERS 45
   I. MOSQUITO-BORNE AND *CULICOIDES*-BORNE VIRAL
     FEVERS 45
     I.A. VENEZUELAN EQUINE ENCEPHALOMYELITIS VIRUS
       DISEASE 45
     I.B. OTHER MOSQUITO-BORNE AND *CULICOIDES*-BORNE
       FEVERS 48
   II. TICKBORNE VIRAL FEVERS 50
   III. PHLEBOTOMINE-BORNE VIRAL FEVERS 52
ARTHROPOD-BORNE VIRAL HEMORRHAGIC FEVERS 54
   I. MOSQUITO-BORNE DISEASES 54
   II. TICKBORNE DISEASES 54
     II.A. CRIMEAN-CONGO HEMORRHAGIC FEVER 54
     II.B. OMSK HEMORRHAGIC FEVER 56
     KYASANUR FOREST DISEASE 56
ASCARIASIS 58
ASPERGILLOSIS 60

BABESIOSIS 62
BALANTIDIASIS 65
BARTONELLOSIS 66
BLASTOMYCOSIS 68
BOTULISM AND INTESTINAL BOTULISM 70
BRUCELLOSIS... 75
CAMPYLOBACTER ENTERITIS 79
CANDIDIASIS 81
CAPILLARIASIS 84
    I. CAPILLARIASIS DUE TO *CAPILLARIA PHILIPPINENSIS*..... 84
    II. CAPILLARIASIS DUE TO *CAPILLARIA HEPATICA* 85
    III. PULMONARYCAPILLARIASIS 87
CAT-SCRATCH DISEASE.. 87
    OTHER INFECTIONS ASSOCIATED WITH ANIMAL BITES 89
CHANCROID 90
CHICKENPOX/HERPES ZOSTER.. 92
CHLAMYDIAL INFECTIONS 97
    GENITAL INFECTIONS, CHLAMYDIAL 97
    URETHRITIS, NONGONOCOCCAL AND NONSPECIFIC 100
CHOLERA AND OTHER VIBRIOSES.. 100
    I. *VIBRIO CHOLERAE* SEROGROUPS O1 AND O139 100
    II. *VIBRIO CHOLERAE* SEROGROUPS
        OTHER THAN 01 AND 0139 108
    III. *VIBRIO* PARAHAEMOLYTICUS ENTERITIS............... 110
    IV. INFECTION WITH VIBRIO VULNIFICUS....................... 111
    V. INFECTION WITH OTHER VIBRIOS 113
CHROMOMYCOSIS... 113
CLONORCHIASIS 114
    OPISTHORCHIASIS 116
COCCIDIOIDOMYCOSIS 117
CONJUNCTIVITIS/KERATITIS 119
    I. ACUTE BACTERIAL CONJUNCTIVITIS 119
    II. KERATOCONJUNCTIVITIS, ADENOVIRAL 122
    III. ADENOVIRAL HEMORRHAGIC CONJUNCTIVITIS 124
        ENTEROVIRAL HEMORRHAGIC CONJUNCTIVITIS............ 124
    IV. CHLAMYDIAL CONJUNCTIVITIS 126
COXSACKIEVIRUS DISEASES 129
    I.A. ENTEROVIRAL VESICULAR PHARYNGITIS 129
    I.B. ENTEROVIRAL VESICULAR STOMATITIS WITH EXANTHEM . 129
    I.C. ENTEROVIRAL LYMPHONODULAR PHARYNGITIS ... 129
    II. COXSACKIEVIRUS CARDITIS 131
CRYPTOCOCCOSIS 132
CRYPTOSPORIDIOSIS 134
    DIARRHEA CAUSED BY *CYCLOSPORA*............................ 137

CYTOMEGALOVIRUS INFECTIONS.. 138
  CYTOMEGALOVIRUS DISEASE 138
  CONGENITAL CYTOMEGALOVIRUS INFECTION......................... 138
DENGUE FEVER 142
  DENGUE HEMORRHAGIC FEVER/DENGUE SHOCK
   SYNDROME 145
DERMATOPHYTOSIS.. 147
  I. TINEA BARBAE AND TINEA CAPITIS 147
  II. TINEA CRURIS AND TINEA CORPORIS............................... 149
  III. TINEA PEDIS 151
  IV. TINEA UNGUIUM 153
DIARRHEA, ACUTE 154
DIARRHEA CAUSED BY *ESCHERICHIA COLI*................................. 155
  I. ENTEROHEMORRHAGIC STRAINS 155
  II. ENTEROTOXIGENIC STRAINS 158
  III. ENTEROINVASIVE STRAINS 160
  IV. ENTEROPATHOGENIC STRAINS....................................... 161
  V. ENTEROAGGREGATIVE *E. COLI* 164
  VI. DIFFUSE-ADHERENCE *E. COLI* 165
DIPHTHERIA 165
DIPHYLLOBOTHRIASIS 171
DRACUNCULIASIS 172
EBOLA-MARBURG VIRAL DISEASES.. 174
ECHINOCOCCOSIS 176
  I. DUE TO *ECHINOCOCCUS GRANULOSUS* 177
  II. DUE TO *ECHINOCOCCUS MULTILOCULARIS*..................... 179
  III. DUE TO *ECHINOCOCCUS VOGELI* 180
EHRLICHIOSIS 181
ENCEPHALOPATHY, SUBACUTE SPONGIFORM 183
  I. CREUTZFELDT-JAKOB DISEASE 183
  II. KURU 186
ENTEROBIASIS 186
ERYTHEMA INFECTIOSUM/ HUMAN PARVOVIRUS INFECTION 189
EXANTHEM SUBITUM 191
FASCIOLIASIS.. 193
FASCIOLOPSIASIS 195
FILARIASIS 197
  DIROFILARIASIS 201
  OTHER NEMATODES PRODUCING MICROFILARIAE IN
   HUMANS... 201
FOODBORNE INTOXICATIONS 202
  I. STAPHYLOCOCCAL FOOD INTOXICATION 203
  II. *CLOSTRIDIUM PERFRINGENS* FOOD INTOXICATION 206
  III. *BACILLUS CEREUS* FOOD INTOXICATION............................ 207

   IV. SCOMBROID FISH POISONING...................................... 209
    V. CIGUATERA FISH POISONING...................................... 209
   VI. PARALYTIC SHELLFISH POISONING 210
  VII. NEUROTOXIC SHELLFISH POISONING 211
 VIII. DIARRHETIC SHELLFISH POISONING 211
   IX. AMNESIC SHELLFISH POISONING 212
    X. PUFFER FISH POISONING (TETRODOTOXIN)................. 212
GASTRITIS CAUSED BY *HELICOBACTER PYLORI* 212
GASTROENTERITIS, ACUTE VIRAL 215
    I. ROTAVIRAL ENTERITIS 215
   II. EPIDEMIC VIRAL GASTROENTEROPATHY 218
GIARDIASIS... 220
GONOCOCCAL INFECTIONS 223
    I. GONOCOCCAL INFECTION 223
   II. GONOCOCCAL CONJUNCTIVITIS (NEONATORUM) 227
GRANULOMA INGUINALE 229
HANTAVIRAL DISEASES 230
    I. HEMORRHAGIC FEVER WITH RENAL SYNDROME 231
   II. HANTAVIRUS PULMONARY SYNDROME...................... 234
HENDRA AND NIPAH VIRAL DISEASES 236
HEPATITIS, VIRAL.. 238
    I. VIRAL HEPATITIS A 238
   II. VIRAL HEPATITIS B 243
  III. VIRAL HEPATITIS C 251
  IV. DELTA HEPATITIS 253
   V. VIRAL HEPATITIS E.. 255
HERPES SIMPLEX AND ANOGENITAL HERPESVIRAL INFECTIONS....... 257
  MENINGOENCEPHALITIS DUE TO CERCOPITHECINE
      HERPES VIRUS 1 261
HISTOPLASMOSIS 262
    I. INFECTION BY *HISTOPLASMA CAPSULATUM* 262
   II. HISTOPLASMOSIS DUBOISII 265
HOOKWORM DISEASE 265
HYMENOLEPIASIS 268
    I. DUE TO *HYMENOLEPIS NANA* 268
   II. DUE TO *HYMENOLEPIS DIMINUTA* 269
  III. DIPYLIDIASIS... 270
INFLUENZA... 270
KAWASAKI SYNDROME 276
LASSA FEVER... 278
LEGIONELLOSIS AND NONPNEUMONIC LEGIONELLOSIS 281
LEISHMANIASIS 284
    I. CUTANEOUS AND MUCOSAL 284
   II. VISCERAL... 287

LEPROSY 289
LEPTOSPIROSIS 293
LISTERIOSIS 296
LOIASIS 299
LYME DISEASE 302
LYMPHOCYTIC CHORIOMENINGITIS.................................... 306
LYMPHOGRANULOMA VENEREUM 308
MALARIA... 310
MALIGNANT NEOPLASMS 323
    I. HEPATOCELLULAR CARCINOMA 324
    II. BURKITT LYMPHOMA... 325
    III. NASOPHARYNGEAL CARCINOMA 325
    IV. MALIGNANCIES POSSIBLY RELATED TO EBV 326
        IV.A. HODGKIN'S DISEASE.. 326
        IV.B. NON-HODGKIN'S LYMPHOMAS 327
    V. KAPOSI'S SARCOMA... 327
    VI. LYMPHATIC TISSUE, MALIGNANCY............................ 329
    VII. CERVICAL CANCER 329
MEASLES.. 330
MELIOIDOSIS 335
    GLANDERS 337
MENINGITIS... 338
    I. VIRAL MENINGITIS 338
    II. BACTERIAL MENINGITIS.. 340
        II.A. MENINGOCOCCAL INFECTION............................ 340
        II.B. *HAEMOPHILUS* MENINGITIS 345
        II.C. PNEUMOCOCCAL MENINGITIS 348
        II.D. NEONATAL MENINGITIS 348
MOLLUSCUM CONTAGIOSUM... 348
MONONUCLEOSIS, INFECTIOUS 350
MUMPS... 353
MYALGIA, EPIDEMIC.. 356
MYCETOMA: ACTINOMYCETOMA AND EUMYCETOMA 357
NAEGLERIASIS AND ACANTHAMEBIASIS 359
NOCARDIOSIS 362
ONCHOCERCIASIS 363
ORF VIRUS DISEASE.. 367
PARACOCCIDIOIDOMYCOSIS 369
PARAGONIMIASIS.. 370
PEDICULOSIS AND PHTHIRIASIS 372
PERTUSSIS AND PARAPERTUSSIS.. 375
PINTA... 379
PLAGUE.. 381
PNEUMONIA... 387

    I. PNEUMOCOCCAL 387
    II. MYCOPLASMAL 391
    III. PNEUMOCYSTIS 392
    IV. CHLAMYDIAL 394
        IV.A. DUE TO *CHLAMYDIA TRACHOMATIS* 394
        IV.B. DUE TO *CHLAMYDIA PNEUMONIAE* 396
    OTHER PNEUMONIAS 398
POLIOMYELITIS, ACUTE 398
PSITTACOSIS.. 405
Q FEVER 407
RABIES... 411
    CHECKLIST FOR TREATMENT OF ANIMAL BITES 417
    RABIES POSTEXPOSURE PROPHYLAXIS GUIDE 419
RAT BITE FEVER 420
    I. STREPTOBACILLOSIS 420
    II. SPIRILLOSIS 421
RELAPSING FEVER 421
RESPIRATORY DISEASE, ACUTE VIRAL.............................. 424
    I. ACUTE VIRAL RHINITIS—THE COMMON COLD 425
    II. ACUTE FEBRILE RESPIRATORY DISEASE 427
RICKETTSIOSES, TICKBORNE... 430
    I. ROCKY MOUNTAIN SPOTTED FEVER....................... 430
    II. BOUTONNEUSE FEVER 432
    III. AFRICAN TICK BITE FEVER...................................... 433
    IV. QUEENSLAND TICK TYPHUS 434
    V. NORTH ASIAN TICK FEVER 434
    VI. RICKETTSIALPOX.. 435
RUBELLA AND CONGENITAL RUBELLA 435
SALMONELLOSIS 440
SCABIES.. 445
SCHISTOSOMIASIS.. 447
SHIGELLOSIS.. 451
SMALLPOX 455
    VACCINIA 457
    MONKEYPOX 458
SPOROTRICHOSIS 459
STAPHYLOCOCCAL DISEASES 460
    I. IN THE COMMUNITY 461
    II. IN HOSPITAL NURSERIES 464
    III. ON HOSPITAL MEDICAL AND SURGICAL WARDS 467
    IV. TOXIC SHOCK SYNDROME 469
STREPTOCOCCAL DISEASES CAUSED BY GROUP A
    (BETA HEMOLYTIC) STREPTOCOCCI 470
    GROUP B STREPTOCOCCAL SEPSIS OF THE NEWBORN 477

DENTAL CARIES OF EARLY CHILDHOOD 477
STRONGYLOIDIASIS 478
SYPHILIS 481
    I. SYPHILIS 481
    II. NONVENEREAL ENDEMIC SYPHILIS 486
TAENIASIS 488
    ASIAN TAENIASIS 491
TETANUS 491
    TETANUS NEONATORUM 495
    TABLE: SUMMARY GUIDE TO TETANUS PROPHYLAXIS
      IN ROUTINE WOUND MANAGEMENT 496
TOXOCARIASIS 497
    GNATHOSTOMIASIS 499
    CUTANEOUS LARVA MIGRANS 500
TOXOPLASMOSIS 500
    CONGENITAL TOXOPLASMOSIS 500
TRACHOMA 504
TRENCH FEVER 506
TRICHINELLOSIS 508
TRICHOMONIASIS 511
TRICHURIASIS 513
TRYPANOSOMIASIS 514
    I. AFRICAN 514
    II. AMERICAN 518
TUBERCULOSIS 521
    DISEASES DUE TO OTHER MYCOBACTERIA 530
TULAREMIA 532
TYPHOID FEVER AND PARATYPHOID FEVER 535
TYPHUS FEVER 541
    I. EPIDEMIC LOUSEBORNE 541
    II. ENDEMIC FLEABORNE 544
    III. SCRUB TYPHUS 545
WARTS, VIRAL 548
YAWS 550
YELLOW FEVER 553
YERSINIOSIS 558
ZYGOMYCOSIS 561
    MUCORMYCOSIS 562
    ENTOMOPHTHORAMYCOSIS 563

ABBREVIATIONS 565
DEFINITIONS 567
INDEX 580
TABLE: IMMUNIZATION SCHEDULE 624

FOREWORD

In the 17th edition of Control of Communicable Diseases Manual (CCDM), the editors have completed extensive revisions and updates of many chapters and have added new chapters and sections to meet the emerging needs of health professionals throughout the world.

The publication started as a small, 3 x 6 inch pamphlet written by Francis Curtis, a health officer in Newton, Massachusetts. While being circulated in New England, the pamphlet caught the attention of Robert Hoyt, a health officer from Manchester, New Hampshire. Hoyt was so impressed with its worth that he presented it to APHA at its annual meeting and recommended that it be published nationally under the auspices of the Association to increase its prestige and influence. The first edition appeared in 1917. It was 30 pages long and listed 38 communicable diseases. Now a 580-page reference work listing more than 136 groups of diseases (and boasting a healthy circulation of 250,000 copies), CCDM has become a classic that sets a standard in public health. Translations have been published in many languages—Spanish, French, Italian, Portuguese, Japanese, Turkish, and Farci.

This versatile manual would not be possible without the dedication of many scientists who contribute their time, knowledge, and expertise to keep the information presented comprehensive and up-to-date. The strongest commendation must be given to the editors for their critical role in guiding this book to completion. During its 82 year history, 4 distinguished epidemiologists have served as editor of CCDM:

Haven Emerson—35 years—editions 1 through 7
John Gordon—15 years—editions 8 through 10
Abram S. Benenson—28 years—editions 11 through 16
James Chin—2 years—17th edition

The new editor, Dr. James Chin is a highly acclaimed international expert on communicable diseases, who has been associated with CCDM for the past three decades. Most recently he has served as associate editor of the 16th edition. He has done exceptional work in maintaining the highest standards of professional excellence in the development of this 17th edition. On behalf of the Association and most importantly the many health professionals who will benefit from this edition, we express our deep and sincere gratitude to Dr. Chin for his outstanding contributions to the Association, to the profession and to global health.

Mohammad N. Akhter, MD, MPH
Executive Vice President
American Public Health Association

PREFACE TO THE SEVENTEENTH EDITION

The *Control of Communicable Diseases Manual* (CCDM)—formerly *Control of Communicable Diseases in Man*—has been revised and republished about every five years by the American Public Health Association (APHA) to provide the most current information and recommendations for communicable disease prevention. The primary aim of CCDM is to provide an accurate, informative text for public health workers in official and voluntary health agencies, including those serving with the armed forces and other governmental agencies, and for health workers in foreign countries. School administrators and students of medicine and public health will also find the material useful. CCDM offers guidance to health workers in developing as well as developed countries.

As a medical epidemiologist who has worked as a researcher, program manager, and teacher of public health surveillance and control of communicable diseases for over four decades, I have been given the privilege of editing this seventeenth and millennium edition of CCDM. I was first invited to serve on the editorial board in 1975 for the twelfth edition when I was the California state epidemiologist responsible for communicable disease control. I continued as an associate editor for the thirteenth (1980), fourteenth (1985), and sixteenth (1995) editions. From 1987 to 1992, I worked for the Global Programme on AIDS (GPA) of the World Health Organization (WHO) in Geneva, Switzerland, and was not able to participate actively in the preparation of the fifteenth (1990) edition.

The five editions of CCDM that I have been involved with span a most exciting period for communicable disease control. In the 1970s, there were premature rumblings about the prospects of eradicating malaria and tuberculosis (TB). In 1976, several "new" infectious diseases were recognized—Legionnaires' disease, toxic shock syndrome, and infant botulism. That same year, "Swine flu" did not appear even though a massive vaccine program was developed in anticipation of its reemergence. The human immunodeficiency virus (HIV) was unknown during the 1970s but was probably spreading silently throughout the world during the mid-to-late 1970s. The last naturally acquired case of smallpox in the world occurred in October 1977, and WHO certified the global eradication two years later. Since then it has been more difficult to eliminate the known official stockpiles of smallpox virus. Now, as we prepare to enter the new millennium, the public health benefits of routine irradiation of ground beef and other foods are being debated just as pasteurization of milk was debated during the early part of the twentieth Century.

During the 1990s, interest and support for communicable disease control have been increasing primarily due to the resurgence of many infectious diseases such as malaria and TB, and the increasing threat of bioterrorism. Perhaps the biggest change in the field of communicable disease control will be in the format and speed of information dissemination. The use of the Internet for communications and publications will continue to increase over the next decade and future publication of CCDM online is almost a certainty. As an interim measure, CCDM was prepared in a CD-ROM format for the sixteenth edition and this may continue for the seventeenth edition. In addition, a CCDM website (http://www.ccdm.org) is being developed to provide current communicable disease prevention and control information and to provide real time updates for all diseases in the seventeenth edition and for any new emerging infectious disease problem.

My task as editor for this millennium edition was made relatively easy because Professor Abram ("Bud") Benenson, my predecessor and mentor, handed me a near perfect manual to maintain and update. The editing of this seventeenth edition was a group effort by a large number of eminent scientists and public health workers who volunteered their valuable time and efforts. The members of the editorial board, selected for their expertise (and that of their associates) on specific diseases, were each assigned chapters for review and updating by themselves or their colleagues. After review by the editor, these chapters were posted on a private CCDM website accessible to all members of the editorial board and to "liaison representatives." These representatives had been designated by various health agencies in the USA (both governmental and nongovernmental), WHO, the Pan American Health Organization (PAHO), and the health departments of Australia, Canada, England, New Zealand, and Scotland.

The many comments and criticisms received, primarily via e-mail, were all considered in preparing the penultimate version. This editorial process was fast and involved a minimal amount of paper and regular mailings. This perhaps helped to conserve a few trees! While this edition presents the composite efforts of many individuals, named and unnamed, in many countries, the ultimate decision about the contents and specific text of this edition was mine. Mine also is the responsibility for any errors or omissions in this millennium edition of CCDM.

James Chin, MD, MPH
Clinical Professor of Epidemiology
School of Public Health
University of California at Berkeley

ACKNOWLEDGMENTS

The assistance that was provided by the APHA staff to keep this edition of CCDM on track and on schedule is gratefully acknowledged. Professor "Bud" Benenson in his "retirement" continued to provide help and guidance in the preparation of this edition. In addition to acknowledging the work of all members of the editorial board and the liaison representatives, including all of their participating colleagues, I need to single out the very active contributions made by staff members of the Centers for Disease Control and Prevention.

Finally, I want to pay special tribute to my editorial assistant, Dr. Florence Morrison. No one should attempt to edit a manual such as CCDM without the assistance of someone like Florence with her vast public health experience and expertise. Her attention to detail and professional understanding of the epidemiology and prevention of communicable diseases were invaluable.

ACKNOWLEDGMENTS

ORGANIZATION AND CONTENTS OF CCDM

Each disease section in CCDM is presented in a standardized format that includes the following information:

Disease name: To avoid confusion based on varying nomenclatures in different languages, each disease is identified by the numeric code assigned by WHO's *International Classification of Diseases*, 9th Revision, Clinical Modification (ICD-9 CM) and 10th Revision, ICD-10.

The English disease names recommended by the Council for International Organizations of Medical Sciences (CIOMS) and the WHO in *International Nomenclature of Diseases,* Volume II (Part 2, Mycoses, 1st edition, 1982, and Part 3, Viral Diseases, 1st edition, 1983) have been used unless the recommended name is too different from that in current use. In that case, the recommended name is shown as the first synonym.

1. **Identification** briefly presents the principal clinical features of the disease and differentiates this disease from others which may have a similar clinical picture. Also noted are appropriate laboratory tests currently used most frequently in diagnostic laboratories for identifying or confirming the etiologic agent.

2. **Infectious agent** identifies the specific pathogen or pathogens that cause the disease; classifies the pathogen(s); and may indicate any of its important characteristics.

3. **Occurrence** provides information on where in the world the disease is known to be prevalent and in what population groups it is most likely to occur. Information on past and current outbreaks may also be included.

4. **Reservoir** indicates the ultimate and/or intermediate human, animal, arthropod, plant, soil, substance—or combination of these—that is the source of infection for a susceptible host.

5. **Mode of Transmission** describes the mechanisms by which an infectious agent is spread to humans. Such mechanisms include direct, indirect, and airborne.

6. **Incubation period** is the interval (in hours, days, or weeks) between the initial, effective exposure to an infectious organism and the first appearance of symptoms of the infection.

7. **Period of communicability** is the time (days, weeks, or months) during which an infectious agent may be transmitted, directly or indirectly, from an infected person to another person; from an

infected animal to humans; or from an infected person to animals or arthropods.

8. **Susceptibility and resistance** provides information on human or animal populations that are at risk either for acquisition of, or resistance to the disease. Information on subsequent immunity is given also.

9. *Methods of control* are described under the following six headings:

A. **Preventive measures:** for individuals and groups.

B. **Control of patient, contacts and the immediate environment:** describes those measures designed to prevent further spread of the disease from infected individuals, and specific or best current treatment to minimize the period of communicability and to reduce morbidity and mortality.

- Recommendations for isolation of patients depend first on "universal precautions," with specific measures cited from the *CDC Guideline for Isolation Precautions in Hospitals* and *CDC Guideline for Infection Control in Hospital Personnel.*

- CCDM is not intended to be a therapeutic guide. However, the most current clinical management, especially of severe diseases and those diseases no longer present in the USA, is presented in section 9B7 of each disease. Specific dosages and clinical management are indicated primarily for those diseases in which delay in instituting therapy might jeopardize the life of the patient.

- Some of the drugs needed for treatment of rare or exotic diseases may not be available commercially within the USA, but may be provided on an Investigational New Drug (IND) basis from CDC (Atlanta).

- Specific details and contact telephone numbers are included in section 9B7 for those diseases where such drugs or biologics may be available. In addition, a list of emergency telephone numbers at CDC is provided in the box below. In general, all such contact with CDC should be through local and state health departments.

C. **Epidemic measures:** describes those procedures of an emergency character designed to limit the spread of a communicable disease that has developed widely in a group or community, or within an area, state or nation.

D. **Disaster implications:** given a disaster, indicates the likelihood that the disease might constitute a major probem if preventive actions are not initiated.

E. **International measures:** outlines those interventions designed to protect populations against the known risk of infection from international sources. This section indicates any special programs, such as WHO Collaborating Centres, which might be operational. These **International Collaborating Centres** can provide national authorities with the services of consultation, collection and analysis of information, assistance in the establishment of standards, production and distribution of standard and reference material, exchange of information, training and organization of collaborative research, and dissemination of information regarding the incidence of specific diseases. WHO should be approached for further details about these Centres.

F. **Bioterrorism measures:** for selected diseases, this new section provides information and guidelines for public health workers who may be confronted with a threatened or actual bioterrorist act with a specific infectious disease agent.

Topic/Disease	Telephone number
CDC Bioterrorism hotline*	(770) 488-7100
CDC Drug Service	(404) 639-3670
Botulism	(404) 639-2206
Rabies	(404) 639-1050
Diphtheria antitoxin	(404) 639-8255

*All suspected incidents of bioterrorism should be reported immediately to the local FBI office. These numbers are available in all telephone directories and can also be obtained by calling 911.

The main CDC telephone number is (404) 639-3311. Usual working hours at CDC, Atlanta are 8:00 AM to 4:30 PM EST; Monday to Friday.

After working hours and on nonworking days (weekends and holidays), the CDC duty officer (404-639-2888) will receive and refer all emergency calls.

SURVEILLANCE AND REPORTING
OF COMMUNICABLE DISEASES

Public health surveillance can be defined as the routine collection, analysis, and dissemination of all data that may be relevant for the prevention and control of a public health problem. Epidemiology is defined as the systematic study of the factors that determine or influence the pattern and prevalence of a disease or a condition in populations. Thus, the control of any communicable disease requires an understanding of the epidemiology of that disease as well as reliable surveillance data pertinent to its prevalence and distribution. Communicable disease reporting is just one part, but an essential component of any comprehensive public health surveillance system.

The growing numbers and potential overcrowding of many human populations can facilitate transmission of communicable diseases from person to person. These factors may also contribute to epidemiologic changes or increased virulence of some infectious disease agents. In addition, the expansion of some populations into new ecologic niches can bring people into contact with new potential disease pathogens and may lead to the emergence of new disease problems.

The first step in the control of any communicable disease, regardless of whether it is a prevalent disease, a newly emerging one, or a disease used for bioterrorism, is prompt recognition and identification. To achieve this goal, an organized system of surveillance for prevalent diseases, known and recognized or new and unknown, is essential. CDC has developed a strategic plan for coping with any anticipated problems that includes the use of sentinel surveillance networks, development of several population-based centers to conduct special surveillance, and related projects that would complement routine public health activities. In addition, a new journal, *Emerging Infectious Diseases*, has been established. CDC and WHO have also significantly increased the electronic transfer of information since the mid-1990s.

However, early detection of the occurrence of any communicable or infectious disease rests on the primary health care worker who sees a case of a known communicable disease, or recognizes the first unusual patient. That physician or other health care worker is obliged to bring this to the attention of the appropriate health officer who then will manage the situation or call for support. This system of passive disease reporting is known to be relatively incomplete and inaccurate, especially for those diseases that may be widely prevalent. This passive reporting system needs to be stimulated periodically to obtain more complete and timely reports on severe communicable diseases that are of major public health concern, such as those infectious diseases caused by agents that may be used for bioterrorism. Nevertheless, communicable disease reporting remains the first line of alert for the prevention and control of communicable diseases: all public health and health care workers should be aware of those diseases that need to be reported as well as how and why they are to be reported.

REPORTING OF COMMUNICABLE DISEASES

The clinician or other responsible health care worker should without delay notify the local health authority that a communicable or a peculiar disease exists within the particular jurisdiction. Administrative regulations that describe which communicable diseases are to be reported and how they should be reported may vary greatly from one region to another because of different conditions and different disease frequencies. This manual presents a basic reporting scheme. The purpose of disease reports is to provide necessary and timely information to permit the institution of appropriate investigation and control measures by responsible health authorities. In addition, the reporting scheme encourages uniformity in morbidity and mortality reporting so that data among different health jurisdictions within a country and among nations can be compared.

A reporting system functions at four levels. The first is the collection of the basic data in the local community where the disease occurs. The data are next assembled at district, state or provincial levels. The third stage is the aggregation of the information under national auspices. Finally, for certain prescribed diseases, report is made by the national health authority to the WHO.

Consideration here is limited to the first level of the reporting system — the collection of basic data at the local level—since that is the fundamental part of any reporting scheme and a primary responsibility of local health workers. The basic data sought at the local level are of two kinds (also see Definitions, Report of a disease):

1. **Report of Cases:** Each local health authority, in conformity with regulations of higher authority, will determine what diseases are to be reported routinely. Procedures should be developed that indicate, who is responsible for reporting, the nature of the report required, and the manner in which reports are forwarded to the next superior jurisdiction.

   Physicians or other responsible health care workers are required to report all notifiable illnesses that come to their attention. In addition, the statutes or regulations of many localities require reporting by hospital, householder or other persons having knowledge of a case of a reportable disease. Within hospitals, a specific officer should be charged with the responsibility for submitting required reports. These may be individual case reports or reports of groups of cases (collective reports).

Case reports of a communicable disease provide minimal identifying data of name, address, diagnosis, age, gender and date of report for each patient, and, in some instances, other suspected cases. Dates of onset and basis for diagnosis are also useful. The right of privacy of the individual must be respected at all levels of the health system.

Collective reports are the number of cases, by diagnosis that occur within a prescribed time and without individual identifying data, e.g., "20 cases of malaria, week ending October 6."

2. **Report of Epidemics:** In addition to individual case reports, any unusual or group expression of illness that may be of public concern (see Definitions, Epidemic) should be reported to the local health authority by the most expeditious means, whether or not that illness is included in the list of diseases officially reportable in the particular locality, and whether it is a well-known identified disease or an indefinite or unknown clinical entity (see Class 4, below).

The diseases listed in this manual are distributed among five classes (see below), according to the practical benefit that can be derived from reporting.

These classes are referred to by number throughout the text under section 9B1 of each disease. The classification scheme provides a basis on which each health jurisdiction may determine its list of regularly reportable diseases. Case finding can be passive, i.e., the physician initiates the report in compliance with custom or regulation, or stimulated passive, when the health officer regularly contacts the clinicians, clinics, or hospitals, to request the desired information. Case finding is active only when the health officer or a staff member of the health department searches the hospital or hospital records to find a current case or cases of a communicable disease.

Class 1: Case Report Universally Required by International Health Regulations or as a Disease under Surveillance by WHO.

This class can be divided into the following types:

1. Those diseases subject to the *International Health Regulations (1969),* Third Annotated Edition 1983, Updated and Reprinted 1992, WHO, Geneva; i.e., the internationally quarantinable diseases—plague, cholera, yellow fever. The Regulations are currently under revision and are expected to be distributed to the World Health Assembly in the year

2002. The key notification change expected is the replacement of the current list of three diseases with a requirement to notify WHO of all disease events of "urgent international public health importance". Criteria to help countries identify which events are urgent and international are being developed and tested.

1A. Diseases under Surveillance by WHO, established by the 22d World Health Assembly—louseborne typhus fever, relapsing fever, paralytic poliomyelitis, malaria and influenza.

An obligatory case report is made to the health authority by telephone, fax, e-mail or other rapid means in an epidemic situation. Collective reports of subsequent cases in a local area on a daily or weekly basis may be requested by the next superior jurisdiction, as for example, in a cholera epidemic. The local health authority forwards the initial report to the next superior jurisdiction by the most expeditious means if it is the first recognized case in the local area or is the first case outside the limits of a local area already reported. Otherwise, reports are submitted weekly by mail or in unusual situations by telephone, fax, or e-mail.

Class 2: Case Report Regularly Required Wherever the Disease Occurs

Two subclasses are recognized based either on the relative urgency for investigation of contacts and source of infection or for starting control measures.

2A. Case report to local health authority by telephone, fax, e-mail or other rapid means. Reports are generally forwarded to next superior jurisdiction weekly by mail—except that the first recognized case in an area or the first case outside the limits of a known affected local area is reported by telephone fax or e-mail — examples are typhoid fever and diphtheria. In addition, infectious diseases caused by agents that may be used by bioterrorists (anthrax, plague, tularemia, botulism, suspected smallpox, etc.) should be reported by telephone as soon as any of these diseases are suspected.

2B. Case report by the most practicable means is forwarded to the next superior jurisdiction as a collective report, weekly by mail. Examples are brucellosis and leprosy.

Class 3: Selectively Reportable in Recognized Endemic Areas

In many states and countries, diseases of this class are not reportable. Reporting may be prescribed in particular regions, states or countries by reason of undue frequency or severity. Three subclasses are recognized: 3A and 3B are useful primarily under conditions of established endemicity as a means to lead toward prompt control measures and to judge the effectiveness of control programs. The main purpose of 3C is to stimulate control measures or to acquire essential epidemiologic data.

> 3A. Case report by telephone, fax, e-mail or other rapid means in specified areas where the disease ranks in importance with Class 2A. These diseases may not be reportable in many countries. Examples are scrub typhus and arenaviral hemorrhagic fever.

> 3B. Case report by most practicable means is forwarded to the next superior jurisdiction as a collective report by mail weekly or monthly; not reportable in many countries; examples—bartonellosis and coccidioidomycosis.

> 3C. Collective report weekly by mail to local health authority is forwarded to next superior jurisdiction by mail weekly, monthly, quarterly, or sometimes annually. Examples are schistosomiasis and fasciolopsiasis.

Class 4: Obligatory Report of Epidemics—No Case Report Required

Prompt report of outbreaks of particular public health importance by telephone, fax, e-mail or other rapid means is forwarded to the next superior jurisdiction. Pertinent data include number of cases, time frame, approximate population involved and apparent mode of spread. Examples are staphylococcal foodborne intoxication, adenoviral keratoconjunctivitis, unidentified syndrome.

Class 5: Official Report Not Ordinarily Justifiable

Diseases of this class are of two general kinds: those typically sporadic and uncommon, often not directly transmissible from person to person (chromoblastomycosis); or those of such epidemiologic nature as to offer no special practical measures for control (common cold).

Diseases are often made reportable but the information gathered is put to no practical use, and with no feedback to those who provided the data. This leads to deterioration in the general level of reporting, even for diseases of much importance. Better case reporting results when official reporting is restricted to those diseases for which control services are provided or potential control procedures are under evaluation, or epidemiologic information is needed for a definite purpose.

James Chin, MD, MPH

James (Jim) Chin is a medical epidemiologist who has worked as a researcher, program manager and teacher of public health surveillance and control of communicable diseases for more than 40 years. He was born in a small village in the Pearl River Delta area of southern China, near the city of Macau. He arrived in the USA in 1937 at the age of four and grew up in the heart of Flatbush, Brooklyn, NY. He graduated from the University of Michigan in 1954 and from the State University of New York, Downstate Medical College in 1958. He received his MPH from the School of Public Health, University of California at Berkeley in 1961 and then joined the Hooper Foundation at the San Francisco Medical Center as an International Research Fellow. He was assigned to the Institute for Medical Research (IMR) in Kuala Lumpur, Malaysia, from 1962 to 1964. After his fellowship, he joined the California State Viral and Rickettsial Diseases Laboratory as a research epidemiologist. He transferred to the Bureau of Communicable Disease Control in the California State Department of Health Services in 1968 as head of the epidemiology unit. He was appointed chief of the bureau in 1971, a position that he held until his early retirement in 1987 to join the World Health Organization (WHO). He was Chief of the Surveillance, Forecasting, and Impact Assessment unit of the Global Programme on AIDS (GPA) in Geneva, Switzerland, until his resignation from GPA/WHO in 1992.

Dr. Chin is board certified in preventive medicine and is an emeritus member of the American Epidemiological Society. He has served on several committees of the Institute of Medicine, National Academy of Sciences. He was a member of the Armed Forces Epidemiological Board, a past president of the Conference of State and Territorial Epidemiologists (CSTE) and a former chairman of the Advisory Committee on Immunization Practices (ACIP). He was the recipient of the 1993 John Snow award from the Epidemiology Section of the American Public Health Association (APHA) for distinguished service and outstanding career contributions to public health epidemiology. Currently, he is a clinical professor of epidemiology at the School of Public Health, University of California at Berkeley, an honorary professor at the University of Hong Kong and an international consultant on the impact of AIDS in developing countries. Dr. Chin and his wife Anne celebrated their 40th wedding anniversary in 1999. They have three children and three grandchildren, and they have recently moved from Berkeley to Stockton, California, to be closer to their grandchildren.

ACQUIRED IMMUNODEFICIENCY
SYNDROME   ICD-9 042–044; ICD-10 B20–B24
(HIV infection, AIDS)

1. Identification—AIDS is a severe disease syndrome that was first recognized in 1981. This syndrome represents the late clinical stage of infection with the human immunodeficiency virus (HIV). Within several weeks to several months after infection with HIV, many persons develop an acute self-limited mononucleosis-like illness lasting for a week or two. Infected persons may then be free of clinical signs or symptoms for many months or years before other clinical manifestations develop. The severity of subsequent HIV related opportunistic infections or cancers is, in general, directly correlated with the degree of immune system dysfunction. More than a dozen opportunistic infections and several cancers were considered to be sufficiently specific indicators of the underlying immunodeficiency for inclusion in the initial case definition of AIDS developed by CDC in 1982. These diseases, if diagnosed by standard histologic and/or culture techniques, were accepted as meeting the surveillance definition of AIDS developed by CDC, if other known causes of immunodeficiency had been ruled out.

In 1987, this definition was revised to include additional indicator diseases and to accept as a presumptive diagnosis some of the indicator diseases if laboratory tests showed evidence of HIV infection. In 1993, CDC again revised the surveillance definition of AIDS to include additional indicator diseases. In addition, all HIV infected persons with a CD4+ cell count of less than 200/cu mm or a CD4+ T-lymphocyte percentage of total lymphocytes less than 14%, regardless of clinical status, are regarded as AIDS cases. Aside from the low CD4 count criteria, CDC's 1993 definition has been generally accepted for clinical use in most developed countries, but it remains too complex for developing countries. Developing countries often lack adequate laboratory facilities for the histologic or culture diagnosis of the specified surrogate indicator diseases. WHO revised an African AIDS case definition for use in developing countries in 1994: it incorporates HIV serologic testing, if available, and includes a few indicator diseases as diagnostic in seropositive individuals. The clinical manifestations of HIV in infants and young children overlap with failure to thrive, inherited immunodeficiencies and other childhood health problems. CDC and WHO have published pediatric AIDS case definitions.

The proportion of HIV infected persons who, in the absence of anti-HIV treatment, will ultimately develop AIDS has been estimated to be over 90%. In the absence of effective anti-HIV treatment, the AIDS case-fatality rate is very high: most (80%–90%) patients in developed countries died within 3–5 years after the diagnosis of AIDS. However, routine use of prophylactic drugs to prevent *Pneumocystis carinii* pneumonia and other opportunistic infections in the USA and most developed countries was able to delay the development of AIDS and death significantly prior to the routine availability of effective anti-HIV treatment.

Serologic tests for antibodies to HIV have been available commercially since 1985. The most commonly used screening test (EIA or ELISA) is highly sensitive and specific. However, when this test is reactive, it must be supplemented by an additional test, such as the Western blot or indirect fluorescent antibody (IFA) test. A nonreactive supplemental test negates the initial reactive EIA test; a positive reaction supports it, and an indeterminate result in the Western blot test calls for further evaluation. WHO recommends as an alternative to the routine use of Western blots and the IFA, the use of another EIA test that is methodologically and/or antigenically independent of the initial EIA tests. Because of the extreme personal significance of a positive HIV antibody test, it is recommended that an initial positive test be confirmed with a second specimen from the patient so as to eliminate possibilities of mislabelling and transcription errors.

Most persons infected with HIV develop detectable antibodies within 1–3 months after infection; occasionally, there may be a more prolonged interval of up to 6 months, with only very rare instances of individuals developing antibodies after 6 months. Other tests to detect HIV infection during the period after infection but prior to seroconversion are available, and include tests for circulating HIV antigen (p24) and PCR tests to detect viral nucleic acid sequences. Since the window period between the earliest possible detection of virus and seroconversion is short (less than 2 weeks), diagnosis of HIV infection with these tests is rare. However, these tests are particularly helpful in diagnosing HIV infection in young babies born to HIV infected women since passively transferred maternal anti-HIV antibodies often cause anti-HIV EIA tests in these infants to be falsely positive even up to the age of 15 months. The absolute T-helper cell (CD4+) count or percentage is used most often to evaluate the severity of HIV infection and to help clinicians make decisions about therapy.

2. Infectious agent—Human immunodeficiency virus (HIV), a retrovirus. Two types have been identified: type 1 (HIV-1) and type 2 (HIV-2). These viruses are serologically and geographically relatively distinct but have similar epidemiologic characteristics. The pathogenicity of HIV-2 is lower than that of HIV-1.

3. Occurrence—AIDS was first recognized as a distinct clinical entity in 1981; in retrospect, however, isolated cases occurred during the 1970s in the USA and in several other areas of the world (Haiti, Africa and Europe). By late 1999, over 700,000 cases of AIDS had been reported in the USA. Although the USA has recorded the largest number of cases, the estimated cumulative and annual AIDS case rates are much higher in most sub-Saharan African countries. Worldwide, WHO estimates that about 13 million AIDS cases (with about two thirds in sub-Saharan Africa) had occurred by 1999.

In the USA, the distribution of AIDS cases by risk behaviors or factors has shifted over the past decade. Although the AIDS epidemic in the USA continues to affect primarily men who have sex with men, the largest increases in rates of reported AIDS cases during the latter half of the 1990s have been among women and minority populations. In 1993 AIDS emerged as the leading cause of death in Americans aged 25–44, but it dropped to second place after unintentional injuries in 1996. However, HIV infection still remains the leading cause of death for black men and women aged 25–44. The reductions in AIDS incidence and deaths in North America since the mid-1990s are largely attributable to more effective antiretroviral therapy, although prevention efforts and the natural evolution of the epidemic have played some role. HIV/AIDS associated with injecting drug use continues to play a central role in the HIV epidemic that affects minorities of color in the USA. Heterosexual transmission of HIV is steadily increasing in the USA and is the predominant mode of HIV transmission throughout the developing world. The immense disparity in access to antiretroviral therapy between developed and developing countries is illustrated by the decrease in annual AIDS deaths in all developed countries since the mid-1990s compared with the steeply rising annual AIDS deaths in most developing countries with high HIV prevalence.

In the USA and other western developed countries, annual HIV incidence decreased markedly before the mid-1980s and has remained relatively low since then. However, in the most severely affected countries in sub-Saharan Africa, annual HIV incidence has continued almost unabated at high levels through the 1980s and 1990s. Outside sub-Saharan Africa, high HIV prevalence rates (more than 1%) in the total 15–49 year old population have been noted only in a few countries in the Caribbean and in south and southeast Asia. Of the estimated 33.4 million persons living with HIV/AIDS around the world in 1999, there were an estimated 22.5 million in sub-Saharan Africa, 6.7 million in south and southeast Asia, 1.4 million in Latin America and 665,000 in the USA. Globally, AIDS has caused more than 14 million deaths, including 2.5 million in 1998. HIV-1 is the most prevalent HIV type throughout the world; HIV-2 has been found primarily in west Africa, with some cases in countries that are linked epidemiologically to west Africa.

4. Reservoir—Humans.

5. Mode of transmission—HIV can be transmitted from person to person through sexual contact; the sharing of HIV contaminated needles and syringes; transfusion of infected blood or its components; and the transplantation of HIV infected tissues or organs. While the virus has occasionally been found in saliva, tears, urine and bronchial secretions, transmission after contact with these secretions has not been reported. The risk of HIV transmission via sexual intercourse is much lower than most other sexually transmitted agents. However, the presence of a concurrent sexually transmitted disease, especially an ulcerative one like chancroid, can greatly facilitate HIV transmission. The primary determinants of sexual transmission of HIV are the patterns and prevalence of sexual risk behaviors such as having unprotected sexual intercourse with many concurrent or overlapping sexual partners. No laboratory or epidemiologic evidence suggests that biting insects have transmitted HIV infection. The risk of transmission from oral sex is not easily quantifiable, but is presumed to be low.

From 15% to 30% of infants born to HIV positive mothers are infected before, during or shortly after birth: treatment of pregnant women with antivirals such as zidovudine results in a marked reduction of infant infections. Breast feeding by HIV infected women can transmit infection to their infants and can account for up to half of mother to child HIV transmission. After direct exposure of health care workers to HIV infected blood through injury with needles and other sharp objects, the rate of seroconversion is less than 0.5%, much lower than the risk of hepatitis B virus infection (about 25%) after similar exposures.

6. Incubation period—Variable. Although the time from infection to the development of detectable antibodies is generally 1–3 months, the time from HIV infection to diagnosis of AIDS has an observed range of less than 1 year to 15 years or longer. Without effective anti-HIV treatment, about half of infected adults will develop AIDS within 10 years after infection. The median incubation period in infected infants is shorter than in adults. The increasing availability of effective anti-HIV therapy since the mid-1990s has significantly reduced the development of AIDS in the USA and most other developed countries.

7. Period of communicability—Unknown; presumed to begin early after onset of HIV infection and extend throughout life. Epidemiologic evidence suggests that infectiousness increases with increasing immune deficiency, clinical symptoms and presence of other STDs. Epidemiologic studies indicate that infectiousness is high during the initial period after infection.

8. Susceptibility and resistance—Unknown, but susceptibility is presumed to be general: race, gender and pregnancy do not appear to affect susceptibility to HIV infection or AIDS. The presence of other STDs, especially those with ulcerations, may increase susceptibility, as may the absence of male circumcision. This latter factor may be related to the general level of penile hygiene. Whether Africans progress from HIV infection to AIDS more rapidly than other populations continues to be studied. The only accepted factor that significantly affects progression from HIV infection to the development of AIDS is age at initial infection. Adolescent and adult males and females who acquire HIV infection at an early age progress to AIDS more slowly than those infected at an older age.

Potential interactions between HIV and other infectious disease agents have caused great medical and public health concern. The only major interaction identified so far is with *Mycobacterium tuberculosis* (*Mtbc*) infection. Persons with latent *Mtbc* infection who are also infected with HIV develop clinical tuberculosis (TB) at an increased rate. Instead of a 10% lifetime risk of developing TB, 60%–80% of adults with dual infections may develop TB. This interaction has resulted in a parallel pandemic of TB: in some urban sub-Saharan African populations where 10%–15% of the adult population have dual infections (HIV and *Mtbc*), annual TB rates increased 5–10 fold during the latter half of the 1990s. No conclusive data indicate that any infection, including *Mtbc* infection, accelerates progression to AIDS in HIV infected persons.

9. **Methods of control—**

  A. ***Preventive measures:*** HIV/AIDS prevention program can be effective only with full political and community commitment to change and/or reduce high HIV risk behaviors.

   1) Public and school health education must stress that having multiple and especially concurrent and/or overlapping sexual partners and sharing drug paraphernalia increase the risk of HIV infection. Students must also be taught the skills needed to avoid or reduce risky behaviors. Programs for school aged youth should be developed to address the needs and developmental levels of students as well as those who do not attend school. The specific needs of minorities, persons with different primary languages and those with visual or hearing impairments must also be addressed.

   2) The only sure way to avoid infection through sex is to abstain from sexual intercourse or to engage in mutually monogamous sexual intercourse with someone known to be uninfected. In other situations, latex condoms must be used correctly every time a person has vaginal, anal or oral sex. Latex condoms with water based lubricants have been shown to reduce the risk of sexual transmission.

   3) Expansion of facilities for treating drug users would reduce HIV transmission. Programs that instruct needle users in decontamination methods and needle exchange programs have been evaluated and shown to be effective.

   4) Anonymous and/or confidential HIV counseling and testing sites are in operation in all states of the USA. Counseling, voluntary HIV testing and medical referrals should be offered routinely: in STD, tuberculosis and drug treatment clinics; in clinics offering prenatal care or family planning services; in facilities that offer services to gay men; and in communities where HIV seroprevalence is high. Sexually active persons should be advised to seek prompt treatment for STDs.

   5) All pregnant women should be counseled about HIV early in pregnancy and encouraged to be tested for HIV infection as a routine part of standard antenatal care. Those found to be

HIV positive should be evaluated to assess their need for zidovudine (ZDV) therapy to prevent in utero and perinatal HIV transmission.

6) Regulations have been established by the U.S. Food and Drug Administration (FDA) to prevent HIV contamination of plasma and blood. All donated units must be tested for HIV antibody; only donations testing negative can be used. People who have engaged in behaviors that place them at increased risk of HIV infection must not donate plasma, blood, organs for transplantation, tissue or cells (including semen for artificial insemination). Organizations (including sperm banks, milk banks or bone banks) that collect plasma, blood or organs should inform potential donors of this recommendation and must test all donors. When possible, donations of sperm, milk or bone should be frozen and stored for 3–6 months. Donors who test negative after that interval can be considered not to have been infected at the time of donation.

7) Physicians should adhere strictly to medical indications for transfusions. The use of autologous transfusions should be encouraged.

8) Only clotting factor products that have been screened and treated to inactivate HIV should be used.

9) Care should be taken in handling, using and disposing of needles or other sharp instruments. Health care workers should wear latex gloves, eye protection and other personal protective equipment in order to avoid contact with blood or fluids that are visibly bloody. Any patient's blood on the worker's skin should be washed off with soap and water without delay. These precautions should be taken in the care of **all** patients and in all laboratory procedures ("universal precautions").

10) WHO recommends immunization of asymptomatic HIV-infected children with the EPI vaccines; those who are symptomatic should not receive BCG vaccine. In the USA, BCG and oral polio vaccines are not recommended for HIV infected children regardless of symptoms; live Measles-Mumps-Rubella vaccines are recommended for all HIV infected children.

B. Control of patient, contacts and the immediate environment:

1) Report to local health authority: Official report of AIDS cases is obligatory in all health jurisdictions in the USA and in most countries. Many states in the USA have also implemented reporting of HIV infections. Official report may be required in some countries or provinces, Class 2B (see Communicable Disease Reporting).

2) Isolation: Isolation of the HIV positive individual is unnecessary, ineffective and unjustified. Universal precautions (q.v.) apply to all hospitalized patients. Observe additional precautions appropriate for specific infections that occur in AIDS patients.

3) Concurrent disinfection: Of equipment contaminated with blood or body fluids and with excretions and secretions visibly contaminated with blood and body fluids by using bleach solution or tuberculocidal germicides.

4) Quarantine: None. Patients and their sexual partners should not donate blood, plasma, organs for transplantation, tissues, cells, semen for artificial insemination or breast milk for human milk banks.

5) Immunization of contacts: None.

6) Investigation of contacts and source of infection: In the USA, notification of sexual and needle sharing partners should, whenever possible, be made by the HIV infected individual. Provider referral is justified only when the patient, after due counseling, still refuses to notify his/her partner, and when the health care provider is certain that no harm will be done to the index case if the partner is notified. Care must be taken to protect patient confidentiality.

7) Specific treatment: Early diagnosis of infection and referral for medical evaluation are indicated. Consult more current sources of information for appropriate drugs, schedules and doses. Periodic updates of HIV/AIDS treatment guidelines are available from the CDC National AIDS Clearinghouse (1-800-458-5231) and are posted on the Clearinghouse World Wide Web site (http://www.cdcnpin.org).

   a) Prior to the development of relatively effective antiretroviral treatment, routinely available in the USA around the mid-1990s, treatment was available only for the opportunistic diseases that resulted from HIV infection. Prophylactic use of oral TMP-SMX, with aerosolized pentamidine as a less effective backup, is recommended to prevent *P. carinii* pneumonia. All HIV infected persons should receive tuberculin skin tests and be evaluated for active disease. If active TB is found, patients should be placed on antituberculous therapy. If no active TB is found, patients who are tuberculin positive or are anergic but were recently exposed should be offered preventive therapy with isoniazid for 12 months.

   b) Decisions to either initiate or change antiretroviral therapy should be guided by monitoring the laboratory parameters of both plasma HIV RNA (viral load) and CD4+ T cell count and by assessing the clinical condition of the patient. Results of these two laboratory tests provide important information about the virologic and immunologic status of the patient and the risk of disease progression to AIDS. Once the decision to initiate antiretroviral therapy has been made, treatment should be aggressive with the goal of maximal viral suppression. In general, a protease inhibitor and two nonnucleoside reverse transcriptase inhibitors should be used initially. Other regimens may be used but are considered less than optimal. Special considerations apply to adolescents and pregnant women, and specific treatment regimens for these patients should be used.

c) Up to mid-1999, the only drug shown to reduce the risk of perinatal HIV transmission was AZT when administered according to the following regimen: administered orally antenatally after 14 weeks gestation and continued throughout pregnancy; intravenously administered during the intrapartum period; and administered orally to the newborn for the first 6 weeks of life. This chemoprophylactic regimen was shown to reduce the risk of perinatal transmission by 66%. A shorter course of AZT treatment had been shown to reduce the risk of perinatal transmission by about 40%.

A study reported out of Uganda in July 1999 found that a single dose of nevirapine given to HIV infected mothers during labor, followed by a single dose given to the newborn within 3 days of birth, gave better results than both the long and short course azidothymidine (AZT) regimens. Just 13.1% of the nevirapine treated infants became infected with HIV, compared with 25.1% of the AZT treated group. Nevirapine is less than $4 a dose, so the prospects of preventing mother to infant transmission of HIV in developing countries may be more feasible in the new millennium. However, development of the necessary HIV testing and counseling services for antenatal females in the poorest developing countries in Africa remains a daunting challenge. In addition, the general lack of anti-HIV treatment for adults means that the number of AIDS related orphans in these countries will increase.

d) Management of health care workers (HCWs) occupationally exposed to blood and other body fluids suspected to contain HIV is complex. The nature of the exposure and factors such as possible pregnancy and drug resistant HIV strains must be considered before HIV postexposure prophylaxis (PEP) is recommended. As of late 1999, recommendations for PEP include a basic 4-week regimen of two drugs (zidovudine and lamivudine) for most HIV exposures, as well as an expanded regimen that includes the addition of a protease inhibitor (indinavir or nelfinavir) for HIV exposures that pose an increased risk of transmission or where resistance to one or more of the antiretroviral agents recommended for PEP is known or suspected. Health care organizations should have protocols that promote and facilitate prompt access to postexposure care and reporting of exposures.

C. Epidemic measures: HIV is currently pandemic, with large numbers of infections reported in the Americas, Europe, Africa and southeast Asia. See 9A, above, for recommendations.

D. Disaster implications: Emergency personnel should follow the same universal precautions as health workers; if latex gloves are not available and skin surfaces contact blood, it should be washed off as soon as possible. Masks, visors and protective clothing are indicated when performing procedures that may involve spurting or splashing of blood or bloody fluids. Emergency transfusion services should use blood donations that are screened for HIV antibody; when it is not possible to test donated blood for HIV antibody, donations should be accepted only from donors who have engaged in no HIV risk behaviors and preferably from donors who have previously tested negative for HIV antibodies.

E. International measures: A global prevention and care program coordinated by WHO was initiated in 1987. Since 1995, the global AIDS program has been coordinated by UNAIDS. Virtually all countries throughout the world have developed an AIDS prevention and care program. Several nations have instituted requirements for AIDS or HIV examinations for entry by foreign travelers (mainly those applying for resident or longer term visas, such as for work or study). WHO and UNAIDS have not endorsed these measures.

ACTINOMYCOSIS   ICD-9 039; ICD-10 A42

1. Identification—A chronic bacterial disease, most frequently localized in the jaw, thorax or abdomen. The lesions are firmly indurated areas of purulence and fibrosis that spread slowly to contiguous tissues; eventually, draining sinuses may be formed that penetrate to the surface. In infected tissue, the organism grows in clusters, called "sulfur granules."

Diagnosis is made by demonstrating slim, nonspore forming, grampositive bacilli, with or without branching, or "sulfur granules" in tissue or pus, and by isolating the microorganisms from samples of appropriate clinical materials not contaminated with normal flora during collection.

The clinical findings and culture allow distinction between actinomycosis and actinomycetoma, which are very different diseases. (See Mycetoma.)

2. Infectious agents—*Actinomyces israelii* is the usual human pathogen; *A. naeslundii, A. meyeri, A. odontolyticus* and *Propionibacterium propionicus* (*Arachnia propionica* or *Actinomyces propionicus*) have also been reported to cause human actinomycosis. Rarely, *A. viscosus* has been reported to cause actinomycosis but has been more reliably established as contributing to the etiology of periodontal disease. All species are gram-positive, nonacid fast, anaerobic to microaerophilic higher bacteria that may be part of the normal oral flora.

3. Occurrence—An infrequent human disease, occurring sporadically throughout the world. All races, both genders and all age groups may be affected; greatest frequency is from 15 to 35 years of age; the ratio of males to females is approximately 2:1. Cases in cattle, horses and other animals are caused by other *Actinomyces* species.

4. Reservoir—Humans are the natural reservoir of *A. israelii* and other agents. In the normal oral cavity, the organisms grow as saprophytes in dental plaque and in tonsillar crypts, without apparent penetration or cellular response in adjacent tissues. Sample surveys in the USA, Sweden and other countries have demonstrated *A. israelii* microscopically in granules from crypts of 40% of extirpated tonsils, and by anaerobic culture, from as many as 30%–48% of specimens of saliva or material from carious teeth.

A. israelii has been found in the vaginal secretions of approximately 10% of women using intrauterine devices. No external environmental reservoir such as straw or soil has been demonstrated.

5. Mode of transmission—Presumably the agent passes by contact from person to person as part of the normal oral flora. From the oral cavity, the organism may be aspirated into the lung or introduced into jaw tissues by injury, by extraction of teeth or by abrasion of the mucosa. Abdominal disease most commonly originates in the appendix. The source of clinical disease is endogenous.

6. Incubation period—Irregular; probably many years after colonization in the oral tissues, and days or months after precipitating trauma and actual penetration of tissues.

7. Period of communicability—Time and manner in which *Actinomyces* and *Arachnia* species become a part of the normal oral flora are unknown; except for rare instances of human bite, infection is unrelated to specific exposure to an infected person.

8. Susceptibility and resistance—Natural susceptibility is low. Immunity following infection has not been demonstrated.

9. **Methods of control** —

A. *Preventive measures:* None, except that maintenance of good oral hygiene, particularly removal of accumulating dental plaque, will reduce risk of oral infection.

B. *Control of patient, contacts and the immediate environment:*

1) Report to local health authority: Official report not ordinarily justifiable, Class 5 (see Communicable Disease Reporting).
2) Isolation: None.
3) Concurrent disinfection: None.
4) Quarantine: None.
5) Immunization of contacts: None.
6) Investigation of contacts and source of infection: Not profitable.
7) Specific treatment: No spontaneous recovery. Prolonged administration of penicillin in high doses is usually effective; tetracycline, erythromycin, clindamycin and cephalosporins are alternatives. Surgical drainage of abscesses is often necessary.

C. *Epidemic measures:* Not applicable, a sporadic disease.

D. *Disaster implications:* None.

E. *International measures:* None.

AMOEBIASIS
(Amebiasis)

ICD-9 006; ICD-10 A06

1. **Identification**—An infection with a protozoan parasite that exists in two forms: the hardy, infective cyst and the more fragile, potentially pathogenic trophozoite. The parasite may act as a commensal or invade the tissues and give rise to intestinal or extraintestinal disease. Most infections are asymptomatic but may become clinically important under certain circumstances. Intestinal disease varies from acute or fulminating dysentery with fever, chills and bloody or mucoid diarrhea (amebic dysentery), to mild abdominal discomfort with diarrhea containing blood or mucus alternating with periods of constipation or remission. Amebic granulomata (ameboma), sometimes mistaken for carcinoma, may occur in the wall of the large intestine in patients with intermittent dysentery or colitis of long duration. Ulceration of the skin, usually in the perianal region, occurs rarely by direct extension from intestinal lesions or amebic liver abscesses; penile lesions may occur in active homosexuals. Dissemination via the

bloodstream may occur and produce abscess of the liver or, less commonly, of the lung or brain.

Amebic colitis is often confused with various forms of inflammatory bowel disease such as ulcerative colitis; special care should be taken to distinguish the two diseases since corticosteroids may exacerbate amebic colitis. Amoebiasis can also mimic numerous other noninfectious and infectious diseases. Conversely, the presence of amebae may be misinterpreted as the cause of diarrhea in a person whose primary enteric illness is the result of another condition.

Diagnosis is made by microscopic demonstration of trophozoites or cysts in fresh or suitably preserved fecal specimens, smears of aspirates or scrapings obtained by proctoscopy or aspirates of abscesses or sections of tissue. The presence of trophozoites containing RBCs is indicative of invasive amoebiasis. Examination should be done on fresh specimens by a trained microscopist since the organism must be differentiated from nonpathogenic amebae and macrophages. Stool antigen detection tests have recently become available, but they do not distinguish pathogenic from nonpathogenic organisms; in the near future, *Entamoeba histolytica*-specific assays should be available. Reference laboratory services may be required. Many serologic tests are available as adjuncts in diagnosing extraintestinal amoebiasis, such as liver abscess, where stool examination is often negative. Serologic tests, particularly HIA immunodiffusion and ELISA, are very useful in the diagnosis of invasive disease. Scintillography, ultrasonography and CAT scanning are helpful in revealing the presence and location of an amebic liver abscess, and can be considered diagnostic when associated with a specific antibody response to *E. histolytica*.

2. Infectious agent—*Entamoeba histolytica*, a parasitic organism not to be confused with *E. hartmanni*, *Escherichia coli* or other intestinal protozoa. Differentiation of pathogenic *E. histolytica* from the morphologically identical nonpathogenic *E. dispar* is based on immunologic differences and on isoenzyme patterns. Nine potentially pathogenic and 13 nonpathogenic zymodemes (which are classified as *E. dispar)* have been identified in isolates from five continents. Most asymptomatic cyst passers carry strains of *E. dispar*.

3. Occurrence—Amebiasis is ubiquitous. Invasive amoebiasis is mostly a disease of young adults. Liver abscesses occur predominately in males. Amoebiasis is rare below age 5 years and especially below 2 years, when dysentery is due typically to shigellae. Published prevalence rates of cyst passage, usually based only on the morphology of the cysts, vary widely from place to place. In general, rates are higher in areas with poor sanitation (such as parts of the tropics), in mental institutions and among sexually promiscuous male homosexuals (probably *E. dispar)*. In areas with good sanitation, amebic infections tend to cluster in households and institutions. The proportion of cyst passers who have clinical disease is usually low.

4. Reservoir—Humans; usually a chronically ill or asymptomatic cyst passer.

5. Mode of transmission—Transmission occurs mainly by ingestion of fecally contaminated food or water containing amebic cysts which are relatively chlorine resistant. Transmission may occur sexually by oral-anal contact. Patients with acute amebic dysentery probably pose only limited danger to others because of the absence of cysts in dysenteric stools and the fragility of trophozoites.

6. Incubation period—Variable, from a few days to several months or years; commonly 2–4 weeks.

7. Period of communicability—During the period *E. histolytica*, cysts are passed which may continue for years.

8. Susceptibility and resistance—Susceptibility to infection is general; those harboring *E. dispar* do not develop disease. Susceptibility to reinfection has been demonstrated but is apparently rare.

9. Methods of control —

    A. Preventive measures:

        1) Educate the general public in personal hygiene, particularly in sanitary disposal of feces, and in handwashing after defecation and before preparing or eating food. Disseminate information regarding the risks involved in eating uncleaned or uncooked fruits and vegetables and in drinking water of questionable purity.

        2) Dispose of human feces in a sanitary manner.

        3) Protect public water supplies from fecal contamination. Sand filtration of water removes nearly all cysts and diatomaceous earth filters remove them completely. Chlorination of water as generally practiced in municipal water treatment does not always kill cysts; small quantities of water as in canteens or Lyster bags are best treated with prescribed concentrations of iodine, either liquid (8 drops of 2% tincture of iodine/quart of water or 12.5 ml/liter of a saturated aqueous solution of iodine crystals), or as water purification tablets (a tablet of tetraglycine hydroperiodide, Globaline®, per quart of water). A contact period of at least 10 minutes (30 minutes if cold) should be allowed to elapse before drinking the water. Portable filters with less than 1.0 μm pore sizes are effective. Water of undetermined quality can be made safe by boiling for 1 minute.

        4) Treat known carriers; stress the need for thorough handwashing after defecation to avoid reinfection from an infected domestic resident.

5) Educate high risk groups to avoid sexual practices that may permit fecal-oral transmission.

6) Health agencies should supervise the sanitary practices of people who prepare and serve food in public eating places and the general cleanliness of the premises involved. Routine examination of food handlers as a control measure is impractical.

7) Disinfectant dips for fruits and vegetables are of unproven value in preventing transmission of *E. histolytica.* Thorough washing with potable water and keeping fruits and vegetables dry may help; cysts are killed by desiccation, by temperatures above 50°C (122°F) and by irradiation.

8) Use of chemoprophylactic agents is not advised.

B. *Control of patient, contacts and the immediate environment:*

1) Report to local health authority: In selected endemic areas; in many states (USA) and countries not reportable, Class 3C (see Communicable Disease Reporting).

2) Isolation: For hospitalized patients, enteric precautions in the handling of feces, contaminated clothing and bed linen. Exclusion of individuals infected with *E. histolytica* from food handling and from direct care of hospitalized and institutionalized patients. Release to return to work in a sensitive occupation when chemotherapy is completed.

3) Concurrent disinfection: Sanitary disposal of feces.

4) Quarantine: None.

5) Immunization of contacts: Not applicable.

6) Investigation of contacts and source of infection: Household members and other suspected contacts should have adequate microscopic examination of feces.

7) Specific treatment: Acute amebic dysentery and extraintestinal amoebiasis should be treated with metronidazole (Flagyl®), followed by iodoquinol (Diodoquin®), paromomycin (Humatin®) or diloxanide furoate (Furamide®). Dehydroemetine (Mebadin®), followed by iodoquinol, paromomycin or diloxanide furoate, is a suitable alternative treatment for severe or refractory intestinal disease.

If a patient with a liver abscess continues to be febrile after 72 hours of therapy with metronidazole, nonsurgical aspiration may be indicated. Chloroquine sometimes is added to metronidazole or dehydroemetine for treating a refractory liver abscess. Occasionally, abscesses may require surgical aspiration if there is a risk of rupture or the abscess continues to enlarge despite therapy. Asymptomatic carriers may be treated with iodoquinol, paromomycin or diloxanide furoate.

Metronidazole is not recommended for use during the first trimester of pregnancy; however, there has been no proof of teratogenicity in humans. Dehydroemetine is contraindicated during pregnancy. Diloxanide furoate and dehydroemetine are available from the CDC Drug Service, CDC, Atlanta, telephone 404-639-3670.

C. *Epidemic measures:* Any group of possible cases requires prompt laboratory confirmation to exclude false positive identification of *E. histolytica* or other etiologic agents and epidemiologic investigation to determine source of infection and mode of transmission. If a common vehicle is indicated, such as water or food, appropriate measures should be taken to correct the situation.

D. *Disaster implications:* Disruption of normal sanitary facilities and food management will favor an outbreak of amebiasis, especially in population groups with large numbers of cyst passers.

E. *International measures:* None.

ANGIOSTRONGYLIASIS   ICD-9 128.8; ICD-10 B83.2
(Eosinophilic meningoencephalitis, Eosinophilic meningitis)

1. Identification—A nematode disease of the CNS with predominantly meningeal involvement. Invasion may be asymptomatic or mildly symptomatic; it is more commonly characterized by severe headache, stiffness of the neck and back and various paresthesias. Temporary facial paralysis occurs in 5% of patients. Low grade fever may be present. The worm has been found in the CSF and in the eye. CSF usually exhibits pleocytosis with more than 20% eosinophils; blood eosinophilia is not always present but has reached 82%. Illness may last a few days to several months. Deaths have rarely been reported.

Differential diagnosis includes cerebral cysticercosis, paragonimiasis, echinococcosis, gnathostomiasis, tuberculous meningitis, coccidioidal meningitis, aseptic meningitis and neurosyphilis.

Diagnosis, especially in endemic areas, is suggested by eosinophils in the CSF and a history of eating raw molluscs. Immunodiagnostic tests are presumptive; demonstration of the worms in the CSF or at autopsy is confirmatory.

2. Infectious agent—*Parastrongylus (Angiostrongylus) cantonensis,* a nematode (lungworm of rats). The third-stage larvae in the intermediate host (terrestrial or marine molluscs) are infective for humans.

3. Occurrence—The disease is endemic in Hawaii, Tahiti, many other Pacific islands, Vietnam, Thailand, Malaysia, China, Indonesia, Taiwan, the Philippines and Cuba. The nematode is found as far north as Japan, as far south as Brisbane, Australia, and in Africa as far west as the Ivory Coast and has also been reported in Madagascar, Egypt, Puerto Rico and New Orleans (USA).

4. Reservoir—The rat (*Rattus* and *Bandicota* spp.).

5. Mode of transmission—Ingestion of raw or insufficiently cooked snails, slugs or land planarians, which are intermediate or transport hosts harboring infective larvae. Prawns, fish and land crabs that have ingested snails or slugs may also transport the infective larvae. Lettuce and other leafy vegetables contaminated by small molluscs may serve as a source of infection. The molluscs are infected by first-stage larvae excreted by an infected rodent; when third-stage larvae have developed in the molluscs, rodents (and people) that ingest the molluscs are infected. In the rat, the larvae migrate to the brain and mature to the adult stage; the young adults migrate to the surface of the brain and through the venous system to reach their final site in the pulmonary arteries.

After mating, the female worm deposits eggs that hatch in terminal branches of the pulmonary arteries; the first-stage larvae enter the bronchial system, pass up the trachea, are swallowed and passed in the feces. In people, the cycle rarely goes beyond the CNS stage.

6. Incubation period—Usually 1–3 weeks; it may be longer or shorter.

7. Period of communicability—Not transmitted from person to person.

8. Susceptibility and resistance—Susceptibility to infection is general. Malnutrition and debilitating diseases may contribute to an increase in severity, even to a fatal outcome.

9. Methods of control—

   A. Preventive measures:

   1) Educate the general public in preparation of raw foods and both aquatic and terrestrial snails.
   2) Control rats.
   3) Boil snails, prawns, fish and crabs for 3–5 minutes, or freeze at −15°C (5°F) for 24 hours; this is effective in killing the larvae.
   4) Avoid eating raw foods that have been contaminated by snails or slugs; thorough cleaning of lettuce and other greens to eliminate molluscs and their products does not always eliminate infective larvae. Radiation pasteurization would be effective.

B. Control of patient, contacts and the immediate environment:

1) Report to local health authority: Official report not ordinarily justifiable, Class 5 (see Communicable Disease Reporting).
2) Isolation: None.
3) Concurrent disinfection: Not necessary.
4) Quarantine: None.
5) Immunization of contacts: Not applicable.
6) Investigation of contacts and source of infection: The source of food involved and its preparation should be investigated.
7) Specific treatment: Mebendazole and albendazole were effective in treating children in Taiwan.

C. Epidemic measures: Any grouping of several cases in a particular geographic area or institution warrants prompt epidemiologic investigation.

D. Disaster implications: None.

E. International measures: None.

ABDOMINAL
ANGIOSTRONGYLIASIS   ICD-9 128.8
INTESTINAL
ANGIOSTRONGYLIASIS   ICD-10 B81.3

Since 1967, a syndrome similar to appendicitis has been recognized in Costa Rica, predominantly among children under the age of 13, with abdominal pain and tenderness in the right iliac fossa and flank, fever, anorexia, vomiting, abdominal rigidity, a tumor-like mass in the right lower quadrant and pain on rectal examination. Leukocytosis is generally between 20,000 and 30,000/cu mm (SI units: 20–30 × 10^9/L), with eosinophils ranging from 11% to 61%. On surgery, yellow granulations are found in the subserosa of the intestinal wall, and eggs and larvae of *Parastrongylus (Angiostrongylus) costaricensis* are found in lymph nodes, intestinal wall and omentum; adult worms are found in the small arteries, generally in the ileocecal area. The infection has been recognized in people in Central and South America and in the USA.

The reservoir of this parasite is a rodent (the cotton rat, *Sigmodon hispidus,* among which the worm is present in southern USA); slugs are the usual intermediate hosts. The adults live in the mesenteric arteries in the cecal area, and the eggs are carried into the intestinal wall. On embryonation, the first-stage larvae migrate to the lumen, are excreted in the feces and are ingested by a slug. Within the slug, the larvae develop to the third stage, which is infective for rats and people. The infective larvae are found in the slug's slime (mucus) left on soil or other surfaces. When this slime or the tiny slugs are ingested by people, the infective larvae penetrate the gut wall, maturing in the lymphatic nodes and vessels. The adult worms migrate to the mesenteric arterioles of the ileocecal region where oviposition occurs. In people, most of the eggs and larvae degenerate and cause a granulomatous reaction. There is no specific treatment; surgical intervention is sometimes necessary.

ANISAKIASIS   ICD-9 127.1; ICD-10 B81.0

1. Identification—A parasitic disease of the human GI tract usually manifested by cramping abdominal pain and vomiting, that results from the ingestion of uncooked or undertreated marine fish containing larval ascaridoid nematodes. The motile larvae burrow into the stomach wall producing acute ulceration with nausea, vomiting and epigastric pain, sometimes with hematemesis. They may migrate upward and attach in the oropharynx, causing cough. In the small intestine, they cause eosinophilic abscesses, and the symptoms may mimic appendicitis or regional enteritis. At times they perforate into the peritoneal cavity; rarely they involve the large bowel.

Diagnosis is made by recognition of the 2-cm-long larvae invading the oropharynx or by visualizing the larvae by gastroscopic examination or in surgically removed tissue. Serological tests are under development.

2. Infectious agents—Larval nematodes of the subfamily Anisakinae, genera *Anisakis* and *Pseudoterranova.*

3. Occurrence—The disease occurs in individuals who eat uncooked and inadequately treated (frozen, salted, marinated, smoked) saltwater fish, squid or octopus. This is common in Japan (sushi and sashimi), the Netherlands (herring), Scandinavia (gravlax) and on the Pacific coast of Latin America (ceviche). Over 12,000 cases have been described in Japan. Formerly, the disease was frequently seen in the Netherlands. Cases are now seen with increasing frequency throughout western Europe and the USA, with the growing consumption of raw fish.

4. Reservoir—Anisakinae are widely distributed in nature, but only certain of those that are parasitic in sea mammals constitute a major threat to humans. The natural life cycle involves transmission of larvae by predation from small crustaceans to squid, octopus or fish, then to sea mammals, with people as incidental hosts.

5. Mode of transmission—The infective larvae live in the abdominal mesenteries of fish; often after death of their host they invade the body muscles of the fish. When ingested by people and liberated by digestion in the stomach, they may penetrate the gastric or intestinal mucosa.

6. Incubation period—Gastric symptoms may develop within a few hours after ingestion. Symptoms referable to the small and large bowel occur within a few days or weeks, depending on the size and location of the larvae.

7. Period of communicability—Direct transmission from person to person does not occur.

8. Susceptibility and resistance—Apparently universal susceptibility.

9. Methods of control —

    A. Preventive measures:

        1) Avoid ingestion of inadequately cooked marine fish. Heating to 60°C (140°F) for 10 minutes, blast-freezing to −35°C (−31°F) or below for 15 hours or freezing by regular means at −23°C (−10°F) for at least 7 days kills the larvae. The latter control method is used with success in the Netherlands. Irradiation effectively kills the parasite.

        2) Cleaning (evisceration) of fish as soon as possible after they are caught reduces the number of larvae penetrating into the muscles from the mesenteries.

        3) Candling is recommended for fishery products in which parasites can be visualized.

    B. Control of patient, contacts and the immediate environment:

        1) Report to local health authority: Not ordinarily justifiable, Class 5 (see Communicable Disease Reporting). However, a case or cases recognized in an area not previously known to be involved, or any in an area where control measures are in effect, should be reported.

        2) Isolation: None.

        3) Concurrent disinfection: None.

        4) Quarantine: None.

        5) Immunization of contacts: None.

        6) Investigation of contacts and source of infection: None. Examination of others possibly exposed at the same time may be productive.

        7) Specific treatment: Gastroscopic removal of larvae; excision of lesions.

    C. Epidemic measures: None.

    D. Disaster implications: None.

    E. International measures: None.

ANTHRAX   ICD-9 022; ICD-10 A22
(Malignant pustule, Malignant edema, Woolsorter disease, Ragpicker disease)

1. Identification—An acute bacterial disease that usually affects the skin, but which may very rarely involve the oropharynx, mediastinum or intestinal tract. In cutaneous anthrax, itching of an exposed skin surface first occurs, followed by a lesion that becomes papular, then vesicular and in 2–6 days develops into a depressed black eschar. The eschar is usually surrounded by moderate to severe and very extensive edema, sometimes with small secondary vesicles. Pain is unusual and, if present, is due to edema or secondary infection. The head, forearms and hands are common sites of infection. The lesion has been confused with human orf (see Orf virus disease). Untreated infections may spread to regional lymph nodes and to the bloodstream with an overwhelming septicemia. The meninges can become involved. Untreated cutaneous anthrax has a case-fatality rate between 5% and 20%, but with effective antibiotic therapy, few deaths occur. The lesion evolves through typical local changes even after the initiation of antibiotic therapy.

Initial symptoms of inhalation anthrax are mild and nonspecific and may include fever, malaise and mild cough or chest pain; acute symptoms of respiratory distress, x-ray evidence of mediastinal widening, fever and shock follow in 3–5 days, with death shortly thereafter. Intestinal anthrax is rare and more difficult to recognize, except that it tends to occur in explosive food poisoning outbreaks; abdominal distress is followed by fever, signs of septicemia and death in the typical case. An oropharyngeal form of primary disease has been described.

Laboratory confirmation is made by demonstration of the causative organism in blood, lesions or discharges by direct polychrome methylene blue (M'Fadyean)–stained smears or by culture or inoculation of mice, guinea pigs or rabbits. Rapid identification of the organism by using immunodiagnostic testing, ELISA and PCR may be available in certain reference laboratories.

2. Infectious agent—*Bacillus anthracis,* a Gram-positive, encapsulated, spore forming, nonmotile rod.

3. Occurrence—Primarily a disease of herbivores; humans and carnivores are incidental hosts. Anthrax is an infrequent and sporadic human infection in most industrialized countries. It is an occupational hazard primarily of workers who process hides, hair (especially from goats), bone and bone products and wool; and of veterinarians and agriculture and wildlife workers who handle infected animals. Human anthrax is endemic in those agricultural regions of the world where anthrax in animals is common; these include countries in South and Central America, southern and eastern Europe, Asia and Africa. New areas of infection in livestock may develop through introduction of animal feed containing contaminated bone meal. Environmental events such as floods may provoke epizootics. Anthrax is considered a leading potential agent in bioterrorism or biowarfare and, as such, could present in epidemiologically unusual circumstances.

4. Reservoir—Animals (normally herbivores, both livestock and wildlife) shed the bacilli in terminal hemorrhages or spilt blood at death. On exposure to the air, the vegetative forms sporulate, and the spores of *B. anthracis,* which are very resistant to adverse environmental conditions and disinfection, may remain viable in contaminated soil for many years. *B. anthracis* is a soil commensal in many parts of the world. Bacterial growth and spore density in soil are enhanced by flooding or other ecological conditions. Soil can also be contaminated by vultures, which spread the organism from one area to another after feeding on anthrax infected carcasses. Dried or otherwise processed skins and hides of infected animals may harbor the spores for years and are the fomites by which the disease is spread worldwide.

5. Mode of transmission—Cutaneous infection is by contact with tissues of animals (cattle, sheep, goats, horses, pigs and others) dying of the disease; possibly by biting flies that had partially fed on such animals; by contact with contaminated hair, wool, hides or products made from them, such as drums, brushes or rugs; or by contact with soil associated with infected animals or contaminated bone meal used in gardening. Inhalation anthrax results from inhalation of spores in risky industrial processes— such as tanning hides and processing wool or bone—where aerosols of *B. anthracis* spores may be produced. Intestinal and oropharyngeal anthrax arise from ingestion of contaminated undercooked meat; there is no evidence that milk from infected animals transmits anthrax. The disease spreads among grazing animals through contaminated soil and feed; among omnivorous and carnivorous animals through contaminated meat, bone meal or other feeds; and among wildlife from feeding on carcasses infected with anthrax. Accidental infections may occur among laboratory workers.

In 1979, an outbreak of largely inhalation anthrax occurred in Yekaterinburg (Sverdlovsk), Russia, in which 66 individuals were documented to have died of anthrax and 11 infected persons were known to have survived; many other cases are presumed to have occurred. Investigations disclosed that the cases occurred as the result of a plume emanating from a biological research institute and led to the conclusion that the outbreak had resulted from an accidental aerosol generated in work related to biological warfare studies.

6. Incubation period—From 1 to 7 days, although incubation periods up to 60 days are possible. (In the Sverdlovsk outbreak, incubation periods extended up to 43 days.)

7. Period of communicability—Transmission from person to person is very rare. Articles and soil contaminated with spores may remain infective for decades.

8. Susceptibility and resistance—Uncertain; there is some evidence of inapparent infection among people in frequent contact with the infectious agent; second attacks can occur, but reports are rare.

9. Methods of control—

A. Preventive measures:

1) Immunize high risk persons with a cell-free vaccine prepared from a culture filtrate containing the protective antigen (available in the USA from the Bioport Corporation, 3500 N. Martin Luther King, Jr., Boulevard, Lansing MI 48909). Evidence indicates that this vaccine is effective in preventing cutaneous and inhalational anthrax; it is recommended for laboratory workers who routinely work with *B. anthracis* and workers who handle potentially contaminated industrial raw materials. It may also be used to protect military personnel against potential exposure to anthrax used as a biological warfare agent. Annual booster injections are recommended if the risk of exposure continues.

2) Educate employees who handle potentially contaminated articles about modes of anthrax transmission, care of skin abrasions and personal cleanliness.

3) Control dust and properly ventilate work areas in hazardous industries, especially those that handle raw animal materials. Maintain continuing medical supervision of employees and provide prompt medical care of all suspicious skin lesions. Workers should wear protective clothing and have adequate facilities for washing and changing clothes after work. Locate eating facilities away from places of work. Vaporized formaldehyde has been used for terminal disinfection of textile mills contaminated with *B. anthracis*.

4) Thoroughly wash, disinfect or sterilize hair, wool and bone meal or other feed of animal origin prior to processing.

5) Do not sell the hides of animals exposed to anthrax or use their carcasses as food or feed supplements (i.e., as bone or blood meal).

6) If anthrax is suspected, do not necropsy the animal but aseptically collect a blood sample for culture. Avoid contamination of the area. If a necropsy is inadvertently performed, autoclave, incinerate or chemically disinfect/fumigate all instruments or materials.

Because the anthrax spores may survive for decades if the carcasses are buried, the preferred disposal technique is to incinerate the carcasses at the site of death or to remove them to a rendering plant, ensure no contamination en route to the plant. Should these methods be impossible, deeply bury carcasses at the site of death, if possible; do not burn them on open fields. Decontaminate soil seeded by carcasses or discharges with 5% lye or anhydrous calcium oxide (quicklime). Deeply buried carcasses should be covered with quicklime.

7) Control effluents and trade wastes from rendering plants that handle potentially infected animals and those from factories that manufacture products from hair, wool, bones or hides likely to be contaminated.

8) Promptly immunize and annually reimmunize all animals at risk. Treat symptomatic animals with penicillin or tetracyclines; immunize these animals after cessation of therapy. They should not be used for food until a few months have passed. Treatment in lieu of immunization may be used for animals exposed to a discrete source of infection, such as contaminated commercial feed.

B. Control of patient, contacts and the immediate environment:

1) Report to local health authority: Case report obligatory in most states and countries, Class 2A (see Communicable Disease Reporting). Also report to the appropriate livestock or agriculture authority. Even a single case of human anthrax, especially of the inhalational variety, is so unusual that it should be reported immediately to both public health and law enforcement authorities for consideration of a bioterrorist source.

2) Isolation: Standard precautions for the duration of illness for cutaneous and inhalation anthrax. Antibiotic therapy sterilizes a skin lesion within 24 hours, but the lesion progresses through its typical cycle of ulceration, sloughing and resolution.

3) Concurrent disinfection: Of discharges from lesions and articles soiled therewith. Hypochlorite is sporicidal and good when organic matter is not overwhelming and the item is not corrodable; hydrogen peroxide, peracetic acid or glutaraldehyde may be alternatives; formaldehyde, ethylene oxide and cobalt irradiation have been used. Spores require steam sterilization, autoclaving or burning to ensure complete destruction. Fumigation and chemical disinfection may be used for valuable equipment. Terminal cleaning.

4) Quarantine: None.

5) Immunization of contacts: None.

6) Investigation of contacts and source of infection: Search for history of exposure to infected animals or animal products and trace to place of origin. In a manufacturing plant, inspect for adequacy of preventive measures as outlined in 9A, above. As mentioned in 9B1, a potential bioterrorist source may need to be ruled out for all human cases of anthrax, especially for those cases with no obvious occupational source of infection.

7) Specific treatment: Penicillin is the drug of choice for cutane-

ous anthrax and is given for 5–7 days. Tetracyclines, erythromycin and chloramphenicol are also effective. The U.S. military recommends parenteral ciprofloxacin or doxycycline for inhalational anthrax; the duration of therapy is not well defined.

C. *Epidemic measures:* Outbreaks may be an occupational hazard of animal husbandry. The occasional epidemics in the USA are local industrial outbreaks among employees who work with animal products, especially goat hair. Outbreaks related to handling and consuming meat from infected cattle have occurred in Asia, Africa and the former Soviet Union.

D. *Disaster implications:* None, except in case of floods in previously infected areas.

E. *International measures:* Sterilize imported bone meal before use as animal feed. Disinfect wool, hair and other products when indicated and practical.

F. *Bioterrorism measures:* During 1998, more than two dozen anthrax threats were made in the USA. None of these threats was real. The general procedures in the USA for dealing with these civilian threats include the following:

1) Anyone who receives a threat about dissemination of anthrax organisms should notify the local office of the Federal Bureau of Investigation (FBI) immediately.
2) In the USA, the FBI has primary responsibility for the investigation of such biological threats, and all other agencies are to cooperate and provide assistance as requested by the FBI.
3) Local and state health departments should be notified also and be ready to provide any public health management and follow-up that may be needed.
4) Persons who may have been exposed to anthrax are not contagious, so quarantine is not appropriate.
5) Persons who may have been exposed should be advised to await laboratory results and need not be placed on chemoprophylaxis. If they become ill before laboratory results are available, they should immediately contact their local health department and proceed to a predetermined emergency care unit, where they should inform the attending staff of their potential exposure.
6) If the threat of exposure to aerosolized anthrax is credible or confirmed, persons at risk should begin postexposure prophylaxis with both an appropriate antibiotic (fluoroquinolones are the drugs of choice; doxycycline is an alternative) and vaccine. Postexposure immunization with an inactivated, cell-free anthrax vaccine is indicated in conjunction with

chemoprophylaxis following a proven biologic incident. Immunization is recommended because of the uncertainty of when or if inhaled spores may germinate. Postexposure immunization consists of three injections: as soon as possible after exposure and at 2 and 4 weeks after exposure. This vaccine has not been evaluated for safety and efficacy in children less than 18 years of age or adults 60 years of age or older.

7) All first responders should follow local protocols for incidents involving biological hazards.

8) Responders can be protected from anthrax spores by donning splash protection, gloves and a full face respirator with high-efficiency particle air (HEPA) filters (Level C) or self-contained breathing apparatus (SCBA) (Level B).

9) Persons who may have been exposed and are potentially contaminated should be decontaminated with soap and copious amounts of water in a shower. Usually no bleach solutions are required. A 1:10 dilution of household bleach (i.e., a final hypochlorite concentration of 0.5%) should be used only if there is gross contamination with the agent and an inability to remove the materials through soap and water decontamination. The use of bleach decontamination is recommended only after soap and water decontamination, and the solution should be rinsed off after 10 to 15 minutes.

10) All persons who are to be decontaminated should remove their clothing and personal effects and place all items in plastic bags, which should be labeled clearly with the owner's name, contact telephone number and inventory of the bag's contents. Personal items may be kept as evidence in a criminal trial or returned to the owner if the threat is unsubstantiated.

11) If the suspect envelope or package associated with an anthrax threat remains sealed (not opened), then first responders should not take any action other than notifying the FBI and packaging the evidence. Quarantine, evacuation, decontamination and chemoprophylaxis efforts are NOT indicated if the envelope or package remains sealed. For incidents involving possibly contaminated letters, the environment in direct contact with the letter or its contents should be decontaminated with a 0.5% hypochlorite solution following a crime scene investigation. Personal effects may be decontaminated similarly.

12) Technical assistance can be provided immediately by contacting the National Response Center at 800-424-8802 or the local Weapons of Mass Destruction Coordinator of the FBI.

ARENAVIRAL HEMORRHAGIC FEVERS IN SOUTH AMERICA	ICD-9 078.7; ICD-10 A96
JUNÍN (ARGENTINIAN) HEMORRHAGIC FEVER	ICD-10 A96.0
MACHUPO (BOLIVIAN) HEMORRHAGIC FEVER	ICD-10 A96.1
GUANARITO (VENEZUELAN) HEMORRHAGIC FEVER	ICD-10 A96.8
SABIÁ (BRAZILIAN) HEMORRHAGIC FEVER	ICD-10 A96.8

1. Identification—Acute febrile viral illnesses; duration is 7–15 days. Onset is gradual with malaise, headache, retroorbital pain, conjunctival injection and sustained fever and sweats, followed by prostration. There may be petechiae and ecchymoses, accompanied by erythema of the face, neck and upper thorax. An enanthem with petechiae on the soft palate is frequent. Severe infections result in epistaxis, hematemesis, melena, hematuria and gingival hemorrhage; encephalopathies, intention tremors and depressed deep tendon reflexes are frequent. Bradycardia and hypotension with clinical shock are common findings, and leukopenia and thrombocytopenia are characteristic. Moderate albuminuria is present, with many cellular and granular casts and vacuolated epithelial cells in the urine. Case-fatality rates range from 15% to 30% or more.

Diagnosis is made by isolation of virus or detection of antigen in blood or organs; by PCR, or serologically by IgM capture ELISA; or detection of neutralizing antibody rises or increasing titers by ELISA or IFA. Laboratory studies for virus isolation and neutralizing antibody tests require BSL-4.

2. Infectious agents—The Tacaribe complex of arenaviruses: Junín for the Argentine disease; the closely related Machupo virus for the Bolivian; Guanarito virus for the Venezuelan; and the Sabiá virus for the Brazilian. (These viruses are related to the viruses of Lassa fever and lymphocytic choriomeningitis.)

3. Occurrence—Argentine hemorrhagic fever was first described among corn harvesters in Argentina in 1955. About 200–300 cases or more were reported from endemic areas of the Argentine pampas each year prior to widespread immunization; incidence has been around 100 cases or fewer in recent years. Disease occurs primarily from March to October (autumn and winter). It occurs more frequently in males than in females, and mainly in those aged 15 to 60 years.

A similar disease, Bolivian hemorrhagic fever, caused by the related virus, occurs sporadically or in epidemics in small villages of rural northeastern Bolivia. In July–September 1994, there were 9 cases with 7 deaths.

In 1989, an outbreak of severe hemorrhagic illness occurred in the municipality of Guanarito, Venezuela; 104 cases with 26 deaths occurred between May 1990 and March 1991 among rural residents in Guanarito and neighboring areas. Cases have since been reported intermittently, and the virus is still present in rodents.

Sabiá virus caused a fatal illness with hemorrhage and jaundice in Brazil in 1990, a laboratory infection in Brazil in 1992 and a laboratory infection treated with ribavirin in the USA in 1994.

4. Reservoir—In Argentina, wild rodents of the pampas (primarily *Calomys musculinus)* are the hosts for Junín virus. In Bolivia, *C. callosus* is the reservoir animal. Cane rats *(Zygodontomys brevicauda)* are implicated as the likely reservoir of Guanarito virus. The reservoir of Sabiá virus is not known, although a rodent host is presumed.

5. Mode of transmission—Transmission to humans occurs primarily by inhalation of small particle aerosols derived directly from rodent excreta containing virus, saliva or from rodents disrupted by mechanical harvesters. Virus deposited in the environment may also be infective when secondary aerosols are generated by farming and grain processing, when ingested or by contact with cuts or abrasions. While uncommon, person to person transmission of Machupo virus has been documented in health care and family settings.

6. Incubation period—Usually 7–16 days.

7. Period of communicability—Not often directly transmitted from person to person, although this has occurred in both Argentine and Bolivian diseases.

8. Susceptibility and resistance—All ages appear to be susceptible, but protective immunity of unknown duration follows infection. Subclinical infections occur.

9. Methods of control—

    A. *Preventive measures:* Specific rodent control in houses has been successful in Bolivia. In Argentina, human contact most commonly occurs in the fields, and rodent dispersion makes control more difficult. An effective live attenuated Junín vaccine has been administered to more than 150,000 individuals in Argentina; it is unlicensed in the USA. In experimental animals, this vaccine is effective against Machupo but not Guanarito virus.

    B. *Control of patient, contacts and the immediate environment:*

        1) Report to local health authority: In selected endemic areas; in most countries not a reportable disease, Class 3A (see Communicable Disease Reporting).

2) Isolation: Strict isolation during the acute febrile period. Respiratory protection may be desirable along with other barrier methods.

3) Concurrent disinfection: Of sputum and respiratory secretions, and blood contaminated materials.

4) Quarantine: None.

5) Immunization of contacts: None.

6) Investigation of contacts and source of infection: Monitoring and, where feasible, control of rodents.

7) Specific treatment: Specific immune plasma given within 8 days of onset is effective in the treatment of Argentine disease. Ribavirin is likely to be useful in all four diseases.

C. Epidemic measures: Rodent control; consider immunization.

D. Disaster implications: None.

E. International measures: None.

ARTHROPOD-BORNE VIRAL DISEASES
(Arboviral Diseases)

Introduction

Numerous arboviruses are known to produce clinical and subclinical infection in humans. There are four main clinical syndromes:

1. an acute CNS illness ranging in severity from mild aseptic meningitis to encephalitis, with coma, paralysis and death;

2. acute benign fevers of short duration, with and without an exanthem; on occasion some may give rise to a more serious illness with CNS involvement or hemorrhages;

3. hemorrhagic fevers, which include acute febrile diseases with extensive hemorrhagic involvement, external or internal, frequently serious, and associated with capillary leakage, shock and high case-fatality rates (all may cause liver damage, but hepatic damage is most severe in yellow fever and is accompanied by frank jaundice); and

4. polyarthritis and rash, with or without fever and of variable duration, benign or with arthralgic sequelae lasting several weeks to months.

These clinical features are the basis of presentation of these diseases.

Most of these viruses are maintained in zoonotic cycles. Humans are usually an unimportant host in maintaining the cycle; infections in humans are incidental and are acquired most frequently during blood feeding by an infected arthropod vector. In only a few cases can humans serve as the principal source of virus amplification and vector infection, such as dengue and yellow fever. Most of the viruses are transmitted by mosquitoes, while the rest are transmitted by ticks, sand flies or biting midges. Laboratory infections may occur, including infections by aerosols.

Although the agents differ, these diseases share common epidemiologic features (related primarily by their vectors) in their transmission cycles that are important in control. Consequently, the selected diseases under each clinical syndrome are arranged in four groups: mosquito-borne and midgeborne; tickborne; sand fly borne; and unknown. Diseases of major importance are described individually or in groups with similar clinical and epidemiologic features.

Viruses believed to be associated with human disease are listed in the accompanying table with type of vector, predominant character of recognized disease and geographic distribution. In some instances, observed cases of disease due to particular viruses are too few to be certain of the usual clinical course. Some viruses capable of causing disease have been recognized only through laboratory acquired exposure. Viruses in which evidence of human infection is based solely on serologic survey are not included; otherwise, the number would be much greater. Those that cause diseases covered in subsequent chapters are marked on the table by an asterisk; some of the less important or less well studied are not discussed in the text.

Over 100 viruses currently classified as arboviruses produce disease in humans. Most of these are further classified by antigenic relationships, morphology and replicative mechanisms into families and genera, of which Togaviridae (*Alphavirus*), Flaviviridae (*Flavivirus*) and Bunyaviridae (*Bunyavirus, Phlebovirus*) are the best known. These genera contain some agents that cause predominantly encephalitis, while others cause predominantly febrile illnesses. Alphaviruses and bunyaviruses are usually mosquito-borne; flaviviruses are either mosquito- or tickborne, with some flaviviruses having no recognized vectors; phleboviruses are generally transmitted by sand flies, with the exception of Rift Valley fever, which is transmitted by mosquitoes. Other viruses of the family Bunyaviridae and of several other groups produce principally febrile diseases or hemorrhagic fevers and may be transmitted by mosquitoes, ticks, sand flies or midges.

DISEASES IN HUMANS CAUSED BY ARTHROPOD-BORNE VIRUSES

Virus Family, Genus, Group	Name of Virus	Vector	Disease in Humans	Where Found
TOGAVIRIDAE *Alphavirus*				
	*Barmah Forest	Mosquito	Fever, arthritis, rash	Australia
	*Chikungunya	Mosquito	Fever, arthritis, rash (hemorrhage rare)	Africa, SE Asia, Philippines
	*Eastern equine encephalomyelitis	Mosquito	Encephalitis	Americas
	Everglades	Mosquito	Fever, encephalitis	Florida (USA)
	*Mayaro (Uruma)	Mosquito	Fever, arthritis, rash	S America
	Mucambo	Mosquito	Fever	S America
	*O'nyong-nyong	Mosquito	Fever, arthritis, rash	Africa
	*Ross River	Mosquito	Fever, arthritis, rash	Australia, S Pacific
	Semliki Forest	Mosquito	Encephalitis	Africa
	*Sindbis (Ockelbo, Babanki)	Mosquito	Fever, arthritis, rash	Africa, India, SE Asia, Europe, Philippines, Australia, Russia
	Tonate	Mosquito	Fever	S America
	*Venezuelan equine encephalomyelitis	Mosquito	Fever, encephalitis	Americas
	*Western equine encephalomyelitis	Mosquito	Fever, encephalitis	Americas

FLAVIVIRIDAE
Flavivirus

*Banzi	Mosquito	Fever	Africa
Bussuquara	Mosquito	Fever	S America
*Dengue 1, 2, 3 and 4	Mosquito	Fever, hemorrhage, rash	Throughout tropics
Edge Hill	Mosquito	Fever, arthritis	Australia
Ilheus	Mosquito	Fever, encephalitis	Central & S America
*Japanese encephalitis	Mosquito	Encephalitis, fever	Asia, Pacific islands, northern Australia
Karshi	Tick	Fever, encephalitis	Asia
Kokobera	Mosquito	Fever, arthritis	Australia
Koutango	Mosquito	Fever, rash	Africa
*Kunjin	Mosquito	Fever, encephalitis	Australia, Sarawak
*Kyasanur Forest disease	Tick	Hemorrhage, fever, meningoencephalitis	India
*Louping ill	Tick	Encephalitis	UK, western Europe
*Murray Valley encephalitis	Mosquito	Encephalitis	Australia, New Guinea
Negishi	Unknown	Encephalitis	Japan
*Omsk hemorrhagic fever	Tick	Hemorrhage, fever	Russia
*Powassan	Tick	Encephalitis	Canada, USA, Russia
*Rocio	Mosquito	Encephalitis	Brazil
Sepik	Mosquito	Fever	New Guinea
*Spondweni	Mosquito	Fever	Africa
*St. Louis encephalitis	Mosquito	Encephalitis, hepatitis	Americas
*Tickborne encephalitis			
*European subtype	Tick	Encephalitis, paralysis	Europe
*Far Eastern subtype	Tick	Encephalitis	Europe, Asia

*Asterisked groups and viruses are discussed in the text. See index for page numbers.

DISEASES IN HUMANS CAUSED BY ARTHROPOD-BORNE VIRUSES

Virus Family, Genus, Group	Name of Virus	Vector	Disease in Humans	Where Found
FLAVIVIRIDAE *Flavivirus (cont.)*				
	Usutu	Mosquito	Fever, rash	Africa
	Wesselsbron	Mosquito	Fever	Africa, SE Asia
	*West Nile	Mosquito	Fever, encephalitis, rash	Africa, Indian subcontinent, Middle East, CIS, Europe
	*Yellow fever	Mosquito	Hemorrhagic fever	Africa, S & Central America
	*Zika	Mosquito	Fever	Africa, SE Asia
BUNYAVIRIDAE *Bunyavirus* Anopheles A group				
	Tacaiuma	Mosquito	Fever	S America
*Group C				
	Apeu	Mosquito	Fever	S America
	Caraparu	Mosquito	Fever	S and Central America
	Itaqui	Mosquito	Fever	S America
	Madrid	Mosquito	Fever	Panama
	Marituba	Mosquito	Fever	S America
	Murutucu	Mosquito	Fever	S America
	Nepuyo	Mosquito	Fever	S and Central America
	Oriboca	Mosquito	Fever	S America
	Ossa	Mosquito	Fever	Panama
	Restan	Mosquito	Fever	Trinidad, Suriname

BUNYAVIRIDAE
Bunyavirus (cont.)

Bunyamwera group

Batai	Mosquito	Fever	Europe, Asia
*Bunyamwera	Mosquito	Fever, rash	Africa
Fort Sherman	Mosquito	Fever	Central America
Germiston	Mosquito	Fever, rash	Africa
Ilesha	Unknown	Fever, rash, hemorrhage	Africa
Shokwe	Mosquito	Fever	Africa
Tucunduba	Mosquito	Encephalitis	Brazil
Tensaw	Mosquito	Encephalitis	N America
Wyeomyia	Mosquito	Fever	S America, Panama
Xingu	Unknown	Fever, hepatitis	Brazil

Bwamba group

*Bwamba	Mosquito	Fever, rash	Africa
Pongola	Mosquito	Fever, arthritis	Africa

California group

*California encephalitis	Mosquito	Encephalitis	USA
Guaroa	Mosquito	Fever	S America, Panama
Inkoo	Mosquito	Fever, encephalitis	Scandinavia, CIS
*Jamestown Canyon	Mosquito	Encephalitis	USA, Canada
*LaCrosse	Mosquito	Encephalitis	USA
*Snowshoe hare	Mosquito	Encephalitis	USA, Canada, China, Russia
Tahyna	Mosquito	Fever	Europe, Africa, Asia

*Asterisked groups and viruses are discussed in the text. See index for page numbers.

DISEASES IN HUMANS CAUSED BY ARTHROPOD-BORNE VIRUSES

Virus Family, Genus, Group	Name of Virus	Vector	Disease in Humans	Where Found
BUNYAVIRIDAE				
Bunyavirus (cont.)				
California group *(cont.)*	Trivittatus	Mosquito	Fever	N America
Guama group	Catu	Mosquito	Fever	S America
	Guama	Mosquito	Fever	S America
Mapputta group	GanGan	Mosquito	Fever, arthritis	Australia
	Trubanaman	Mosquito	Fever, arthritis	Australia
Simbu group	*Oropouche	*Culicoides*	Fever, meningitis	S America, Panama
	Shuni	Mosquito, *Culicoides*	Fever	Africa, Asia
Phlebovirus				
(*Sand fly fever group)	Alenquer	Unknown	Fever	S America
	Candiru	Unknown	Fever	S America
	Chagres	Phlebotomine	Fever	Central America
	Morumbi	Unknown	Fever	Brazil
	Sand fly Naples type	Phlebotomine	Fever	Europe, Africa, Asia
	Punta Toro	Phlebotomine	Fever	Panama
	Rift Valley fever	Mosquito	Fever, hemorrhage, encephalitis, retinitis	Africa
	Sand fly Sicilian type	Phlebotomine	Fever	Europe, Africa, Asia
	Serra Norte	Unknown	Fever	Brazil
	Toscana	Phlebotomine	Aseptic meningitis	Italy, Portugal

BUNYAVIRIDAE
Nairovirus

Virus	Vector	Disease	Location
*Nairobi sheep disease	Tick	Fever	Africa, India
*Dugbe	Tick	Fever	Africa
*Crimean-Congo hemorrhagic fever	Tick	Hemorrhagic fever	Europe, Africa, central Asia, Middle East

Unclassified

Virus	Vector	Disease	Location
Bangui	Unknown	Fever, rash	Africa
*Bhanja	Tick	Fever	Africa, Europe, Asia
Issyk-Kul (Keterah)	Tick	Fever	Asia, CIS
Kasokero	Unknown	Fever	Africa
Nyando	Mosquito	Fever	Africa
Tamdy	Tick	Fever	Uzbekistan, CIS
Tataguine	Mosquito	Fever, rash	Africa
Wanowrie	Tick	Fever, hemorrhage	Middle East, Asia

REOVIRIDAE
Orbivirus

Group	Virus	Vector	Disease	Location
*Changuinola group	Changuinola	Phlebotomine	Fever	Central America
*Kemerovo group	Kemerovo	Tick	Fever	Russia
	Lipovnik	Tick	Fever, meningitis	Europe
*Colorado tick fever	Colorado tick fever	Tick	Fever	USA, Canada

*Asterisked groups and viruses are discussed in the text. See index for page numbers.

DISEASES IN HUMANS CAUSED BY ARTHROPOD-BORNE VIRUSES

Virus Family, Genus, Group	Name of Virus	Vector	Disease in Humans	Where Found
RHABDOVIRIDAE				
Ungrouped	Orungo	Mosquito	Fever	Africa
Vesicular stomatitis group	*Vesicular stomatitis, Indiana & New Jersey	Phlebotomine	Fever, encephalitis	Americas
	Vesicular stomatitis, Alagoas	Phlebotomine	Fever	S America
	*Chandipura	Mosquito	Fever	India, Africa
	Piry	Unknown	Fever	S America
	Jurona	Mosquito	Fever	Brazil
LeDantec group	LeDantec	Unknown	Encephalitis	Senegal
ORTHOMYXOVIRIDAE	Dhori	Tick	Fever	Africa, Europe, Asia
	*Thogoto	Tick	Meningitis	Africa, Europe
NOT CLASSIFIED	*Quaranfil	Tick	Fever	Africa

*Asterisked groups and viruses are discussed in the text. See index for page numbers.

APHA

ARTHROPOD-BORNE VIRAL ARTHRITIS AND RASH   ICD-9 066.3; ICD-10 B33.1
(Polyarthritis and rash, Ross River fever, Epidemic polyarthritis)
CHIKUNGUNYA VIRUS DISEASE   ICD-10 A92.0
MAYARO VIRUS DISEASE   ICD-10 A92.8
(Mayaro fever, Uruma fever)
O'NYONG-NYONG FEVER   ICD-10 A92.1
SINDBIS (OCKELBO) VIRUS DISEASE AND OTHERS   ICD-10 A92.8
(Pogosta disease, Karelian fever)

1. Identification—A self-limiting febrile viral disease characterized by arthalgia or arthritis, primarily in the wrist, knee, ankle and small joints of the extremities, which lasts from days to months. In many patients, the onset of arthritis is followed in 1-10 days by a maculopapular rash, usually nonpruritic, affecting mainly the trunk and limbs. Buccal and palatal enanthema may occur. The rash resolves within 7-10 days, and is followed by a fine desquamation. Fever is sometimes absent. Cervical lymphadenopathy occurs frequently. Paresthesias and tenderness of palms and soles are present in a small percentage of cases.

Rash is also common in infections by Mayaro, Sindbis, chikungunya and o'nyong-nyong viruses. Polyarthritis is a characteristic feature of infections with chikungunya, Sindbis and Mayaro viruses.

Minor hemorrhages have been attributed to chikungunya virus disease in southeast Asia and India (see Dengue Hemorrhagic Fever). In chikungunya virus disease, leukopenia is common; convalescence is often prolonged.

Serologic tests show a rise in titer to alphaviruses; the virus may be isolated from the blood of acutely ill patients in newborn mice, mosquitoes or cell culture.

2. Infectious agents—Ross River and Barmah Forest viruses; Sindbis, Mayaro, chikungunya and o'nyong-nyong viruses cause similar illnesses.

3. Occurrence—Major outbreaks of Ross River virus disease (epidemic polyarthritis) have occurred in Australia in the state of Victoria and in south Australia, coastal New South Wales, western Australia, Northern Territory and Queensland, chiefly from January to May. Sporadic cases occur in other coastal regions of Australia and New Guinea. In 1979, a major outbreak occurred in Fiji and spread to other Pacific islands, including Tonga and the Cook Islands, with 15,000 cases in American Samoa in 1979-80. Barmah Forest virus infection has been reported in Queensland, the Northern Territory and western Australia. Chikungunya virus is found in Africa, India, southeast Asia and the Philippine Islands; Sindbis virus occurs throughout the Eastern Hemisphere. O'nyong-nyong virus is known only from Africa; epidemics in 1959-63 and 1996-97 involved millions of cases throughout east Africa. Mayaro occurs in northern South America and Trinidad.

4. Reservoir—Unknown for most viruses. Transovarian transmission of Ross River virus has been demonstrated in *Aedes vigilax*, making an insect reservoir a possibility. Similar transmission cycles may occur with other viruses of the group. Birds are a source of mosquito infection for Sindbis virus.

5. Mode of transmission—Ross River virus is transmitted by *Culex annulirostris, Ae. vigilax, Ae. polynesiensis* and other *Aedes* spp. of mosquitoes; chikungunya virus by *Aedes aegypti* and possibly others; o'nyong-nyong virus by *Anopheles* spp.; Sindbis virus by various *Culex* spp., especially *C. univittatus*, and *C. morsitans* and *Ae. communis*; Mayaro virus by *Mansonia* and *Haemagogus* spp.

6. Incubation period—Three to eleven days.

7. Period of communicability—No evidence of direct transmission from person to person.

8. Susceptibility and resistance—Recovery is universal and followed by lasting homologous immunity; second attacks are unknown. Inapparent infections are common, especially in children, among whom the overt disease is rare. In epidemic polyarthritis, arthritis occurs most frequently among adult females and in people with HLA DR7 Gm $a^+x^+b^+$ phenotypes.

9. Methods of control—

> **A. Preventive measures:** The general measures applicable to mosquito-borne viral encephalitides (see Arthropod-Borne Viral Encephalitides, section I9A, 1–5 and 8).
>
> **B. Control of patient, contacts and the immediate environment:**
> 1) Report to local health authority: In selected endemic areas; in many countries, not a reportable disease, Class 3B (see Communicable Disease Reporting).
> 2) Isolation: To avoid further transmission, protect patients from mosquitoes.
> 3) Concurrent disinfection: None.
> 4) Quarantine: None.
> 5) Immunization of contacts: None.
> 6) Investigation of contacts and source of infection: Search for unreported or undiagnosed cases where the patient lived during the 2 weeks prior to onset; check all family members serologically.
> 7) Specific treatment: None.

C. Epidemic measures: Same as for arthropod-borne viral fevers (see Dengue Fever, 9C).

D. Disaster implications: None.

E. International measures: WHO Collaborating Centres.

ARTHROPOD-BORNE VIRAL ENCEPHALITIDES
I. MOSQUITO-BORNE VIRAL ENCEPHALITIDES   ICD-9 062

JAPANESE ENCEPHALITIS	ICD-10 A83.0
WESTERN EQUINE ENCEPHALITIS	ICD-10 A83.1
EASTERN EQUINE ENCEPHALITIS	ICD-10 A83.2
ST. LOUIS ENCEPHALITIS	ICD-10 A83.3
MURRAY VALLEY ENCEPHALITIS (AUSTRALIAN ENCEPHALITIS)	ICD-10 A83.4
LACROSSE ENCEPHALITIS	ICD-10 A83.5
CALIFORNIA ENCEPHALITIS	ICD-10 A83.5
ROCIO ENCEPHALITIS	ICD-10 A83.6
JAMESTOWN CANYON ENCEPHALITIS	ICD-10 A83.8
SNOWSHOE HARE ENCEPHALITIS	ICD-10 A83.8

1. Identification—A group of acute inflammatory viral diseases of short duration involving parts of the brain, spinal cord and meninges. Signs and symptoms of these diseases are similar but vary in severity and rate of progress. Most infections are asymptomatic; mild cases often occur as febrile headache or aseptic meningitis. Severe infections are usually marked by acute onset, headache, high fever, meningeal signs, stupor, disorientation, coma, tremors, occasional convulsions (especially in infants) and spastic (but rarely flaccid) paralysis. Case-fatality rates range from 0.3% to 60%, with the rates due to Japanese (JE), Murray Valley (MV) and eastern equine encephalomyelitis (EEE) among the highest. Neurologic sequelae occur with variable frequency depending on age and infecting agent; they tend to be most severe in infants infected with JE, western equine encephalomyelitis (WEE) and EEE viruses. Mild leukocytosis is usual in these mosquito-borne diseases; leukocytes in the CSF, predominantly lymphocytes, range from 50 to 500/cu mm (SI units: 50 to 500×10^6/L) and may be 1,000/cu mm or greater (SI units: $1,000 \times 10^6$/L or greater) in infants infected with EEE virus. The elderly are at greatest risk of encephalitis with St. Louis encephalitis (SLE) or EEE virus infection, while children under 15 years of age are at greatest risk from LaCrosse virus infection and may develop seizures.

These diseases require differentiation from the tickborne encephalitides (see below); encephalitic and nonparalytic poliomyelitis; rabies; mumps meningoencephalitis; lymphocytic choriomeningitis; aseptic meningitis due to enteroviruses; herpes encephalitis; postvaccinal or postinfection encephalitides; and bacterial, mycoplasmal, protozoal, leptospiral and mycotic meningitides or encephalitides. Venezuelan equine encephalomyelitis, Rift Valley fever and West Nile viruses produce primarily arthropod-borne viral fever (see Arthropod-Borne Viral Fevers), but may sometimes cause encephalitis.

Identification is made by demonstrating specific IgM in acute-phase serum or CSF, or antibody rises between early and late specimens of serum by neutralization, CF, HI, FA, ELISA or other serologic tests. Cross reactions may occur within a virus group. Virus may occasionally be isolated by inoculation of suckling mice or cell culture with the brain tissue of fatal cases, rarely from blood or CSF after symptoms have appeared; histopathologic changes are not specific for individual viruses.

2. Infectious agents—Each disease is caused by a specific virus in one of three groups: EEE and WEE in the alphaviruses (Togaviridae, *Alphavirus*); JE, Kunjin, MV encephalitis, SLE and Rocio encephalitis in the flaviviruses (Flaviviridae, *Flavivirus*); and LaCrosse, California encephalitis, Jamestown Canyon and snowshoe hare viruses in the California group of bunyaviruses (Bunyaviridae, *Bunyavirus*).

3. Occurrence—EEE is recognized in eastern and north central USA and adjacent Canada, in scattered areas of Central and South America and in the Caribbean islands; WEE in western and central USA, Canada and parts of South America; JE in western Pacific islands from Japan to the Philippines, rarely cases have occurred on Badu Island in the Torres Strait and in far North Queensland, Australia and in many areas of eastern Asia from Korea to Indonesia, China and India; Kunjin and MV encephalitis in parts of Australia and New Guinea; SLE in most of the USA, in Ontario (Canada) and in Trinidad, Jamaica, Panama and Brazil; Rocio encephalitis in Brazil; LaCrosse encephalitis in the USA from Minnesota and Texas east to New York and Georgia; snowshoe hare encephalitis in Canada, China and Russia. Cases due to these viruses occur in temperate latitudes in summer and early fall and are commonly limited to areas and years of high temperature and many mosquitoes.

4. Reservoir—California group viruses overwinter in *Aedes* eggs; the true reservoir or means of winter carryover for other viruses is unknown, possibly birds, rodents, bats, reptiles, amphibians or survival in mosquito eggs or adults, with the mechanisms probably differing for each virus.

5. Mode of transmission—By the bite of infective mosquitoes. Most important vectors are:

• For EEE in the USA and Canada, probably *Culiseta melanura* from bird to bird, and one or more *Aedes* and *Coquillettidia* spp. from birds or other animals to humans;

• For WEE in western USA and Canada, *Culex tarsalis;*

• For JE, *C. tritaeniorhynchus, C. vishnui* complex and in the tropics, *C. gelidus;*

• For MV, probably *C. annulirostris;*

• For SLE in the USA, *C. tarsalis,* the *C. pipiens-quinquefasciatus* complex and *C. nigripalpus;*

• For LaCrosse, *Ae. triseriatus.*

Mosquitoes, if not transovarianly infected, acquire virus, such as La-Crosse virus, from wild birds or small mammals, but pigs, as well as birds, are important for JE. LaCrosse virus is transovarianly and venereally transmitted in *Ae. triseriatus* mosquitoes.

6. Incubation period—Usually 5–15 days.

7. Period of communicability—Not directly transmitted from person to person. Virus is not usually demonstrable in the blood of humans after onset of disease. Mosquitoes remain infective for life. Viremia in birds usually lasts 2–5 days, but may be prolonged in bats, reptiles and amphibia, particularly if interrupted by hibernation. Horses develop active disease with the two equine viruses and with JE, but viremia is rarely present in high titer or for long periods; therefore, humans and horses are uncommon sources of mosquito infection.

8. Susceptibility and resistance—Susceptibility to clinical disease is usually highest in infancy and old age; inapparent or undiagnosed infection is more common at other ages. Susceptibility varies with virus, e.g., LaCrosse encephalitis is usually a disease of children, while severity of SLE increases with age. Infection results in homologous immunity. In highly endemic areas, adults are largely immune to local strains by reason of mild and inapparent infection; susceptibles are mainly children.

9. Methods of control—

A. Preventive measures:

1) Educate the public as to the modes of spread and control.
2) Destroy larvae and eliminate breeding places of known and suspected vector mosquitoes, e.g., destroy or spray tires to prevent breeding of the LaCrosse vector.
3) Kill mosquitoes by space and residual spraying of human habitations (also see Malaria, 9A1–5).
4) Screen sleeping and living quarters; use mosquito bed nets.
5) Avoid exposure to mosquitoes during hours of biting, or use repellents (see Malaria, 9A2–4).

6) In endemic areas, immunize domestic animals or house them away from living quarters, e.g., pigs in JE endemic areas.

7) Mouse brain inactivated vaccine against JE encephalitis is used for children in Japan, Korea, Thailand, India and Taiwan. This vaccine is commercially available in the USA and is recommended for those traveling to endemic areas for extended visits to rural areas. Live attenuated and formalin inactivated primary hamster kidney cell vaccines are licensed and widely used in China.

For those under continued intensive exposure in laboratory situations, EEE and WEE vaccines (inactivated, dried) are available from U.S. Army Medical Research and Materiel Command, ATTN: MCMR-UMP, Fort Detrick, Frederick, MD 21702-5009 (telephone 301-619-2051).

8) Protect accidentally exposed laboratory workers passively with human or animal immune serum.

B. Control of patient, contacts and the immediate environment:

1) Report to local health authority: Case report obligatory in most states (USA) and in some countries, Class 2A (see Communicable Disease Reporting). Report under the appropriate disease; or as "encephalitis, other forms"; or as "aseptic meningitis," with etiology or clinical type specified when known.

2) Isolation: None; virus is not usually found in blood, secretions or discharges during clinical disease. Enteric precautions (see Definitions) are appropriate until enterovirus meningoencephalitis (see Viral Meningitis) is ruled out.

3) Concurrent disinfection: None.

4) Quarantine: None.

5) Immunization of contacts: None.

6) Investigation of contacts and source of infection: Search for missed cases and the presence of vector mosquitoes; test for viremia in both febrile and asymptomatic family members. Primarily a community vector control problem (see 9C, below).

7) Specific treatment: None.

C. Epidemic measures:

1) Identification of infection among horses or birds and recognition of human cases in the community have epidemiologic value by indicating frequency of infection and areas involved. Immunization of horses probably does not limit spread of the virus in the community; immunization of pigs against JE should have a significant effect.

2) Fogging or spraying from aircraft with suitable insecticides has shown promise for aborting urban epidemics of SLE.

D. Disaster implications: None.

E. International measures: Spray with insecticide those airplanes arriving from recognized areas of prevalence. WHO Collaborating Centres.

II. TICKBORNE VIRAL ENCEPHALITIES   ICD-9 063; ICD-10 A84

FAR EASTERN TICKBORNE ENCEPHALITIS	ICD-10 A84.0
(Russian spring-summer encephalitis)	
CENTRAL EUROPEAN TICKBORNE ENCEPHALITIS	ICD-10 A84.1
LOUPING ILL	ICD-10 A84.8
POWASSAN VIRUS ENCEPHALITIS	ICD-10 A84.8

1. Identification—A group of viral diseases clinically resembling the mosquito-borne encephalitides except that the Far Eastern tickborne subtype (FE) is often associated with focal epilepsy, flaccid paralysis (particularly of the shoulder girdle) and other residua. Central European tickborne encephalitis (CEE), also called diphasic milk fever or diphasic meningoencephalitis, produces a milder disease but has a longer course, averaging 3 weeks. The initial febrile stage of CEE is not associated with symptoms referable to the CNS, and the second phase of fever and meningoencephalitis follows 4-10 days after apparent recovery; fatality and severe residua are less frequent than for the FE tickborne disease. Powassan encephalitis (PE) has a similar clinical course with an approximate 10% case-fatality rate and approximately 50% neurologic sequelae among survivors. Louping ill in humans also has a diphasic pattern and is relatively mild.

Specific identification is made by demonstration of specific IgM in acute phase serum or CSF, by serologic tests of paired sera, or by isolation of virus from blood during acute illness or from brain postmortem by inoculation of suckling mice or cell culture. Common serologic tests do not differentiate members of this group but do distinguish the group from most other similar diseases.

2. Infectious agents—A complex within the flaviviruses; minor antigenic differences exist, more with Powassan than others, but viruses causing these diseases are closely related.

3. Occurrence—Disease of the CNS caused by this virus complex is distributed spottily over much of the former Soviet Union, other parts of eastern and central Europe, Scandinavia and the UK. In general, the FE subtype has been found predominantly in the far eastern region of the former Soviet Union; CEE predominates in Europe, while louping ill occurs chiefly in the British Isles and Ireland, but recently has been recognized in western Europe. Powassan virus is present in Canada, the USA and Russia. Seasonal incidence depends on density of the tick vectors. *Ixodes persulcatus* in eastern Asia is usually active in spring and early summer; bites from *I. ricinus* occur in Europe in both early summer and early autumn; and in the USA and Canada, human bites by *I. cookei* peak from June to September.

Areas of highest incidence are those where humans have intimate association with large numbers of infected ticks, generally in rural or forested areas, but also in some urban populations. Local epidemics of CEE have occurred among people consuming unpasteurized milk and dairy products from goats and sheep, thus the name "diphasic milk fever." The age pattern varies widely in different regions and is influenced by opportunity for exposure to ticks, consumption of milk from infected animals or previously acquired immunity. Laboratory infections are common, some with serious sequelae, including death.

4. Reservoir—The tick or ticks and mammals in combination, appear to be the true reservoir; transovarian tick passage of some tickborne encephalitis viruses has been demonstrated. Sheep and deer are the primary vertebrate hosts for louping ill, while rodents and other small mammals and birds serve as sources of tick infections with FE, CEE and PE viruses.

5. Mode of transmission—By the bite of infective ticks or by consumption of milk from certain infected animals. *Ixodes persulcatus* is the principal vector in eastern Russia, and *I. ricinus* in western Russia and other parts of Europe; the latter is also the vector of louping ill of sheep in Scotland. *I. cookei* is the principal vector in eastern Canada and USA. Larval ticks ingest virus by feeding on infected vertebrates, including rodents, other mammals or birds. CEE may be acquired by consumption of infected raw milk.

6. Incubation period—Usually 7–14 days.

7. Period of communicability—Not directly transmitted from person to person. A tick infected at any stage remains infective for life. Viremia in a variety of vertebrates may last for several days; in humans, up to 7–10 days.

8. Susceptibility and resistance—Both genders and all ages are susceptible. Infection, whether inapparent or overt, leads to immunity.

9. Methods of control—

A. Preventive measures:

1) See Lyme Disease, 9A, for measures against ticks.

2) Inactivated virus vaccines have been used extensively in Europe and the former Soviet Union with reported safety and effectiveness.

3) Boil or pasteurize milk of susceptible animals in areas where diphasic meningoencephalitis (CEE) occurs.

B. Control of patient, contacts and the immediate environment:

1) Report to local health authority: In selected endemic areas; in most countries, not a reportable disease, Class 3B (see Communicable Disease Reporting).

2) Isolation: None, after tick removal.

3) Concurrent disinfection: None.

4) Quarantine: None.

5) Immunization of contacts: None.

6) Investigation of contacts and source of infection: Search for missed cases, presence of tick vectors and animals excreting virus in milk.

7) Specific treatment: None.

C. Epidemic measures: See Lyme Disease, 9C.

D. Disaster implications: None.

E. International measures: WHO Collaborating Centres.

ARTHROPOD-BORNE VIRAL FEVERS
I. MOSQUITO-BORNE AND *CULICOIDES*-BORNE VIRAL FEVERS:
(Yellow fever and dengue are presented separately.)
I.A. VENEZUELAN EQUINE ENCEPHALOMYELITIS VIRUS DISEASE   ICD-9 066.2; ICD-10 A92.2
(Venezuelan equine encephalitis, Venezuelan equine fever)

1. Identification—Clinical manifestations of this viral infection are influenza-like, with an abrupt onset of severe headache, chills, fever, myalgia, retroorbital pain, nausea and vomiting. Conjunctival and pharyngeal congestion are the only physical signs. Most infections are relatively mild, with symptoms lasting 3-5 days. Some cases may have a diphasic fever course; after a few days of fever, particularly in children, CNS involvement may appear and range from somnolence to frank encephalitis with disorientation, convulsions, paralysis, coma and death. During the 1971 Texas outbreak, 3 of 40 patients studied had severe CNS involvement, with sequelae of personality change and/or paralysis.

Presumptive diagnosis is made on clinical and epidemiologic grounds (exposure in an area where an equine epizootic is in progress) and confirmed by virus isolation, rise in antibody titer or detection of specific IgM. Virus can be isolated in cell culture or in newborn mice from blood and nasopharyngeal washings during the first 72 hours of symptoms; acute and convalescent sera drawn 10 days apart can demonstrate rising antibody titers. Laboratory infections may occur when proper containment facilities are not used.

2. Infectious agent—Venezuelan equine encephalomyelitis (VEE) virus, an alphavirus (Togaviridae, *Alphavirus*), with enzootic subtypes and epizootic varieties of subtype 1.

3. Occurrence—Endemic in northern South America, Trinidad and Central America. The disease appears as epizootics, principally in northern and western South America; the epizootic in 1970–71 spread through Central America into the USA.

4. Reservoir—Enzootic subtypes of VEE are maintained in a rodent mosquito cycle. Epizootic varieties of subtype 1 are believed to arise periodically from enzootic VEE 1D viruses in northern South America. During outbreaks, epizootic VEE virus is transmitted in a cycle involving horses, which serve as the major source of virus, to mosquitoes, which in turn infect humans. Humans also develop sufficient viremia to serve as hosts in a human mosquito human transmission cycle.

5. Mode of transmission—By the bite of an infected mosquito. VEE viruses have been isolated from *Culex (Melanoconion), Aedes, Mansonia, Psorophora, Haemagogus, Sabethes, Deinocerites* and *Anopheles* mosquitoes and possibly ceratopogonid gnats. Laboratory infection by aerosol transmission is common; there is no evidence of transmission from horses to humans.

6. Incubation period—Usually 2–6 days; can be as short as 1 day.

7. Period of communicability—Infected humans and horses are infectious for mosquitoes for up to 72 hours; infected mosquitoes probably transmit virus throughout life.

8. Susceptibility and resistance—Susceptibility is general. Mild infections and subsequent immunity occur frequently in endemic areas. Children are at greatest risk for developing CNS infection.

9. **Methods of control** —

A. *Preventive measures:*

1) Use general mosquito control procedures.
2) Avoid forested endemic areas, especially at night.
3) Investigational live attenuated virus (TC-83) and inactivated vaccines for VEE have been used effectively to protect laboratory workers and other adults at high risk (available from the U.S. Army Medical Research and Materiel Command, ATTN: MCMR-UMP, Fort Detrick, Frederick, MD 21702-5009 (telephone 301-619-2051). The attenuated vaccine proved to be effective in protecting horses during the 1970–71 epizootic; control of infection in horses effectively prevented additional human cases. Vaccine for use in horses is commercially available.

B. *Control of patient, contacts and the immediate environment:*

1) Report to local health authority: In selected endemic areas; in most countries, not a reportable disease, Class 3B (see Communicable Disease Reporting).
2) Isolation: Blood and body fluid precautions. Patients should be treated in a screened room or in quarters treated with a residual insecticide for at least 5 days after onset, or until afebrile.
3) Concurrent disinfection: None.
4) Quarantine: None.
5) Immunization of contacts: None.
6) Investigation of contacts and source of infection: Search for unreported or undiagnosed cases.
7) Specific treatment: None.

C. *Epidemic measures:*

1) Determine extent of the infected areas; immunize horses and/or restrict their movement from the affected area.
2) Use approved mosquito repellents for those exposed.
3) Conduct a community survey to determine density of vector mosquitoes, their breeding places and effective control measures.
4) Identify infected horses, prevent mosquitoes from feeding on them and intensify mosquito control efforts in the affected area.

D. *Disaster implications:* None.

E. *International measures:* Immunize animals and restrict their movement from epizootic areas to areas free of the disease.

I.B. OTHER MOSQUITO-BORNE
  AND *CULICOIDES*-BORNE
  FEVERS   ICD-9 066.3
BUNYAMWERA VIRAL FEVER   ICD-10 A92.8
BWAMBA VIRUS DISEASE   ICD-10 A92.8
RIFT VALLEY FEVER   ICD-10 A92.4
WEST NILE FEVER   ICD-10 A92.3
GROUP C VIRUS DISEASE   ICD-10 A92.8
OROPOUCHE VIRUS DISEASE   ICD-10 A93.0

1. Identification—A group of viruses that cause febrile illnesses usually lasting a week or less, many of which are dengue-like (see table in the arbovirus introduction for mosquito-borne viruses). Initial symptoms include fever, headache, malaise, arthralgia or myalgia, and occasionally nausea and vomiting; generally, there is some conjunctivitis and photophobia. Fever may or may not be diphasic. Rash is common in infections with West Nile virus.

Meningoencephalitis is an occasional complication of West Nile and Oropouche virus infections. Persons with Rift Valley fever (RVF) may develop retinitis, encephalitis or hepatitis associated with hemorrhage that may be fatal. Several group C viruses are reported to produce weakness in the lower limbs; they are rarely fatal. Epidemics of RVF and Oropouche fever may involve thousands of patients.

Serologic tests differentiate other fevers of viral or unknown origin, but in general, viruses within the same genus are difficult to distinguish serologically. In some cases, virus isolation is possible from blood drawn during the febrile period by inoculation into suckling mice or cell culture. Laboratory infections may occur with many of these viruses.

2. Infectious agents—Each disease is caused by a distinct virus with the same name as the disease. West Nile, Banzi, Kunjin, Spondweni and Zika viruses are flaviviruses; the group C bunyaviruses are Apeu, Caraparu, Itaqui, Madrid, Marituba, Murutucu, Nepuyo, Oriboca, Ossa and Restan. Oropouche is a bunyavirus of the Simbu group. RVF is a phlebovirus. Others in smaller groups are listed in the introductory table.

3. Occurrence—West Nile virus has caused outbreaks in Egypt, Israel, India, France, Romania, Czech Republic, and is widespread in parts of Africa, the northern Mediterranean area and western Asia; Rift Valley, Bwamba and Bunyamwera fevers thus far have been identified only in Africa. Group C virus fevers occur in tropical South America, Panama and Trinidad. Oropouche fever is found in Trinidad, Panama, Peru and Brazil; Kunjin virus in Australia. Seasonal incidence depends on vector density. Occurrence is primarily rural, although occasionally RVF, Oropouche and West Nile have been involved in explosive urban and suburban outbreaks.

4. Reservoir—Unknown for many of these viruses; some may be maintained in a continuous vertebrate mosquito cycle in tropical environments. Oropouche virus may be transmitted by *Culicoides*. Birds are a source of mosquito infection for West Nile virus; rodents serve as reservoirs for group C viruses.

5. Mode of transmission—In most instances, by bite of an infective mosquito as follows:

• For West Nile, *Culex univittatus* in southern Africa, *C. modestus* in France and *C. pipiens molestus* in Israel;

• For Bunyamwera, *Aedes* spp.;

• For Group C viruses, species of *Aedes* and *Culex (Melanoconion);*

• For Rift Valley (in sheep and other animals), potential vectors include various *Aedes* mosquitoes; *Ae. mcintoshi* may be infected transovarially and account for maintenance of RVF virus in enzootic foci.

Many human infections of RVF are associated with the handling of animal tissues during necropsy or butchering. *Culex pipiens* was implicated in a 1977 epidemic of RVF in Egypt with at least 600 deaths; mechanical transmission by hematophagous flies and transmission by aerosols or contact with highly infective blood may contribute to RVF outbreaks. Other arthropods may be vectors, such as *Culicoides paraensis* for the Oropouche virus.

6. Incubation period—Usually 3-12 days.

7. Period of communicability—Not directly transmitted from person to person. Infected mosquitoes probably transmit virus throughout life. Viremia, essential for vector infection, occurs with many of these viruses during early clinical illness in humans.

8. Susceptibility and resistance—Susceptibility appears to be general, in both sexes and throughout life. Inapparent infections and mild disease are common. Infection leads to immunity; susceptibles in highly endemic areas are mainly young children.

9. Methods of control—

A. Preventive measures:

1) Follow the general measures applicable to mosquito-borne viral encephalitides (see 9A1-6 and 9A8). For RVF, precautions in care and handling of infected animals and their products, as well as human acute phase blood, are important.

2) An experimental inactivated cell culture RVF vaccine is available for humans; live and inactivated vaccines are available for sheep, goats and cattle.

B. *Control of patient, contacts and the immediate environment:*

1) Report to local health authority: In selected endemic areas; in most countries, not a reportable disease, Class 3B (see Communicable Disease Reporting). For RVF, notify WHO, FAO and the International Office of Epizootics in Paris.
2) Isolation: Blood and body fluid precautions. Keep patient in screened room or in quarters treated with an insecticide for at least 5 days after onset or until afebrile. Blood of RVF patients may be infectious.
3) Concurrent disinfection: None.
4) Quarantine: None.
5) Immunization of contacts: None.
6) Investigation of contacts and source of infection: Determine patient's place of residence during fortnight before onset. Search for unreported or undiagnosed cases.
7) Specific treatment: None.

C. *Epidemic measures:*

1) Use approved mosquito repellents for people exposed to bites of vectors.
2) Do not slaughter sick or dying domestic animals suspected of being infected with RVF.
3) Determine density of vector mosquitoes; identify and destroy their breeding places.
4) Immunize sheep, goats and cattle against RVF.
5) Identification of infected sheep and other animals (Rift Valley) and serologic surveys of birds (West Nile) or rodents (group C viruses) provide information regarding the prevalence of infection and areas involved.

D. *Disaster implications:* None.

E. *International measures:* For RVF, immunize animals and restrict their movement from enzootic areas to clean areas; do not butcher sick animals; for others, none except enforcement of international agreements designed to prevent transfer of mosquitoes by ships, airplanes and land transport. WHO Collaborating Centres.

II. TICKBORNE VIRAL FEVERS   ICD-9 066.1
COLORADO TICK FEVER AND   ICD-10 A93.2
OTHER TICKBORNE FEVERS   ICD-10 A93.8

1. Identification—Colorado tick fever (CTF) is an acute febrile (often diphasic) viral disease with infrequent rash. After initial onset, a brief remission is usual, followed by a second bout of fever lasting 2–3 days; neutropenia and thrombocytopenia almost always occur on the fourth to fifth day of fever. Characteristically, CTF is a moderately severe disease, with occasional encephalitis, myocarditis or tendency to bleed. Deaths are rare. Bhanja virus can cause severe neurologic disease and death; CNS infections also occur with Kemerovo and Thogoto viruses (the latter may cause hepatitis).

Laboratory confirmation of CTF is made by isolation of virus from blood inoculated into suckling mice or cell cultures or by demonstration of antigen in erythrocytes by IF (CTF virus may persist in erythrocytes for up to 120 days). IFA detects serum antibodies as early as 10 days after onset of illness. Diagnostic methods for confirming other tickborne viral fevers vary only slightly, except that serum is used for virus isolation instead of erythrocytes.

2. Infectious agents—Colorado tick fever, Nairobi sheep disease (Ganjam), Kemerovo, Lipovnik, Quaranfil, Bhanja, Thogoto and Dugbe viruses.

3. Occurrence—Colorado tick fever is endemic in the mountainous regions above 5,000 feet in the western USA and Canada. Virus has been isolated from *Dermacentor andersoni* ticks in Alberta and British Columbia. It occurs most frequently in those with recreational or occupational exposure (hiking, fishing) in enzootic loci; seasonal incidence parallels the period of greatest tick activity (April–June in the Rocky Mountains of the USA). (Geographic distribution of other viruses is shown in the introductory table.)

4. Reservoir—Reservoirs for CTF include small mammals such as ground squirrels, porcupines, chipmunks and *Peromyscus* spp.; also ticks, principally *D. andersoni.*

5. Mode of transmission—By bite of an infective tick. Immature ticks *(D. andersoni)* acquire CTF virus by feeding on viremic animals; they pass the virus transstadially and transmit virus to humans when feeding as adult ticks.

6. Incubation period—Usually 4–5 days.

7. Period of communicability—Not directly transmitted from person to person except by transfusion. The wildlife cycle is maintained by ticks, which remain infective throughout life. Virus is present in blood during the febrile stage and in CTF, in erythrocytes from 2 to 16 weeks or more after onset.

8. Susceptibility and resistance—Susceptibility apparently is universal. Second attacks are rare.

9. **Methods of control—**

A. *Preventive measures:* Personal protective measures to avoid tick bites; control of ticks and rodent hosts (see Lyme Disease, 9A).

B. *Control of patient, contacts and the immediate environment:*

1) Report to local health authority: In endemic areas (USA); in most states and countries, not a reportable disease, Class 3B (see Communicable Disease Reporting).
2) Isolation: Blood and body fluid precautions. No blood donations for 4 months.
3) Concurrent disinfection: None; remove ticks from patients.
4) Quarantine: None.
5) Immunization of contacts: None.
6) Investigation of contacts and source of infection: Identification of tick infested areas.
7) Specific treatment: None.

C. *Epidemic measures:* Not applicable.

D. *Disaster implications:* None.

E. *International measures:* WHO Collaborating Centres.

III. PHLEBOTOMINE-BORNE VIRAL FEVERS

SAND FLY FEVER   ICD-9 066.0; ICD-10 A93.1
(Phlebotomus fever, Papatasi fever)

CHANGUINOLA VIRUS DISEASE   ICD-9 066.0; ICD-10 A93.8
(Changuinola fever)

VESICULAR STOMATITIS VIRUS DISEASE   ICD-9 066.8; ICD-10 A93.8
(Vesicular stomatitis fever)

1. **Identification**—A group of arboviral diseases with headache; fever of 38.3°C–39.5°C (101°F–103°F), sometimes higher; retrobulbar pain on motion of the eyes; injected sclerae; malaise; nausea and pain in the limbs and back. Pharyngitis, oral mucosal vesicular lesions and cervical adenopathy are characteristic of vesicular stomatitis virus (VSV) infections. Leukopenia is usual on the fourth to fifth day after onset of fever. Symptoms may be alarming, but death is very rare. Complete recovery may be preceded by prolonged mental depression. Encephalitis may occur following Toscana and Chandipura virus infections.

A presumptive diagnosis is based on the clinical picture and the occurrence of multiple similar cases. Diagnoses may be confirmed serologically by detection of specific IgM antibodies or by antibody titer rise, or by isolation of virus from blood inoculated into newborn mice or cell culture; for VSV infections, from throat swabs and vesicular fluid.

2. Infectious agents—The sand fly fever group of viruses (Bunyaviridae, *Phlebovirus*); at least seven related immunologic types (Naples, Sicilian, Candiru, Chagres, Alenquer, Toscana and Punta Toro) have been isolated from humans and differentiated. In addition, Changuinola virus (an orbivirus) and VSV of the Indiana type (a rhabdovirus), both of which produce febrile disease in humans, have been isolated from *Lutzomyia* spp. sand flies. Chandipura virus is a rhabdovirus.

3. Occurrence—A disease of subtropical and tropical areas with long periods of hot, dry weather in Europe, Asia and Africa, and rainforests in Western Hemisphere tropics, distributed in a belt extending around the Mediterranean and eastward into Myanmar (Burma) and China. The disease is seasonal in temperate zones north of the equator, occurring between April and October, and is prone to affect military personnel and travelers from nonendemic areas.

4. Reservoir—Principal reservoir is the sand fly, in which the virus is maintained transovarianly. Arboreal rodents and nonhuman primates may harbor VSV. Rodents (gerbils) have been implicated as a reservoir for Eastern Hemisphere sand fly viruses.

5. Mode of transmission—By bite of an infective sand fly. The vector of the classic virus is a small, hairy, blood-sucking midge *(Phlebotomus papatasi,* the common sand fly), which bites at night and has a limited flight range. Sand flies of the genus *Sergentomyia* have also been found to be infected and may be vectors. Members of the genus *Lutzomyia* are involved in Central and South America.

6. Incubation period—Up to 6 days, usually 3–4 days, rarely less.

7. Period of communicability—Virus is present in the blood of an infected person at least 24 hours before and 24 hours after onset of fever. Phlebotomines become infective about 7 days after biting an infected person and remain so for their normal life span of about 1 month.

8. Susceptibility and resistance—Susceptibility is essentially universal; homologous acquired immunity is probably lasting. Relative resistance of native populations in sand fly areas is probably attributable to infection early in life.

9. Methods of control —

    A. Preventive measures: Personal protective measures to prevent sand fly feeding; control of sand flies is the principal objective (see Leishmaniasis, Cutaneous and Mucosal, 9A2).

B. *Control of patient, contacts and the immediate environment:*

1) Report to local health authority: In selected endemic areas; in most countries, not a reportable disease, Class 3C (see Communicable Disease Reporting).
2) Isolation: None; prevent access of sand flies to infected individuals for the first few days of illness by very fine screening or mosquito bed nets (10–12 mesh/cm or 25–30 mesh/inch, aperture size not more than 0.085 cm or 0.035 inch) and by spraying quarters with insecticide.
3) Concurrent disinfection: None; destroy sand flies in residences.
4) Quarantine: None.
5) Immunization of contacts: Not currently available.
6) Investigation of contacts and source of infection: In the Eastern Hemisphere, search for breeding areas of sand flies around dwellings, especially in rubble heaps, in masonry cracks and under stones.
7) Specific treatment: None.

C. *Epidemic measures:*

1) Educate the public about conditions leading to infection and the importance of preventing sand fly bites by use of repellents, particularly after sundown.
2) Use insecticides to control sand flies in and about human habitations, communitywide.

D. *Disaster implications:* None.

E. *International measures:* WHO Collaborating Centres.

ARTHROPOD-BORNE VIRAL HEMORRHAGIC FEVERS
I. MOSQUITO-BORNE DISEASES
(Dengue hemorrhagic fever and yellow fever are presented separately.)
II. TICKBORNE DISEASES
II.A. CRIMEAN-CONGO HEMORRHAGIC FEVER   ICD-9 065.0; ICD-10 A98.0
(Central Asian hemorrhagic fever)

1. Identification—A viral disease with sudden onset of fever, malaise, weakness, irritability, headache, severe pain in limbs and loins and marked anorexia. Vomiting, abdominal pain and diarrhea occur occasionally. Flush on face and chest and conjunctival injection develop early. Hemorrhagic enanthem of soft palate, uvula and pharynx, and a fine petechial rash spreading from the chest and abdomen to the rest of the body are generally associated with the disease; occasionally, large purpuric areas are observed.

There may be bleeding from gums, nose, lungs, uterus and intestine, but in large amounts only in serious or fatal cases, often associated with severe liver damage. Hematuria and albuminuria are common but usually not massive. Fever is constantly elevated for 5–12 days or may be biphasic; it falls by lysis. Convalescence is prolonged. Other findings are leukopenia, with lymphopenia more marked than neutropenia. Thrombocytopenia is common. The reported case-fatality rate ranges from 2% to 50%. In Russia, there are estimated to be five infections for each hemorrhagic case.

Diagnosis is made by isolation of virus from blood by inoculation of cell cultures or suckling mice or by PCR. Serologic diagnosis is by ELISA, reverse passive HI, IFA, CF, immunodiffusion or plaque-reduction neutralization test. Specific IgM may be present during the acute phase; convalescent sera often have low neutralization antibody titers.

2. Infectious agent—The Crimean-Congo hemorrhagic fever virus (Bunyaviridae, *Nairovirus*).

3. Occurrence—Observed in the steppe regions of western Crimea, on the Kersch Peninsula, in Kazakhstan and Uzbekistan, in the Rostov and Astrakhan regions of Russia, as well as in Albania and Bosnia-Herzogovina, Bulgaria, Iraq, the Arabian Peninsula, Pakistan, western China, tropical Africa and South Africa. Most patients are animal husbandry workers or medical personnel. Seasonal occurrence in Russia is from June to September, the period of vector activity. Virus or antibodies in humans have been observed in several areas of central and east Africa; hemorrhagic fever cases have been reported from South Africa and Mauritania (west Africa).

4. Reservoir—In nature, believed to be hares, birds and *Hyalomma* spp. of ticks in Eurasia and South Africa; reservoir hosts remain undefined in tropical Africa, but *Hyalomma* and *Boophilus* ticks, and insectivores and rodents may be involved. Domestic animals (sheep, goats and cattle) may act as amplifying hosts.

5. Mode of transmission—By bite of infective adult *Hyalomma marginatum* or *H. anatolicum*. Immature ticks are believed to acquire infection from the animal hosts and by transovarian transmission. Nosocomial infection of medical workers, occurring after exposure to blood and secretions from patients, has been important in recent outbreaks; tertiary cases have occurred in family members of medical workers. Infection is also associated with butchering infected animals.

6. Incubation period—Usually 1 to 3 days, with a range of 1–12 days.

7. Period of communicability—Highly infectious in the hospital setting. Nosocomial infections are common after exposure to blood and secretions.

8. Susceptibility and resistance—Immunity after infection probably lasts for life.

9. Methods of control—

    A. Preventive measures: See Lyme Disease, 9A, for preventive measures against ticks. An inactivated mouse brain vaccine has been used in eastern Europe and the former Soviet Union. No vaccine is available in the USA.

    B. Control of patient, contacts and the immediate environment:

        1) Report to local health authority: In selected epidemic areas; in most countries, not a reportable disease, Class 3B (see Communicable Disease Reporting).

        2) Isolation: Blood and body fluid precautions.

        3) Concurrent disinfection: Bloody discharges are infective; decontaminate by heat or chlorine disinfectants.

        4) Quarantine: None.

        5) Immunization: None, except in eastern Europe.

        6) Investigation of contacts and source of infection: Search for missed cases and the presence of infective animals and possible vectors.

        7) Specific treatment: Intravenous ribavirin and convalescent plasma with a high neutralizing antibody titer are regarded as useful.

    C. Epidemic measures: See Lyme Disease, 9C.

    D. Disaster implications: None.

    E. International measures: WHO Collaborating Centres.

II.B. OMSK HEMORRHAGIC FEVER   ICD-9 065.1; ICD-10 A98.1
KYASANUR FOREST DISEASE   ICD-9 065.2; ICD-10 A98.2

1. Identification—These two viral diseases have marked similarities: Onset is sudden with chills, headache, fever, pain in lower back and limbs and severe prostration, often associated with conjunctivitis, diarrhea and vomiting by the third or fourth day. A papulovesicular eruption on the soft palate, cervical lymphadenopathy and conjunctival suffusion are usually present. Confusion and encephalopathic symptoms may occur in patients with Kyasanur Forest disease (KFD); often there is a biphasic course of illness and fever, and the CNS abnormalities develop after an afebrile period of 1–2 weeks.

Severe cases are associated with hemorrhages but with no cutaneous rash. Bleeding occurs from gums, nose, GI tract, uterus and lungs (but rarely from the kidneys), sometimes for many days and, when severe, results in shock and death; shock may also occur without manifest hemorrhage. The febrile period ranges from 5 days to 2 weeks, at times with a secondary rise in the third week. Estimated case-fatality rate is from 1% to 10%. Leukopenia and thrombocytopenia are marked. Convalescence tends to be slow and prolonged.

Diagnosis is made by isolation of virus from blood in suckling mice or cell cultures (virus may be present up to 10 days following onset) or by serologic tests.

2. Infectious agents—The Omsk hemorrhagic fever (OHF) and KFD viruses are closely related; they belong to the tickborne encephalitis-louping ill complex of flaviviruses and are similar antigenically to the other viruses in the complex.

3. Occurrence—In the Kyasanur Forest of the Shimoga and Kanara districts of Karnataka, India, principally in young adult males exposed in the forest during the dry season, from November to June. In 1983, there were 1,155 cases with 150 deaths, the largest epidemic of KFD ever reported. OHF occurs in the forest steppe regions of western Siberia, within the Omsk, Novosibirsk, Kurgan and Tjumen regions. The Novosibirsk district reported 2 to 41 cases per year between 1989 and 1998, mostly in muskrat trappers. Seasonal occurrence in each area coincides with vector activity. Laboratory infections are common with both viruses.

4. Reservoir—In KFD, probably rodents, shrews and monkeys; in OHF, rodents, muskrats and ticks.

5. Mode of transmission—By bite of infective (especially nymphal) ticks, probably *Haemaphysalis spinigera* in KFD. In OHF, infective ticks possibly are *Dermacentor reticulatus (pictus)* and *D. marginatus;* direct transmission from muskrat to human occurs, with disease in the families of muskrat trappers.

6. Incubation period—Usually 3–8 days.

7. Period of communicability—Not directly transmitted from person to person. Infected ticks remain so for life.

8. Susceptibility and resistance—All ages and genders are probably susceptible; previous infection leads to immunity.

9. Methods of control—See Tickborne Viral Encephalitides and Lyme Disease, 9. A formalinized mouse-brain virus vaccine has been reported for

OHF; tickborne encephalitis vaccine also has been used to protect against OHF without proof of efficacy. An experimental vaccine has been used to prevent KFD in endemic areas of India.

ASCARIASIS　　　　　　　　　　ICD-9 127.0; ICD-10 B77
(Roundworm infection, Ascaridiasis)

1. Identification—A helminthic infection of the small intestine generally associated with few or no symptoms. Live worms, passed in stools or occasionally from the mouth, anus, or nose, are often the first recognized sign of infection. Some patients have pulmonary manifestations (pneumonitis, Löffler syndrome) caused by larval migration (mainly during reinfections) and characterized by wheezing, coughing, fever, blood eosinophilia and pulmonary infiltration. Heavy parasite burdens may aggravate nutritional deficiency. Serious complications, sometimes fatal, include bowel obstruction by a bolus of worms, particularly in children; or obstruction of a hollow viscus, such as bile duct, pancreatic duct or appendix, by one or more adult worms. Reports of ascaris pancreatitis are increasing.

Diagnosis is made by identifying eggs in feces or adult worms passed from the anus, mouth or nose. Intestinal worms may be visualized by radiologic and sonographic techniques; pulmonary involvement may be confirmed by identifying ascarid larvae in the sputum or gastric washings.

2. Infectious agent—*Ascaris lumbricoides,* the large intestinal roundworm of humans. *A. suum,* a similar parasite of pigs, rarely, if ever, develops to maturity in humans, although it may cause larva migrans.

3. Occurrence—Common and worldwide, with greatest frequency in moist tropical countries where prevalence often exceeds 50%. The prevalence and intensity of infection are usually highest in children between 3 and 8 years. In the USA, *Ascaris* is most commonly detected in recent immigrants from developing countries.

4. Reservoir—Humans; ascarid eggs in soil.

5. Mode of transmission—By ingestion of infective eggs from soil contaminated with human feces or from uncooked produce contaminated with soil containing infective eggs, but not directly from person to person or from fresh feces. Transmission takes place mainly in the vicinity of the home, where children, in the absence of sanitary facilities, fecally pollute the area; heavy infections in children are frequently the result of ingesting soil. Contaminated soil may be carried long distances on feet or footwear into houses and conveyances; transmission of infection by dust is also possible.

Eggs reach the soil in the feces, then undergo development (embryonation); at summer temperatures they become infective after 2-3 weeks and may then remain infective for several months or years in favorable soil. Ingested embryonated eggs hatch in the intestinal lumen; the larvae penetrate the gut wall and reach the lungs via the circulatory system. Larvae grow and develop in the lungs; 9-10 days after infection they pass into the alveoli, ascend the trachea, and are swallowed to reach the small intestine 14-20 days after infection, where they grow to maturity, mate and begin egg laying 45-60 days after ingestion of the embryonated eggs. Eggs passed by gravid females are discharged in feces.

6. Incubation period—The life cycle requires 4-8 weeks to be completed.

7. Period of communicability—As long as mature fertilized female worms live in the intestine. Usual life span of adult worms is 12 months; maximum may be up to 24 months. The female worm can produce more than 200,000 eggs a day. Under favorable conditions, embryonated eggs can remain viable in soil for years.

8. Susceptibility and resistance—Susceptibility is general.

9. Methods of control—

A. Preventive measures:

1) Educate the public in the use of toilet facilities.
2) Provide adequate facilities for proper disposal of feces and prevent soil contamination in areas immediately adjacent to houses, particularly in children's play areas.
3) In rural areas, construct privies that prevent dissemination of ascarid eggs through overflow, drainage or otherwise. Treating human feces by composting for later use as fertilizer may not kill all eggs.
4) Encourage satisfactory hygienic habits on the part of children; in particular, train them to wash hands before eating and handling food.
5) In endemic areas, protect food from dirt. Food that has been dropped on the floor should not be eaten unless washed or reheated.

B. Control of patient, contacts and the immediate environment:

1) Report to local health authority: Official report not ordinarily justifiable, Class 5 (see Communicable Disease Reporting).
2) Isolation: None.
3) Concurrent disinfection: Sanitary disposal of feces.

4) Quarantine: None.

5) Immunization of contacts: None.

6) Investigation of contacts and source of infection: Determine others who should be treated. Environmental sources of infection should be sought, particularly on premises of affected families.

7) Specific treatment: Mebendazole (Vermox®) and albendazole (Zentel®) (also efficacious against *Trichuris trichiura* and hookworm, see Trichuriasis and Hookworm Disease); both are contraindicated during pregnancy. Erratic migration of ascarid worms has been reported following mebendazole therapy; however, this may also occur with other medications, or spontaneously in heavy infections. Pyrantel pamoate (Antiminth®, Combantrin®) is also effective in a single dose (also against hookworm, but not against *T. trichiura*).

C. *Epidemic measures:* Survey for prevalence in highly endemic areas, educate the community in environmental sanitation and in personal hygiene and provide treatment facilities.

D. *Disaster implications:* None.

E. *International measures:* None.

ASPERGILLOSIS   ICD-9 117.3; ICD-10 B44

1. Identification—A fungal disease that may present with a variety of clinical syndromes produced by several of the *Aspergillus* species. Patients with chronic lung disease (especially asthma, but also chronic obstructive pulmonary disease or cystic fibrosis) and allergy to the aspergilli may develop bronchial damage and intermittent bronchial plugging, a condition called allergic bronchopulmonary aspergillosis (ABPA). Saprophytic endobronchial colonization in patients with bronchitis or bronchiectasis may cause clumps of hyphae to form within ectatic bronchi, or a large mass of hyphae may fill a previously existing cavity (i.e., fungus ball or aspergilloma). An *Aspergillus* species may appear as a concomitant organism in a bacterial lung abscess or empyema.

Invasive aspergillosis may occur, particularly in patients receiving cytotoxic or immunosuppressive therapy; it may disseminate to the brain, kidneys and other organs and is often fatal. Invasion of blood vessels with thrombosis and infarction is characteristic of infection in immunosuppressed patients.

The organisms may infect the implantation site of a cardiac prosthetic valve. *Aspergillus* species are the most common causes of otomycosis; the fungi may colonize or cause invasive infection of the paranasal sinuses.

Growing on certain foods, many isolates of *A. flavus* (and occasionally other species) will produce aflatoxins or other mycotoxins; these cause disease in animals and fish and are highly carcinogenic for experimental animals. An association between high aflatoxin levels in foods and hepatocellular cancer has been noted in Africa and southeast Asia.

The diagnosis of ABPA is suggested by wheal-and-flare responses to scratch or intradermal tests with *Aspergillus* antigens, episodes of bronchial plugging, eosinophilia, serum precipitating antibodies against *Aspergillus*, elevated serum concentration of IgE and transient pulmonary infiltrates (with or without central bronchiectasis). Saprophytic endobronchial colonization is diagnosed by culture or microscopic demonstration of *Aspergillus* mycelia in sputum or in plugs of expectorated hyphae. Serum precipitins to antigens of *Aspergillus* species are usually present. Fungus balls of the lung can usually be diagnosed by chest x-ray and medical history. Diagnosis of invasive aspergillosis depends on microscopic demonstration of the *Aspergillus* mycelia in infected tissue; confirmation by culture is definitive and differentiates the disease from the histologically similar presentations caused by other fungi.

2. Infectious agents—*Aspergillus fumigatus* and *A. flavus* are the most common causes of aspergillosis in humans, although other species have also been implicated. *A. fumigatus* causes most cases of fungus ball; *A. niger* is the usual cause of otomycosis.

3. Occurrence—Worldwide; uncommon and sporadic; no distinctive differences in incidence by race or gender.

4. Reservoir—*Aspergillus* species are ubiquitous in nature, particularly in decaying vegetation, such as in piles of leaves or compost piles. Conidia are commonly present in the air both outdoors and indoors and in all seasons of the year.

5. Mode of transmission—Inhalation of airborne conidia.

6. Incubation period—Probably a few days to weeks.

7. Period of communicability—Not transmitted from person to person.

8. Susceptibility and resistance—The ubiquity of *Aspergillus* species and the usual occurrence of the disease as a secondary infection suggest a high degree of resistance by healthy people. Susceptibility is increased by immunosuppressive or cytotoxic therapy, and invasive disease is seen primarily in those with prolonged neutropenia. Patients with HIV infection or chronic granulomatous disease of childhood are also susceptible.

9. Methods of control—

A. Preventive measures: High efficiency particulate air (HEPA) filtered room air can decrease the incidence of invasive aspergillosis in hospitalized patients with profound and prolonged neutropenia.

B. Control of patient, contacts and the immediate environment:

1) Report to local health authority: Official report not ordinarily justifiable, Class 5 (see Communicable Disease Reporting).
2) Isolation: None.
3) Concurrent disinfection: Ordinary cleanliness. Terminal cleaning.
4) Quarantine: None.
5) Immunization of contacts: None.
6) Investigation of contacts: Not ordinarily indicated.
7) Specific treatment: ABPA is treated with corticosteroid suppression and usually requires prolonged therapy. Surgical resection, if possible, is the treatment of choice for aspergilloma. Amphotericin B (Fungizone® or a lipid formation) IV is also useful in tissue invasive forms. Itraconazole may be useful in some of the more slowly progressing and more immunocompetent cases. Immunosuppressive therapy should be discontinued or reduced as much as possible. Endobronchial colonization should be treated by measures to improve bronchopulmonary drainage.

C. Epidemic measures: Not generally applicable; a sporadic disease.

D. Disaster implications: None.

E. International measures: None.

BABESIOSIS   ICD-9 088.8; ICD-10 B60.0

1. Identification—A potentially severe and sometimes fatal disease caused by infection with a protozoan parasite of RBCs. The clinical syndrome may include fever, chills, myalgia, fatigue and jaundice secondary to a hemolytic anemia that may last from several days to a few months. Seroprevalence studies indicate that most infections are asymptomatic. In some cases, parasitemia without symptoms may last for months or even years. Dual infection with *Borrelia burgdorferi,* causal agent of Lyme disease, is known to occur and may increase the severity of both diseases.

Diagnosis is made by identification of the parasite within RBCs on a thick or thin blood film. Demonstration of specific antibodies by serologic analysis (IFA babesial DNA (PCR)) or isolation of the parasite in appropriate laboratory animals provides supportive evidence for the diagnosis. Differentiation from *Plasmodium falciparum* on blood film examination may be difficult in patients who have been in malarious areas or who may have acquired infection by blood transfusion; if diagnosis is uncertain, manage as if it were a case of malaria and send thick and thin blood films to an appropriate reference laboratory.

2. Infectious agents—A number of different species are known to have caused disease in humans. *Babesia microti* is the most common in the eastern and midwestern USA, while *Babesia* isolate type WA1 parasites are most common on the west coast. *B. divergens* is the most common species in Europe.

3. Occurrence—Worldwide in scattered locations. In the USA, the geographic distribution of *B. microti* infection has increased along with the widening range of the tick vector, *Ixodes scapularis* (formerly called *I. dammini*). Babesiosis is endemic on Nantucket and other islands in Massachusetts, Block Island, Shelter Island, eastern Long Island and southern Connecticut. Infection has also been reported from Wisconsin and Minnesota. Human cases due to *Babesia* isolate type WA1 have been reported in California and Washington state. Other species have caused human infection in Missouri and Mexico. In Europe, human infections caused by *B. divergens* have been reported from France, Ireland, Scotland, Spain, Sweden, Russia and Yugoslavia. Human infections with less well characterized species of *Babesia* have been reported from China, Taiwan, Egypt, the Canary Islands and South Africa.

4. Reservoir—Rodents for *B. microti* and cattle for *B. divergens*. Reservoir for *Babesia* isolate type WA1 and MO1 (Missouri) are unknown.

5. Mode of transmission—*B. microti* is transmitted primarily during the summer months by the bite of nymphal *Ixodes* ticks *(I. scapularis)* that have fed on infected deer mice *(Peromyscus leucopus)* and other small mammals (e.g., voles, *Microtus pennsylvanicus*). The adult tick is normally found on deer (which are not infected by the parasite) but may also parasitize and be spread by a variety of mammalian and avian hosts. The vector of *B. divergens* in Europe appears to be *I. ricinus*. Occasionally, cases of babesiosis have been reported to have been transmitted by blood transfusion from asymptomatic but parasitemic donors. Patients usually do not recall a tick bite. Two cases of mother to infant transmission have been reported.

6. Incubation period—Variable; 1 week to 8 weeks has been reported after discrete exposures. Recrudescence of symptoms after prolonged asymptomatic parasitemia may occur months to more than a year after initial exposure.

7. Period of communicability—Not transmitted from person to person except by blood transfusion. Asymptomatic blood donors have been shown to be infectious for as long as 12 months after initial infection.

8. Susceptibility and resistance—Susceptibility to *B. microti* is assumed to be universal; immunocompromised, asplenic and elderly persons are at particular risk of symptomatic infection.

9. Methods of control—

A. Preventive measures: Educate the public about the mode of transmission and means for personal protection. Control rodents around human habitation and use tick repellents.

B. Control of patient, contacts and the immediate environment:

1) Report to local health authority: Report newly suspected cases by telephone, particularly in areas not previously known to be endemic, Class 3B (see Communicable Disease Reporting).
2) Isolation: Blood and body fluid precautions.
3) Concurrent disinfection: None.
4) Quarantine: None.
5) Protection of contacts: None, but household members possibly exposed at the same time as the patient should be evaluated for infection and observed for fever.
6) Investigation of contacts and source of infection: Cases occurring in a new area deserve careful study. Blood donors in transfusion related cases should be investigated promptly and deferred from future donations.
7) Specific treatment: The combination of clindamycin and quinine has been effective in experimental animal studies and in most patients with *B. microti* infections who have received this drug combination. Infection does not respond to chloroquine. Azithromycin either alone or in combination with quinine or with clindamycin and doxycycline has been effective in some cases, and azithromycin in combination with atovaquone shows promise in experimental animals. Pentamidine in combination with TMP-SMX was effective in one reported case of *B. divergens*. Exchange transfusion may be required in patients with a high proportion of parasitized RBCs. Dialysis may be necessary for patients with renal failure.

C. Epidemic measures: None.

D. Disaster implications: None.

E. International measures: None.

BALANTIDIASIS   ICD-9 007.0; ICD-10 A07.0
(Balantidiosis, Balantidial dysentery)

1. Identification—A protozoan infection of the colon characteristically producing diarrhea or dysentery, accompanied by abdominal colic, tenesmus, nausea and vomiting. Occasionally the dysentery resembles that due to amebiasis, with stools containing much blood and mucus but relatively little pus. Peritoneal or urogenital invasion is rare.

Diagnosis is made by identifying the trophozoites or cysts of *Balantidium coli* in fresh feces, or trophozoites in material obtained by sigmoidoscopy.

2. Infectious agent—*Balantidium coli,* a large ciliated protozoan.

3. Occurrence—Worldwide; the incidence of human disease is low. Waterborne epidemics occasionally occur in areas of poor environmental sanitation. Environmental contamination with swine feces may result in a higher incidence. Laboratory pigs may carry this parasite. A large epidemic occurred in frontier areas of Ecuador in 1978.

4. Reservoir—Swine and possibly other animals, such as rats and nonhuman primates.

5. Mode of transmission—By ingestion of cysts from feces of infected hosts; in epidemics, mainly by fecally contaminated water. Sporadic transmission is by transfer of feces to mouth by hands or by contaminated water or food.

6. Incubation period—Unknown; may be only a few days.

7. Period of communicability—As long as the infection persists.

8. Susceptibility and resistance—People appear to have a high natural resistance. In individuals debilitated from other diseases the infection may be serious and even fatal.

9. Methods of control—

    A. Preventive measures:

        1) Educate the general public in personal hygiene.
        2) Educate and supervise food handlers via health agencies.
        3) Dispose of feces in a sanitary manner.
        4) Minimize contact with hog feces.
        5) Protect public water supplies against contamination with hog feces. Diatomaceous earth and sand filters remove all cysts, but ordinary water chlorination does not destroy cysts. Small quantities of water are best treated by boiling.

B. *Control of patient, contacts and the immediate environment:*

1) Report to local health authority: Official report not ordinarily justifiable, Class 5 (see Communicable Disease Reporting).
2) Isolation: None.
3) Concurrent disinfection: Sanitary disposal of feces.
4) Quarantine: None.
5) Immunization of contacts: Not applicable.
6) Investigation of contacts and source of infection: Microscopic examination of feces of household members and suspected contacts. Also investigate contact with hogs; consider treating infected pigs with tetracycline.
7) Specific treatment: Tetracyclines eliminate infection; metronidazole (Flagyl®) may also be effective.

C. *Epidemic measures:* Any grouping of several cases in an area or institution requires prompt epidemiologic investigation, especially of environmental sanitation.

D. *Disaster implications:* None.

E. *International measures:* None.

BARTONELLOSIS   ICD-9 088.0; ICD-10 A44
(Oroya fever, Verruga peruana, Carrión disease)

1. Identification—A bacterial infection with two markedly different clinical forms: a febrile anemia (Oroya fever, ICD-10 A44.0) and a benign dermal eruption (Verruga peruana, ICD-10 A44.1). Asymptomatic infection and a carrier state may occur. Oroya fever is characterized by irregular fever, headache, myalgia, arthralgia, pallor, severe hemolytic anemia (macrocytic or normocytic and usually hypochromic) and generalized nontender lymphadenopathy. Verruga peruana has a preeruptive stage characterized by shifting pain in muscles, bones and joints; the pain, often severe, lasts minutes to several days at any one site. The dermal eruption may be miliary with widely disseminated, small, hemangioma-like nodules, or nodular with fewer but larger deep-seated lesions, most prominent on the extensor surfaces of the limbs. Individual nodules, particularly near joints, may develop into tumor-like masses with an ulcerated surface.

Verruga peruana may be preceded by Oroya fever or by an asymptomatic infection, with an interval of weeks to months between the stages. The case-fatality rate of untreated Oroya fever ranges from 10% to 90%; death is often associated with protozoal and bacterial superinfections, including salmonella septicemia. Verruga peruana has a prolonged course but seldom results in death.

Diagnosis is made by demonstration of the infectious agent adherent to or within RBCs during the acute stage by Giemsa staining, in sections of skin lesions during the eruptive stage or by blood culture on special media during either stage. PCR and a number of serologic techniques have been used to establish the diagnosis.

2. Infectious agent—*Bartonella bacilliformis*.

3. Occurrence—Limited to mountain valleys of Peru, Ecuador and southwest Colombia, between altitudes of 2,000 and 9,200 ft (600 to 2,800 m) above sea level, where the sand fly vector is present; no special predilection for age, race or gender.

4. Reservoir—Humans with the agent present in the blood. In endemic areas, the asymptomatic carrier rate may reach 5%. There is no known animal reservoir.

5. Mode of transmission—By the bite of sand flies of the genus *Lutzomyia*. Species are not identified for all areas; *Lutzomyia verrucarum* is important in Peru. These insects feed only from dusk to dawn. Blood transfusion, particularly during the Oroya fever stage, may transmit infection.

6. Incubation period—Usually 16-22 days, but occasionally 3-4 months.

7. Period of communicability—Not directly transmitted from person to person, other than by transfused blood. Humans are infectious for the sand fly for a long period; the agent may be present in blood weeks before and up to several years after clinical illness. Duration of infectivity of the sand fly is unknown.

8. Susceptibility and resistance—Susceptibility is general, but the disease is milder in children than in adults. Inapparent infections and carriers are known. Recovery from untreated Oroya fever almost invariably gives permanent immunity to this form; the Verruga stage may recur.

9. Methods of control—

   A. Preventive measures:

      1) Control sand flies (see Leishmaniasis, Cutaneous, 9A).
      2) Avoid known endemic areas after sundown; otherwise apply insect repellent to exposed parts of the body and use fine mesh bed netting.
      3) Blood from residents of an endemic area should not be used for transfusions until it has tested negative.

B. *Control of patient, contacts and the immediate environment:*

1) Report to local health authority: In selected endemic areas; in most countries not a reportable disease, Class 3B (see Communicable Disease Reporting).
2) Isolation: Blood and body fluid precautions. The infected individual should be protected from bites of sand flies (see 9A, above).
3) Concurrent disinfection: None.
4) Quarantine: None.
5) Immunization of contacts: None.
6) Investigation of contacts and source of infection: Identification of sand flies, particularly in localities where the infected person was exposed after sundown during the preceding 3–8 weeks.
7) Specific treatment: Penicillin, streptomycin, chloramphenicol and tetracyclines are all effective in reducing fever and bacteremia. Ampicillin and chloramphenicol are also effective against the frequent secondary complication, salmonellosis.

C. *Epidemic measures:* Intensify case finding and systematically spray houses with a residual insecticide.

D. *Disaster implications:* Only if refugee centers are established in an endemic locus.

E. *International measures:* None.

BLASTOMYCOSIS   ICD-9 116.0; ICD-10 B40
(North American blastomycosis, Gilchrist disease)

1. Identification—Blastomycosis is a granulomatous mycosis, primarily of the lungs and skin. Pulmonary blastomycosis may be acute or chronic. Acute infection is rarely recognized but presents with the sudden onset of fever, cough and a pulmonary infiltrate on chest x-ray. The acute disease resolves spontaneously after 1–3 weeks of illness. During or after the resolution of the pneumonia, some patients exhibit extrapulmonary infection. More commonly, there is an indolent onset that evolves into the chronic disease.

Cough and chest aching may be mild or absent so that patients may present with infection already spread to other sites, particularly skin, and less often to bone, prostate or epididymis. Skin lesions begin as erythematous papules that become verrucous, crusted or ulcerated and spread slowly. Most commonly, lesions are located on the face and distal extremities. Weight loss, weakness and low-grade fever are often present. Pulmonary lesions may cavitate. The course of untreated disseminated or chronic pulmonary blastomycosis is eventual progression and usually, death.

Direct microscopic examination of unstained smears of sputum and material from lesions shows characteristic "broad-based" budding forms of the fungus, often dumbbell in shape, which can be isolated by culture. Serologic test results are not useful.

2. Infectious agent—*Blastomyces dermatitidis (Ajellomyces dermatitidis)*, a dimorphic fungus that grows as a yeast in tissue and in enriched culture media at 37°C (98.6°F), and as a mold at room temperature (25°C/77°F).

3. Occurrence—Uncommon. Occurs sporadically in central and south-eastern USA, Canada, Africa (Zaire, Tanzania, South Africa), India, Israel and Saudi Arabia. Rare in children; more frequent in males than females. Disease in dogs is frequent; it has also been reported in cats, a horse, a captive African lion and a sea lion.

4. Reservoir—Moist soil, particularly wooded areas along waterways and undisturbed places, i.e., under porches or sheds.

5. Mode of transmission—Conidia, typical of the mold or saprophytic growth form, inhaled in spore laden dust.

6. Incubation period—Indefinite; probably a few weeks or less to months. For symptomatic infections, median is 45 days.

7. Period of communicability—Not transmitted directly from people or animals to people.

8. Susceptibility and resistance—Unknown. Inapparent pulmonary infections are probable but of undetermined frequency. There is evidence that cell mediated immunity plays a role in controlling lung infection. The rarity of the natural disease and of laboratory acquired infections suggests people are relatively resistant.

9. Methods of control —

  A. *Preventive measures:* Unknown.

  B. *Control of patient, contacts and the immediate environment:*

  1) Report to local health authority: Official report not ordinarily justifiable, Class 5 (see Communicable Disease Reporting).
  2) Isolation: None.
  3) Concurrent disinfection: Sputum, discharges and all contaminated articles. Terminal cleaning.
  4) Quarantine: None.

5) Immunization of contacts: None.

6) Investigation of contacts and source of infection: Not profitable unless clusters of disease occur.

7) Specific treatment: Itraconazole is the drug of choice, but amphotericin B (Fungizone®) is indicated in patients severely ill or with brain lesions.

C. Epidemic measures: Not applicable, a sporadic disease.

D. Disaster implications: None.

E. International measures: None.

BOTULISM
INTESTINAL BOTULISM, formerly
INFANT BOTULISM   ICD-9 005.1; ICD-10 A05.1

1. Identification—There are three forms of botulism—foodborne (the classic form), wound and intestinal (infant and adult) botulism. The site of toxin production is different for each of the forms but all share the flaccid paralysis that results from botulinum neurotoxin. Intestinal botulism has been proposed as the new designation for what had been called infant botulism. This new name has not been officially accepted as of mid-1999, but will be generally used in this chapter instead of infant botulism.

Foodborne botulism is a severe intoxication resulting from ingestion of preformed toxin present in contaminated food. The illness is characterized by acute bilateral cranial nerve impairment and descending weakness or paralysis. Visual difficulty (blurred or double vision), dysphagia and dry mouth are often the first complaints. These symptoms may extend to a symmetrical flaccid paralysis in a paradoxically alert person. Vomiting and constipation or diarrhea may be present initially. Fever is absent unless a complicating infection occurs. The case-fatality rate in the USA is 5%–10%. Recovery may take months.

In **wound botulism** the same clinical picture is seen after the causative organism contaminates a wound in which anaerobic conditions develop.

Intestinal (infant) botulism is the most common form of botulism in the USA; it results from ingestion of *Clostridium botulinum* spores with subsequent outgrowth and in-vivo toxin production in the large intestine. It affects infants under 1 year of age almost exclusively, but can affect adults who have altered GI anatomy and microflora. The illness typically begins with constipation, followed by lethargy, listlessness, poor feeding, ptosis, difficulty swallowing, loss of head control, hypotonia extending to generalized weakness (the "floppy baby") and, in some cases, respiratory insufficiency and arrest. Infant botulism has a wide spectrum of clinical severity, ranging from mild illness with gradual onset to sudden infant death; some studies suggest that it may cause an estimated 5% of cases of sudden infant death syndrome (SIDS). The case-fatality rate of hospitalized cases in the USA is less than 1%; without access to hospitals with pediatric intensive care units, more would die.

Diagnosis of foodborne botulism is made by demonstration of botulinum toxin in serum, stool, gastric aspirate or incriminated food; or by culture of *C. botulinum* from gastric aspirate or stool in a clinical case. Identification of organisms in a suspected food is helpful but not diagnostic because botulinum spores are ubiquitous; the presence of toxin in a suspected contaminated food source is more significant. The diagnosis may be accepted in a person with the clinical syndrome who had consumed a food item incriminated in a laboratory confirmed case. Wound botulism is diagnosed by toxin in serum or by positive wound culture. Electromyography with rapid repetitive stimulation can be useful in corroborating the clinical diagnosis for all forms of botulism.

The diagnosis of intestinal botulism is established by identification of *C. botulinum* organisms and/or toxin in patient's feces or in autopsy specimens. Toxin is rarely detected in the sera of patients.

2. Infectious agent—Foodborne botulism is caused by toxins produced by *Clostridium botulinum,* a spore forming obligate anaerobic bacillus. A few nanograms of the toxin can cause illness. Most human outbreaks are due to types A, B, E and rarely to type F. Type G has been isolated from soil and autopsy specimens but an etiologic role in botulism has not been established. Type E outbreaks are usually related to fish, seafood and meat from marine mammals.

Toxin is produced in improperly processed, canned, low acid or alkaline foods, and in pasteurized and lightly cured foods held without refrigeration, especially in airtight packaging. The toxin is destroyed by boiling; inactivation of spores requires much higher temperatures. Type E toxin can be produced slowly at temperatures as low as 3°C (37.4°F), which is lower than that of ordinary refrigeration.

Most cases of infant botulism have been caused by type A or B. A few cases (toxin types E and F) have been reported from neurotoxigenic clostridial species *C. butyricum* and *C. baratii,* respectively.

3. Occurrence—Worldwide; sporadic cases, family and general outbreaks occur where food products are prepared or preserved by methods that do not destroy the spores and permit toxin formation. Cases rarely result from commercially processed products; outbreaks have occurred from contamination through cans damaged after processing. Cases of intestinal botulism have been reported from five continents: Asia, Australia, Europe, and North and South America. The actual incidence and distribution of intestinal botulism are unknown because physician awareness and diagnostic testing remain limited, as demonstrated by a review of intestinal botulism cases reported between 1976, when it was first recognized in

California, and the beginning of 1999. Of the 1,700 cumulative global case total, over 1,400 were reported by the USA, with close to half of those cases reported by California. Internationally, about 150 cases have been detected in Argentina; less than 20 each in Australia and Japan; less than 15 in Canada; and about 30 from Europe (mostly Italy and the UK), with scattered reports from Chile, China, Israel and Yemen.

4. Reservoir—Spores are ubiquitous in soil worldwide; they are frequently recovered from agricultural products, including honey. Spores are also found in marine sediments and in the intestinal tract of animals, including fish.

5. Mode of transmission—Foodborne botulism is acquired by ingestion of food in which toxin has been formed, predominantly after inadequate heating during preservation and without subsequent adequate cooking. Most poisonings in the USA are due to home canned vegetables and fruits; meat is an infrequent vehicle. Several outbreaks have recently occurred following consumption of uneviscerated fish. Cases associated with baked potatoes and improperly handled commercial potpies have been reported. One recent outbreak was attributed to sautéed onions, two others to minced garlic in oil. Some of these recent outbreaks originated in restaurants. Newer varieties of certain garden foods such as tomatoes, formerly considered too acidic to support growth of *C. botulinum*, may no longer be low hazard foods for home canning.

In Canada and Alaska, outbreaks have been associated with seal meat, smoked salmon and fermented salmon eggs. In Europe, most cases are due to sausages and smoked or preserved meats; in Japan, to seafood. These differences have been attributed in part to the greater use of sodium nitrite for preserving meats in the USA.

Wound botulism cases often result from contamination of the wounds by ground-in soil or gravel or from improperly treated open fractures. Wound botulism has been reported among chronic drug abusers (primarily in dermal abscesses from subcutaneous injection of heroin and also from sinusitis in cocaine "sniffers").

Intestinal botulism arises from ingestion of botulinum spores that then germinate in the colon, rather than by ingestion of preformed toxin. Possible sources of spores for infants are multiple, and include foods and dust. Honey, fed on occasion to infants, can contain *C. botulinum* spores.

6. Incubation period—Neurologic symptoms of foodborne botulism usually appear within 12–36 hours, sometimes several days, after eating contaminated food. In general, the shorter the incubation period, the more severe the disease and the higher the case-fatality rate. The incubation period of intestinal botulism in infants is unknown, since the precise time that the infant ingested the causal botulinum spores cannot be determined.

7. Period of communicability—Despite excretion of *C. botulinum* toxin and organisms at high levels (ca. 10^6 organisms/g) in the feces of intestinal botulism patients for weeks to months after onset of illness, no instance of secondary person to person transmission has been documented. Foodborne botulism patients typically excrete the toxin and organisms for shorter periods.

8. Susceptibility and resistance—Susceptibility is general. Almost all patients hospitalized with intestinal botulism have been between 2 weeks and 1 year of age; 94% were less than 6 months, and the median age at onset was 13 weeks. Cases of intestinal botulism have occurred in all major racial and ethnic groups. Adults with special bowel problems leading to unusual GI flora (or with a flora unintentionally altered by antibiotic treatment for other purposes) may be susceptible to intestinal botulism.

9. Methods of control—

   A. *Preventive measures:*

   1) Ensure effective control of processing and preparation of commercially canned and preserved foods.
   2) Educate those concerned with home canning and other food preservation techniques regarding the proper time, pressure and temperature required to destroy spores, the need for adequately refrigerated storage of incompletely processed foods, and the effectiveness of boiling, with stirring, home canned vegetables for at least 10 minutes to destroy botulinum toxins.
   3) *C. botulinum* may or may not cause container lids to bulge and the contents to have "off-odors." Other contaminants can also cause cans or bottle lids to bulge. Bulging containers should not be opened, and foods with off-odors should not be eaten or "taste tested." Commercial cans with bulging lids should be returned unopened to the vendor.
   4) Although *C. botulinum* spores are ubiquitous, identified sources such as honey, should not be fed to infants.

   B. *Control of patient, contacts and the immediate environment:*

   1) Report to local health authority: Case report of suspected and confirmed cases obligatory in most states and countries, Class 2A (see Communicable Disease Reporting); immediate telephone report indicated.
   2) Isolation: Not required, but handwashing is indicated after handling soiled diapers.
   3) Concurrent disinfection: The implicated food(s) should be detoxified by boiling before discarding, or the containers broken and buried deeply in soil to prevent ingestion by animals. Contaminated utensils should be sterilized by boiling

or by chlorine disinfection to inactivate any remaining toxin. Usual sanitary disposal of feces from infant cases. Terminal cleaning.

4) Quarantine: None.

5) Management of contacts: None for simple direct contacts. Those who are known to have eaten the incriminated food should be purged with cathartics, given gastric lavage and high enemas and kept under close medical observation. The decision to provide presumptive treatment with polyvalent (equine AB or ABE) antitoxin to asymptomatic exposed individuals should be weighed carefully: balance the potential protection when antitoxin is administered early (within 1–2 days after eating the implicated meal) against the risk of adverse reactions and sensitization to horse serum.

6) Investigation of contacts and source of toxin: Study recent food history of those ill, and recover all suspected foods for appropriate testing and disposal. Search for other cases of botulism to rule out foodborne botulism.

7) Specific treatment: Intravenous administration as soon as possible of 1 vial of polyvalent (AB or ABE) botulinum antitoxin, available from CDC, Atlanta, through state health departments is considered a part of routine treatment (the emergency telephone number at CDC for botulism calls during regular office hours is 404-639-2206; and after hours and on weekends is 404-639-2888). Serum should be collected to identify the specific toxin before antitoxin is administered, but antitoxin should not be withheld pending test results. Most important is immediate access to an intensive care unit so that respiratory failure, the usual cause of death, can be anticipated and managed promptly. For wound botulism, in addition to antitoxin, the wound should be debrided and/or drainage established, and appropriate antibiotics (e.g., penicillin) administered.

In intestinal botulism, meticulous supportive care is essential. Equine botulinum antitoxin is not used because of the hazard of sensitization and anaphylaxis. An investigational human derived botulinal immune globulin (BIG) is currently available for the treatment only of infant botulism patients under an FDA approved open-label Treatment Investigational New Drug protocol from the California Department of Health Services. Information on BIG for the "empiric" treatment of suspected intestinal botulism in infants can be obtained from the California Department of Health Services at 510-540-2646 (24-hour line). Antibiotics do not improve the course of the disease, and aminoglycoside antibiotics in particular may worsen it by causing a synergistic neuromuscular blockade. Thus, antibiotics should be used only to treat secondary infections. Assisted respiration may be required.

C. *Epidemic measures:* Suspicion of a single case of botulism should immediately raise the question of a group outbreak involving a family or others who have shared a common food. Home preserved foods should be the prime suspect until ruled out, although restaurant foods or widely distributed commercially preserved foods are occasionally identified as the source of intoxication and pose a far greater threat to the public health.

In addition, because recent outbreaks have implicated unusual food items, even theoretically unlikely foods should be considered. When any food is implicated by epidemiologic or laboratory findings, immediate recall of the product is necessary, as is immediate search for people who shared the suspected food and for any remaining food from the same source. Any remaining food may be similarly contaminated; such food, if found, should be submitted for laboratory examination. Sera, gastric aspirates and stool from patients and (when indicated) from others exposed but not ill should be collected and forwarded immediately to a reference laboratory before administration of antitoxin.

D. *Disaster implications:* None.

E. *International measures:* Commercial products may have been distributed widely; international efforts may be required to recover and test implicated foods. International common source outbreaks have occurred.

F. *Bioterrorism measures:* Botulinum toxins can be easily used by terrorists. Although the greatest threat may be via aerosol use, the more common threat may be via its use in food and drink. The occurrence of even a single case of botulism, especially if there is no obvious source of an improperly preserved food should raise the possibility of deliberate use of botulinum toxin. All such cases should be reported immediately so that appropriate investigations can be initiated without delay.

BRUCELLOSIS   ICD-9 023; ICD-10 A23
(Undulant fever, Malta fever, Mediterranean fever)

1. Identification—A systemic bacterial disease with acute or insidious onset, characterized by continued, intermittent or irregular fever of variable duration; headache; weakness; profuse sweating; chills; arthralgia; depression; weight loss and generalized aching. Localized suppurative infections of organs, including the liver and spleen, may occur; subclinical disease has been reported, and chronic localized infections can occur. The disease may last for several days, months or occasionally a year or more if not adequately treated.

Osteoarticular complications are seen in 20%-60% of cases; sacroiliitis is the most frequent joint manifestation. Genitourinary involvement is reported in 2%-20% of cases, with orchitis and epididymitis most common. Recovery is usual but disability is often pronounced. The case-fatality rate of untreated brucellosis is 2% or less and usually results from endocarditis caused by *Brucella melitensis* infections. Part or all of the original syndrome may reappear as relapses. A neurotic symptom complex is sometimes misdiagnosed as chronic brucellosis.

Laboratory diagnosis is made by appropriate isolation of the infectious agent from blood, bone marrow or other tissues, or from discharges of the patient. Serologic tests in experienced laboratories are valuable, especially when paired sera show a rise in antibody titer. Interpretation of serologic tests in chronic and recurrent cases is especially difficult since titers are usually low. Tests measuring IgG antibody may be useful, particularly in chronic cases, since active infection is associated with a titer rise. Specific serologic techniques are needed for *B. canis* antibodies, which do not cross react with the other species.

2. Infectious agents—*Brucella abortus,* biovars 1-6 and 9; *B. melitensis,* biovars 1-3; *B. suis,* biovars 1-5; and *B. canis.*

3. Occurrence—Worldwide, especially in Mediterranean countries of Europe and North and east Africa, Middle Eastern countries, India, central Asia, Mexico, and Central and South America. The sources of infection and the responsible organism vary according to geographic area. Brucellosis is predominantly an occupational disease of those working with infected animals or their tissues, especially farm workers, veterinarians and abattoir workers; hence it is more frequent among males. Sporadic cases and outbreaks occur among consumers of raw milk and milk products (especially unpasteurized soft cheese) from cows, sheep and goats. Isolated cases of infection with *B. canis* occur in animal handlers from contact with dogs. Currently reported incidence in the USA is less than 120 cases annually; worldwide, the disease is often unrecognized and unreported.

4. Reservoir—Cattle, swine, goats and sheep. Infection may occur in bison, elk, caribou and some species of deer. *B. canis* is an occasional problem in laboratory dog colonies and kennels; a small percentage of pet dogs and a higher proportion of stray dogs have positive *B. canis* antibody titers. Coyotes have been found to be infected.

5. Mode of transmission—By contact with tissues, blood, urine, vaginal discharges, aborted fetuses and especially placentas (through breaks in the skin), and by ingestion of raw milk and dairy products (unpasteurized cheese) from infected animals. Airborne infection of animals occurs in pens and stables, and of humans in laboratories and abattoirs. A small number of cases result from accidental self-inoculation of strain 19 Brucella vaccine; the same risk is present when Rev-1 vaccine is handled.

6. Incubation period—Highly variable and difficult to ascertain; usually 5–60 days; 1–2 months commonplace; occasionally several months.

7. Period of communicability—No evidence of communicability from person to person.

8. Susceptibility and resistance—Severity and duration of clinical illness are subject to wide variation. Duration of acquired immunity is uncertain.

9. Methods of control—Ultimate control of human brucellosis rests on the elimination of the disease among domestic animals.

A. Preventive measures:

1) Educate the public (especially tourists) not to drink untreated milk or eat products made from unpasteurized or otherwise untreated milk.
2) Educate farmers and workers in slaughterhouses, meat processing plants and butcher shops as to the nature of the disease and the risk in the handling of carcasses and products of potentially infected animals, and the proper operation of abattoirs to reduce exposure (especially appropriate ventilation).
3) Educate hunters to use barrier precautions (gloves, clothing) in dressing feral swine and to bury the remains.
4) Search for infection among livestock by serologic test and by ELISA or ring test of cows' milk; eliminate infected animals by segregation and/or slaughter. Infection among swine usually requires slaughter of the herd. In areas of high prevalence, immunize young goats and sheep with live attenuated Rev-1 strain of *B. melitensis,* and calves and sometimes adult animals with strain 19, *B. abortus.* Since 1996, the recombinant RB51 vaccine has largely replaced the use of strain 19 for immunization of cattle against *B. abortus.* RB51 vaccine appears to be less virulent for humans than strain 19.
5) While evidence for its efficacy has not been proven in clinical trials, it is recommended that persons inadvertently inoculated with strain 19 or Rev-1 vaccines be given doxycycline 100 mg twice daily, combined with rifampin 600–900 mg once daily for 21 days; for conjunctival inoculations, prophylaxis should be maintained for 4–6 weeks.

6) Pasteurize milk and dairy products from cows, sheep and goats. Boiling milk is effective when pasteurization is impossible.

7) Exercise care in handling and disposal of placenta, discharges and fetus from an aborted animal. Disinfect contaminated areas.

B. *Control of patient, contacts and the immediate environment:*

1) Report to local health authority: Case report obligatory in most states and countries, Class 2B (see Communicable Disease Reporting).

2) Isolation: Draining and secretion precautions if there are draining lesions; otherwise none.

3) Concurrent disinfection: Of purulent discharges.

4) Quarantine: None.

5) Immunization of contacts: None.

6) Investigation of contacts and source of infection: Trace infection to the common or individual source, usually infected domestic goats, swine or cattle, or raw milk or dairy products from cows and goats. Test suspected animals and remove reactors.

7) Specific treatment: A combination of rifampin (600–900 mg daily) or streptomycin (1 g daily), and doxycycline (200 mg daily) for at least 6 weeks is the treatment of choice. In severely ill, toxic patients, corticosteroids may be helpful. If possible, tetracycline should be avoided in children less than 7 years old to avoid tooth staining. TMP-SMX is effective, but relapses are common (30%). Relapses occur in about 5% of patients treated with doxycycline and rifampin and are due to sequestered rather than resistant organisms; patients should be retreated with the original regimen. Arthritis may occur in recurrent cases.

C. *Epidemic measures:*
Search for common vehicle of infection, usually raw milk or milk products, especially cheese, from an infected herd. Recall incriminated products; stop production and distribution unless pasteurization is instituted.

D. *Disaster implications:* None.

E. *International measures:*
Control of domestic animals and animal products in international trade and transport. WHO Collaborating Centres.

CAMPYLOBACTER ENTERITIS

ICD-9 008.4; ICD-10 A04.5

(Vibrionic enteritis)

1. Identification—An acute zoonotic bacterial enteric disease of variable severity characterized by diarrhea, abdominal pain, malaise, fever, nausea and vomiting. The illness is frequently over within 2–5 days and usually lasts no more than 10 days. Prolonged illness may occur in adults; relapses can occur. Gross or occult blood in association with mucus and WBCs is often present in liquid stools. A typhoid-like syndrome or reactive arthritis may occur, and rarely, febrile convulsions, Guillain-Barré syndrome or meningitis. Some cases mimic acute appendicitis. Many infections are asymptomatic.

Diagnosis is based on isolation of the organisms from stool using selective media, reduced oxygen tension and an incubation temperature of 43°C (109.4°F). Visualization of motile and curved, spiral or S-shaped rods similar to those of *Vibrio cholerae* by phase contrast or darkfield microscopy of stool can provide rapid presumptive evidence for *Campylobacter* enteritis.

2. Infectious agents—*Campylobacter jejuni* and, less commonly, *C. coli* are the usual causes of *Campylobacter* diarrhea in humans. A variety of 20 or more biotypes and serotypes occur; their identification may be helpful for epidemiologic purposes. Other *Campylobacter* organisms, including *C. laridis* and *C. fetus* ssp. *fetus,* have also been associated with diarrhea in normal hosts.

3. Occurrence—These organisms are an important cause of diarrheal illness in all parts of the world and all age groups, causing 5%–14% of diarrhea worldwide. They are an important cause of travelers' diarrhea. In developed countries; children (less than 5 years) and young adults have the highest incidence of illness. In developing countries, illness is confined largely to children under 2 years of age, especially among infants. Common source outbreaks have occurred, most often associated with foods, especially undercooked chicken, unpasteurized milk and nonchlorinated water; these occur in spring and fall. The largest number of sporadic cases in temperate areas occur in the warmer months.

4. Reservoir—Animals, most frequently poultry and cattle. Puppies, kittens, other pets, swine, sheep, rodents and birds may also be sources of human infection. Most raw poultry meat is contaminated with *C. jejuni.*

5. Mode of transmission—By ingestion of the organisms in undercooked chicken and pork, contaminated food and water, or raw milk; from contact with infected pets (especially puppies and kittens), farm animals or infected infants. Contamination of milk most frequently occurs from fecal carrier cattle; people and food can be contaminated from poultry, especially from common cutting boards. Person to person transmission appears to be uncommon with *C. jejuni.*

6. Incubation period—Usually 2 to 5 days, with a range of 1–10 days, depending on dose ingested.

7. Period of communicability—Throughout the course of infection; usually from several days to several weeks. Individuals not treated with antibiotics may excrete organisms for as long as 2–7 weeks. The temporary carrier state is probably of little epidemiologic importance, except in infants and others who are incontinent of stool. Chronic infection of poultry and other animals constitutes the primary source of infection.

8. Susceptibility and resistance—Immune mechanisms are not well understood, but lasting immunity to serologically related strains follows infection. In developing countries, most people develop immunity in the first 2 years of life.

9. Methods of control—

    A. Preventive measures:

        1) Use irradiated foods or cook thoroughly all foodstuffs derived from animal sources, particularly poultry. Avoid recontamination from uncooked foods within the kitchen after cooking is completed.

        2) Pasteurize all milk and chlorinate or boil water supplies.

        3) Implement comprehensive control programs and hygienic measures (change of boots and clothes; thorough cleaning and disinfection) to prevent spread of organisms in poultry and animal farms.

        4) Recognize, prevent and control *Campylobacter* infections among domestic animals and pets. Puppies and kittens with diarrhea are possible sources of infection; erythromycin may be used to treat their infections, reducing risk of transmission to children. Stress handwashing after animal contact.

        5) Minimize contact with poultry and its feces; wash hands when this cannot be avoided.

    B. Control of patient, contacts and the immediate environment:

        1) Report to local health authority: Obligatory case report in most states and some countries, Class 2B (see Communicable Disease Reporting).

        2) Isolation: Enteric precautions for hospitalized patients. Exclude symptomatic individuals from food handling or care of people in hospitals, custodial institutions and day care centers;

exclusion of asymptomatic convalescent stool positive individuals is indicated only for those with questionable handwashing habits. Stress proper handwashing.

3) Concurrent disinfection: Of feces and articles soiled therewith. In communities with a modern and adequate sewage disposal system, feces can be discharged directly into sewers without preliminary disinfection. Terminal cleaning.

4) Quarantine: None.

5) Immunization of contacts: None is available.

6) Investigation of contacts and source of infection: Useful only to detect outbreaks; investigate outbreaks to identify the implicated food, water or raw milk to which others may have been exposed.

7) Specific treatment: None generally indicated except rehydration and electrolyte replacement (see Cholera, 9B7). *C. jejuni* or *C. coli* organisms are susceptible in vitro to a number of antimicrobial agents, including erythromycin, tetracyclines and quinolones, but these agents are of value only early in the illness and when the identity of the infecting organism is known, or to eliminate the carrier state.

*C. **Epidemic measures:*** Groups of cases, such as in a classroom, should be reported immediately to the local health authority, with search for vehicle and mode of spread.

*D. **Disaster implications:*** A risk when mass feeding and poor sanitation coexist.

*E. **International measures:*** WHO Collaborating Centres.

CANDIDIASIS   ICD-9 112; ICD-10 B37
(Moniliasis, Thrush, Candidosis)

1. Identification—A mycosis usually confined to the superficial layers of skin or mucous membranes, that presents clinically as oral thrush, intertrigo, vulvovaginitis, paronychia or onychomycosis. Ulcers or pseudomembranes may be formed in the esophagus, stomach or intestine. Candidemia most commonly arises from intravascular catheters and may produce lesions in many organs, such as kidney, spleen, lung, liver, eye, meninges, brain and native cardiac valves or around prosthetic cardiac valves.

Diagnosis requires evaluation of both laboratory and clinical evidence of candidiasis. The single most valuable laboratory test is microscopic demonstration of pseudohyphae and/or yeast cells in infected tissue or body fluids. Culture confirmation is important, but isolation from sputum, bronchial washings, stool, urine, mucosal surfaces, skin or wounds is not proof of a causal relationship to the disease. Severe or recurrent oropharyngeal infection in an adult with no obvious underlying cause should suggest the possibility of HIV infection.

2. Infectious agents—*Candida albicans, C. tropicalis, C. dubliniensis* and occasionally other species of *Candida. Candida (Torulopsis) glabrata* is distinguished from other causes of candidiasis by lack of pseudohyphae formation in tissue.

3. Occurrence—Worldwide. The fungus *C. albicans* is often part of the normal human flora.

4. Reservoir—Humans.

5. Mode of transmission—By contact with secretions or excretions of mouth, skin, vagina and feces, from patients or carriers; by passage from mother to neonate during childbirth; and by endogenous spread.

6. Incubation period—Variable, 2–5 days for thrush in infants.

7. Period of communicability—Presumably while lesions are present.

8. Susceptibility and resistance—The frequent isolation of *Candida* species from sputum, throat, feces and urine in the absence of clinical evidence of infection suggests a low level of pathogenicity or widespread immunity. Oral thrush is a common, usually benign condition during the first few weeks of life. Clinical disease occurs when host defenses are low. Local factors contributing to superficial candidiasis include interdigital intertrigo and paronychia on hands with excessive water exposure (as among cannery and laundry workers) and intertrigo in moist skin folds of obese individuals. Repeated clinical skin or mucosal eruptions are common.

Prominent among systemic factors predisposing to superficial candidiasis are diabetes mellitus, therapy with broad-spectrum antibiotics or supraphysiologic doses of adrenal corticosteroids, and HIV infection. Women in the third trimester of pregnancy are prone to vulvovaginal candidiasis. Factors predisposing to deep candidiasis include immunosuppression, indwelling intravenous catheters, neutropenia, hematologic malignancies and very low birthweight in neonates. Urinary tract candidiasis usually arises as a complication of prolonged catheterization of the bladder or renal pelvis. Most adults and older children have a delayed dermal hypersensitivity to the fungus and possess humoral antibodies.

9. Methods of control —

A. *Preventive measures:* Detect early and treat locally any infection in the mouth, esophagus or urinary bladder of those with predisposing systemic factors (see 8, above) to prevent systemic spread. Fluconazole chemoprophylaxis decreases the incidence of deep candidiasis during the first 2 months following allogeneic bone marrow transplantation.

B. *Control of patient, contacts and the immediate environment:*

1) Report to local health authority: Official report not ordinarily justifiable, Class 5 (see Communicable Disease Reporting).
2) Isolation: None.
3) Concurrent disinfection: Of secretions and contaminated articles.
4) Quarantine: None.
5) Immunization of contacts: None.
6) Investigation of contacts and source of infection: Not profitable in sporadic cases.
7) Specific treatment: Ameliorating the underlying causes of candidiasis often facilitates cure, e.g., removal of indwelling central venous catheters. Topical nystatin or an azole (miconazole, clotrimazole, ketoconazole, fluconazole) is useful in many forms of superficial candidiasis. Oral clotrimazole (Mycelex®) troches or nystatin suspension is effective for treatment of oral thrush. Itraconazole suspension (Sporanox®) or fluconazole (Diflucan®) is effective in oral and esophageal candidiasis. Vaginal infection may be treated with oral fluconazole or topical clotrimazole, miconazole, butoconazole, terconazole, tioconazole or nystatin. Amphotericin B (Fungizone®) IV, with or without 5-fluorocytosine, is the drug of choice for visceral or invasive candidiasis. Lipid formulations of amphotericin B are probably also effective.

C. *Epidemic measures:* Outbreaks are most frequently due to contaminated intravenous solutions and thrush in newborn nurseries. Concurrent disinfection and terminal cleaning should be practiced with care comparable to that used for epidemic diarrhea in hospital nurseries (see Diarrhea, section IV, 9A).

D. *Disaster implications:* None.

E. *International measures:* None.

CAPILLARIASIS

Three types of nematodes of the superfamily Trichuroidea, genus *Capillaria,* produce disease in humans.

I. CAPILLARIASIS DUE TO *CAPILLARIA PHILIPPINENSIS*   ICD-9 127.5; ICD-10 B81.1
(Intestinal capillariasis)

1. Identification—First described on Luzon, Philippines, in 1963, the disease is clinically an enteropathy with massive protein loss and a malabsorption syndrome that lead to progressive weight loss and extreme emaciation. Fatal cases are characterized by the presence of great numbers of parasites in the small intestine together with ascites and pleural transudate. Case-fatality rates of 10% have been reported. Subclinical cases also occur, but usually become symptomatic in time.

Diagnosis is made on clinical findings plus the identification of eggs or larval or adult parasites in the stool. The eggs resemble those of *Trichuris trichiura.* Jejunal biopsy may reveal the worms in the mucosa.

2. Infectious agent—*Capillaria philippinensis.*

3. Occurrence—Intestinal capillariasis is endemic in the Philippine Islands and in Thailand; a few cases have been reported from Japan, Korea, Taiwan and Egypt. Single cases have been reported from Iran, India, Indonesia and Colombia. The disease has reached epidemic proportions on Luzon, where more than 1,800 cases have been seen since 1967. In one village, one third of the population acquired the infection. Males between the ages of 20 and 45 appear to be particularly at risk.

4. Reservoir—Unknown; thought to be aquatic birds. Fish are considered to serve as intermediate hosts.

5. Mode of transmission—A history of ingestion of raw or inadequately cooked small fish eaten whole is usually obtained from patients. Experimentally, infective larvae develop in the intestines of freshwater fish that ingest eggs; monkeys, Mongolian gerbils and some birds fed these fish become infected, and the parasite matures within their intestines.

6. Incubation period—Unknown in humans; in animal studies, about a month or more.

7. Period of communicability—Not transmitted directly from person to person.

8. Susceptibility and resistance—Susceptibility appears to be general in those geographic areas in which the parasite is prevalent. Attack rates are often high.

9. **Methods of control—**

A. *Preventive measures:*

  1) Do not eat uncooked fish or other aquatic animal life in known endemic areas.
  2) Provide adequate facilities for the disposal of feces.

B. *Control of patient, contacts and the immediate environment:*

  1) Report to local health authority: Case report by most practicable means, Class 3B (see Communicable Disease Reporting).
  2) Isolation: None.
  3) Concurrent disinfection: None. Sanitary disposal of feces.
  4) Quarantine: None.
  5) Immunization of contacts: None.
  6) Investigation of contacts and source of infection: Fecal examination of all members of family groups and others with common exposure to raw or undercooked fish, with treatment of infected individuals.
  7) Specific treatment: Mebendazole (Vermox®) or albendazole (Zentel®) is the drug of choice.

C. *Epidemic measures:* Prompt investigation of cases and contacts with treatment of cases as indicated. Education on the need to cook all fish.

D. *Disaster implications:* None.

E. *International measures:* None.

II. CAPILLARIASIS DUE TO
CAPILLARIA HEPATICA   ICD-9 128.8; ICD-10 B83.8
(Hepatic capillariasis)

1. Identification—An uncommon and occasionally fatal disease in humans due to the presence of adult *Capillaria hepatica* in the liver. The picture is that of an acute or subacute hepatitis with marked eosinophilia resembling that of visceral larva migrans; the organism can disseminate to the lungs and other viscera.

Diagnosis is made by demonstrating eggs or the parasite in a liver biopsy or at necropsy.

2. Infectious agent—*Capillaria hepatica (Hepaticola hepatica).*

3. Occurrence—Since it was recognized as a human disease in 1924, about 30 cases have been reported from North and South America, Turkey, Switzerland, Czechoslovakia, Yugoslavia, Italy, Africa, Hawaii, India, Japan and Korea.

4. Reservoir—Primarily an infection of rats (as many as 86% were infected in some reports) and other rodents, but also seen in a large variety of domestic and wild mammals. The adult worms live and produce eggs in the liver.

5. Mode of transmission—The adult worms produce fertilized eggs that remain in the liver until the death of the host animal. When infected liver is eaten, the eggs are freed by digestion, reach the soil in the feces and develop to the infective stage in 2-4 weeks. When a suitable host ingests these embryonated eggs, they hatch in the intestine and the larvae migrate through the wall of the gut and are transported via the portal system to the liver, where they mature and produce eggs. Spurious infection in humans may be detected when eggs are found in the stool after infected liver, raw or cooked, has been eaten; since these eggs are not embryonated, infection cannot be established.

6. Incubation period—From 3 to 4 weeks.

7. Period of communicability—Not directly transmitted from person to person.

8. Susceptibility and resistance—Susceptibility is universal; malnourished children are more often infected.

9. Methods of control—

   A. Preventive measures:

     1) Avoid ingestion of dirt directly (pica) or in contaminated food or water or on hands.
     2) Protect water supplies and food from soil contamination.

   B. Control of patient, contacts and the immediate environment:

     1) Report to local health authority: Official report not ordinarily justifiable, Class 5 (see Communicable Disease Reporting).
     2) Isolation: None.
     3) Concurrent disinfection: None.
     4) Quarantine: None.
     5) Immunization of contacts: None.
     6) Investigation of contacts and source of infection: Not applicable.
     7) Specific treatment: Thiabendazole (Mintezol®) and albendazole (Zentel®) are effective in killing the worms in the liver.

   C. Epidemic measures: Not applicable.

   D. Disaster implications: None.

   E. International measures: None.

III. PULMONARY
CAPILLARIASIS   ICD-9 128.8; ICD-10 B 83.8

A pulmonary disease manifested by fever, cough and asthmatic breathing, caused by *Capillaria aerophila (Thominx aerophila)*, a nematode parasite of cats, dogs and other carnivorous mammals. Pneumonitis may be severe; heavy infections may be fatal. The worms live in tunnels in the epithelial lining of the trachea, bronchi and bronchioles; fertilized eggs are sloughed into the air passages, coughed up, swallowed and discharged from the body in the feces. In the soil, larvae develop in the eggs and remain infective for a year or longer. Infection is acquired by people, mostly children, by ingesting infective eggs in soil or in soil contaminated food or water. Eggs may appear in the sputum in 4 weeks; symptoms may appear earlier or later. Human cases have been recorded from the former Soviet Union (8 cases), Morocco and Iran (1 each); animal infection has been reported in North and South America, Europe, Asia and Australia.

CAT-SCRATCH DISEASE   ICD-9 078.3; ICD-10 A28.1
(Cat-scratch fever, Benign lymphoreticulosis)

1. Identification—Cat-scratch disease (CSD) is a subacute, usually self-limited bacterial disease characterized by malaise, granulomatous lymphadenitis and variable patterns of fever. It is often preceded by a cat scratch, lick or bite that produces a red papular lesion. Involvement of a regional lymph node follows, usually within 2 weeks, and may progress to suppuration. The papule at the inoculation site can be located in 50%–90% of cases. Parinaud oculoglandular syndrome after inoculation of the eye and neurologic complications, such as encephalopathy and optic neuritis, can occur. Prolonged high fever may be accompanied by osteolytic lesions and/or hepatic and splenic granulomata. Bacteremia, peliosis hepatis and bacillary angiomatosis are seen as manifestations of infection with this group of organisms in immunocompromised persons, particularly HIV infection.

CSD can be clinically confused with other diseases that cause regional lymphadenopathies, such as tularemia, brucellosis, tuberculosis, plague and pasteurellosis (see below).

Diagnosis is based on a consistent clinical picture combined with serologic evidence of antibody to *Bartonella*. A titer of 1:64 or greater by IFA assay is considered positive.

Histopathologic examination of the involved lymph nodes may reveal consistent characteristics, but is not diagnostic. Pus obtained from lymph nodes is usually bacteriologically sterile by conventional techniques; however, after prolonged incubation on rabbit blood agar in 5% CO_2 at

36°C (96.8°F), *Bartonella* has been grown from some lymph node aspirates.

2. Infectious agent—*Bartonella* (formerly *Rochalimaea*) *henselae* has been implicated epidemiologically, bacteriologically and serologically as the etiologic agent of most CSD, as well as of bacillary angiomatosis, peliosis hepatis and bacteremia. Related *Bartonellae,* such as *B. quintana,* may also produce illnesses among immunocompromised hosts, but do not cause CSD. *Afipia felis,* a previously described candidate organism, is felt to play a minor role, if any, in CSD.

3. Occurrence—Worldwide, but uncommon. Prospective surveillance in one state (USA) found an annual incidence of 4.0 cases/100,000 population. Genders are equally affected, and CSD is more common in children and young adults. Familial clustering occurs rarely. The majority of cases are seen during late summer, fall and winter months.

4. Reservoir—Domestic cats are vectors and reservoirs for *B. henselae;* there is no evidence of clinical illness in cats even when chronic bacteremia has been demonstrated.

5. Mode of transmission—Most patients (more than 90%) give a history of scratch, bite, lick or other exposure to a healthy, usually young cat (often a kitten). Dog scratch or bite, monkey bite or contact with rabbits, chickens or horses has been reported prior to the syndrome, but cat involvement was not excluded in all cases. Cat fleas transmit *B. henselae* readily among cats, but as of late 1999 they have not been shown to play a role in direct transmission of *B. henselae* to humans.

6. Incubation period—Variable, usually 3–14 days from inoculation to primary lesion and 5–50 days from inoculation to lymphadenopathy.

7. Period of communicability—Not directly transmitted from person to person.

8. Susceptibility and resistance—Unknown.

9. Methods of control —

A. *Preventive measures:* Thorough cleaning of cat scratches and bites may be helpful. Flea control is very important.

B. *Control of patient, contacts and the immediate environment:*

1) Report to local health authority: Official report not ordinarily justifiable, Class 5 (see Communicable Disease Reporting).
2) Isolation: None.
3) Concurrent disinfection: Of discharges from purulent lesions.
4), 5) and 6) Quarantine, Immunization of contacts and Investigation of contacts and source of infection: Not applicable.

7) Specific treatment: Therapeutic effectiveness of antibiotics is currently unclear in CSD. Most commonly used antibiotics, such as rifampin, erythromycin and doxycycline, are effective in the disseminated forms of infection seen in AIDS cases. Treatment of uncomplicated CSD in immunocompetent patients is not indicated. However, all immunocompromised patients should be treated for 1–3 months. Needle aspiration of suppurative lymphadenitis may be required for relief of pain, but incisional biopsy of lymph nodes should be avoided.

C. **Epidemic measures:** Not applicable.

D. **Disaster implications:** None.

E. **International measures:** None.

OTHER INFECTIONS ASSOCIATED WITH ANIMAL BITES

Other diseases that result from animal bites include: pasturellosis from cats and less often from dogs and other animals; B-virus (cercopithecine herpesvirus-1) from monkey bites (see under *Herpes simplex*); tularemia; *Streptobacillus moniliformis* (rat bite fever); plague; tetanus; and rabies. Animal bites may also transmit pathogens, such as streptococci and staphylococci, that result in pyogenic infections in addition to anaerobes and *Acinetobacter* species.

Pasteurellosis (ICD-9 027.2; ICD-10 A28.0) is caused by *Pasteurella multocida* and *P. haemolytica*. Carriage has been noted in the respiratory tract and oropharynx of a large percentage of healthy cats, dogs and other animals. Human infection is usually secondary to a cat or dog bite and is manifested as a cellulitis with swelling and pain out of proportion to the visible lesion; lymphadenopathy and sepsis can occur. Onset of symptoms usually occurs less than 24 hours after a cat or dog bite. Chronic respiratory tract disease also occurs among elderly patients with underlying disease. The organism is susceptible to penicillin, the drug of choice; a tetracycline is an effective alternate therapeutic agent. First generation cephalosporins are not generally active against *Pasteurella*. Augmentin is a reasonable choice for bites in general, since it covers pasteurella, strep, staph and anareobes.

Capnocytophaga canimorsus, formerly known as CDC group DF-2 (ICD-9 027.8), can cause febrile illnesses in patients with impaired immune systems who have been licked, bitten or scratched by dogs or cats. Cellulitis, fever, septicemia, purulent meningitis, endocarditis or septic arthritis appear after 1–5 days; case-fatality rates reported in high risk groups vary from 4% to 27%. Splenectomy, chronic pulmonary disease and alcoholism are predisposing factors; the incidence is higher in men and those over 40. Diagnosis is made by finding Gram-negative bacilli within neutrophils and by isolating the etiologic organism. A related but less virulent organism, *C. cynodegmi* can be isolated from wound infections that follow a dog bite or a cat scratch. Both of these organisms are frequently present in the mouths of healthy dogs and cats. Penicillin G, the antibiotic of choice for these infections, should be given prophylactically to high risk individuals bitten by a dog or cat.

CHANCROID   ICD-9 099.0; ICD-10 A57
(Ulcus molle, Soft chancre)

1. Identification—An acute bacterial infection localized in the genital area and characterized clinically by single or multiple painful, necrotizing ulcers at the site of infection, frequently accompanied by painful swelling and suppuration of regional lymph nodes. Minimally symptomatic lesions may occur on the vaginal wall or cervix; asymptomatic infections may occur in women. Extragenital lesions have been reported. Chancroid ulcers, like other genital ulcers, are associated with increased risk of HIV infection.

Diagnosis is made by isolation of the organism from lesion exudate on a selective medium that incorporates vancomycin into chocolate, rabbit or horse blood agar enriched with fetal calf serum. Gram stains of lesion exudate may suggest the diagnosis if numerous gram-negative coccobacilli are seen "streaming" between leukocytes. PCR and immunofluorescence for direct detection of organism in ulcers, and serology, are available on a research basis.

2. Infectious agent—*Haemophilus ducreyi*, the Ducrey bacillus.

3. Occurrence—More often diagnosed in men, especially those who frequent prostitutes. Most prevalent in tropical and subtropical regions of the world, where the incidence may be higher than that of syphilis and may approach that of gonorrhea in men. The disease is much less common in temperate zones and may occur in small outbreaks. In the USA, outbreaks and some endemic transmission have occurred, principally among migrant farm workers and poor inner city residents.

4. Reservoir—Humans.

5. Mode of transmission—By direct sexual contact with discharges from open lesions and pus from buboes. Autoinoculation to nongenital sites may occur in infected people. Sexual abuse must be considered when chancroid is found in children beyond the neonatal period.

6. Incubation period—From 3 to 5 days, up to 14 days.

7. Period of communicability—Until healed and as long as the infectious agent persists in the original lesion or discharging regional lymph nodes, which lasts for several weeks or months without antibiotic treatment. Antibiotic therapy eradicates *H. ducreyi* and lesions heal in 1–2 weeks.

8. Susceptibility and resistance—Susceptibility is general; the uncircumcised are at higher risk than the circumcised. There is no evidence of natural resistance.

9. Methods of control—

> **A. Preventive measures:**
>
> > 1) Preventive measures are those for syphilis (see Syphilis, 9A).
> > 2) Follow all patients with nonherpetic genital ulcerations serologically for syphilis and HIV.
>
> **B. Control of patient, contacts and the immediate environment:**
>
> > 1) Report to local health authority: Case report obligatory in many states and countries, Class 2B (see Communicable Disease Reporting).
> > 2) Isolation: None; avoid sexual contact until all lesions are healed.
> > 3) Concurrent disinfection: None.
> > 4) Quarantine: None.
> > 5) Immunization of contacts: None.
> > 6) Investigation of contacts and source of infection: Examine and treat all sexual contacts within 10 days before onset of symptoms. Women without visible signs may rarely be carriers. Sexual contacts even without signs should receive prophylactic treatment.
> > 7) Specific treatment: Ceftriaxone, erythromycin, azithromycin or, for adults only, ciprofloxacin is the recommended drug. Alternatives include amoxicillin with clavulanic acid. Fluctuant inguinal nodes should be aspirated through intact skin to prevent spontaneous rupture.
>
> **C. Epidemic measures:** Persistent occurrence or an increased incidence is an indication for more rigid application of measures outlined in 9A and 9B, above. When compliance with the treatment schedule (9B7) is a problem, consideration should be given to a single dose of ceftriaxone or azithromycin. Empirical therapy to high risk groups with or without lesions, including prostitutes, clinic patients reporting prostitute contact, and clinic patients with genital ulcers and negative darkfields may be required to control an outbreak.
>
> **D. Disaster implications:** None.
>
> **E. International measures:** See Syphilis, 9E.

CHICKENPOX/HERPES
ZOSTER   ICD-9 052–053; ICD-10 B01–B02
(Varicella/Shingles)

1. Identification—Chickenpox (varicella) is an acute, generalized viral disease with sudden onset of slight fever, mild constitutional symptoms and a skin eruption that is maculopapular for a few hours, vesicular for 3–4 days and leaves a granular scab. The vesicles are monolocular and collapse on puncture, in contrast to the multilocular, noncollapsing vesicles of smallpox. Lesions commonly occur in successive crops, with several stages of maturity present at the same time; they tend to be more abundant on covered than on exposed parts of the body. Lesions may appear on the scalp, high in the axilla, on mucous membranes of the mouth and upper respiratory tract and on the conjunctivae; they tend to occur in areas of irritation, such as sunburn or diaper rash. They may be so few as to escape observation. Mild, atypical and inapparent infections occur. Occasionally, especially in adults, the fever and constitutional manifestations may be severe.

The case-fatality rate in the USA is lower for children than for adults. One out of every 100,000 children with varicella (aged 5–9, the lowest risk group) will die from varicella, compared with 1 out of every 5,000 adults. Serious complications of varicella include pneumonia (viral and bacterial), secondary bacterial infections, hemorrhagic complications and encephalitis. Children with acute leukemia, including those in remission after chemotherapy, are at increased risk of disseminated disease, fatal in 5%–10% of cases. Neonates who develop varicella between ages 5 and 10 days are at increased risk of developing severe generalized chickenpox, as are those whose mothers develop the disease 5 days prior to or within 2 days after delivery. Prior to the availability of effective viral therapies, the fatality rate was up to 30%, but it is likely lower now. Infection early in pregnancy may be associated with congenital varicella syndrome in 0.7% of cases, and infection occurring at 13–20 weeks gestation may be associated with a 2% risk. Clinical chickenpox was a frequent antecedent of Reye syndrome prior to the identification of the association of Reye syndrome with aspirin use for viral infections.

Herpes zoster (shingles) is a local manifestation of reactivation of latent varicella infection in the dorsal root ganglia. Vesicles with an erythematous base are restricted to skin areas supplied by sensory nerves of a single or associated group of dorsal root ganglia. Lesions may appear in crops in irregular fashion along nerve pathways, are usually unilateral, deeper seated and more closely aggregated than those of chickenpox; histologically they are identical. Severe pain and paresthesia are common, and as many as 30% of the elderly may suffer postherpetic neuralgia. The incidence of both zoster and postherpetic neuralgia increase with increasing age, and there is some evidence that almost 10% of children being treated for a malignant neoplasm are prone to develop zoster; persons with HIV infection are also at increased risk for zoster. In the immunosuppressed and those with diagnosed malignancies, extensive chickenpox-like lesions may appear outside the dermatome; this may also occur in otherwise normal individuals with fewer lesions. Intrauterine infection and varicella before 2 years of age are also associated with zoster at an early age. Occasionally, a varicelliform eruption follows some days after herpes zoster, and rarely there is a secondary eruption of zoster after chickenpox.

Laboratory tests—such as visualization of the virus by EM; isolation of virus in cell cultures; demonstration of viral antigen in smears using FA, of viral DNA by PCR or of a rise in serum antibodies—are not routinely required but are useful in complicated cases and in epidemiologic studies. In the vaccine era, viral strain identification testing to differentiate vaccine virus from wild virus may be needed in certain situations (e.g., to document whether herpes zoster in a vaccine recipient is due to vaccine or wild virus). A number of antibody assays are now commercially available; however, these tests are not sensitive enough to be used for post immunization testing of immunity. Multinucleated giant cells may be detected in Giemsa-stained scrapings from the base of a lesion; these are not found in vaccinia lesions but do occur in herpes simplex lesions. Thus, they are not specific for varicella infections, and with the availability of rapid direct fluorescent antibody testing, they now have limited value in clinical testing.

2. Infectious agent—Human (alpha) herpesvirus 3 (varicella-zoster virus, VZV), a member of the *Herpesvirus* group.

3. Occurrence—Worldwide. Infection with human (alpha) herpesvirus 3 is nearly universal. In temperate climates, at least 90% of the population has had chickenpox by age 15 and at least 95% by young adulthood. In temperate zones, chickenpox occurs most frequently in winter and early spring. The epidemiology of varicella in tropical countries differs from temperate climates, with a higher proportion of cases occurring among adults. Zoster occurs more commonly in older people.

4. Reservoir—Humans.

5. Mode of transmission—From person to person by direct contact, droplet or airborne spread of vesicle fluid or secretions of the respiratory tract of chickenpox cases or of vesicle fluid of patients with herpes zoster; indirectly through articles freshly soiled by discharges from vesicles and mucous membranes of infected people. In contrast to vaccinia and variola, scabs from varicella lesions are not infective. Chickenpox is one of the most readily communicable of diseases, especially in the early stages of the eruption; zoster has a much lower rate of transmission (varicella seronegative contacts develop chickenpox). Susceptibles have about an 80%-90% risk of infection after household exposure to varicella.

6. Incubation period—From 2 to 3 weeks; commonly 14-16 days; may be prolonged after passive immunization against varicella (see 9A2, below) and in the immunodeficient.

7. Period of communicability—As long as 5 but usually 1–2 days before onset of rash, and continuing until all lesions are crusted (usually about 5 days). Contagiousness may be prolonged in patients with altered immunity. The secondary attack rate among susceptible siblings is 70%–90%. Patients with zoster may be sources of infection for a week after the appearance of their vesiculopustular lesions. Susceptible individuals should be considered to be infectious 10–21 days following exposure.

8. Susceptibility and resistance—Susceptibility to chickenpox is universal among those not previously infected; ordinarily a more severe disease of adults than of children. Infection usually confers long immunity; second attacks are rare but have been documented in immunocompetent persons; subclinical reinfection is common. Viral infection remains latent, and disease may recur years later as herpes zoster in about 15% of older adults, and sometimes in children.

Neonates whose mothers are not immune and patients with leukemia may suffer severe, prolonged or fatal chickenpox. Adults with cancer—especially of lymphoid tissue, with or without steroid therapy—immunodeficient patients and those on immunosuppressive therapy may have an increased frequency of severe zoster, both localized and disseminated.

9. Methods of control—

A. Preventive measures:

1) A live attenuated varicella virus vaccine (Varivax®) was licensed for use in the USA in 1995. A single 0.5 ml SC dose is recommended for routine immunization of children aged 12 to 18 months and for immunization of children up to 12 years of age who have not had varicella. This vaccine had a cumulative efficacy estimated at 70%–90% in preventing varicella in children followed for up to 6 years. Postlicensure effectiveness estimates ranged from about 85%–90% for prevention of all disease and 100% for prevention of moderate or severe disease. If an immunized person does get varicella, it is usually a very mild case with fewer lesions (usually less than 50, which are frequently not vesicular), mild or no fever and shorter duration of illness. If administered within 3 days of exposure, varicella vaccine is likely to prevent or at least significantly modify disease in a case contact. The vaccine may be used to protect children and adolescents with lymphoblastic leukemia in remission; 2 doses 4–8 weeks apart are needed. Vaccine is provided free for these patients under an investigational protocol through the VARIVAX Coordinating Center, at 215-283-0897.

Varicella vaccine is recommended for susceptible persons more than 13 years. Priority groups for adult immunization include persons who have close contact with persons at high risk for serious complications, persons who live or work in environments where transmission of VZV is likely (e.g., teachers of young children, day care employees and residents and staff members in institutional settings), persons who live and work in environments where transmission can occur (e.g., college students, inmates and staff members of correctional institutions and military personnel), nonpregnant women of childbearing age, adolescents and adults living in households with children and international travelers. Persons more than 13 years old require 2 doses of vaccine 4–8 weeks apart. A mild varicella-like rash at the site of injection or at distant sites has been observed in about 2%–4% of children and about 5% of adults. The vaccine may cause herpes zoster later in life, although the rate seems to be lower than that after natural disease. The duration of immunity is unknown, but antibodies have persisted for at least 10 years in the USA. However, persistence of antibody has occurred in the presence of circulating wild virus.

2) Protect high risk individuals who cannot be immunized, such as nonimmune neonates and the immunodeficient, from exposure by immunizing household or other close contacts.

3) Varicella-zoster immune globulin (VZIG), prepared from the plasma of normal blood donors with high antibody titer to VZV, is effective in modifying or preventing disease if given within 96 hours after exposure (see 9B5, below).

B. Control of patient, contacts and the immediate environment:

1) Report to local health authority: In many states (USA) and countries, not a reportable disease; varicella related deaths became nationally notifiable in the USA on January 1, 1999; Class 3C (see Communicable Disease Reporting).

2) Isolation: Exclude children from school, medical offices, emergency rooms or public places until vesicles become dry, usually after 5 days in unimmunized children and 1–4 days with breakthrough varicella in immunized children; exclude infected adults from the workplace and avoid contact with susceptibles. In the hospital, strict isolation is appropriate because of the risk of serious varicella in susceptible immuno-compromised patients.

3) Concurrent disinfection: Articles soiled by discharges from the nose and throat.

4) Quarantine: Usually none. However, in a hospital where susceptible children with known recent exposure must remain for medical reasons, the risk of spread to steroid treated or immunodeficient patients may justify quarantine of known

contacts for a period of at least 10–21 days after exposure (up to 28 days if VZIG has been given).

5) Protection of contacts: Vaccine is recommended for use in susceptible persons following exposure to varicella. Data from household, hospital and community settings indicate that varicella vaccine is effective in preventing illness or modifying varicella severity if used within 3 days, and possibly up to 5 days, of exposure.

VZIG given within 96 hours of exposure may prevent or modify disease in susceptible close contacts of cases. VZIG is available from Blood Service Regional Offices of the American Red Cross or through a central ordering number in the USA (617-461-0891) for certain high risk persons exposed to chickenpox. It is indicated for newborns of mothers who develop chickenpox within 5 days prior to or within 48 hours after delivery. There is no assurance that administration of VZIG to a pregnant woman will prevent congenital malformations in the fetus, but it may modify the severity of varicella in the pregnant woman.

Antiviral drugs such as acyclovir, appear to be useful in prevention or modification of varicella in exposed individuals if given within a week of exposure. A dose of 80 mg/kg/day in 4 divided doses has been used, but there is as yet no regimen generally recommended for this purpose.

6) Investigation of contacts and source of infection: A source of infection may be a case of varicella or herpes zoster. All contacts of the source, especially those ineligible for postexposure immunization, such as pregnant women and those at high risk for severe disease (immunocompromised individuals and neonates whose mothers have symptoms of varicella within 5 days before and 2 days after delivery), should be evaluated promptly for consideration of VZIG administration. Infectious patients should be isolated until all lesions are crusted; exposed susceptibles eligible for immunization should receive vaccine immediately to control or prevent an outbreak.

7) Specific treatment: While both vidarabine (adenine arabinoside, Ara-A®) and acyclovir (Zovirax®) are effective in treating varicella-zoster infections, the latter is generally considered the antiviral agent of choice for treatment of varicella. For herpes zoster, newer analogues with improved absorption after oral administration are available (valacyclovir and famcyclovir). These medications may shorten the duration of symptoms and pain of zoster in the normal older patient, especially if administered within 24 hours of rash onset.

C. Epidemic measures: Outbreaks of varicella are common in schools, day care and institutional settings, and may be protracted, disruptive and associated with complications. Infectious cases should be isolated and susceptible contacts immunized promptly (or referred to their health care provider for immunization) to control an outbreak. Those persons ineligible for immunization, such as susceptible pregnant females and those at high risk for severe disease (as above), should be evaluated immediately for consideration of VZIG administration.

D. Disaster implications: Outbreaks of chickenpox may occur among children when crowded together in emergency housing situations.

E. International measures: Same as for C above.

CHLAMYDIAL INFECTIONS

As laboratory techniques improve, chlamydial organisms are increasingly implicated as causes of human disease. Chlamydiae are obligate intracellular bacteria that differ from viruses and rickettsiae but, like the latter, are sensitive to broad-spectrum antimicrobials. Those that cause human disease are classified into three species:

1) *Chlamydia psittaci,* the etiologic agent of psittacosis (q.v.);

2) *C. trachomatis,* including serotypes that cause trachoma (q.v.), genital infections (see below), chlamydial conjunctivitis (q.v.) and infant pneumonia (q.v.), and other serotypes that cause lymphogranuloma venereum (q.v.); and

3) *C. pneumoniae,* the cause of respiratory disease including pneumonia (q.v.) and implicated in coronary artery disease.

Chlamydiae are now increasingly recognized as important pathogens responsible for a number of sexually transmitted infections, with infant eye and lung infections consequent to maternal genital infection.

GENITAL INFECTIONS, CHLAMYDIAL   ICD-9 099.8; ICD-10 A56

1. Identification—Sexually transmitted genital infection is manifested in males primarily as a urethritis, and in females as a mucopurulent cervicitis. Clinical manifestations of urethritis are often difficult to distinguish from gonorrhea and include mucopurulent discharges of scanty or moderate quantity, urethral itching, and burning on urination. Asymptomatic infection may be found in 1%–25% of sexually active men. Possible complications or sequelae of male urethral infections include epididymitis, infertility and Reiter syndrome. In homosexual men, receptive anorectal intercourse may result in chlamydial proctitis.

In the female, the clinical manifestations may be similar to those of gonorrhea and frequently present as a mucopurulent endocervical discharge, with edema, erythema and easily induced endocervical bleeding caused by inflammation of the endocervical columnar epithelium. However, up to 70% of sexually active women with chlamydial infections are asymptomatic. Complications and sequelae include salpingitis with subsequent risk of infertility, ectopic pregnancy or chronic pelvic pain. Asymptomatic chronic infections of the endometrium and fallopian tubes may lead to the same outcome. Less frequent manifestations include bartholinitis, urethral syndrome with dysuria and pyuria, perihepatitis (Fitz-Hugh-Curtis syndrome) and proctitis. Infection during pregnancy may result in premature rupture of membranes and preterm delivery, and conjunctival and pneumonic infection of the newborn. Endocervical chlamydial infection has been associated with increased risk of acquiring HIV infection.

Chlamydial infections may be acquired concurrently with gonorrhea and persist after the gonorrhea has been successfully treated. Because gonococcal and chlamydial cervicitis are often difficult to distinguish clinically, treatment for both organisms is recommended when one is suspected. However, treatment for gonorrhea is not always needed when *C. trachomatis* is diagnosed.

Diagnosis of nongonococcal urethritis (NGU) or cervicitis is usually based on the failure to demonstrate *Neisseria gonorrhoeae* by smear and culture; chlamydial etiology is confirmed by examination of intraurethral or endocervical swab material by direct IF test with monoclonal antibody, EIA, DNA probe, nucleic acid amplification test (NAAT) or cell culture. NAATs can be used with urine specimens. The intracellular organisms are less readily recoverable from the discharge itself. For other agents, see Urethritis, Nongonococcal, below.

2. Infectious agent—*Chlamydia trachomatis,* immunotypes D through K, has been identified in approximately 35%–50% of NGU cases in the USA.

3. Occurrence—Common worldwide; in the USA, Canada, Australia and Europe, recognition has increased steadily in the last two decades.

4. Reservoir—Humans.

5. Mode of transmission—Sexual intercourse.

6. Incubation period—Poorly defined, probably 7–14 days or longer.

7. Period of communicability—Unknown. Relapses are probably common.

8. Susceptibility and resistance—Susceptibility is general. No acquired immunity has been demonstrated; cellular immunity is immunotype specific.

9. **Methods of control —**

A. Preventive measures:

1) Health and sex education; same as for syphilis (see Syphilis, 9A), with emphasis on use of a condom when engaging in sexual intercourse.
2) Screening of sexually active adolescent girls should be routine. Screening of adult women should also be considered if they are less than 25 years of age, have multiple or new sex partners, and/or use barrier contraceptives inconsistently. Newer tests for *C. trachomatis* infection which enable screening of adolescent and young adult males, as well, may be used with urine specimens.

B. Control of patient, contacts and the immediate environment:

1) Report to local health authority: Case report is required in most states in the USA, Class 2B (see Communicable Disease Reporting).
2) Isolation: Universal precautions, as appropriate for hospitalized patients. Appropriate antibiotic therapy renders discharges noninfectious; patients should refrain from sexual intercourse until treatment of index patient and current sexual partners is completed.
3) Concurrent disinfection: Care in disposal of articles contaminated with urethral and vaginal discharges.
4) Quarantine: None.
5) Immunization of contacts: Not applicable.
6) Investigation of contacts and source of infection: Prophylactic treatment of sexual partners is recommended. As a minimum, concurrent treatment of regular sex partners is a practical approach to management. If neonates born to infected mothers have not received systemic treatment, chest x-ray at 3 weeks of age and again after 12–18 weeks may be considered to exclude subclinical chlamydial pneumonia.
7) Specific treatment: Doxycycline (PO), 100 mg twice daily for 7 days or tetracycline (PO), 500 mg, 4 times daily for 7 days. Erythromycin is an alternative drug and is the drug of choice for the newborn and for women with a known or suspected pregnancy. Azithromycin (PO), 1 g in a single dose, is also effective.

C. Epidemic measures: None.

D. Disaster implications: None.

E. International measures: None.

URETHRITIS, NONGONOCOCCAL
AND NONSPECIFIC   ICD-9 099.4; ICD-10 N34.1
(NGU, NSU)

While chlamydiae are the most frequently isolated etiologic agents in cases of gonococcus negative urethritis, other agents are involved in a significant number of cases. *Ureaplasma urealyticum* is considered the etiologic agent in approximately 10%–20% of NGU cases; *Herpesvirus simplex* type 2 and *Trichomonas vaginalis* are rarely implicated. If laboratory facilities for demonstration of chlamydia are not available, all cases of NGU (together with their sexual partners) are best managed as though their infections were chlamydia, especially since many chlamydia negative cases also respond to antibiotic therapy.

CHOLERA AND OTHER VIBRIOSES   ICD-9 001; ICD-10 A00
I. *VIBRIO CHOLERAE* SEROGROUPS
O1 AND O139

1. Identification—An acute bacterial enteric disease characterized in its severe form by sudden onset, profuse painless watery stools, nausea and vomiting early in the course of illness, and, in untreated cases, rapid dehydration, acidosis, circulatory collapse, hypoglycemia in children, and renal failure. Asymptomatic infection is much more frequent than clinical illness, especially with organisms of the El Tor biotype; mild cases with only diarrhea are common, particularly among children. In severe untreated cases (cholera gravis), death may occur within a few hours, and the case-fatality rate may exceed 50%; with proper treatment, the rate is less than 1%.

Diagnosis is confirmed by isolating *Vibrio cholerae* of the serogroup O1 or O139 from feces. If laboratory facilities are not nearby or immediately available, Cary Blair transport medium can be used to transport or store a fecal or rectal swab. For clinical purposes, a quick presumptive diagnosis can be made by darkfield or phase microscopic visualization of the vibrios moving like "shooting stars," inhibited by preservative free, serotype specific antiserum. For epidemiologic purposes, a presumptive diagnosis can be based on the demonstration of a significant rise in titer of antitoxic and vibriocidal antibodies. In nonendemic areas, isolated organisms from initial suspected cases should be confirmed by appropriate biochemical and serologic reactions and by testing the organisms for cholera toxin production or for the presence of cholera toxin genes. In epidemics, once laboratory confirmation and antibiotic sensitivity have been established, all cases need not be laboratory confirmed.

2. Infectious agent—*Vibrio cholerae* serogroup O1 includes two biotypes—classical and El Tor—each of which includes organisms of

Inaba, Ogawa and (rarely) Hikojima serotypes. *V. cholerae* O139 also causes typical cholera. The clinical pictures of illness caused by *V. cholerae* O1 of either biotype and *V. cholerae* O139 are similar because an almost identical enterotoxin is elaborated by these organisms. In any single epidemic, one particular type tends to be dominant; currently the El Tor biotype is predominant. In some areas of India and Bangladesh a proportion of clinical cholera is caused by *V. cholerae* O139 and some cases of *V. cholerae* O1 of classical biotype have been observed in Bangladesh during the past decade.

Vibrios that are biochemically indistinguishable but do not agglutinate in *V. cholerae* serogroup O1 antiserum (non-O1 strains, formerly known as nonagglutinable vibrios [NAGs] or noncholera vibrios [NCVs]) are now included in the species *V. cholerae*. Some strains elaborate cholera enterotoxin but most do not. Prior to 1992, non-O1 strains were recognized to cause sporadic cases and rare outbreaks of diarrheal disease, but were not associated with large epidemics.

However, in late 1992, large-scale epidemics of severe dehydrating diarrhea, typical of cholera, were reported in India and Bangladesh. The causative organism was a new serogroup of *V. cholerae* O139, which elaborates the same cholera toxin but differs from O1 strains in lipopolysaccharide (LPS) structure and in producing capsular antigen. The clinical and epidemiologic picture of illness caused by this organism is typical of cholera, and cases should be reported as cholera. The epidemic O139 strain, which possesses the virulence factors of *V. cholerae* O1 El Tor was apparently derived by a deletion in the genes that encode the O1 lipopolysaccharide antigen of an El Tor strain followed by the acquisition of a large fragment of new DNA encoding the enzymes that allow synthesis of O139 lipopolysaccharide and capsule. The reporting of nontoxinogenic *V. cholerae* O1 or of non-O1 *V. cholerae* infections, other than O139, as cholera is inaccurate and leads to confusion.

3. Occurrence—During the 19th century, pandemic cholera spread repeatedly from the Ganges delta of India to most of the world. During the first half of the 20th century, the disease was confined largely to Asia, except for a severe epidemic in Egypt in 1947. During the latter half of the 20th century, the epidemiology of cholera has been marked by three major observations: 1) the relentless global spread of the seventh pandemic of cholera caused by *V. cholerae* O1 El Tor; 2) recognition that environmental reservoirs of cholera exist and include one along the Gulf of Mexico coast of the USA; and 3) the appearance for the first time of large explosive epidemics of cholera gravis caused by *V. cholerae* organisms of a serogroup other than O1 (*V. cholerae* O139).

Since 1961, *V. cholerae* of the El Tor biotype has spread from Indonesia through most of Asia into eastern Europe. In 1970 this biotype was introduced into west Africa and spread rapidly throughout that continent to become endemic in many African countries. Epidemics occurred in the Iberian Peninsula and Italy in the 1970s. El Tor cholera returned to South

America in 1991 after a century of absence, and caused explosive epidemics along the Pacific coast of Peru. From Peru it spread rapidly to neighboring countries and by 1994, approximately one million cholera cases had been recorded in Latin America. Notably, although the clinical disease was as severe as seen in other regions of the world, the overall case fatality in Latin America was kept remarkably low (about 1%) except in highly rural areas in the Andes and Amazon region where patients were often far from medical care.

A particularly explosive outbreak of El Tor cholera occurred among Rwandan refugees in Goma, Zaire in July, 1994, that resulted in approximately 70,000 cases and 12,000 deaths over the course of little more than one month. In total, 384,403 cases and 10,692 deaths were reported to WHO in 1994 by 94 countries. The global case fatality rate in 1994 was 2.8%, varying from 1% in the Americas, to 1.3% in Asia and 5% in Africa. These variations reflect differences in reporting and in access to appropriate treatment, and do not reflect alterations in virulence.

Except for two laboratory acquired cases, there was no known indigenous cholera in the Western Hemisphere between 1911 and 1973, when a case due to *V. cholerae* El Tor Inaba occurred in Texas with no known source. In 1978, and in the early 1990s there were additional sporadic *V. cholerae* O1 El Tor Inaba infections in Louisiana and Texas. The occurrence of these cases from the Gulf coast over many years, all due to a single indigenous strain led to the identification of an environmental reservoir of *V. cholerae* O1 El Tor Inaba in the Gulf of Mexico.

In October 1992, cholera outbreaks occurred simultaneously in several sites in Tamilnadu State, India. Strains isolated from these outbreaks did not agglutinate in O1 antisera nor were they typable with any of the standard panel of 138 non-O1 *V. cholerae* antisera. The new serogroup, designated O139 Bengal, spread rapidly throughout the region over the next few months affecting several hundred thousand persons. During this epidemic period, *V. cholerae* O139 almost completely replaced *V. cholerae* O1 strains in hospitalized cholera patients and in samples of surface water. The epidemic continued to spread through 1994, with cases of O139 cholera reported from 11 countries in Asia. This new strain was soon introduced into other continents by infected travelers, but secondary spread outside of Asia has not been reported. In the early 1990s it was believed that the O139 epidemics in Asia might be the beginning of an eighth pandemic of cholera. However, not only did O139 not spread to cause epidemic disease in Africa and South America, it greatly diminished in India and Bangladesh, and disappeared from areas to which it had spread and did not account for more than 5-10% of cases anywhere. Cholera O139 may in the future cause large explosive epidemics in another region of the world and therefore requires continued international surveillance.

Since cholera returned to Latin America in the early 1990s, cases of traveler's cholera have greatly increased. Moreover, by using optimized bacteriologic methods (TCBS medium) several prospective studies have demonstrated that the incidence of traveler's cholera in USA and Japanese travelers is considerably higher than had been previously estimated.

4. Reservoir—Humans; observations in the USA, Bangladesh and Australia over the past two decades have clearly demonstrated that environmental reservoirs exist, apparently in association with copepods or other zooplankton in brackish water or estuaries.

5. Mode of transmission—Through ingestion of food or water contaminated directly or indirectly with feces or vomitus of infected persons. El Tor and O139 organisms can persist in water for long periods. When epidemic El Tor cholera appeared in Latin America in explosive fashion in 1991, faulty municipal water systems, contaminated surface waters, and unsafe domestic water storage methods resulted in extensive waterborne transmission of cholera. Beverages prepared with contaminated water and sold by street vendors, ice and even commercial bottled water were incriminated. Cooked grains with sauces have been incriminated as vehicles in cholera transmission. *V. cholerae* introduced by a food handler into one of these foods and stored unrefrigerated can increase by several logs within 8-12 hours. Vegetables and fruit "freshened" with untreated sewage wastewater have also served as vehicles of transmission. Outbreaks or epidemics as well as sporadic cases are often attributed to raw or undercooked seafood. Sometimes these vehicles come from polluted waters as in outbreaks on Guam, Kiribati, Portugal, Italy and Ecuador. In other instances, as in the USA, sporadic cases of cholera follow the ingestion of raw or inadequately cooked seafood from nonpolluted waters. The Louisiana and Texas cases have been traced to eating shellfish from coastal and estuarine waters where a natural reservoir of *V. cholerae* O1, serotype Inaba, appears to exist in an estuarine environment not characterized by sewage contamination. Clinical cholera in endemic areas is usually confined to the lowest socioeconomic groups.

6. Incubation period—From a few hours to 5 days, usually 2-3 days.

7. Period of communicability—Presumably as long as stools are positive, usually only a few days after recovery. Occasionally the carrier state may persist for several months. Antibiotics known to be effective against the infecting strains (e.g., tetracycline against the O139 strain and most O1 strains) shorten the period of communicability. Very rarely, chronic biliary infection that lasts for years has been observed in adults associated with intermittent shedding of vibrios in the stool.

8. Susceptibility and resistance—Variable; gastric achlorhydria increases risk of illness, and breast fed infants are protected. Cholera gravis due to the El Tor biotype and O139 vibrio occurs significantly more often among persons with blood group O. Infection with either *V. cholerae* O1 or O139 results in a rise in agglutinating and antitoxic antibodies, and increased resistance to reinfection. Serum vibriocidal antibodies, which are readily detected following O1 infection (but for which comparably specific, sensitive and reliable assays are not available for O139 infection), are the best immunologic correlate of protection against O1 cholera. Field studies show that an initial clinical infection by *V. cholerae* O1 of the classical biotype confers protection against either classical or El Tor biotypes; in contrast an initial clinical infection caused by biotype El Tor results in only a modest level of long-term protection that is limited to El Tor infections. In endemic areas, most people acquire antibodies by early adulthood. However, infection with O1 strains affords no protection against O139 infection and vice versa. In experimental challenge studies in volunteers, an initial clinical infection due to *V. cholerae* O139 confered significant protection against diarrhea upon rechallenge with *V. cholerae* O139.

9. Methods of control—

A. *Preventive measures:*

1) See Typhoid fever, 9A1–7.
2) Active immunization with the current killed whole cell vaccine given parenterally is of little practical value in epidemic control or management of contacts to cases. These vaccines have been shown to provide partial protection (50%) of short duration (3–6 months) in highly endemic areas and do not prevent asymptomatic infection; they are not recommended. Two oral vaccines that provide significant protection for several months against cholera caused by O1 strains have become available in a number of countries: One is a single-dose live vaccine (strain CVD 103-HgR, available under the trade names Orachol® in Europe and Mutacol in Canada, SSVI); the other is a nonliving vaccine consisting of inactivated vibrios plus B-subunit of the cholera toxin, given on a 2-dose schedule (Dukoral, SBL). As of late 1999, these vaccines were not licensed in the USA.
3) Measures that inhibit or otherwise compromise the movement of people, foods or other goods are not justified.

B. *Control of patient, contacts and the immediate environment:*

1) Report to local health authority: Case report universally required by *International Health Regulations* (1969), Third Annotated Edition 1983, Updated and Reprinted 1992, WHO, Geneva; Class 1 (see Communicable Disease Reporting).
2) Isolation: Hospitalization with enteric precautions is desirable for severely ill patients; strict isolation is not necessary. Less severe cases can be managed on an outpatient basis with oral rehydration and an appropriate antimicrobial agent. Crowded cholera wards can be operated without hazard to staff and

visitors when effective handwashing and basic procedures of cleanliness are practiced. Fly control should be practiced.

3) Concurrent disinfection: Of feces and vomitus and of linens and articles used by patients, by heat, carbolic acid or other disinfectant. In communities with a modern and adequate sewage disposal system, feces can be discharged directly into the sewers without preliminary disinfection. Terminal cleaning.

4) Quarantine: None.

5) Management of contacts: Surveillance of persons who shared food and drink with a cholera patient for 5 days from last exposure. If there is evidence or high likelihood of secondary transmission within households, household members should be given chemoprophylaxis; in adults, tetracycline (500 mg 4 times daily) or doxycycline (a single daily dose of 300 mg) for 3 days, unless local strains are known or believed to be tetracycline resistant. Children may also be given tetracycline (50 mg/kg/day in 4 divided doses) or doxycycline (a single dose of 6 mg/kg) for 3 days; with such short courses of tetracyclines, staining of teeth is not a problem. Alternative prophylactic agents that may be useful where *V. cholerae* O1 strains are resistant to tetracycline include: furazolidone (Furox-one®) (100 mg 4 times daily for adults and 1.25 mg/kg 4 times daily for children); erythromycin (pediatric dosage 40 mg/kg/day in 4 divided doses; adult dosage 250 mg 4 times daily); TMP-SMX (320 mg TMP and 1600 mg SMX twice daily for adults and 8 mg/kg TMP and 40 mg/kg SMX daily in 2 divided doses for children); or ciprofloxacin (500 mg twice daily for adults). TMP-SMX is not useful for *V. cholerae* O139 infections as these strains are resistant to this antimicrobial. Mass chemoprophylaxis of whole communities is never indicated and can lead to antibiotic resistance. Immunization of contacts is not indicated.

6) Investigation of contacts and source of infection: Investigate possibilities of infection from polluted drinking water and contaminated food. Meal companions for the 5 days prior to onset should be interviewed. A search by stool culture for unreported cases is recommended only among household members or those exposed to a possible common source in a previously uninfected area.

7) Specific treatment: These are three mainstays in the treatment of patients with cholera: 1) aggressive rehydration therapy; 2) administration of effective antibiotics; and 3) treatment of complications. Aggressive rehydration by oral and intravenous routes to repair fluid and electrolyte deficits and to replace the prodigious ongoing diarrheal losses is the cornerstone of cholera therapy. Appropriate antimicrobials are an important adjunct to fluid therapy, as they diminish the volume and

duration of purging and rapidly curtail the excretion of vibrios, thereby diminishing the chance of secondary transmission. Finally, as rehydration therapy becomes increasingly effective, patients who survive from hypovolemic shock and severe dehydration manifest certain complications such as hypoglycemia that must be recognized and treated promptly. If these basic guidelines are adhered to, case fatality, even during explosive outbreaks in developing countries can be kept to less than 1%.

In initiating prompt aggressive fluid therapy with volumes of electrolyte solution adequate to correct dehydration, acidosis and hypokalemia most patients with mild or moderate fluid loss can be treated entirely with oral rehydration using solutions that contain glucose 20 g/L (or sucrose 40 g/L or cooked rice powder 50 g/L); NaCl (3.5 g/L); KCl (1.5 g/L); and trisodium citrate dihydrate (2.9 g/L) or $NaHCO_3$ (2.5 g/L). Mild and moderate volume depletion should be corrected with oral solutions by replacing, over 4–6 hours, a volume matching the estimated fluid loss (approximately 5% of body weight for mild and 7% for moderate dehydration). Continuing losses are replaced by giving, over 4 hours, a volume of oral solution 1.5 times the stool volume lost in the previous 4 hours.

Patients in shock should be given rapid IV rehydration with a balanced multielectrolyte solution containing approximately 130 mEq/L of Na^+, 25–48 mEq/L of bicarbonate, acetate or lactate ions, and 10–15 mEq/L of K^+. Useful solutions include Ringer's lactate or WHO "diarrhea treatment solution" (4 g NaCl, 1 g KCl, 6.5 g sodium acetate and 8 g glucose/L), and "Dacca solution" (5 g NaCl, 4 g $NaHCO_3$ and 1 g KCl/L), which can be prepared locally in an emergency. The initial fluid replacement should be 30 ml/kg in the first hour for infants and in the first 30 minutes for persons over 1 year of age, after which the patient should be reassessed. After circulatory collapse has been effectively reversed, most patients can be switched to oral rehydration to complete the 10% initial fluid deficit replacement and to match continuing fluid loss.

Appropriate antimicrobial agents can shorten the duration of diarrhea, reduce the volume of rehydration solutions required, and shorten the duration of vibrio excretion. Adults are given tetracycline 500 mg 4 times a day, and children 12.5 mg/kg 4 times daily, for 3 days. When tetracycline resistant strains of *V. cholerae* are prevalent, alternative antimicrobial regimens include TMP-SMX (320 mg trimethoprim and 1600 mg sulfamethoxazole twice daily for adults and 8 mg/kg trimethoprim and 40 mg/kg sulfamethoxazole daily in 2 divided doses for children, for 3 days); furazolidone (100 mg 4 times daily for adults and 1.25 mg/kg 4 times daily for children, for 3 days); or erythromycin (250 mg 4 times daily for adults and 10 mg/kg 3 times daily for children, for 3 days). Ciprofloxacin, 250 mg once daily for three days, is also a useful regimen for adults. *V. cholerae* O139 strains are resistant to TMP-SMX. Since individual strains of *V. cholerae* O1 or O139 may be resistant to any of these antimicrobials, knowledge of the sensitivity of local strains to these agents, if available, should be used to guide the choice of the antimicrobial therapy.

C. Epidemic measures:

1) Educate the population at risk concerning the need to seek appropriate treatment without delay.
2) Provide effective treatment facilities.
3) Adopt emergency measures to ensure a safe water supply. Chlorinate public water supplies, even if the source water appears to be uncontaminated. Chlorinate or boil water used for drinking, cooking and washing dishes and food containers unless the water supply is adequately chlorinated and subsequently protected from contamination.
4) Ensure careful preparation and supervision of food and drinks. After cooking or boiling, protect against contamination by flies and unsanitary handling; leftover foods should be thoroughly reheated before ingestion. Persons with diarrhea should not prepare food or haul water for others. Food served at funerals of cholera victims may be particularly hazardous and should be discouraged during epidemics.
5) Initiate a thorough investigation designed to find the vehicle and circumstances (time, place, person) of transmission, and plan control measures accordingly.
6) Provide appropriate safe facilities for sewage disposal.
7) Parenteral whole cell vaccine is not recommended.
8) If local conditions are relatively settled, the new oral cholera vaccines can serve as an additional adjunct measure to aid in cholera control. However, these vaccines should not be used in chaotic situations or where there is a severe shortage of water that interferes with the provision of oral rehydration therapy.

D. Disaster implications:
Risk of outbreaks is high in areas where cholera is endemic if large groups of people are crowded together without adequate food handling or sanitary facilities.

E. International measures:

1) Governments are required to report by telegraph to WHO and adjacent countries the first imported, first transferred or first

nonimported case of cholera due to *V. cholerae* O1 or O139 in an area previously free of the disease. In the USA, clinicians and microbiologists report suspected cases to their state epidemiologist; state health departments then notify the CDC, which confirms the case and notifies WHO.

2) Measures applicable to ships, aircraft and land transport arriving from cholera areas are specified in *International Health Regulations* (1969), Third Annotated Edition 1983, Updated and Reprinted 1992, WHO, Geneva.

3) International travelers: Immunization with the parenteral whole cell vaccine is not recommended by WHO for travel from country to country in any part of the world and is not officially required by any country. Immunization with either of the new oral vaccines is recommended for individuals from industrialized countries traveling to areas of endemic or epidemic cholera. In those countries where the new oral vaccines are already licensed, immunization is particularly recommended for travelers who have known risk factors such as individuals with hypochlorhydria (consequent to partial gastrectomy or medication) or cardiac disease (e.g., arrhythmias), the elderly, or any individuals of blood group O. As of late 1999, these vaccines were not licensed in the USA. *International Health Regulations* state that "... a person on an international voyage, who has come from an infected area within the incubation period of cholera and who has symptoms indicative of cholera, may be required to submit to stool examination."

4) WHO Collaborating Centres.

II. *VIBRIO CHOLERAE* SEROGROUPS OTHER THAN O1 AND O139   ICD-9 005.8; ICD-10 A05.8

1. Identification—Of the more than 100 *V. cholerae* serogroups that exist, only O1 and O139 are associated with the epidemiologic features and clinical syndrome of cholera. However, organisms of *V. cholerae* serogroups other than O1 and O139 have been associated with sporadic cases and small outbreaks of gastroenteritis. They have also rarely been isolated from patients with septicemic disease (usually immunocompromised hosts).

2. Infectious agent—*V. cholerae* pathogens of serogroups other than O1 and O139. As with all *V. cholerae*, growth is enhanced in an environment of 1% NaCl. Rarely do non-O1/non-O139 *V. cholerae* strains elaborate cholera toxin or harbor the colonization factors of O1 and O139 epidemic strains. Some non-O1/non-O139 strains make a heat stable enterotoxin (so-called NAG-ST). Epidemiologic and volunteer challenge studies have documented the pathogenicity of strains that produce NAG-ST. The non-O1/non-O139 strains isolated from blood of septicemic patients have been heavily encapsulated.

3. Occurrence—Non-O1/non-O139 *V. cholerae* strains are associated with 2%-3% of cases (including travelers) of diarrheal illness in tropical developing countries. Isolation rates are higher in coastal areas.

4. Reservoir—Non-O1/non-O139 *V. cholerae* are found in aquatic environments worldwide, particularly in mildly brackish waters where they constitute autochthonous flora. Although these organisms are halophilic, they can also proliferate in fresh water (e.g., lakes). Vibrio counts vary with season and peak in warm seasons. In brackish waters they are found adherent to chitinous zooplankton and shellfish.

5. Mode of transmission—Cases of non-O1/non-O139 gastroenteritis are usually linked to consumption of raw or undercooked seafood, particularly shellfish. In tropical endemic areas, some infections may be due to ingestion of surface waters. Wound infections arise from environmental exposure, usually to brackish water or from occupational accidents among fishermen, shellfish harvesters, etc. In high risk hosts septicemia may result from a wound infection or from ingestion of contaminated seafood.

6. Incubation period—Short. From 12 to 24 hours in outbreaks and an average of 10 hours in experimental challenge of volunteers (range 5.5 to 96 hours).

7. Period of communicability—It is not known whether in nature these infections can be transmitted from person to person or by humans contaminating food vehicles. If the latter indeed occurs the period of potential communicability would likely be limited to the period of vibrio excretion, usually several days.

8. Susceptibility and resistance—All humans are believed to be susceptible to gastroenteritis if they ingest a sufficient number of non-O1/non-O139 *V. cholerae* in an appropriate food vehicle or to develop a wound infection if the wound is exposed to vibrio containing water or shellfish. Septicemia develops only in abnormal hosts such as those who are immunocompromised, have chronic liver disease or severe malnutrition.

9. Methods of control—

   A. Preventive measures:

      1) Educate consumers about the risks associated with eating raw seafood unless it has been irradiated.

      2) Educate seafood handlers and processors on the following preventive measures:

   a) Ensure that cooked seafood reaches temperatures adequate
      to kill the organism by heating for 15 minutes at 70°C/
      158°F (organisms may survive at 60°C/140°F for up to 15
      minutes and at 80°C/176°F for several minutes).
   b) Handle cooked seafood in a manner that precludes contamination from raw seafood or contaminated seawater.
   c) Keep all seafood, raw and cooked, adequately refrigerated
      before eating.
   d) Avoid use of seawater in food handling areas, e.g., on cruise
      ships.

   B., C. and D. Control of patient, contacts and immediate environment; Epidemic measures and Disaster implications: See Staphylococcal food intoxication (section I, 9B except for B2, 9C and 9D). Isolation: Enteric precautions.

Patients with liver disease or who are immunosuppressed (by treatment or underlying disease) and alcoholics should be warned not to eat raw seafood. When disease occurs in these individuals, a history of eating seafood and especially the presence of bullous skin lesions justify early institution of antibiotic therapy, with a combination of oral minocycline (100 mg every 12 h) and intravenous cefotaxime (2 grams every 8 h) as the treatment regimen of choice. Tetracyclines and ciprofloxacin are also effective.

III. *VIBRIO PARAHAEMOLYTICUS* ENTERITIS   ICD-9 005.4; ICD-10 A05.3
(*Vibrio parahaemolyticus* infection)

   1. Identification—An intestinal disorder characterized by watery diarrhea and abdominal cramps in the majority of cases, and sometimes with nausea, vomiting, fever and headache. Occasionally, a dysentery-like illness is observed with bloody or mucoid stools, high fever and high WBC count. Typically, it is a disease of moderate severity lasting 1–7 days; systemic infection and death rarely occur.

   Diagnosis is confirmed by isolating the Kanagawa positive vibrios from the patient's stool on appropriate media; or identifying 10^5 or more organisms per gram of an epidemiologically incriminated food (usually seafood).

   2. Infectious agent—*Vibrio parahaemolyticus*, a halophilic vibrio. Twelve different "O" antigen groups and approximately 60 different "K" antigen types have been identified. Pathogenic strains are generally (but not always) capable of producing a characteristic hemolytic reaction (the "Kanagawa phenomenon").

   3. Occurrence—Sporadic cases and common-source outbreaks have been reported from many parts of the world, particularly Japan, southeast Asia and the USA. Several large foodborne outbreaks have occurred in the USA in which undercooked seafood was the food vehicle. Cases occur primarily in warm months. Some recent outbreaks have been due to Kanagawa negative, urease positive strains.

4. Reservoir—Marine coastal environs are the natural habitat. During the cold season, organisms are found in marine silt; during the warm season, they are found free in coastal waters and in fish and shellfish.

5. Mode of transmission—Ingestion of raw or inadequately cooked seafood, or any food contaminated by handling raw seafood, or by rinsing with contaminated water.

6. Incubation period—Usually between 12 and 24 hours, but can range from 4 to 30 hours.

7. Period of communicability—Not communicable from person to person.

8. Susceptibility and resistance—Most people are probably susceptible.

9. Methods of control—

A. Preventive measures: The same as those for prevention of non O1/non O139 *V. cholerae* infections.

B., C. and D. Control of patient, contacts and immediate environment; Epidemic measures and Disaster implications: See Staphylococcal food intoxication (section I, 9B except for B2, 9C and 9D). Isolation: Enteric precautions.

IV. INFECTION WITH *VIBRIO VULNIFICUS*   ICD-9 005.8; ICD-10 A05.8

1. Identification—Infection with *Vibrio vulnificus* produces septicemia in persons with chronic liver disease, chronic alcoholism or hemochromatosis; or those who are immunosuppressed. The disease appears 12 hours to 3 days after eating raw or undercooked seafood, especially oysters. One third of patients are in shock when they present for care or develop hypotension within 12 hours after hospital admission. Three quarters of patients have distinctive bullous skin lesions; thrombocytopenia is common and there is often evidence of disseminated intravascular coagulation. Over 50% of patients with primary septicemia die; the mortality rate exceeds 90% among those who become hypotensive. *V. vulnificus* can also infect wounds sustained in coastal or estuarine waters; wounds range from mild, self-limited lesions to rapidly progressive cellulitis and myositis that can mimic clostridial myonecrosis in the rapidity of spread and destructiveness.

2. Infectious agent—A halophilic, usually lactose positive (85% of isolates) marine *Vibrio* that is biochemically quite similar to *V. parahaemolyticus*. Confirmation of species identity sometimes requires use of DNA probes or numerical taxonomy in a reference laboratory. *V. vulnificus* expresses a polysaccharide capsule, of which there are multiple antigenic types on its surface.

3. Occurrence—*V. vulnificus* is the most common agent of serious infections caused by the genus *Vibrio* in the USA. In coastal areas the annual incidence of *V. vulnificus* disease is about 0.5 cases per 100,000 population; approximately 2/3 of these cases are primary septicemia. *V. vulnificus* cases have been reported from many areas of the world (e.g., Japan, Korea, Taiwan, Israel, Spain, Turkey).

4. Reservoir—*V. vulnificus* is a free living autochtonous flora of estuarine environments. It is recovered from estuarine waters and from shellfish, particularly oysters. During warm summer months this *Vibrio* can be isolated routinely from most cultured oysters.

5. Mode of transmission—Among persons of high risk, including those who are immunocompromised or have chronic liver disease, infection is acquired by the ingestion of raw or undercooked seafood. In contrast, in immunocompetent normal hosts, wound infections typically occur after exposure to estuarine water (e.g., boating accidents) or from occupational wounds (oyster shuckers, fishermen).

6. Incubation period—Usually 12 to 72 hours after eating raw or undercooked seafood.

7. Period of communicability—This is not considered to be an infection that is transmitted from person to person, either directly or via contamination of food except as described in I.5 above.

8. Susceptibility and resistance—Persons with cirrhosis, hemachromatosis and other chronic liver disease and immunocompromised hosts (from either underlying disease or medication) are at greatly increased risk for the septicemic form of disease. Based on data from the Florida State Health Department for the period 1981–1992, the annual incidence of *V. vulnificus* illness among adults with liver disease who ate raw oysters was 7.2 per 100,000 versus 0.09 per 100,000 for adults without known liver disease.

9. **Methods of control**—

    A. Preventive measures: The same as those for prevention of non-O1/non-O139 *V. cholerae* infections.

V. INFECTION WITH OTHER VIBRIOS   ICD-9 005.8; ICD-10 A05.8

Infection with certain other *Vibrio* species has been associated with diarrheal disease. These include *V. cholerae* of serogroups other than O1, *V. mimicus* (some strains elaborate an enterotoxin indistinguishable from that produced by *V. cholerae* O1 and O139), *V. fluvialis*, *V. furnissii*, and *V. hollisae*. Septicemic disease in hosts with underlying liver disease, severe malnutrition or immuno-competence has rarely been associated with *V. hollisae. V. alginolyticus* and *V. damsela* have been associated with wound infections.

CHROMOMYCOSIS   ICD-9 117.2; ICD-10 B43
(Chromoblastomycosis, Dermatitis verrucosa)

1. **Identification**—A chronic spreading mycosis of the skin and subcutaneous tissues, usually of a lower extremity. Progression to contiguous tissues is slow, over a period of years, with eventual large verrucous or even cauliflower-like masses and lymphatic stasis. Rarely a cause of death.

Microscopic examination of scrapings or biopsies from lesions reveals characteristic large, brown, thick walled, rounded cells that divide by fission in two planes. Confirmation of the diagnosis should be made by biopsy and attempted cultures of the fungus.

2. **Infectious agents**—*Phialophora verrucosa, Fonsecaea (Phialophora) pedrosoi, F. compacta, Cladosporium carrionii, Rhinocladiella aquaspersa, Botryomyces caespitatus, Exophiala spinifera* and *Exophiala jeanselmei.*

3. **Occurrence**—Worldwide; sporadic cases in widely scattered areas, but mainly Central America, Caribbean islands, southern USA, South America, South Pacific islands, Australia, Japan, Madagascar and Africa. Primarily a disease of rural, barefooted agricultural workers in tropical regions, probably because of more frequent penetrating wounds of feet

and limbs not protected by shoes or clothing. The disease is most common in men aged 30–50 years; women are rarely infected.

4. Reservoir—Wood, soil and decaying vegetation.

5. Mode of transmission—Minor penetrating trauma, usually a sliver of contaminated wood or other material.

6. Incubation period—Unknown; probably months.

7. Period of communicability—Not transmitted from person to person.

8. Susceptibility and resistance—Unknown, but rarity of disease and absence of laboratory acquired infections suggest that humans are relatively resistant.

9. Methods of control—

   A. *Preventive measures:* Protect against small puncture wounds by wearing shoes or protective clothing.

   B. *Control of patient, contacts and the immediate environment:*

   1) Report to local health authority: Official report not ordinarily justifiable, Class 5 (see Communicable Disease Reporting).
   2) Isolation: None.
   3) Concurrent disinfection: Of discharges from lesions and articles soiled therewith.
   4) Quarantine: None.
   5) Immunization of contacts: Not applicable.
   6) Investigation of contacts and source of infection: Not indicated.
   7) Specific treatment: Oral 5-fluorocytosine or itraconazole benefits some patients. Large lesions may respond better when 5-fluorocytosine is combined with amphotericin B (Fungizone®) IV. Small lesions are sometimes cured by excision.

   C. *Epidemic measures:* Not applicable; a sporadic disease.

   D. *Disaster implications:* None.

   E. *International measures:* None.

CLONORCHIASIS   ICD-9 121.1; ICD-10 B66.1
(Chinese or oriental liver fluke disease)

1. Identification—A trematode disease of the bile ducts. Clinical complaints may be slight or absent in light infections; symptoms result from local irritation of bile ducts by the flukes. Loss of appetite, diarrhea and a sensation of abdominal pressure are common early symptoms.

Rarely, bile duct obstruction producing jaundice may be followed by cirrhosis, enlargement and tenderness of the liver, and progressive ascites and edema. It is a chronic disease, sometimes of 30 years or longer duration, but not often a direct or contributing cause of death and often completely asymptomatic. However, it is a significant risk factor for development of cholangiocarcinoma.

Diagnosis is made by finding the characteristic eggs in feces or duodenal drainage fluid, to be differentiated from those of other flukes. Serologic diagnosis by ELISA can be performed.

2. Infectious agent—*Clonorchis sinensis,* the Chinese liver fluke.

3. Occurrence—Highly endemic in southeast China, but present throughout the country except in the northwest; occurs in Japan, Taiwan, Korea, Vietnam and probably in Laos and Cambodia, principally in the Mekong River delta. In other parts of the world, imported cases may be recognized in immigrants from Asia. In most endemic areas highest prevalence is among adults over the age of 30.

4. Reservoir—Humans, cats, dogs, swine, rats and other animals.

5. Mode of transmission—People are infected by eating raw or undercooked freshwater fish containing encysted larvae. During digestion, larvae are freed from cysts and migrate via the common bile duct to biliary radicles. Eggs deposited in the bile passages are evacuated in feces. Eggs in feces contain fully developed miracidia; when ingested by a susceptible operculate snail (e.g., *Parafossarulus),* they hatch in its intestine, penetrate the tissues and asexually generate larvae (cercariae) that emerge into the water. On contact with a second intermediate host (about 110 species of freshwater fish belonging mostly to the family Cyprinidae), cercariae penetrate the host fish and encyst, usually in muscle, occasionally on the underside of scales. The complete life cycle, from person to snail to fish to person, requires at least 3 months.

6. Incubation period—Unpredictable, as it varies with the number of worms present; flukes reach maturity within 1 month after encysted larvae are ingested.

7. Period of communicability—Infected individuals may pass viable eggs for as long as 30 years; infection is not directly transmitted from person to person.

8. Susceptibility and resistance—Susceptibility is universal.

9. Methods of control—

    A. Preventive measures:

        1) Thoroughly cook or irradiate all freshwater fish. Freezing at -10°C (14°F) for at least 5 days or storage for several weeks in

a saturated salt solution has been recommended but remains unproven.

2) In endemic areas, educate the public to the dangers of eating raw or improperly treated fish and the necessity for sanitary disposal of feces to avoid contaminating sources of food fish. Prohibit disposal of night soil and animal waste (excreta) in fishponds.

B. Control of patient, contacts and the immediate environment:

1) Report to local health authority: Official report not ordinarily justifiable, Class 5 (see Communicable Disease Reporting).
2) Isolation: None.
3) Concurrent disinfection: Sanitary disposal of feces.
4) Quarantine: None.
5) Immunization of contacts: Not applicable.
6) Investigation of contacts and source of infection: Of the individual case, not usually indicated. A community problem (see 9C, below).
7) Specific treatment: The drug of choice is praziquantel (Biltricide®).

C. Epidemic measures: Locate source of infected fish. Shipments of dried or pickled fish are the likely source in nonendemic areas; fresh or chilled freshwater fish from endemic areas are flown daily to the USA.

D. Disaster implications: None.

E. International measures: Control of fish or fish products imported from endemic areas.

OPISTHORCHIASIS ICD-9 121.0; ICD-10 B66.0

Opisthorchiasis is caused by small liver flukes of cats and some other fish eating mammals. *Opisthorchis felineus* occurs in Europe and Asia, and has infected 2 million people in the former Soviet Union; *O. viverrini* is endemic in southeast Asia, especially Thailand, where approximately 8 million are infected. These worms are the leading cause of cholangiocarcinoma throughout the world; in northern Thailand, rates are as high as 85/10,000 population. The biology of these flatworms, the characteristics of the disease and methods of control are essentially the same as those for clonorchiasis, above. Eggs cannot be easily distinguished from those of *Clonorchis*.

COCCIDIOIDOMYCOSIS ICD-9 114; ICD-10 B38
(Valley fever, San Joaquin fever, Desert fever, Desert rheumatism, Coccidioidal granuloma)

1. Identification—A deep mycosis that generally begins as a respiratory infection. The primary infection may be entirely asymptomatic or resemble an acute influenzal illness with fever, chills, cough and (rarely) pleuritic pain. About one fifth of clinically recognized cases (an estimated 5% of all primary infections) develop erythema nodosum, most frequently in Caucasian females and rarest in African-American males. Primary infection may heal completely without detectable residuals; may leave fibrosis, a pulmonary nodule that may or may not have calcified areas; leave a persistent thin-walled cavity; or most rarely, may progress to the disseminated form of the disease.

Disseminated coccidioidomycosis is a progressive, frequently fatal but uncommon granulomatous disease characterized by lung lesions and abscesses throughout the body, especially in subcutaneous tissues, skin, bone and the CNS. Coccidioidal meningitis resembles tuberculous meningitis but runs a more chronic course. An estimated 1/1,000 cases of symptomatic coccidioidomycosis become disseminated.

Diagnosis is made by demonstrating the fungus by microscopic examination or culture of sputum, pus, urine, CSF or biopsies of skin lesions or organs. (Handling cultures of the mold form is extremely hazardous and must be carried out in a BSL-2 or BSL-3 facility.) A positive skin test to spherulin appears from 2-3 days to 3 weeks after onset of symptoms. Precipitin and CF tests are usually positive within the first 3 months of clinical disease. The precipitin test detects IgM antibody, which appears 1-2 weeks after symptoms appear and lasts for 3-4 months. Complement fixation tests detect mostly IgG antibody, which appears 1-2 months after clinical symptoms start and persists for 6-8 months. Serial skin and serologic tests may be necessary to confirm a recent infection or indicate dissemination; skin tests are often negative in disseminated disease, and serologic tests may be negative in the immunocompromised.

2. Infectious agent—*Coccidioides immitis,* a dimorphic fungus. It grows in soil and culture media as a saprophytic mold that reproduces by arthroconidia; in tissues and under special conditions of culture, the parasitic form grows as spherical cells (spherules) that reproduce by endospore formation.

3. Occurrence—Primary infections are common only in arid and semiarid areas of the Western Hemisphere: in the USA, from California to southern Texas; in northern Argentina, Paraguay, Colombia, Venezuela, Mexico and Central America. Elsewhere, dusty fomites from endemic areas can transmit infection; disease has occurred in people who have merely traveled through endemic areas. The disease affects all ages, both genders, and all races. More than half of patients with symptomatic infection are between 15 and 25 years of age; males are affected much more frequently than females, probably because of occupational exposure. Infection is most frequent in summers following a rainy winter or spring, especially after wind and dust storms. It is an important disease among migrant workers, archeologists and military personnel from nonendemic areas who move into endemic areas. Since 1991, a marked increase of coccidioidomycosis has been reported in California.

4. Reservoir—Soil; especially in and around Indian middens and rodent burrows, in regions with appropriate temperature, moisture and soil requirements ("Lower Sonoran Life Zone"); infects humans, cattle, cats, dogs, horses, burros, sheep, swine, wild desert rodents, coyotes, chinchillas, llamas and other animal species.

5. Mode of transmission—Inhalation of the infective arthroconidia from soil and in laboratory accidents from cultures. While the parasitic form is normally not infective, accidental inoculation of infected pus or culture suspension into the skin or bone can result in granuloma formation.

6. Incubation period—In primary infection, 1 to 4 weeks. Dissemination may develop insidiously, sometimes without recognized symptoms of primary pulmonary infection and years after the primary infection.

7. Period of communicability—Not directly transmitted from humans or animals to humans. *C. immitis* on casts and dressings may rarely change from the parasitic to the infective saprophytic form after 7 days.

8. Susceptibility and resistance—Frequency of subclinical infection is indicated by the high prevalence of positive coccidioidin or spherulin reactors in endemic areas; recovery is generally followed by solid, lifelong immunity. However, reactivation can occur in those who become immunosuppressed therapeutically or by HIV infection. Susceptibility to dissemination is much greater in African Americans, Filipinos and other Asians, pregnant women and those with AIDS or other types of immunosuppression. Isolated coccidioidal meningitis cases are more common in Caucasian males.

9. Methods of control—

    A. Preventive measures:

        1) In endemic areas: Plant grass, oil unpaved airfields, and use other dust control measures (including face masks, air-conditioned cabs and wetting soil).

        2) Individuals from nonendemic areas should preferably not be recruited to dusty occupations, such as road building. Skin testing could be used to screen out susceptibles.

    B. Control of patient, contacts and the immediate environment:

        1) Report to local health authority: Case report of recognized cases, especially outbreaks, in selected endemic areas (USA);

in many countries, not a reportable disease, Class 3B (see Communicable Disease Reporting).

2) Isolation: None.
3) Concurrent disinfection: Of discharges and soiled articles. Terminal cleaning.
4) Quarantine: None.
5) Immunization of contacts: None.
6) Investigation of contacts and source of infection: Not recommended except in cases appearing in nonendemic areas, where residence, work exposure and travel history should be obtained.
7) Specific treatment: Primary coccidioidomycosis usually resolves spontaneously without therapy. Amphotericin B (Fungizone®) IV is beneficial in severe infections. Fluconazole is currently the agent of choice for meningeal infection. Ketoconazole and itraconazole have been useful in chronic, nonmeningeal coccidioidomycosis.

C. Epidemic measures: Outbreaks occur when groups of susceptibles are infected by airborne conidia. Dust control measures should be instituted where practicable (see 9A1, above).

D. Disaster implications: Possible hazard if large groups of susceptibles are forced to move through or to live under dusty conditions in areas where the fungus is prevalent.

E. International measures: None.

F. Bioterroism measures: C. immitis arthrospores have potential use as a bioterrorist weapon. See Anthrax, section F, for general measures to be taken when confronted with a threat of C. immitis arthrospores.

CONJUNCTIVITIS/
KERATITIS
ICD-9 372.0–372.3, 370;
ICD-10 H10, H16

I. ACUTE BACTERIAL
CONJUNCTIVITIS ICD-9 372.0; ICD-10 H10.0
(Pinkeye, "Sticky eye,"Brazilian purpuric fever [ICD-10 A48.4])

1. Identification—A clinical syndrome beginning with lacrimation, irritation and hyperemia of the palpebral and bulbar conjunctivae of one or both eyes, followed by edema of lids and mucopurulent discharge. In severe cases, ecchymoses of the bulbar conjunctiva and marginal infiltration of the cornea with photophobia may occur. Nonfatal (except as noted below), the disease has a clinical course that may last from 2 days to 2–3 weeks; many patients have no more than hyperemia of the conjunctivae and slight exudate for a few days.

Occasional cases of systemic disease have occurred among children in several communities in Brazil, 1–3 weeks after conjunctivitis due to a unique invasive clone of *Haemophilus influenzae* biogroup *aegyptius*. This severe illness, Brazilian purpuric fever (BPF), has had a 70% case-fatality rate among more than 100 cases recognized over a wide geographic area of Brazil including four states; it may be clinically indistinguishable from meningococcemia. The etiologic agent has been isolated from conjunctival, pharyngeal and blood cultures.

Confirmation of clinical diagnosis by microscopic examination of a stained smear or culture of the discharge is required to differentiate bacterial from viral or allergic conjunctivitis, or infection by adenovirus or enterovirus. Inclusion conjunctivitis (see below), trachoma and gonococcal conjunctivitis are described separately.

2. Infectious agents—*Haemophilus influenzae* biogroup *aegyptius* (Koch-Weeks bacillus) and *Streptococcus pneumoniae* appear to be the most important; *H. influenzae* type b, *Moraxella* and *Branhamella* spp., *Neisseria meningitidis* and *Corynebacterium diphtheriae* may also produce the disease. *H. influenzae* biogroup *aegyptius,* gonococci (see Gonoccocal Infections), *S. pneumoniae, S. viridans,* various gram-negative enteric bacilli and, rarely, *Pseudomonas aeruginosa* may produce the disease in newborn infants.

3. Occurrence—Widespread and common throughout the world, particularly in warmer climates; frequently epidemic. In the USA, infection with *H. influenzae* biogroup *aegyptius* is confined largely to southern rural areas extending from Georgia to California, primarily during summer and early autumn; in North Africa and the Middle East, infection occurs as seasonal epidemics. Infection due to other organisms occurs throughout the world, often in association with acute viral respiratory disease during cold seasons. BPF has been restricted essentially to Brazil; two cases that occurred in Australia were similar clinically, but the organism differed from the Brazilian strain.

4. Reservoir—Humans. Carriers of *H. influenzae* biogroup *aegyptius* and *S. pneumoniae* are common in many areas during interepidemic periods.

5. Mode of transmission—Contact with discharges from the conjunctivae or upper respiratory tracts of infected people; from contaminated fingers, clothing and other articles, including shared eye makeup applicators, multiple dose eye medications and inadequately sterilized instruments such as tonometers. The organisms may be mechanically transmitted by eye gnats or flies in some areas, but their importance as vectors is undetermined and probably differs from area to area.

6. Incubation period—Usually 24–72 hours.

7. Period of communicability—During the course of active infection.

8. Susceptibility and resistance—Children under 5 are most often affected; incidence decreases with age. The very young, the debilitated and the aged are particularly susceptible to staphylococcal infections. Immunity after attack is low grade and varies with the infectious agent.

9. Methods of control—

A. *Preventive measures:* Personal hygiene, hygienic care and treatment of affected eyes.

B. *Control of patient, contacts and the immediate environment:*

1) Report to local health authority: Obligatory report of epidemics; no case report for classic disease, Class 4; for systemic disease, Class 2A (see Communicable Disease Reporting).
2) Isolation: Drainage and secretion precautions. Children should not attend school during the acute stage.
3) Concurrent disinfection: Of discharges and soiled articles. Terminal cleaning.
4) Quarantine: None.
5) Immunization of contacts: None.
6) Investigation of contacts and source of infection: Usually not profitable for conjunctivitis; should be undertaken for BPF.
7) Specific treatment: Local application of an ointment or drops containing a sulfonamide such as sodium sulfacetamide, gentamicin or combination antibiotics such as polymyxin B with neomycin or trimethoprim is generally effective. For BPF, systemic treatment is required; isolates are sensitive to both ampicillin and chloramphenicol and resistant to TMP-SMX. Oral rifampin (20 mg/kg/day for 2 days) may be more effective than local chloramphenicol in eradication of the BPF clone and may be useful in prevention of BPF among children with BPF clone conjunctivitis. (See Gonococcal Conjunctivitis, 9B7.)

C. *Epidemic measures:*

1) Prompt and adequate treatment of patients and their close contacts.
2) In areas where insects are suspected of mechanically transmitting infection, measures to prevent access of eye gnats or flies to eyes of sick and well people.
3) Insect control, according to the suspected vector.

D. *Disaster implications:* None.

E. *International measures:* None.

II. KERATOCONJUNCTIVITIS, ADENOVIRAL ICD-9 077.1; ICD-10 B30.0

(Epidemic keratoconjunctivitis [EKC], Shipyard conjunctivitis, Shipyard eye)

1. Identification—An acute viral disease of the eye, with unilateral or bilateral inflammation of conjunctivae and edema of the lids and periorbital tissue. Onset is sudden with pain, photophobia, blurred vision and occasionally low grade fever, headache, malaise and tender preauricular lymphadenopathy. Approximately 7 days after onset in about half the cases, the cornea exhibits several small round subepithelial infiltrates that may eventually form punctate erosions that stain with fluorescein. Duration of acute conjunctivitis is about 2 weeks, although the keratitis may continue to evolve, leaving discrete subepithelial opacities that may interfere with vision for a few weeks. In severe cases permanent scarring may result.

Diagnosis is confirmed by recovery of virus from appropriate cell cultures inoculated with eye swabs or conjunctival scrapings; virus may be visualized by FA staining of scrapings or by IEM; viral antigen may be detected by ELISA testing. Type specific titer rises can be determined in serum neutralization or HAI tests.

2. Infectious agents—In the USA, typically adenovirus types 8, 19 and 37 are responsible, though other adenovirus types have been involved. Most severe disease has been found in infections caused by types 8, 5 and 19.

3. Occurrence—Presumably worldwide. Both sporadic cases and large outbreaks have occurred in Asia, Hawaii, North America and Europe.

4. Reservoir—Humans.

5. Mode of transmission—Direct contact with eye secretions of an infected person and, indirectly, through contaminated surfaces, instruments or solutions. In industrial plants, epidemics are centered in first-aid stations and dispensaries where treatment is frequently administered for minor trauma to the eye; transmission then occurs through fingers, instruments and other contaminated items. Similar outbreaks have originated in eye clinics and medical offices. When dispensary and clinic personnel acquire the disease, they may act as sources of infection. Family spread is common, with children typically introducing the infection.

6. Incubation period—The incubation period is between 5 and 12 days, but in many instances this duration is exceeded.

7. Period of communicability—From late in the incubation period to 14 days after onset. Prolonged viral shedding has been reported.

8. Susceptibility and resistance—There is usually complete type specific immunity after adenoviral infections. Trauma, even minor, and eye manipulation increase the risk of infection.

9. Methods of control—

A. *Preventive measures:*

1) Educate patients about personal cleanliness and the risk associated with use of common towels and toilet articles. Educate patients to minimize hand-to-eye contact.
2) Avoid communal eyedroppers, medicines, eye makeup, instruments or towels.
3) In ophthalmologic procedures in dispensaries, clinics and offices, asepsis should include vigorous handwashing before examining each patient and systematic sterilization of instruments after use; high-level disinfection (see Definitions) is recommended for instruments that will have contact with the conjunctivae or eyelids. Gloves should be worn for examining eyes of patients with possible or confirmed EKC. Any ophthalmic medicines or droppers that have come in contact with eyelids or conjunctivae should be discarded. Medical personnel with overt conjunctivitis should not have any physical contact with patients.
4) With persistent outbreaks, patients with EKC should be seen in physically separated facilities.
5) Use safety measures such as goggles in industrial plants.

B. *Control of patient, contacts and the immediate environment:*

1) Report to local health authority: Obligatory report of epidemics; no individual case report, Class 4 (see Communicable Disease Reporting).
2) Isolation: Drainage and secretion precautions; patients should use separate towels and linens during the acute stage. Infected medical personnel or patients should not come in contact with uninfected patients.
3) Concurrent disinfection: Of conjunctival and nasal discharges and articles soiled therewith. Terminal cleaning.
4) Quarantine: None.
5) Immunization of contacts: None.
6) Investigation of contacts and source of infection: In outbreaks, the source of infection should be identified and precautions taken to prevent further transmission.
7) Specific treatment: None during the acute phase. If the residual opacities interfere with the patient's ability to work, topical corticosteroids may be administered by a qualified ophthalmologist.

C. Epidemic measures:

1) Strictly apply recommendations in 9A, above.
2) Organize convenient facilities for prompt diagnosis, which eliminates or minimizes contact between infected and uninfected individuals.

D. Disaster implications: None.

E. International measures: WHO Collaborating Centres.

III. ADENOVIRAL HEMORRHAGIC CONJUNCTIVITIS   ICD-9 077.2; ICD-10 B30.1

(Pharyngoconjunctival fever)

ENTEROVIRAL HEMORRHAGIC CONJUNCTIVITIS   ICD-9 077.4; ICD-10 B30.3

(Apollo 11 disease, Acute hemorrhagic conjunctivitis)

1. Identification—In adenoviral conjunctivitis, lymphoid follicles usually develop, the conjunctivitis lasts 7–15 days and there are frequently small subconjunctival hemorrhages. In one adenoviral syndrome, pharyngoconjunctival fever (PCF), there is upper respiratory disease and fever with minor degrees of corneal epithelial inflammation (epithelial keratitis).

In enteroviral acute hemorrhagic conjunctivitis (AHC), onset is sudden with redness, swelling and pain often in both eyes; the course of the inflammatory disease is 4–6 days, during which time subconjunctival hemorrhages appear on the bulbar conjunctiva as petechiae that enlarge to form confluent subconjunctival hemorrhages. The large hemorrhages gradually resolve over 7–12 days. In large outbreaks of enteroviral AHC, there has been a low incidence of polio-like paralysis, including cranial nerve palsies, lumbosacral radiculomyelitis and lower motor neuron paralysis. The neurologic complications start a few days to a month after the conjunctivitis and often leave some residual weakness.

Laboratory confirmation of adenovirus infections is made by isolation of the virus from conjunctival swabs in cell culture, by detection of viral antigens by IF, by identification of viral nucleic acid with a DNA probe and by a rising antibody titer. Enterovirus infection is diagnosed by isolation of the agent, immunofluorescence, demonstration of a rising antibody titer or PCR.

2. Infectious agents—Adenoviruses and picornaviruses. Most adenoviruses can cause PCF, but types 3, 4 and 7 are the most common causes; adenovirus PCF outbreaks have occurred from poorly chlorinated swimming pools.

The most prevalent picornavirus type has been designated as enterovirus 70; this and a variant of coxsackievirus A24 have caused large outbreaks of AHC.

3. Occurrence—PCF occurs during outbreaks of adenovirus associated respiratory disease or as summer epidemics associated with swimming pools. AHC was first recognized in Ghana in 1969 and Indonesia in 1970; since then numerous epidemics have occurred in many tropical areas of Asia, Africa, Central and South America, the Caribbean, the Pacific islands and parts of Florida and Mexico. An outbreak in American Samoa in 1986 due to coxsackievirus A24 variant was estimated to have attacked 48% of the population. Smaller outbreaks have occurred in some European countries, usually associated with eye clinics. Cases have also occurred among southeast Asian refugees arriving in the USA and travelers returning to the USA from areas with AHC epidemics.

4. Reservoir—Humans.

5. Mode of transmission—By direct or indirect contact with discharge from infected eyes. Person to person transmission is most noticeable in families, where high attack rates often occur. Adenovirus can be transmitted in poorly chlorinated swimming pools and has been reported as "swimming pool conjunctivitis"; it is also transmitted by respiratory droplets. The large epidemics of AHC in developing countries are associated with overcrowding and low hygienic standards. Schoolchildren have been implicated in the rapid dissemination of AHC throughout a community.

6. Incubation period—For adenovirus infection, 4-12 days with an average of 8 days. For picornavirus infection, 12 hours to 3 days.

7. Period of communicability—Adenovirus infections may be communicable up to 14 days after onset, picornavirus at least 4 days after onset.

8. Susceptibility and resistance—Infection can occur at all ages. Reinfections and/or relapses have been reported. The role and duration of the immune response are not yet clear.

9. Methods of control —

A. *Preventive measures:* Since there is no effective treatment, prevention is critical. Personal hygiene should be emphasized, including no sharing of towels and avoidance of overcrowding. Maintain strict asepsis in eye clinics; wash hands before examining each patient. Eye clinics must ensure proper high level disinfection of potentially contaminated equipment. Closing schools may be indicated. Adequately chlorinate swimming pools.

B. Control of patient, contacts and the immediate environment:

1) Report to local health authority: Obligatory report of epidemics; no case report, Class 4 (see Communicable Disease Reporting).
2) Isolation: Drainage and secretion precautions; it is desirable to restrict contact with cases while disease is active; e.g., children should not attend school.
3) Concurrent disinfection: Of conjunctival discharges and articles and equipment soiled by them. Terminal cleaning.
4) Quarantine: None.
5) Immunization of contacts: None.
6) Investigation of contacts and source of infection: Locate other cases to determine whether a common source of infection is involved.
7) Specific treatment: None.

C. Epidemic measures:

1) Organize adequate facilities for the diagnosis and symptomatic treatment of cases.
2) Improve standard of hygiene and limit overcrowding wherever possible.

D. Disaster implications: None.

E. International measures: WHO Collaborating Centres.

IV. CHLAMYDIAL CONJUNCTIVITIS   ICD-9 077.0; ICD-10 A74.0
(Inclusion conjunctivitis, Paratrachoma, Neonatal inclusion blennorrhea, "Sticky eye")
(See separate chapter for Trachoma.)

1. Identification—In the newborn, an acute conjunctivitis with purulent discharge, usually recognized within 5–12 days after birth. The acute stage usually subsides spontaneously in a few weeks, but inflammation of the eye may persist for as long as a year or more if untreated and result in mild scarring of the conjunctivae and infiltration of the cornea (micropannus). Chlamydial pneumonia (see Pneumonia, Chlamydial) occurs in some infants with concurrent nasopharyngeal infection. Gonococcal infection must be ruled out.

In children and adults, an acute follicular conjunctivitis is seen typically with preauricular lymphadenopathy on the involved side, hyperemia, infiltration and a slight mucopurulent discharge, often with superficial corneal involvement. In adults, there may also be a chronic phase with scant discharge and symptoms that sometimes persist for a year or longer if untreated. The agent may cause symptomatic infection of the urethral epithelium in men and women and the cervix in women with or without associated conjunctivitis.

Laboratory methods to assist diagnosis include isolation in cell culture, antigen detection using IF staining of direct smears, EIA methods, or DNA probe.

2. Infectious agents—*Chlamydia trachomatis* of serovars D through K. Feline strains of *C. psittaci* have caused acute follicular keratoconjunctivitis in humans.

3. Occurrence—Sporadic cases of conjunctivitis are reported throughout the world among sexually active adults. Neonatal conjunctivitis due to *C. trachomatis* is common and occurs in 15%–35% of newborns exposed to maternal infection. Among adults with genital chlamydial infection, 1/300 develop chlamydial eye disease.

4. Reservoir—Humans for *C. trachomatis;* cats for *C. psittaci.*

5. Mode of transmission—The agent is generally transmitted during sexual intercourse; the genital discharges of infected people are infectious. In the newborn, conjunctivitis is usually acquired by direct contact with infectious secretions during transit through the birth canal. In-utero infection may also occur. The eyes of adults become infected by the transmission of genital secretions to the eye, usually by the fingers. Occasionally older children may acquire conjunctivitis from infected newborns or other household members; they should be assessed for sexual abuse. Outbreaks reported among swimmers in nonchlorinated pools have not been confirmed by culture and may be due to adenooviruses or other known causes of "swimming pool conjunctivitis."

6. Incubation period—In newborns, 5–12 days with a range from 3 days to 6 weeks; 6–19 days for adults.

7. Period of communicability—While genital or ocular infection persists; carriage on mucous membranes has been observed as long as 2 years after birth.

8. Susceptibility and resistance—There is no evidence of resistance to reinfection, although the severity of the disease may be decreased.

9. Methods of control —

  A. Preventive measures:

   1) Correct and consistent use of condoms to prevent sexual transmission and prompt treatment of persons with chlamydial urethritis and cervicitis.
   2) General preventive measures are those for other STDs (see Syphilis, 9A).

3) Identification of infection in pregnant women with high risk for infection, by culture or antigen detection, is critical. Treatment of cervical infection in pregnant women will prevent subsequent transmission to the infant. Erythromycin base, 500 mg 4 times daily for 7 days, is usually effective, but frequent GI side effects interfere with compliance.

4) Routine prophylaxis for gonococcal ophthalmia neonatorum should be practiced. The method of choice is either a single application into the eyes of the newborn of a 2.5% solution of povidone-iodine, tetracycline 1% eye ointment, erythromycin 0.5% eye ointment or silver nitrate 1% eye drops within 1 hour after delivery. All methods give comparable results in preventing gonococcal conjunctivitis; in field studies povidone-iodine was significantly more effective in preventing neonatal eye infections. Ocular prophylaxis does not prevent nasopharyngeal colonization and risk of subsequent chlamydial pneumonia. Penicillin is ineffective against chlamydiae.

B. Control of patient, contacts and the immediate environment:

1) Report to local health authority: Case report of neonatal cases obligatory in many states (USA) and countries, Class 2B (see Communicable Disease Reporting).

2) Isolation: Drainage and secretion precautions for the first 96 hours after starting treatment.

3) Concurrent disinfection: Aseptic techniques and handwashing by personnel appear to be adequate to prevent nursery transmission.

4) Quarantine: None.

5) Immunization of contacts: Not applicable.

6) Investigation of contacts and source of infection: All sexual contacts of adult cases, and mothers and fathers of neonatally infected infants should be examined and treated. Infected adults should also be investigated for evidence of ongoing infection with gonorrhea and syphilis.

7) Specific treatment: For ocular and genital infections of adults, a tetracycline, erythromycin or ofloxacin is effective when given by mouth for 2 weeks. Azithromycin is an effective single dose therapy.

Oral treatment of neonatal ocular infections with erythromycin for 2 weeks is recommended to eliminate the risk of chlamydial pneumonia as well; the dose is 10 mg/kg, given every 12 hours during the first week of life and every 8 hours thereafter.

C. Epidemic measures: Sanitary control of swimming pools; ordinary chlorination suffices.

D. Disaster implications: None.

E. International measures: WHO Collaborating Centres.

COXSACKIEVIRUS DISEASES ICD-9 074; ICD-10 B34.1

The coxsackieviruses, which are members of the enterovirus group of the family Picornaviridae, are the causal agents of a group of diseases discussed here, as well as epidemic myalgia, enteroviral hemorrhagic conjunctivitis and meningitis (see each disease under its individual listing); and coxsackievirus carditis (see below). They cause disseminated disease in newborns, and there is evidence suggesting their involvement in the etiology of juvenile onset, insulin-dependent diabetes.

I.A. ENTEROVIRAL VESICULAR PHARYNGITIS ICD-9 074.0; ICD-10 B08.5
(Herpangina, Aphthous pharyngitis)

I.B. ENTEROVIRAL VESICULAR STOMATITIS WITH EXANTHEM ICD-9 074.3; ICD-10 B08.4
(Hand, foot and mouth disease)

I.C. ENTEROVIRAL LYMPHONODULAR PHARYNGITIS ICD-9 074.8; ICD-10 B08.8
(Acute lymphonodular pharyngitis, Vesicular pharyngitis)

1. Identification—Vesicular pharyngitis (herpangina) is an acute, self-limited, viral disease characterized by sudden onset, fever, sore throat and small (1-2 mm), discrete, grayish papulovesicular pharyngeal lesions on an erythematous base, which gradually progress to slightly larger ulcers. These lesions, which usually occur on the anterior pillars of the tonsillar fauces, soft palate, uvula and tonsils, may be present for 4-6 days after the onset of illness. No fatalities have been reported. In one series, febrile convulsions occurred in 5% of cases.

Vesicular stomatitis with exanthem (hand, foot and mouth disease) differs from vesicular pharyngitis in that oral lesions are more diffuse and may occur on the buccal surfaces of the cheeks and gums and on the sides of the tongue. Papulovesicular lesions, which may persist from 7 to 10 days, also occur commonly as an exanthem, especially on the palms, fingers and soles; occasionally maculopapular lesions appear on the buttocks. Although the disease is usually self-limited, rare cases in infants have been fatal.

Acute lymphonodular pharyngitis also differs from vesicular pharyngitis in that the lesions are firm, raised, discrete, whitish to yellowish nodules, surrounded by a 3 to 6 mm zone of erythema. They occur predominantly on the uvula, anterior tonsillar pillars and posterior pharynx, with no exanthem.

Stomatitis due to herpes simplex virus requires differentiation; it has larger, deeper, more painful ulcerative lesions, commonly located in the front of the mouth. These diseases are not to be confused with vesicular stomatitis caused by the vesicular stomatitis virus, normally of cattle and horses, which in humans usually occurs in dairy workers, animal husbandrymen and veterinarians. Foot-and-mouth disease of cattle, sheep and swine rarely affects laboratory workers handling the virus; however, humans can be a mechanical carrier of the virus and the source of animal outbreaks. A virus not serologically differentiable from coxsackievirus B-5 causes vesicular disease in swine, which may be transmitted to humans.

Differentiation of the related but distinct coxsackievirus syndromes is facilitated during epidemics. Virus may be isolated from lesions and nasopharyngeal and stool specimens in cell cultures and/or suckling mice. Since many serotypes may produce the same syndrome and common antigens are lacking, serologic diagnostic procedures are not routinely available unless virus is isolated for use in the serologic tests.

2. Infectious agents—For vesicular pharyngitis, coxsackievirus, group A, types 1–10, 16 and 22. **For vesicular stomatitis,** coxsackievirus, group A, type A16 predominantly and types 4, 5, 9 and 10; group B, types 2 and 5; and (less often) enterovirus 71. **For acute lymphonodular pharyngitis,** coxsackievirus, group A, type 10. Other enteroviruses have occasionally been associated with these diseases.

3. Occurrence—Probably worldwide for vesicular pharyngitis and vesicular stomatitis, both sporadically and in epidemics; greatest incidence is in summer and early autumn; occurs mainly in children under 10 years, but adult cases (especially in young adults) are not unusual. Isolated outbreaks of acute lymphonodular pharyngitis, predominantly in children, may occur in summer and early fall. These diseases frequently occur in outbreaks among groups of children (e.g., in nursery schools, child care centers).

4. Reservoir—Humans.

5. Mode of transmission—Direct contact with nose and throat discharges and feces of infected people (who may be asymptomatic) and by aerosol droplet spread; no reliable evidence of spread by insects, water, food or sewage.

6. Incubation period—Usually 3–5 days for vesicular pharyngitis and vesicular stomatitis; 5 days for acute lymphonodular pharyngitis.

7. Period of communicability—During the acute stage of illness and perhaps longer, since these viruses persist in stool for several weeks.

8. Susceptibility and resistance—Susceptibility to infection is universal. Immunity to the specific etiologic virus is probably acquired by clinical or inapparent infection; duration unknown. Second attacks may occur with group A coxsackievirus of a different serologic type.

9. Methods of control—

    A. Preventive measures: Reduce person to person contact, where practicable, by measures such as crowd reduction and ventilation. Promote handwashing and other hygienic measures in the home.

    B. Control of patient, contacts and the immediate environment:

      1) Report to local health authority: Obligatory report of epidemics; no case report, Class 4 (see Communicable Disease Reporting).

      2) Isolation: Enteric precautions.

      3) Concurrent disinfection: Of nose and throat discharges. Wash or discard articles soiled therewith. Give careful attention to prompt handwashing when handling discharges, feces and articles soiled therewith.

      4) Quarantine: None.

      5) Immunization of contacts: None.

      6) Investigation of contacts and source of infection: Of no practical value except to detect other cases in groups of preschool children.

      7) Specific treatment: None.

    C. Epidemic measures: Give general notice to physicians of increased incidence of the disease, together with a description of onset and clinical characteristics. Isolate diagnosed cases and all children with fever, pending diagnosis, with special attention to respiratory secretions and feces.

    D. Disaster implications: None.

    E. International measures: WHO Collaborating Centres.

II. COXSACKIEVIRUS CARDITIS   ICD-9 074.2; ICD-10 B33.2
(Viral carditis, Enteroviral carditis)

1. Identification—An acute or subacute viral myocarditis or pericarditis which occurs as a manifestation (occasionally associated with other manifestations) of infection with enteroviruses, especially group B coxsackievirus.

The myocardium is affected, particularly in neonates, in whom fever and lethargy may be followed rapidly by heart failure with pallor, cyanosis, dyspnea, tachycardia and enlargement of heart and liver. Heart failure may be progressive and fatal, or recovery may take place over a few weeks; some cases run a relapsing course over months and may show residual heart damage. In young adults, pericarditis is the more common manifestation, with acute chest pain, disturbance of heart rate and rhythm, and often dyspnea. It may mimic myocardial infarction but is frequently associated with pulmonary or pleural manifestations. The disease may be associated with aseptic meningitis, hepatitis, orchitis, pancreatitis or epidemic myalgia (see Myalgia, Epidemic).

A diagnosis is usually made by serologic studies or by isolation of the virus from feces, but such results are not conclusive; a significant rise in specific antibody titers is diagnostic. Virus is rarely isolated from pericardial fluid, myocardial biopsy or postmortem heart tissue, but such an isolation provides a definitive diagnosis.

2. Infectious agents—Group B coxsackievirus (types 1–5); occasionally group A coxsackievirus (types 1, 4, 9, 16, 23) and other enteroviruses.

3. Occurrence—An uncommon disease, mainly sporadic, but increased during epidemics of group B coxsackievirus infection. Institutional outbreaks, with high case-fatality rates in newborns, have been described in maternity units.

4., 5., 6., 7., 8. and **9. Reservoir, Mode of transmission, Incubation period, Period of communicability, Susceptibility and resistance** and **Methods of control**—Same as for epidemic myalgia (q.v.).

CRYPTOCOCCOSIS ICD-9 117.5; ICD-10 B45
(Torula)

1. Identification—A deep mycosis usually presenting as a subacute or chronic meningitis; infection of lungs, kidneys, prostate and bone may occur. The skin may show acneiform lesions, ulcers or subcutaneous tumor-like masses. Occasionally, *Cryptococcus neoformans* may act as an endobronchial saprophyte in patients with other lung diseases. Untreated meningitis terminates fatally within weeks to months.

Diagnosis of cryptococcal meningitis is aided by visualizing encapsulated budding forms on microscopic examination of CSF mixed with India ink; urine or pus may also contain these forms. Tests for antigen in serum and CSF are often helpful. Diagnosis is confirmed by histopathology or by culture (media containing cycloheximide inhibit *C. neoformans* and should not be used). Mayer's mucicarmine stains most cryptococci in tissue deep red, aiding histopathologic diagnosis.

2. Infectious agents—*Cryptococcus neoformans* var. *neoformans* and *C. neoformans* var. *gattii;* the latter is more frequent in tropical or subtropical climates. The perfect (sexual) states of these fungi are called *Filobasidiella neoformans* var. *neoformans* and *F. neoformans* var. *bacillispora.*

3. Occurrence—Sporadic cases occur in all parts of the world. Mainly adults are infected, males more frequently than females. Patients with far advanced HIV infection have increased susceptibility to cryptococcosis, almost always variety *neoformans.* Infection also occurs in cats, dogs, horses, cows, monkeys and other animals.

4. Reservoir—Saprophytic growth in the external environment. The variety *neoformans* can be isolated consistently from old pigeon nests and pigeon droppings and from soil in many parts of the world. The variety *gattii* has been isolated from foliage and bark of certain species of eucalyptus trees.

5. Mode of transmission—Presumably by inhalation.

6. Incubation period—Unknown. Pulmonary disease may precede brain infection by months or years.

7. Period of communicability—Not transmitted directly from person to person, or between animals and people.

8. Susceptibility and resistance—All races are susceptible; however, the frequency of *C. neoformans* in the external environment and the rarity of infection suggest that humans have appreciable resistance. Susceptibility is increased during corticosteroid therapy, immune deficiency disorders (especially AIDS) and disorders of the reticuloendothelial system, particularly Hodgkin's disease and sarcoidosis.

9. Methods of control —

    A. Preventive measures: While there have been no case clusters traced to exposure to them, the ubiquity of *C. neoformans* in weathered pigeon droppings suggests that removal of large accumulations should be preceded by chemical decontamination, such as by an iodophor, or thorough wetting to prevent aerosolization of the agent.

    B. Control of patient, contacts and the immediate environment:

        1) Report to local health authority: Official report required in some jurisdictions as a possible manifestation of AIDS, Class 2B (see Communicable Disease Reporting).

2) Isolation: None.
3) Concurrent disinfection: Of discharges and contaminated dressings. Terminal cleaning.
4) Quarantine: None.
5) Immunization of contacts: None.
6) Investigation of contacts and source of infection: None.
7) Specific treatment: Amphotericin B (Fungizone®) IV is effective in many cases; 5-fluorocytosine is useful in combination with amphotericin B. The combination is often the therapy of choice but has substantial toxicity. In AIDS patients cryptococcosis is difficult to cure; fluconazole is useful after an initial course of amphotericin B and is continued indefinitely.

C. Epidemic measures: None.

D. Disaster implications: None.

E. International measures: None.

CRYPTOSPORIDIOSIS   ICD-9 136.8; ICD-10 A07.2

1. Identification—A parasitic infection of medical and veterinary importance that affects epithelial cells of the human GI, biliary and respiratory tracts, as well as over 45 different vertebrate species including poultry and other birds, fish, reptiles, small mammals (rodents, cats, dogs) and large mammals (particularly cattle and sheep). Asymptomatic infections are common and constitute a source of infection for others. The major symptom in human patients is diarrhea, which may be profuse and watery, preceded by anorexia and vomiting in children. The diarrhea is associated with cramping abdominal pain. General malaise, fever, anorexia, nausea and vomiting occur less often. Symptoms often wax and wane but remit in fewer than 30 days in most immunologically healthy people. Immunodeficient people, especially AIDS patients, may be unable to clear the parasite, and the disease has a prolonged and fulminant clinical course contributing to death. Symptoms of cholecystitis may occur in biliary tract infections; the relationship between respiratory tract infections and clinical symptoms is unclear.

Diagnosis is generally made by identification of oocysts in fecal smears or of life cycle stages of the parasites in intestinal biopsy sections. Oocysts are small (4-6 μm) and may be confused with yeast unless appropriately stained. Most commonly used stains include auramine–rhodamine, a modified acid–fast, and safranin–methylene blue. Additionally, new and more sensitive immunobased ELISA assays have recently become available.

A fluorescein tagged monoclonal antibody is useful for detecting oocysts in both stool and environmental samples. Infection with this organism is not easily detected unless looked for specifically. Serologic assays may be helpful in epidemiologic studies, but when the antibody appears and how long it lasts after infection are not known.

2. Infectious agent—*Cryptosporidium parvum,* a coccidian protozoa, is the species associated with human infection.

3. Occurrence—Worldwide. *Cryptosporidium* oocysts have been identified in human fecal specimens from more than 50 countries on six continents. In developed areas such as the USA and Europe, prevalence of infection was found in less than 1% to 4.5% of individuals surveyed by stool examination. In developing regions, the prevalence is significantly higher; the range is from 3% to 20%. Children under 2 years of age, animal handlers, travelers, men who have sex with many other men and close personal contacts of infected individuals (families, health care and day care workers) are particularly likely to be infected. Outbreaks have been reported in day care centers around the world. Outbreaks have also been associated with: drinking water (at least three major outbreaks involved public water supplies); recreational use of water including waterslides, swimming pools and lakes; and drinking unpasteurized apple cider that had been contaminated with cow manure.

4. Reservoir—Humans, cattle and other domestic animals.

5. Mode of transmission—Fecal-oral, which includes person to person, animal to person, waterborne, and foodborne transmission. The parasite infects intestinal epithelial cells and multiplies initially by schizogony, followed by a sexual cycle resulting in oocysts in the feces that can survive under adverse environmental conditions for long periods of time. Oocysts are highly resistant to chemical disinfectants used to purify drinking water. One or more autoinfective cycles may occur in humans.

6. Incubation period—Not precisely known; 1-12 days is the likely range, with an average of about 7 days.

7. Period of communicability—Oocysts, the infectious stage, appear in the stool at the onset of symptoms and are infectious immediately upon excretion. Oocysts continue to be excreted in the stool for several weeks after symptoms resolve; outside the body, they may remain infective for 2-6 months in a moist environment.

8. Susceptibility and resistance—People with intact immune function may have asymptomatic or self-limited symptomatic infections; it is not clear whether reinfection and latent infection with reactivation can occur. Individuals with impaired immunity generally clear their infections when the causes of immunosuppression (including malnutrition or intercurrent viral infections such as measles) are removed. In those with AIDS (q.v.), even though the clinical course may vary and asymptomatic periods may occur, the infection usually persists throughout the illness; approximately 2% of AIDS patients reported to CDC were infected with cryptosporidiosis when AIDS was diagnosed; hospital experience indicates that 10%–20% of AIDS patients develop infection at some time during their illness.

9. Methods of control—

A. *Preventive measures:*

1) Educate the public in personal hygiene.
2) Dispose of feces in a sanitary manner; use care in handling animal or human excreta.
3) Have those in contact with calves and other animals with diarrhea (scours) wash their hands carefully.
4) Boil drinking water supplies for 1 minute; chemical disinfectants are not effective against oocysts. Only filters capable of removing particles 0.1–1.0 µm in diameter should be considered.
5) Remove infected persons from jobs that require handling food that will not be subsequently cooked.
6) Exclude infected children from day care facilities until diarrhea stops.

B. *Control of patient, contacts and the immediate environment:*

1) Report to local health authority: Case report by most practicable means, Class 3B (see Communicable Disease Reporting).
2) Isolation: For hospitalized patients, enteric precautions in the handling of feces, vomitus and contaminated clothing and bed linen; exclusion of symptomatic individuals from food handling and from direct care of hospitalized and institutionalized patients; release to return to work in sensitive occupations when asymptomatic. Stress proper handwashing.
3) Concurrent disinfection: Of feces and articles soiled therewith. In communities with modern and adequate sewage disposal systems, feces can be discharged directly into sewers without preliminary disinfection. Terminal cleaning. Heating to 45°C (113°F) for 5–20 minutes, 60°C (140°F) for 2 minutes, or chemical disinfection with 10% formalin or 5% ammonia solution is effective.
4) Quarantine: None.
5) Immunization of contacts: None.
6) Investigation of contacts and source of infection: Microscopic examination of feces of household members and other suspected contacts, especially those who are symptomatic. Contact with cattle or domestic animals warrants investigation. If

waterborne transmission is suspected, large volume water sampling filters can be employed to look for oocysts in the water.

7) Specific treatment: No treatment other than rehydration, when indicated, has been proven to be effective; administration of passive antibodies and antibiotics is under study. If the individual is taking immunosuppressive drugs, these should be stopped or reduced if possible.

C. *Epidemic measures:* Investigate clustered cases in an area or institution epidemiologically to determine source of infection and mode of transmission; search for a common vehicle, such as recreational water, drinking water, raw milk or other potentially contaminated food or drink, and institute applicable prevention or control measures. Control of person to person or animal to person transmission requires special emphasis on personal cleanliness and sanitary disposal of feces.

D. *Disaster implications:* None.

E. *International measures:* None.

DIARRHEA CAUSED BY
CYCLOSPORA   ICD-10 A07.8

This diarrheal disease is caused by a newly identified coccidian protozoa (*Cyclospora cayetanensis*). This clinical syndrome consists of watery diarrhea (6 or more stools/day), nausea, anorexia, abdominal cramping, fatigue and weight loss; fever is rare. The median incubation period is about 1 week. *Cyclospora* can invade the jejunal epithelium and produce enteritis. Diarrhea in the immunocompetent can be prolonged but is self-limited, and lasts 9–43 days according to various reports; mean duration of organism shedding was 23 days in Peruvian children. In the immunocompromised, diarrhea lasted for months in some patients. It has also been associated with prolonged diarrhea in travelers to Asia, the Caribbean, Mexico and Peru.

Diagnosis is made by identification of the 8–9 mm size oocysts, about twice the size of *Cryptosporidium parvum* in wet mount under phase contrast microscopy. A modified acid-fast stain can be used. Organisms fluoresce under ultraviolet illumination.

Transmission appears to be primarily waterborne, and occurs either through drinking or swimming in contaminated water; but there have been international outbreaks involving thousands of persons traced to raspberries from Guatemala that occurred in at least 3 successive years during the late 1990s. Other vehicles have included basil and lettuce. Outbreaks have a seasonal pattern, with warmer months predominating in reported cases. The way in which the produce was contaminated was not determined for any of the outbreaks, in part because methods for detecting *Cyclospora* on produce and in other environmental samples are insensitive to low levels of the parasite. Produce should be washed thoroughly before it is eaten; however, this practice does not eliminate the risk of *Cyclospora*. Health care providers should consider the diagnosis of *Cyclospora* infection in persons with prolonged diarrheal illness and request stool specimens so that specific tests for this parasite can be made.

Cyclosporiasis can be treated with a 7 day course of oral trimethoprim (TMP)-sulfamethoxazole (SMX) (for adults, 160 mg TMP plus 800 mg SMX twice daily; for children, 5 mg/kg TMP plus 25 mg/kg SMX twice daily). In patients who are not treated, illness can be protracted, with remitting and relapsing symptoms. Treatment regimens for patients who cannot tolerate sulfa drugs have not been identified.

As of mid 1998, five states and one municipality in the USA had mandated reporting of this disease. In mid 1998, the Council of State and Territorial Epidemiologists passed a resolution recommending that cyclosporiasis be made a nationally notifiable disease in the USA. In jurisdictions where formal reporting mechanisms are not yet established, clinicians and laboratorians who identify cases of cyclosporiasis unrelated to travel outside North America are encouraged to inform the appropriate local, provincial, territorial, or state health departments. In Canada, these agencies are encouraged to contact the Division of Disease Surveillance, Bureau of Infectious Diseases, Laboratory Center for Disease Control, telephone (613) 941-1288; and, in the USA, CDC's Division of Parasitic Diseases, National Center for Infectious Diseases, telephone (770) 488-7760.

CYTOMEGALOVIRUS INFECTIONS

While infection with cytomegalovirus (CMV) is very common, it produces symptomatic disease relatively rarely; when it does, the manifestations vary depending on the age and immunocompetence of the individual at the time of infection.

CYTOMEGALOVIRUS DISEASE
ICD-9 078.5; ICD-10 B25

CONGENITAL CYTOMEGALOVIRUS INFECTION
ICD-9 771.1; ICD-10 P35.1

1. Identification—The most severe form of this viral disease develops in 5%-10% of infants infected in utero. These infants have signs and symptoms of severe generalized infection, especially involving the CNS and liver. Lethargy, convulsions, jaundice, petechiae, purpura, hepatosplenomegaly, chorioretinitis, intracerebral calcifications and pulmonary infiltrates occur in varying degrees. Survivors exhibit mental retardation, microcephaly, motor disabilities, hearing loss and evidence of chronic liver disease. Death may occur in utero; the neonatal case-fatality rate is high for severely affected infants. Although neonatal CMV infection occurs in only 0.3%–1% of births, 90%–95% of these intrauterine infections are inapparent; however, about 15–25% of these infants eventually manifest some degree of neurosensory disability. Fetal infection may occur during either primary or reactivated maternal infections, but primary infections carry a much higher risk for symptomatic disease and sequelae. Seronegative newborns who receive blood transfusions from seropositive donors may also develop severe disease.

Infection acquired later in life is generally inapparent but may cause a syndrome clinically and hematologically similar to Epstein-Barr virus mononucleosis, but distinguishable by virologic or serologic tests and the absence of heterophile antibodies. CMV causes up to 10% of all cases of mononucleosis seen among university students and hospitalized adults aged 25–34 years. CMV is the most common cause of posttransfusion mononucleosis following transfusion to nonimmune individuals; many posttransfusion infections are clinically inapparent. Disseminated infection, with pneumonitis, retinitis, GI tract disorders (gastritis, enteritis, colitis) and hepatitis, occurs in immunodeficient and immunosuppressed patients; this is a serious manifestation of AIDS.

CMV is also the most common cause of posttransplant infection, both for solid organ and bone marrow transplants; in the former, this is particularly so with a seronegative recipient and a seropositive (carrier) donor, whereas reactivation is a common cause of disease after bone marrow transplant. In both cases, the rate of serious disease is about 25%.

Diagnosis in the newborn is made by virus isolation or PCR, usually from urine. Diagnosis of CMV disease in the adult is made difficult by the high frequency of asymptomatic and relapsing infections. Multiple modalities for diagnosis should always be used if possible. Virus isolation, CMV antigen detection (which can be done within 24 hours) and CMV DNA detection by PCR or in situ hybridization can be used to demonstrate virus in organs, blood, respiratory secretions or urine. Serologic studies should be done to demonstrate the presence of CMV specific IgM antibody or a fourfold rise in antibody titer. Interpretation of the results requires knowledge of the clinical and epidemiologic background of the patient.

2. **Infectious agent**—Human (beta) herpesvirus 5 (human CMV), a member of the subfamily Betaherpesvirus of the family Herpesviridae; includes several antigenically related strains.

3. **Occurrence**—Worldwide. In the USA, intrauterine infection occurs

in 0.5% to 1% of pregnancies. Infection is acquired early in life in developing countries. The prevalence of serum antibodies in adults varies from 40% in highly developed countries to almost 100% in developing countries; it is inversely related to socioeconomic status within the USA and is higher in women than in men. In the UK, prevalence of antibodies is related to race rather than social class. In various population groups, 8%–60% of infants begin shedding virus in the urine during their first year of life as a result of infection acquired from the mother's cervix or breast milk.

4. Reservoir—Humans are the only known reservoir of human CMV; strains found in many animal species are not infectious for humans.

5. Mode of transmission—Intimate exposure by mucosal contact with infectious tissues, secretions and excretions. CMV is excreted in urine, saliva, breast milk, cervical secretions and semen during primary and reactivated infections. The fetus may be infected in utero from either a primary or reactivated maternal infection; serious fetal infection with manifest disease at birth occurs most commonly during a mother's primary infection, but infection (usually without disease) may develop even when maternal antibodies existed prior to conception. Postnatal infection occurs more commonly in infants born to mothers shedding CMV in cervical secretions at delivery; thus, transmission of the virus from the infected cervix at delivery is a common means of neonatal infection. Virus can be transmitted to infants through infected breast milk, an important source of infection but not disease. Viremia may be present in asymptomatic people, so the virus may be transmitted by blood transfusion, probably associated with leukocytes. CMV is excreted by a large number of children in day care centers, which may represent a community reservoir. Transmission through sexual intercourse is also common and is reflected by almost universal infection of men who have many male sexual partners.

6. Incubation period—Illness following a transplant or transfusion with infected blood begins within 3–8 weeks. Infection acquired during birth is first demonstrable 3–12 weeks after delivery.

7. Period of communicability—Virus is excreted in urine and saliva for many months and may persist or be episodic for several years following primary infection. After neonatal infection, virus may be excreted for 5–6 years. Adults appear to excrete virus for shorter periods, but the virus persists as a latent infection. Less than 3% of healthy adults are pharyngeal excreters. Excretion recurs with immunodeficiency and immunosuppression.

8. Susceptibility and resistance—Infection is ubiquitous. Fetuses, patients with debilitating diseases, those on immunosuppressive drugs and especially organ allograft recipients (kidney, heart, bone marrow) and patients with AIDS are more susceptible to overt and severe disease.

9. **Methods of control—**

   A. *Preventive measures:*

   1) Take care in handling diapers; wash hands after diaper changes and toilet care of newborns and infants.
   2) Women of childbearing age who work in hospitals (especially delivery and pediatric wards) should use "universal precautions"; in day care centers and preschools (especially those with mentally retarded populations), observe strict standards of hygiene such as handwashing.
   3) Avoid transfusing neonates of seronegative mothers with blood from CMV seropositive donors.
   4) Avoid transplanting organ tissues from CMV seropositive donors to seronegative recipients. If unavoidable, hyperimmune IG or prophylactic administration of antivirals may be helpful.

   B. *Control of patient, contacts and the immediate environment:*

   1) Report to local health authority: Official report not ordinarily justifiable, Class 5 (see Communicable Disease Reporting).
   2) Isolation: None. Secretion precautions may be applied while in the hospital for patients known to be excreting virus.
   3) Concurrent disinfection: Discharges from hospitalized patients and articles soiled therewith.
   4) Quarantine: None.
   5) Immunization of contacts: None commercially available.
   6) Investigation of contacts and source of infection: None, because of the high prevalence of asymptomatic shedders in the population.
   7) Specific treatment: Ganciclovir, IV and PO, and foscarnet IV have been approved for the treatment of CMV retinitis in immunocompromised persons. These drugs may also be helpful, especially when combined with anti-CMV immune globulin, for pneumonitis and possibly GI disease in immunocompromised persons.

   C. *Epidemic measures:* None.

   D. *Disaster implications:* None.

   E. *International measures:* None.

DENGUE FEVER
ICD-9 061; ICD-10 A90
(Breakbone fever)

1. Identification—An acute febrile viral disease characterized by sudden onset, fever for 3–5 days (rarely more than 7 and often biphasic), intense headache, myalgia, arthralgia, retroorbital pain, anorexia, GI disturbances and rash. Early generalized erythema occurs in some cases. A generalized maculopapular rash usually appears about the time of defervescence. Minor bleeding phenomena, such as petechiae, epistaxis or gum bleeding may occur at any time during the febrile phase. Dark skinned races frequently have no visible rash. With underlying conditions, adults may have major bleeding phenomena, such as GI hemorrhage in peptic ulcer cases or menorrhagia. Dengue infections with increased vascular permeability, unusual bleeding manifestations and involvement of specific organs are presented below under dengue hemorrhagic fever (DHF). Recovery may be associated with prolonged fatigue and depression. Lymphadenopathy and leukopenia with relative lymphocytosis are usual; thrombocytopenia (less than 100×10^3/cu mm; SI units less than 100×10^9/L) and elevated transaminases occur less frequently. Epidemics are explosive, but fatalities in the absence of dengue hemorrhagic fever are rare.

Differential diagnosis includes all epidemiologically relevant diseases listed under arthropod-borne viral fevers, yellow fever, measles, rubella, malaria, leptospirosis and other systemic febrile illnesses, especially those accompanied by rash.

HI, CF, IgG and IgM ELISA, and neutralization tests are diagnostic aids. IgM antibody, indicating current or recent infection, is usually detectable by day 6–7 after onset of illness. Virus is isolated from blood by inoculation of mosquitoes, or into mosquito or vertebrate cell cultures, then identified with serotype specific monoclonal antibodies.

2. Infectious agent—The viruses of dengue fever are flaviviruses and include serotypes 1, 2, 3 and 4 (dengue-1, -2, -3, -4). The same viruses are responsible for dengue hemorrhagic fever (see below).

3. Occurrence—Dengue viruses of multiple types are now endemic in most countries in the tropics. In Asia, dengue viruses are highly endemic in southern China and Hainan, Vietnam, Laos, Cambodia (Kampuchea), Thailand, Myanmar (Burma), India, Pakistan, Sri Lanka, Indonesia, the Philippines, Malaysia and Singapore; and with lower endemicity in New Guinea, Bangladesh, Nepal, Taiwan and much of the Pacific. Dengue viruses of several types have circulated in Queensland, northern Australia, since 1981.

Dengue-1, -2, -3 and -4 are now endemic in Africa. In large areas of west Africa, dengue viruses are probably transmitted epizootically in monkeys; urban dengue involving humans is also common in this area. In recent years, outbreaks of dengue fever have occurred on the east coast of Africa from Mozambique to Ethiopia and on offshore islands such as the Seychelles and Comoros, with a small number of dengue and DHF-like cases reported from Saudi Arabia.

In the Americas, successive introduction and circulation of all four serotypes in the Caribbean and Central and South America have occurred since 1977 and extended into Texas in 1980, 1986, 1995 and 1997. As of the late 1990s, two or more dengue viruses are endemic or periodically epidemic in Mexico, virtually all of the Caribbean, and Central America, Colombia, Bolivia, Ecuador, Peru, Venezuela, the Guyanas, Suriname, Brazil, Paraguay, and Argentina. Epidemics may occur wherever vectors are present and virus is introduced, whether in urban or rural areas.

4. Reservoir—The viruses are maintained in a human *Aedes aegypti* mosquito cycle in tropical urban centers; a monkey mosquito cycle serves as a reservoir in southeast Asia and west Africa.

5. Mode of transmission—By the bite of infective mosquitoes, principally *Ae. aegypti*. This is a day biting species, with increased biting activity for 2 hours after sunrise and several hours before sunset. Both *Ae. aegypti* and *Ae. albopictus* are found in urban settings; both are present within the USA. *Ae. albopictus,* which is abundant in much of Asia, is less anthropophilic than *Ae. aegypti* and hence is a less efficient epidemic vector. In Polynesia, one of the *Ae. scutellaris* spp. complex serves as the vector. In Malaysia, *Ae. niveus* complex and in west Africa *Ae. furcifer-taylori* complex mosquitoes are involved in enzootic monkey mosquito transmission.

6. Incubation period—From 3 to 14 days, commonly 4–7 days.

7. Period of communicability—Not directly transmitted from person to person. Patients are infective for mosquitoes from shortly before to the end of the febrile period, usually a period of 3–5 days. The mosquito becomes infective 8–12 days after the viremic blood meal and remains so for life.

8. Susceptibility and resistance—Susceptibility in humans is apparently universal, but children usually have a milder disease than adults. Recovery from infection with one serotype provides lifelong homologous immunity but does not provide protection against other serotypes and may exacerbate subsequent infections (see Dengue hemorrhagic fever, below).

9. Methods of control—

    A. Preventive measures:

        1) Educate the public on personal measures for eliminating or destroying mosquito larval habitats and protecting against day

biting mosquitoes by using screening, protective clothing and repellents (see Malaria, 9A3 and 9A4).

2) Survey community to determine the density of vector mosquitoes, to identify larval habitats (which for *Ae. aegypti* are usually artificial or natural water holding containers close to or within human habitations (e.g., old tires, flower pots, water storage containers) and to promote and implement plans for their elimination.

B. Control of patient, contacts and the immediate environment:

1) Report to local health authority: Obligatory report of epidemics; case reports, Class 4 (see Communicable Disease Reporting).

2) Isolation: Blood precautions. Until the fever subsides, prevent access of day biting mosquitoes to patients by screening the sickroom or using a mosquito bednet, preferably insecticide impregnated for febrile patients, or by spraying quarters with a knockdown adulticide or residual insecticide.

3) Concurrent disinfection: None.

4) Quarantine: None.

5) Immunization of contacts: None. If dengue occurs near possible jungle foci of yellow fever, immunize the population against yellow fever because the urban vector for the two diseases is the same.

6) Investigation of contacts and source of infection: Determine patient's place of residence during the 2 weeks before onset of illness and search for unreported or undiagnosed cases.

7) Specific treatment: None, supportive. Aspirin is contraindicated.

C. Epidemic measures:

1) Search for and destroy *Aedes* species of mosquitoes in places of human habitation, and eliminate or apply larvicide to all potential larval habitats of *Ae. aegypti.*

2) Use mosquito repellents for people exposed to vector mosquitoes.

D. Disaster implications: Epidemics can be extensive and may affect a high percentage of the population.

E. International measures: Enforce international agreements designed to prevent the spread of *Ae. aegypti* via ships, airplanes and land transport from areas where infestation exists. Improve international surveillance and exchange of data between countries. WHO Collaborating Centres.

DENGUE HEMORRHAGIC FEVER/DENGUE SHOCK SYNDROME (DHF/DSS)\   ICD-9 065.4; ICD-10 A91

1. Identification—A severe mosquito transmitted viral illness endemic in much of south and southeast Asia, the Pacific and Latin America; it is characterized by increased vascular permeability, hypovolemia and abnormal blood clotting mechanisms. It is recognized principally in children, but occurs also in adults. The WHO case definition for DHF is: (1) fever or history of recent fever; (2) thrombocytopenia; platelet count equal to or less than 100×10^3/cu mm (SI units equal to or less than 100×10^9/L); (3) hemorrhagic manifestations such as a positive tourniquet test, petechiae or overt bleeding phenomena; and (4) evidence of plasma leakage due to increased vascular permeability. Usually a 20% or greater increase in the hematocrit is observed compared with recovery value or pleural or abdominal effusions diagnosed by ultrasound, tomography or X-ray. Dengue shock syndrome (DSS) includes the more severe DHF patients plus signs of shock: (1) rapid, weak pulse; (2) narrow pulse pressure (less than 20 mm Hg); (3) hypotension for age; and (4) cold, clammy skin and restlessness. Prompt oral or intravenous fluid therapy may reduce hematocrit rise and require alternate observations to document increased plasma leakage.

Illness is biphasic; it begins abruptly with fever and, in children, with mild upper respiratory complaints, often anorexia, facial flush and mild GI disturbances. Coincident with defervescence and decreasing platelet count, the patient's condition suddenly worsens, with marked weakness, severe restlessness, facial pallor and often diaphoresis, severe abdominal pain and circumoral cyanosis. The liver may be enlarged, usually 2 or more days after defervescence.

Hemorrhagic phenomena are seen frequently and include scattered petechiae, a positive tourniquet test, easy bruisability, and less frequently, epistaxis, bleeding at venipuncture sites and gum bleeding. GI hemorrhage is an ominous prognostic sign that usually follows a prolonged period of shock. In severe cases, findings include accumulation of fluids in serosal cavities, low serum albumin, elevated transaminases, a prolonged prothrombin time and low levels of C3 complement protein. DHF cases manifesting severe liver damage with or without encephalopathy have been observed during large epidemics of dengue-3 in Indonesia and Thailand. Case-fatality rates in untreated or mistreated shock have been as high as 40%–50%; with good physiologic fluid replacement therapy, rates should be 1%–2%.

Serologic tests show a rise in antibody titer against dengue viruses. IgM antibody, indicating a current or recent flavivirus infection, is usually detectable by day 6–7 after onset of illness. Virus can be isolated from blood during the acute febrile stage of illness by inoculation of mosquitoes or cell cultures. Isolation from organs at autopsy is difficult, but chances are improved by mosquito inoculation. Virus specific nucleic acid sequences may be detected by PCR.

(Infection with dengue viruses with or without hemorrhagic manifestations is covered above. The related yellow fever and other hemorrhagic fevers are presented separately.)

2. Infectious agent—See Dengue Fever, above. All four dengue serotypes can cause DHF/DSS, in descending order of frequency: types 2, 3, 4 and 1.

3. Occurrence—Recent epidemics of DHF have occurred in the Philippines, New Caledonia, Tahiti, China, Vietnam, Laos, Cambodia (Kampuchea), Thailand, Malaysia, Singapore, Indonesia, Myanmar (Burma), Pakistan, India, Sri Lanka, Maldives, Cuba, Venezuela, French Guiana, Suriname, Brazil, Colombia, Nicaragua and Puerto Rico. The largest outbreak reported to date was that in Vietnam in 1987, when approximately 370,000 cases were reported. In tropical Asia, DHF/DSS is observed almost exclusively among children of the indigenous population under 15 years of age. Occurrence is greatest during the rainy season and in areas of high *Ae. aegypti* prevalence.

4., 5., 6. and **7. Reservoir, Mode of transmission, Incubation period** and **Period of communicability**—See Dengue Fever, above.

8. Susceptibility and resistance—The risk factor described best is the circulation of heterologous dengue antibody, acquired passively in infants or actively from an earlier infection. Such antibodies may enhance infection of mononuclear phagocytes through the formation of infectious immune complexes. Geographic origin of dengue strain, age, gender and human genetic susceptibility are also important risk factors.

In the 1981 Cuban outbreak caused by a southeast Asian dengue-2 virus, DHF/DSS was observed 5 times more often in white than in black patients. In Myanmar, East Indians and Burmese were equally susceptible to DHF.

9. Methods of control—

   A. Preventive measures: See Dengue Fever, above.

   B. Control of patient, contacts and immediate environment:

   1), 2), 3), 4), 5) and 6) Report to local health authority, Isolation, Concurrent disinfection, Quarantine, Immunization of contacts and Investigation of contacts and source of infection: See Dengue Fever, above.

   7) Specific treatment: Hypovolemic shock resulting from plasma leakage from an acute increase in vascular permeability often responds to oxygen therapy and rapid replacement with fluid and electrolyte solution (lactated Ringer's solution at 10–20 ml/kg/hour). In more severe cases of shock, plasma and/or

plasma expanders should be used. The rate of fluid and plasma administration must be judged by estimates of loss, usually by microhematocrit. A continued rise in hematocrit value in the presence of vigorous IV fluid administration indicates need for plasma or other colloid. **Care must be taken to watch for and avoid overhydration.** Blood transfusions are indicated only when severe bleeding results in a true falling hematocrit. The use of heparin to manage clinically significant hemorrhage occurring in the presence of well-documented disseminated intravascular coagulation is high risk and of no proven benefit. Fresh plasma, fibrinogen and platelet concentrate may be used to treat severe hemorrhage. Aspirin is contraindicated because of its hemorrhagic potential.

C., D. and *E. Epidemic measures, Disaster implications* and *International measures:* See Dengue Fever, above.

DERMATOPHYTOSIS ICD-9 110; ICD-10 B35
(Tinea, Ringworm, Dermatomycosis, Epidermophytosis, Trichophytosis, Microsporosis)

Dermatophytosis and tinea are general terms, essentially synonymous, applied to mycotic disease of keratinized areas of the body (hair, skin and nails). Various genera and species of fungi known collectively as the dermatophytes are causative agents. The dermatophytoses are subdivided according to the site of infection.

I. TINEA BARBAE AND TINEA CAPITIS ICD-9 110.0; ICD-10 B35.0
(Ringworm of the beard and scalp, Kerion, Favus)

1. Identification—A fungal disease that begins as a small papule and spreads peripherally, leaving scaly patches of temporary baldness. Infected hairs become brittle and break off easily. Occasionally, boggy, raised and suppurative lesions develop, called kerions.

Favus of the scalp (ICD-9 110.9) is a variety of tinea capitis caused by *Trichophyton schoenleinii*. It is characterized by a mousy odor and by formation of small, yellowish, cuplike crusts (scutulae) that look as though they were stuck on the scalp. Affected hairs do not break off but become gray and lusterless and eventually fall out and leave baldness that may be permanent.

Tinea capitis is easily distinguished from piedra, a fungus infection of the hair occurring in South America and some countries of southeast Asia and Africa. Piedra is characterized by black, hard "gritty" nodules on hair shafts, caused by *Piedraia hortai*, or white, soft pasty nodules caused by *Trichosporon beigelii*, now called *T. ovoides* or *T. inkin*.

Examination of the scalp under UV light (Wood's lamp) for yellow-green fluorescence is helpful in diagnosing tinea capitis caused by *Microsporum canis* and *M. audouinii*; *Trichophyton* species do not fluoresce. In infections caused by *Microsporum* spp., microscopic examination of scales and hair in 10% potassium hydroxide or UV microscopy of a calcofluor white preparation reveals characteristic hyaline ectothrix (outside the hair) arthrospores; *Trichophyton* spp. present an endothrix (inside the hair) pattern of invasion. The fungus should be cultured for confirmation of the diagnosis.

2. Infectious agents—Various species of *Microsporum* and *Trichophyton*. Identification of genus and species is important for epidemiologic and prognostic reasons.

3. Occurrence—Tinea capitis caused by *Trichophyton tonsurans* infections is now epidemic in urban areas in eastern USA, Puerto Rico, Mexico and Australia. *M. canis* infections occur in both rural and urban areas wherever infected cats and dogs are present. *M. audouinii* was widespread in the USA in the past, particularly in urban areas; *T. verrucosum* and *T. mentagrophytes* var. *mentagrophytes* infections occur primarily in rural areas where the disease exists in cattle, horses, rodents and wild animals.

4. Reservoir—Humans for *T. tonsurans, T. schoenleinii* and *T. audouinii;* animals, especially dogs, cats and cattle, harbor the other organisms noted above.

5. Mode of transmission—Direct skin to skin or indirect contact, especially from the backs of theater seats, barber clippers, toilet articles such as combs and hairbrushes, or clothing and hats contaminated with hair from infected people or animals.

6. Incubation period—Usually 10 to 14 days.

7. Period of communicability—Viable fungus may persist on contaminated materials for long periods.

8. Susceptibility and resistance—Children below the age of puberty are highly susceptible to *M. canis;* all ages are subject to *Trichophyton* infections. Reinfections are rarely if ever noted.

9. Methods of control—

    A. Preventive measures:

        1) Educate the public, especially parents, to the danger of acquiring infection from infected individuals as well as from dogs, cats and other animals.

2) In the presence of epidemics or in hyperendemic areas where non-*Trichophyton* species are prevalent, survey heads of young children by UV light (Wood's lamp) before they enter school.

B. *Control of patient, contacts and the immediate environment:*

1) Report to local health authority: Obligatory report of epidemics; no individual case report, Class 4 (see Communicable Diesease Reporting). Outbreaks in schools should be reported to school authorities.
2) Isolation: None.
3) Concurrent disinfection: In mild cases, daily washing of the scalp removes loose hair. Use of selenium sulfide shampoos to remove scale is helpful. In severe cases, wash scalp daily and cover hair with a cap. Contaminated caps should be boiled after use.
4) Quarantine: Not practical.
5) Immunization of contacts: None.
6) Investigation of contacts and source of infection: Study household contacts, pets and farm animals for evidence of infection; treat if infected. Some animals, especially cats, may be inapparent carriers.
7) Specific treatment: Griseofulvin (Gris-PEG®) by mouth for at least 4 weeks is treatment of choice. Systemic antibacterial agents are useful if ringworm lesions become secondarily infected by bacteria; in the case of kerions, also use a keratolytic cream and a cotton cover for the scalp. Examine weekly and take cultures; when cultures become negative, complete recovery may be assumed.

C. *Epidemic measures:* In epidemics in schools or other institutions, educate children and parents as to mode of spread, prevention and personal hygiene. Enlist services of physicians and nurses for diagnosis; carry out follow-up surveys.

D. *Disaster implications:* None.

E. *Internatio:ual measures:* None.

II. TINEA CRURIS   ICD-9 110.3; ICD-10 B35.6
(Ringworm of groin and perianal region)
TINEA CORPORIS   ICD-9 110.5; ICD-10 B35.4
(Ringworm of the body)

1. Identification—A fungal disease of the skin other than of the scalp, bearded areas and feet, that characteristically appears as flat, spreading, ring shaped lesions. The periphery is usually reddish, vesicular or pustular and may be dry and scaly or moist and crusted. As the lesion progresses peripherally, the central area often clears, leaving apparently normal skin. Differentiation from inguinal candidiasis is necessary, since treatment differs.

Presumptive diagnosis is made by taking scrapings from the advancing lesion margins, clearing in 10% potassium hydroxide and examining microscopically or by UV microscopy of calcofluor white preparations for segmented, branched hyaline filaments of fungus. Final identification is by culture.

2. Infectious agents—Most species of *Microsporum* and *Trichophyton;* also *Epidermophyton floccosum. Scytalidium dimidiatum* and *S. hyalinum* cause "dry type" tinea corporis in tropical areas.

3. Occurrence—Worldwide and relatively frequent. Males are infected more often than females.

4. Reservoir—Humans, animals and soil; tinea cruris is almost always in males.

5. Mode of transmission—Direct or indirect contact with skin and scalp lesions of infected people, lesions of animals; contaminated floors, shower stalls, benches and similar articles.

6. Incubation period—Usually 4 to 10 days.

7. Period of communicability—As long as lesions are present and viable fungus persists on contaminated materials.

8. Susceptibility and resistance—Susceptibility is widespread, aggravated by friction and excessive perspiration in axillary and inguinal regions, and when environmental temperatures and humidity are high. All ages are susceptible.

9. Methods of control—

A. *Preventive measures:* Launder towels and clothing with hot water and/or fungicidal agent; general cleanliness in showers and dressing rooms of gymnasiums, especially repeated washing of benches; frequent hosing and rapid draining of shower rooms. A fungicidal agent such as cresol should be used to disinfect benches and floors.

B. *Control of patient, contacts and the immediate environment:*

1) Report to local health authority: Obligatory report of epidemics; no individual case report, Class 4 (see Communicable Disease Reporting). Report infections of schoolchildren to school authorities.

2) Isolation: While under treatment, infected children should be excluded from gymnasiums, swimming pools and activities likely to lead to exposure of others.

3) Concurrent disinfection: Effective and frequent laundering of clothing.

4) Quarantine: None.

5) Immunization of contacts: None.

6) Investigation of contacts and source of infection: Examine school and household contacts, household pets and farm animals; treat infections as indicated.

7) Specific treatment: Thorough bathing with soap and water, removal of scabs and crusts and application of an effective topical fungicide such as miconazole, ketoconazole, clotrimazole, econazole, naftifine, terbinafine, tolnaftate or ciclopirox may suffice. Griseofulvin (Gris-PEG®) by mouth is effective; oral itraconazole (Sporanox®) or oral terbinafine (Lamisil®) is also effective.

C. *Epidemic measures:* Educate children and parents about the nature of the infection, its mode of spread and the need to maintain good personal hygiene.

D. *Disaster implications:* None.

E. *International measures:* None.

III. TINEA PEDIS ICD-9 110.4; ICD-10 B35.3
(Ringworm of the foot, Athlete's foot)

1. Identification—This fungal disease presents with characteristic scaling or cracking of the skin, especially between the toes, or blisters containing a thin watery fluid; commonly called athlete's foot. In severe cases, vesicular lesions appear on various parts of the body, especially the hands; these dermatophytids do not contain the fungus but are an allergic reaction to fungus products.

Presumptive diagnosis is verified by microscopic examination of potassium hydroxide- or calcofluor white–treated scrapings from lesions between the toes that reveal septate branching filaments. Clinical appearance of lesions is not diagnostic; final identification is by culture.

2. Infectious agents—*Trichophyton rubrum, T. mentagrophytes* var. *interdigitale* and *Epidermophyton floccosum.*

3. Occurrence—Worldwide; a common disease. Adults are more often affected than children, males more than females. Infections are more frequent and more severe in hot weather.

4. Reservoir—Humans.

5. Mode of transmission—Direct or indirect contact with skin lesions of infected people or contaminated floors, shower stalls and other articles used by infected people.

6. Incubation period—Unknown.

7. Period of communicability—As long as lesions are present and viable spores persist on contaminated materials.

8. Susceptibility and resistance—Susceptibility is variable and infection may be inapparent. Repeated attacks are frequent.

9. Methods of control—

A. *Preventive measures:* Those for tinea corporis, above. Educate the public to maintain strict personal hygiene; take special care in drying between toes after bathing; regularly use a dusting powder containing an effective fungicide on the feet and particularly between the toes. Occlusive shoes may predispose to infection and disease.

B. *Control of patient, contacts and the immediate environment:*

1) Report to local health authority: Obligatory report of epidemics; no individual case report, Class 4 (see Communicable Disease Reporting). Report high incidence in schools to school authorities.
2) Isolation: None.
3) Concurrent disinfection: Boil socks of heavily infected individuals to prevent reinfection.
4) Quarantine: None.
5) Immunization of contacts: None.
6) Investigation of contacts and source of infection: None.
7) Specific treatment: Topical fungicides such as miconazole, clotrimazole, ketoconazole, ciclopirox or tolnaftate. Expose feet to air by wearing sandals; use dusting powders. Griseofulvin (Gris-PEG®) by mouth may be indicated in severe, protracted disease, but is usually less effective than conscientious application of local fungicides.

C. *Epidemic measures:* Thoroughly clean and wash floors of gymnasiums, showers and similar sources of infection; disinfect with a fungicidal agent such as cresol. Educate the public about the mode of spread.

D. *Disaster implications:* None.

E. *International measures:* None.

IV. TINEA UNGUIUM   ICD-9 110.1; ICD-10 B35.1
(Ringworm of the nails, Onychomycosis)

1. Identification—A chronic fungal disease involving one or more nails of the hands or feet. The nail gradually thickens, and becomes discolored and brittle, an accumulation of caseous-appearing material forms beneath the nail or the nail becomes chalky and disintegrates.

Diagnosis is made by microscopic examination of potassium hydroxide preparations of the nail and of detritus beneath the nail for hyaline fungal elements. Etiology should be confirmed by culture.

2. Infectious agents—Various species of *Trichophyton*. Rarely caused by *Epidermophyton floccosum* or *Microsporum* or *Scytalidium* species.

3. Occurrence—Common.

4. Reservoir—Humans; rarely animals or soil.

5. Mode of transmission—Presumably by extensions from skin infections acquired by direct contact with skin or nail lesions of infected people, or from indirect contact (contaminated floors and shower stalls) with a low rate of transmission, even to close family associates.

6. Incubation period—Unknown.

7. Period of communicability—As long as an infected lesion is present.

8. Susceptibility and resistance—Susceptibility variable. Reinfection is frequent.

9. Methods of control—

A. *Preventive measures:* Cleanliness and use of a fungicidal agent such as cresol for disinfecting floors in common use; frequent hosing and rapid draining of shower rooms.

B. *Control of patient, contacts and the immediate environment:*

1) Report to local health authority: Official report not ordinarily justifiable, Class 5 (see Communicable Disease Reporting).
2), 3), 4), 5) and 6) Isolation, Concurrent disinfection, Quarantine, Immunization of contacts and Investigation of contacts and source of infection: Not practical.
7) Specific treatment: Oral itraconazole and terbinafine are the drugs of choice. Griseofulvin (Gris-PEG®) by mouth is less effective. Treatment should be given until nails grow out (about 3–6 months for fingernails, 12–18 months for toenails).

C., D. and E. *Epidemic measures, Disaster implications* and *International measures:* Not applicable.

DIARRHEA, ACUTE   ICD-9 001–009; ICD-10 A00–A09

Diarrhea is often accompanied by other clinical signs and symptoms including vomiting, fever, dehydration and electrolyte disturbances. It is a symptom of infection by many different bacterial, viral and parasitic enteric agents. The specific diarrheal diseases—cholera, shigellosis, salmonellosis, *Escherichia coli* infections, yersiniosis, giardiasis, *Campylobacter* enteritis, cryptosporidiosis and viral gastroenteropathy—are each described in detail under individual listings elsewhere in this book. Diarrhea can also occur in association with other infectious diseases such as malaria and measles, as well as chemical agents. Change in the enteric flora induced by antibiotics may produce acute diarrhea by overgrowth and toxin production by *Clostridium difficile*.

Approximately 70%–80% of the vast number of sporadic diarrheal episodes in people visiting treatment facilities in less developed countries could be diagnosed etiologically if the complete battery of newer laboratory tests were available and utilized. In the USA, where 5 million cases per year are estimated to occur and approximately 4 million are seen by a health care provider, the comparable figure is about 45% of cases. In the USA, the majority of diarrheal illness is caused primarily by viral agents, and the most common cause of gastroenteritis is rotavirus. A smaller proportion of diarrheal disease in the USA is attributed to bacterial pathogens such as *E. coli, Salmonella* and *Shigella* species, *Vibrio* species, and *Cl. difficile*.

From a practical clinical standpoint, diarrheal illnesses can be divided into six clinical presentations:

1) simple diarrhea, managed by oral rehydration with solutions containing water, glucose and electrolytes, with its specific etiology not important in management;

2) bloody diarrhea (dysentery), caused by organisms such as *Shigella, E. coli* O157:H7 and certain other organisms;

3) persistent diarrhea that lasts at least 14 days;

4) severe purging as seen in cholera;

5) minimal diarrhea, associated with vomiting, typical of some viral gastroenteritides; and illness from the toxins, such as those of *Staphylococcus aureus, Bacillus cereus* or *Cl. perfringens;* and

6) hemorrhagic colitis, with watery diarrhea containing gross blood but without fever or fecal leukocytes.

The details pertaining to the individual diseases are presented in separate chapters.

APHA

DIARRHEA CAUSED BY *ESCHERICHIA COLI*
ICD-9 008.0;
ICD-10 A04.0–A04.4

Strains of *Escherichia coli* that cause diarrhea are of six major categories: 1) enterohemorrhagic; 2) enterotoxigenic; 3) enteroinvasive; 4) entero-pathogenic; 5) enteroaggregative; and 6) diffuse-adherent. Each category has a different pathogenesis, possesses distinct virulence properties, and comprises a separate set of O:H serotypes. Differing clinical syndromes and epidemiologic patterns may also be seen.

I. DIARRHEA CAUSED BY ENTEROHEMORRHAGIC STRAINS
ICD-9 008.0; ICD-10 A04.3
(EHEC, Shiga toxin producing *E. coli* [STEC], *E. coli* O157:H7, Verotoxin producing *E. coli*) [VTEC]

1. Identification—This category of diarrheogenic *E. coli* was recognized in 1982 when an outbreak of hemorrhagic colitis occurred in the USA and was shown to be due to an unusual serotype, *E. coli* O157:H7, that had not previously been incriminated as an enteric pathogen. The diarrhea may range from mild and nonbloody to stools that are virtually all blood but contain no fecal leukocytes. The most feared clinical manifestations of EHEC infection are the hemolytic uremic syndrome (HUS) and thrombotic thrombocytopenic purpura (TTP). Approximately 2-7% of subjects who manifest EHEC diarrhea progress to develop HUS. EHEC elaborate potent cytotoxins called Shiga toxins 1 and 2. Shiga toxin 1 is identical to Shiga toxin elaborated by *Shigella dysenteriae* 1; notably, HUS is also a well recognized severe complication of *S. dysenteriae* 1 disease. Previously, these toxins were called verotoxins 1 and 2 or Shiga-like toxins I and II. Elaboration of these toxins depends on the presence of certain phages carried by the bacteria. In addition, EHEC strains harbor a virulence plasmid that is involved in attachment of the bacteria to intestinal mucosa. Most EHEC strains have within their chromosome a pathogenicity island that contains multiple virulence genes encoding proteins that cause attaching and effacing lesions of the human intestinal mucosa.

In North America most strains of the most common EHEC serotype, O157:H7, can be identified in stool cultures by their inability to ferment sorbitol in media such as MacConkey-sorbitol (used to screen for *E. coli* O157:H7). Since it is now recognized that some EHEC strains ferment sorbitol, other techniques to detect EHEC must be employed. These include demonstrating the ability to elaborate Shiga toxins; serotyping to identify characteristics serotypes; or the use of DNA probes that identify the toxin genes, the presence of the EHEC virulence plasmid or specific sequences within the pathogenicity island. Lack of fever in most patients can help to differentiate this from shigellosis and dysentery caused by enteroinvasive strains of *E. coli* or by *Campylobacter*.

2. Infectious agent—While the main EHEC serotype in North America is *E. coli* O157:H7, other serotypes such as O26:H11, O111:H8, O103:H2, O113:H21, and O104:H21 have been implicated.

3. Occurrence—These infections are now recognized to be an important problem in North America, Europe, South Africa, Japan, the southern cone of South America and Australia. Their relative importance in the rest of the world is less well established. Serious outbreaks, including cases of hemorrhagic colitis, HUS, and some deaths, have occurred in the USA from inadequately cooked hamburgers, unpasteurized milk, apple cider (made from apples that were probably contaminated by cow manure) and alfalfa sprouts.

4. Reservoir—Cattle are the most important reservoir of EHEC; humans may also serve as a reservoir for person to person transmission. There is increasing evidence that in North America deer may also serve as a reservoir.

5. Mode of transmission—Transmission occurs mainly by ingestion of contaminated food; as with *Salmonella*, it is most often due to inadequately cooked beef (especially ground beef) and also raw milk and fruit or vegetables contaminated with ruminant feces. As with *Shigella*, transmission also occurs directly from person to person, in families, child care centers and custodial institutions. Waterborne transmission has also been documented; one outbreak was associated with swimming in a crowded lake and one was caused by drinking contaminated unchlorinated municipal water.

6. Incubation period—Typically relatively long, ranging from 2 to 8 days, with a median of 3–4 days.

7. Period of communicability—The duration of excretion of the pathogen, which is typically for a week or less in adults but 3 weeks in one third of children. Prolonged carriage is uncommon.

8. Susceptibility and resistance—The infectious dose is very low. Little is known about differences in susceptibility and immunity. Old age appears to be a risk factor, so hypochlorhydria may be a factor contributing to susceptibility. Children less than 5 years of age are at greatest risk of developing HUS.

9. Methods of control —

    A. Preventive measures: The potential severity of this disease calls for early involvement of the local health authorities to identify the source and apply appropriate specific preventive measures. As soon as the diagnosis is suspected, it is of paramount importance to block person to person transmission by instructing family members in the necessity for frequent (and especially postdefecatory) handwashing with soap and water, disposal of soiled diapers and human waste, and prevention of food and beverage contamination. Measures likely to reduce the incidence of illness include the following:

1) Manage slaughterhouse operations to minimize contamination of meat by animal intestinal contents.
2) Pasteurize milk and dairy products.
3) Irradiate beef, especially ground beef.
4) Heat beef adequately during cooking, especially ground beef. The USDA Food Safety Inspection Service and the 1997 FDA Food Code recommend cooking ground beef to an internal temperature of 155°F (68°C) for at least 15-16 seconds. Reliance on cooking until all pink color is gone is not as reliable as using a meat thermometer.
5) Protect, purify and chlorinate public water supplies; chlorinate swimming pools.
6) Ensure adequate hygiene in childcare centers, especially frequent handwashing with soap and water.

B. *Control of patient, contacts and the immediate environment:*

1) Report to local health authority: Case report of *E. coli* O157:H7 infection is obligatory in many states (USA) and countries, Class 2B (see Communicable Disease Reporting). Recognition and reporting of outbreaks is especially important.
2) Isolation: During acute illness, enteric precautions. Because of the extremely small infective dose, infected patients should not be employed to handle food or to provide child or patient care until 2 successive negative fecal samples or rectal swabs are obtained (collected 24 hours apart and not sooner than 48 hours after the last dose of antimicrobials).
3) Concurrent disinfection: Of feces and contaminated articles. In communities with a modern and adequate sewage disposal system, feces can be discharged directly into sewers without preliminary disinfection. Terminal cleaning.
4) Quarantine: None.
5) Management of contacts: When feasible, contacts with diarrhea should be excluded from food handling and the care of children or patients until the diarrhea ceases and 2 successive negative stool cultures are obtained. All contacts should be carefully indoctrinated in the need for thorough handwashing after defecation and before handling food or caring for children or patients.
6) Investigation of contacts and source of infection: Cultures of contacts should generally be confined to food handlers, attendants and children in child care centers and other situations where the spread of infection is particularly likely.

Culture of suspected foods is relatively nonproductive in sporadic cases.

7) Specific treatment: Fluid and electrolyte replacement is important when diarrhea is watery or there are signs of dehydration (see Cholera, 9B7). The role of antibacterial treatment of infections with *E. coli* O157:H7 and other EHEC is uncertain. Some evidence suggests that treatment with TMP-SMX fluorquinolones and certain other antimicrobials may precipitate complications such as HUS.

C. Epidemic measures:

1) Report at once to the local health authority any group of acute bloody diarrhea cases, even in the absence of specific identification of the causal agent.

2) Search intensively for the specific vehicle (food or water) by which the infection was transmitted, evaluate potential for ongoing person to person transmission, and use the results of epidemiologic investigations to guide specific control measures.

3) Exclude use of and trace the source of suspected food; in large common-source foodborne outbreaks, prompt recall may prevent many cases.

4) If a waterborne outbreak is suspected, issue an order to boil water and chlorinate suspected water supplies adequately under competent supervision or do not use them.

5) If a swimming-associated outbreak is suspected, close pools or beaches until chlorinated or shown to be free of fecal contamination and until adequate toilet facilities are provided to prevent further contamination of water by bathers.

6) If a milkborne outbreak is suspected, pasteurize or boil the milk.

7) Prophylactic administration of antibiotics is not recommended.

8) Publicize the importance of handwashing after defecation; provide soap and individual paper towels if otherwise not available.

D. Disaster implications: A potential problem where personal hygiene and environmental sanitation are deficient (see Typhoid fever, 9D).

E. International measures: WHO Collaborating Centres.

II. DIARRHEA CAUSED BY ENTEROTOXIGENIC STRAINS ICD-9 008.0; ICD-10 A04.1
(ETEC)

1. Identification—A major cause of travelers' diarrhea in people from industrialized countries who visit less developed countries, this bacterial disease is also an important cause of dehydrating diarrhea in infants and children in less developed countries. Enterotoxigenic strains may behave like *Vibrio cholerae* in producing a profuse watery diarrhea without blood or mucus. Abdominal cramping, vomiting, acidosis, prostration and dehydration can occur, and low grade fever may or may not be present; the symptoms usually last fewer than 5 days.

ETEC can be identified by demonstrating enterotoxin production, by immunoassays, bioassays or by DNA probe techniques that identify LT and ST genes (for heat labile and heat stable toxins) in colony blots.

2. Infectious agent—ETEC elaborate a heat labile enterotoxin (LT), a heat stable toxin (ST) or both toxins (LT/ST). The most common O serogroups include O6, O8, O15, O20, O25, O27, O63, O78, O80, O114, O115, O128ac, O148, O153, O159 and O167.

3. Occurrence—An infection primarily of developing countries. During the first 3 years of life, children in developing countries experience multiple ETEC infections which leads to the acquisition of immunity; consequently, illness in older children and adults occurs less frequently. Infection occurs among travelers from industrialized countries who visit less developed countries. Several outbreaks of ETEC infection have occurred recently in the USA.

4. Reservoir—Humans. ETEC infections are largely species specific; people constitute the reservoir for strains causing diarrhea in humans.

5. Mode of transmission—Contaminated food and, less often, contaminated water. Transmission via contaminated weaning foods may be particularly important in infection of infants. Direct contact transmission by fecally contaminated hands is believed to be rare.

6. Incubation period—Incubations as short as 10–12 hours have been observed in outbreaks and in volunteer studies with certain LT-only and ST-only strains. The incubation of LT/ST diarrhea in volunteer studies has usually been 24–72 hours.

7. Period of communicability—For the duration of excretion of the pathogenic ETEC, which may be prolonged.

8. Susceptibility and resistance—Epidemiologic studies and rechallenge studies in volunteers clearly demonstrate that serotype specific immunity is acquired following ETEC infection. Multiple infections with different serotypes are required to develop broad-spectrum immunity against ETEC.

9. Methods of control —

A. *Preventive measures:*

1) For general measures for prevention of fecal-oral spread of infection, see Typhoid fever, 9A.
2) For adult travelers going for short periods of time to high risk areas where it is not possible to obtain safe food or water, the

use of prophylactic antibiotics may be considered; norfloxacin, 400 mg daily, has been shown to be effective. However, a much preferable approach is to initiate very early treatment, beginning with the onset of diarrhea (e.g., after the second or third loose stool). (See section 9B7, below.)

B. *Control of patient, contacts and the immediate environment:*

1) Report to local health authority: Obligatory report of epidemics; no individual case report, Class 4 (see Communicable Disease Reporting).
2) Isolation: Enteric precautions for known and suspected cases.
3) Concurrent disinfection: Of all fecal discharges and soiled articles. In communities with a modern and adequate sewage disposal system, feces can be discharged directly into sewers without preliminary disinfection. Thorough terminal cleaning.
4) Quarantine: None.
5) Immunization of contacts: None.
6) Investigation of contacts and source of infection: Not indicated.
7) Specific treatment: Electrolyte-fluid therapy to prevent or treat dehydration is the most important measure (see Cholera, section 9B7). Most cases do not require any other therapy. For severe travelers' diarrhea in adults, early treatment with loperamide (Imodium®) (not for children) and an antibiotic such as a fluoroquinolone (ciprofloxacin PO 500 mg twice daily) or norfloxacin (PO 400 mg daily) for 5 days. Fluoroquinolones are used as initial therapy because many ETEC strains worldwide are resistant to a variety of other antimicrobials. However, if local strains are known to be sensitive, TMP-SMX (PO) (160 mg-800 mg) twice daily or doxycycline (PO) (100 mg) once daily, for 5 days are useful. Feeding should be continued, according to the patient's appetite.

C. *Epidemic measures:* Epidemiologic investigation may be indicated to determine how transmission is occurring.

D. *Disaster implications:* None.

E. *International measures:* WHO Collaborating Centres.

III. DIARRHEA CAUSED BY ENTEROINVASIVE STRAINS (EIEC)

ICD-9 008.0; ICD-10 A04.2

1. Identification—This inflammatory disease of the gut mucosa and submucosa caused by EIEC strains of *E. coli* closely resembles that produced by *Shigella*. The organisms possess the same plasmid dependent ability to invade and multiply within epithelial cells. However, clinically, the syndrome of watery diarrhea due to EIEC is much more common than dysentery. The O antigens of EIEC may cross-react with *Shigella* O antigens. Illness begins with severe abdominal cramps, malaise, watery stools, tenesmus and fever; in less than 10% of patients, it progresses to the passage of multiple, scanty, fluid stools containing blood and mucus.

EIEC may be suspected by the presence of many fecal leukocytes visible in a stained smear of mucus, a finding also in shigellosis. Tests available in reference laboratories include an immunoassay that detects the plasmid encoded specific outer membrane proteins that are associated with epithelial cell invasiveness; a bioassay (the guinea pig–keratoconjunctivitis test) detects epithelial cell invasiveness; DNA probes detect the enteroinvasiveness plasmid.

2. Infectious agent—Strains of *E. coli* shown to possess enteroinvasiveness dependent on the presence of a large virulence plasmid encoding invasion plasmid antigens. The main O serogroups in which EIEC fall include O28ac, O29, O112, O124, O136, O143, O144, O152, O164 and O167.

3. Occurrence—EIEC infections are endemic in less developed countries, and cause about 1%–5% of diarrheal episodes among people visiting treatment centers. Occasional infections and outbreaks of EIEC diarrhea have been reported in industrialized countries.

4. Reservoir—Humans.

5. Mode of transmission—Scant available evidence suggests that EIEC is transmitted by contaminated food.

6. Incubation period—Incubations as short as 10 and 18 hours have been observed in volunteer studies and outbreaks, respectively.

7. Period of communicability—Duration of excretion of EIEC strains.

8. Susceptibility and resistance—Little is known about susceptibility and immunity to EIEC.

9. Methods of control—Same as for ETEC, above. For the rare cases of severe diarrhea with enteroinvasive strains, as for shigellosis, treat using antimicrobials effective against local *Shigella* isolates.

IV. DIARRHEA CAUSED BY ENTEROPATHOGENIC STRAINS   ICD-9 008.0; ICD-10 A04.0
(EPEC, Enteropathogenic *E. coli* enteritis)

1. Identification—This is the oldest recognized category of diarrhea producing *E. coli*, implicated in 1940s and 1950s studies in which certain O:H serotypes were found to be associated with infant summer diarrhea, outbreaks of diarrhea in infant nurseries, and community epidemics of infant diarrhea. Diarrheal disease in this category is virtually confined to infants less than 1 year of age in whom it causes watery diarrhea with mucus, fever and dehydration. EPEC cause dissolution of the microvilli of enterocytes and initiate attachment of the bacteria to enterocytes. The diarrhea in infants can be both severe and prolonged, and in developing countries may be associated with high case fatality.

EPEC can be tentatively identified by agglutination with antisera that detect EPEC O serogroups, but confirmation requires both O and H typing with high quality reagents. EPEC organisms exhibit localized adherence to HEp-2 cells in cell cultures, a property that requires the presence of an EPEC virulence plasmid. The EPEC adherence factor (EAF) DNA probe detects the EPEC virulence plasmid; there is a 98% correlation between the detection of localized adherence and EAF probe positivity.

2. Infectious agent—The major EPEC O serogroups include O55, O86, O111, O119, O125, O126, O127, O128ab and O142.

3. Occurrence—Since the late 1960s, EPEC has largely disappeared as an important cause of infant diarrhea in North America and Europe. However, it remains a major agent of infant diarrhea in many developing areas, including South America, southern Africa and Asia.

4. Reservoir—Humans.

5. Mode of transmission—By contaminated infant formula and weaning foods. In infant nurseries, transmission by fomites and by contaminated hands can occur if handwashing techniques are compromised.

6. Incubation period—As short as 9–12 hours in adult volunteer studies. It is not known whether the same incubation applies to infants who acquire infection by natural transmission.

7. Period of communicability—Limited to the duration of excretion of EPEC, which may be prolonged.

8. Susceptibility and resistance—Although susceptibility to clinical infection appears to be confined virtually to young infants in nature, it is not known if this is due to immunity or to age related, nonspecific host factors. Since diarrhea can be induced experimentally in some adult volunteers, specific immunity may be important in determining susceptibility. EPEC infection is uncommon in breast fed infants.

9. Methods of control—

A. Preventive measures:

1) Encourage mothers to breast feed their infants exclusively from birth to 4-6 months of age. Provide adequate support for

breast feeding. Help the mother to establish or reestablish breast feeding.

Where available, give newborns pasteurized donor breast milk until they go home if a mother's own breast milk is not available or sufficient. Infant formulas should be held at room temperature only for short periods. Cup feeding is preferred to bottle feeding as early as possible.

2) Practice rooming in for mothers and infants in maternity facilities, unless there is a firm medical indication for separating them. If mother or infant has a GI or respiratory infection, keep the pair together but isolate them from healthy pairs.

In special care facilities, separate infected infants from those who are premature or ill in other ways.

3) Provide individual equipment for each infant, include a thermometer, kept at the bassinet. No common bathing or dressing tables should be used, and no bassinet stands should be used for holding or transporting more than one infant at a time.

4) Prevention of hospital outbreaks depends on handwashing between handling babies and maintaining high sanitary standards in the facilities in which babies are held.

B. *Control of patient, contacts and the immediate environment:*

1) Report to local health authority: Obligatory report of epidemics; no individual case report, Class 4 (see Communicable Disease Reporting). Two or more concurrent cases of diarrhea requiring treatment for these symptoms in a nursery or among those recently discharged are to be interpreted as an outbreak requiring investigation.

2) Isolation: Enteric precautions for known and suspected cases.

3) Concurrent disinfection: Of all fecal discharges and soiled articles. In communities with a modern and adequate sewage disposal system, feces can be discharged directly into sewers without preliminary disinfection. Thorough terminal cleaning.

4) Quarantine: Use enteric precautions and cohort methods (see 9C, below).

5) Immunization of contacts: None.

6) Investigation of contacts and source of infection: Families of discharged babies should be contacted for diarrheal status of the baby (see 9C, below).

7) Specific treatment: Electrolyte-fluid therapy (oral or IV) is the most important measure (see Cholera, 9B7). Most cases do not require any other therapy. For severe enteropathogenic infant diarrhea, oral TMP-SMX (10–50 mg/kg/day) has been shown to ameliorate the severity and duration of diarrheal illness; it should be administered in 3–4 divided doses for 5 days.

However, since many EPEC strains are resistant to a variety of antibiotics, selection should be based on the sensitivity of local isolated strains. Feeding, including breast feeding, should be continued.

C. *Epidemic measures:* For nursery epidemics (see section 9B1, above) the following:

1) All babies with diarrhea should be placed in one nursery under enteric precautions. Admit no more babies to the contaminated nursery. Suspend maternity service unless a clean nursery is available with separate personnel and facilities; promptly discharge infected infants when medically possible. For the babies exposed in the contaminated nursery, provide separate medical and nursing personnel skilled in the care of infants with communicable diseases. Observe contacts for at least 2 weeks after the last case leaves the nursery; promptly remove each new case to one nursery ward used for these infants. Maternity service may be resumed after discharge of all contact babies and mothers, and thorough cleaning and terminal disinfection. Put into practice the recommendations of 9A, above, so far as feasible, in the emergency.
2) Carry out a thorough epidemiologic investigation into the distribution of cases by time, place, person and exposure to risk factors to determine how transmission is occurring.

D. *Disaster implications:* None.

E. *International measures:* WHO Collaborating Centres.

V. DIARRHEA CAUSED BY ENTEROAGGREGATIVE *E. COLI* ICD-9 008.0; ICD-10 A04.4
(EAggEC)

This category of diarrhea producing *E. coli* is an important cause of infant diarrhea in less developed countries where it is the single most common cause of persistent diarrhea in infants. In animal models, these *E. coli* organisms evoke a characteristic histopathology in which EAggEC adhere to enterocytes in thick biofilm of aggregating bacteria and mucus. At present, the most widely available method to identify EAggEC is by the HEp-2 assay, wherein these strains produce a characteristic "stacked brick" aggregative pattern as they attach to one another and to the HEp-2 cells; this is a plasmid dependent characteristic that is mediated by novel fimbriae. Most EAggEC encode one or more cytotoxin/enterotoxin that are believed to be responsible for the watery diarrhea with mucus seen in infants and children infected with this pathogen. A DNA probe has been described. The incubation period is estimated to be 20-48 hours.

1. Identification—This category of diarrhea producing *E. coli* was first associated with infant diarrhea in a study in Chile in the late 1980s. It was subsequently recognized in India as being particularly associated with persistent diarrhea (diarrhea that continues unabated for at least 14 days), an observation that has since been confirmed by reports from Brazil, Mexico and Bangladesh.

2. Infectious agent—EAggEC harbor a virulence plasmid required for expression of the unique fimbriae that encode aggregative adherence and many strains express a cytotoxin/enterotoxin. Among the most common EAggEC O serotypes are O3:H2 and O44:H18. Many EAggEC strains initially appear as rough strains lacking O antigens.

3. Occurrence—Reports associating EAggEC with infant diarrhea, and particularly persistent diarrhea, have come from multiple countries in Latin America and Asia and from the Democratic Republic of Congo (DRC, formerly Zaire) in Africa. Reports from Germany and the United Kingdom suggest that EAggEC may be responsible for a small proportion of diarrheal disease in industrialized countries as well.

VI. DIARRHEA CAUSED BY DIFFUSE-ADHERENCE *E. COLI* ICD-9 008.0; ICD-10 A04.4
(DAEC)

A sixth category of diarrhea producing *E. coli* now recognized is diffuse-adherence *E. coli* (DAEC). The name derives from the characteristic pattern of adherence of these bacteria to HEp-2 cells in tissue culture. DAEC is the least well-defined category of diarrhea causing *E. coli*. Nevertheless, data from several epidemiologic field studies of pediatric diarrhea in less developed countries have found DAEC to be significantly more common in children with diarrhea than in matched controls; other studies have failed to find such a difference. Notably, preliminary evidence suggests that DAEC may be more pathogenic in children of preschool age rather than in infants and toddlers. Two DAEC strains failed to cause diarrhea when fed to volunteers and no outbreaks due to this category have yet been recognized. At present little is known about the reservoir, modes of transmission, host risk factors or period of communicability of DAEC.

DIPHTHERIA ICD-9 032; ICD-10 A36

1. Identification—An acute bacterial disease that primarily involves the tonsils, pharynx, larynx, nose, occasionally other mucous membranes or skin and sometimes the conjunctivae or vagina. The characteristic lesion, caused by liberation of a specific cytotoxin, is an asymmetrical adherent grayish white membrane with surrounding inflammation. The throat is moderately to severely sore in faucial or pharyngotonsillar diphtheria, with cervical lymph nodes somewhat enlarged and tender; in moderate to severe cases, there is marked swelling and edema of the neck with extensive tracheal membranes that progress to airway obstruction.

Nasal diphtheria can be mild and chronic with one sided nasal discharge and excoriations. Inapparent infections (or colonization) outnumber clinical cases. The toxin can cause myocarditis, with heart block and progressive congestive failure beginning about 1 week after onset. Later effects include neuropathies that can mimic Guillain-Barre syndrome. Case-fatality rates of 5%–10% for noncutaneous diphtheria have changed little in 50 years. The lesions of cutaneous diphtheria are variable and may be indistinguishable from, or a component of, impetigo; peripheral effects of the toxin are usually not evident.

Diphtheria should be suspected in the differential diagnosis of bacterial (especially streptococcal) and viral pharyngitis, Vincent's angina, infectious mononucleosis, oral syphilis and candidiasis.

Presumptive diagnosis is based on observation of an asymmetrical, grayish white membrane, especially if it extends to the uvula and soft palate and is associated with tonsillitis, pharyngitis or cervical lymphadenopathy, or a serosanguinous nasal discharge. The diagnosis is confirmed by bacteriologic examination of lesions. If diphtheria is strongly suspected, specific treatment with antibiotics and antitoxin should be initiated while studies are pending and should be continued even in the face of a negative laboratory report.

2. Infectious agent—*Corynebacterium diphtheriae* of gravis, mitis or intermedius biotype. Toxin production results when the bacteria are infected by corynebacteriophage containing the diphtheria toxin gene *tox*. Nontoxigenic strains rarely produce local lesions; however, they have been increasingly associated with infective endocarditis.

3. Occurrence—A disease of colder months in temperate zones, that primarily involves nonimmunized children under 15 years of age; often found among adults in population groups whose immunization was neglected. In the tropics, seasonal trends are less distinct; inapparent, cutaneous and wound diphtheria cases are much more common.

In the USA, from 1980 to 1998, an average of fewer than 4 cases was reported annually; two thirds of the affected people were 20 years of age or older. A massive outbreak of diphtheria began in the Russian Federation in 1990 and spread to all countries of the former Soviet Union and Mongolia. Contributing factors included increased susceptibility among adults due to waning of vaccine induced immunity, failure to fully immunize children due to unwarranted contraindications, antivaccine movements and declining socioeconomic conditions. This epidemic began to decline after reaching a peak in 1995; however, it was responsible for more than

150,000 reported cases and 5,000 deaths between 1990-97. In Ecuador, an outbreak of diphtheria occurred in 1993-94, with about 200 cases, half of whom were 15 years of age or older. In both epidemics, control was achieved by mass immunization activities.

4. Reservoir—Humans.

5. Mode of transmission—Contact with a patient or carrier; more rarely, contact with articles soiled with discharges from lesions of infected people. Raw milk has served as a vehicle.

6. Incubation period—Usually 2-5 days, occasionally longer.

7. Period of communicability—Variable, until virulent bacilli have disappeared from discharges and lesions; usually 2 weeks or less and seldom more than 4 weeks. Effective antibiotic therapy promptly terminates shedding. The rare chronic carrier may shed organisms for 6 months or more.

8. Susceptibility and resistance—Infants born of immune mothers are relatively immune; protection is passive and usually lost before the sixth month. Lifelong immunity is usually, but not always, acquired after disease or inapparent infection. Immunization with toxoid produces prolonged but not lifelong immunity. Serosurveys in the USA indicate that more than 40% of adults lack protective levels of circulating antitoxin; decreasing immunity levels have also been found in Canada, Australia and several European countries. However, many of these older adults may have immunologic memory and would be protected against disease after exposure. In the USA, most children have been immunized; by the second quarter of 1997, 95% of 2 year old children had received 3 doses of diphtheria vaccine. Antitoxic immunity protects against systemic disease but not against colonization in the nasopharynx.

9. Methods of control—

   A. Preventive measures:

   1) Educational measures are important: inform the public, and particularly the parents of young children, of the hazards of diphtheria and the necessity for active immunization.
   2) The only effective control is widespread active immunization with diphtheria toxoid. Immunization should be initiated in infancy with a formulation containing diphtheria toxoid, tetanus toxoid and either acellular pertussis antigens (DtaP, the preferred preparation in the USA) or whole cell pertussis vaccine (DTP). Formulations that combine diphtheria and tetanus toxoid, whole cell pertussis, and *Haemophilus influenzae* type b vaccine (DTP-Hib) are also available.

3) The following schedules are recommended for use in the USA. (Some countries may recommend different ages for specific doses or fewer than 4 doses in the primary series.)

a) For children less than 7 years of age—

A primary series of diphtheria toxoid combined with other antigens, such as DTaP, or DTP-Hib. The first 3 doses are given at 4- to 8-week intervals beginning when the infant is 6–8 weeks old; a fourth dose is given 6–12 months after the third dose. This schedule does not need to be restarted because of any delay in administering the scheduled doses. A fifth dose is given at 4–6 years of age prior to school entry; this dose is not necessary if the fourth dose is given after the fourth birthday. If the pertussis component of DTP is contraindicated, diphtheria and tetanus toxoids for children (DT) should be substituted.

b) For persons 7 years of age and older—

Because adverse reactions may increase with age, a preparation with a reduced concentration of diphtheria toxoid (adult Td) is usually used after the 7th birthday for booster doses. For a previously unimmunized individual, a primary series of 3 doses of adsorbed tetanus and diphtheria toxoids, Td, is given. The first 2 doses are given at 4- to 8-week intervals and the third dose 6 months to 1 year after the second dose. Limited data from Sweden suggest that this regimen may not induce protective antibody levels in most adults, and additional doses may be needed.

c) Active protection should be maintained by administering a dose of Td every 10 years thereafter.

4) Special efforts should be made to ensure that those who are at higher risk of patient exposure, such as health workers, are fully immunized and receive a booster dose of Td every 10 years.

5) For children and adults who are severely immunocompromised or infected with HIV, diphtheria immunization is indicated. Use the same schedule and dose as for immunocompetent persons, even though the immune response may be suboptimal.

B. Control of patient, contacts and the immediate environment:

1) Report to local health authority: Case report is obligatory in most states (USA) and countries, Class 2A (see Communicable Disease Reporting).

2) Isolation: Strict isolation for pharyngeal diphtheria, contact isolation for cutaneous diphtheria, until two cultures from

both throat and nose (and skin lesions in cutaneous diphtheria), taken not less than 24 hours apart, and not less than 24 hours after cessation of antimicrobial therapy, fail to show diphtheria bacilli. Where culture is impractical, isolation may be ended after 14 days of appropriate antibiotic treatment (see 9B7, below).

3) Concurrent disinfection: Of all articles in contact with patient and all articles soiled by discharges of patient. Terminal cleaning.

4) Quarantine: Adult contacts whose occupations involve handling food (especially milk) or close association with nonimmunized children should be excluded from that work until they have been treated as described below and bacteriologic examination proves them not to be carriers.

5) Management of contacts: All close contacts should have cultures taken from the nose and throat and should be kept under surveillance for 7 days. A single dose of benzathine penicillin (IM, see below for doses) or a 7-10 day course of erythromycin (PO) is recommended for all persons with household exposure to diphtheria, regardless of their immunization status. Those who handle food or work with school children should be excluded from work or school until bacteriologic examination proves them not to be carriers. Previously immunized contacts should receive a booster dose of diphtheria toxoid if more than 5 years have elapsed since their last dose, and a primary series should be initiated in nonimmunized contacts; use Td, DT, DTP, DTaP or DTP-Hib vaccine, depending on the contact's age.

6) Investigation of contacts and source of infection: The search for carriers by use of nose and throat cultures, other than among close contacts, is not ordinarily useful or indicated if provisions of 9B5, above, are carried out.

7) Specific treatment: If diphtheria is strongly suspected on the basis of clinical findings, antitoxin (only antitoxin of equine origin is available) should be given immediately after bacteriologic specimens are taken, without waiting for results. Diphtheria antitoxin (DAT) is on the CDC Drug Service formulary as an investigational product. The National Immunization Program (NIP) responds to clinical inquiries for DAT during business hours (8:00 a.m. to 4:30 p.m. EST; Monday-Friday at 404-639-8255). After hours or on weekends and holidays, call the CDC Duty Officer at 404-639-2888. DAT is stored at quarantine stations around the country for rapid distribution. After completion of tests to rule out hypersensitivity, a single dose of 20,000-100,000 units is given IM, depending on the area of involvement and severity of the disease. Intramuscular admin-

istration usually suffices; in severe infections, both IV and IM administration may be indicated. Antibiotics are not a substitute for antitoxin. Procaine penicillin G (IM) (25,000 to 50,000 units/kg/d for children and 1.2 million units/kg/d for adults, in 2 divided doses) or parenteral erythromycin (40-50 mg/kg/d, with a maximum of 2 g/d) has been recommended until the patient can swallow comfortably, at which point erythromycin PO in 4 divided doses or penicillin V PO (125-250 mg 4 times daily) may be substituted for a recommended total treatment period of 14 days. Some erythromycin resistant strains have been identified, but they are uncommon and not a public health problem. Newer macrolide antibiotics, including azithromycin and clarithromycin, should be effective for erythromycin susceptible strains, but these antibiotics do not offer any substantial advantage over erythromycin.

Prophylactic treatment of carriers: A single dose of benzathine penicillin G (IM) (600,000 units for persons less than 6 years of age and 1.2 million units for persons 6 years of age or older) or a 7-10 day course of erythromycin (PO) (40 mg/kg/d for children and 1 g/d for adults) has been recommended.

C. *Epidemic measures:*

1) Immunize the largest possible proportion of the population group involved, emphasize protection of infants and preschool children. In an epidemic involving adults, immunize groups that are most affected and at high risk. Repeat immunization procedures 1 month later to provide at least 2 doses to recipients.

2) Identify close contacts and define population groups at special risk. In areas with appropriate facilities, carry out a prompt field investigation of reported cases to verify the diagnosis and to determine the biotype and toxigenicity of *C. diphtheriae*.

D. *Disaster implications:* Outbreaks can occur when social or natural conditions lead to crowding of susceptible groups, especially infants and children. This frequently occurs when there are large-scale movements of susceptible populations.

E. *International measures:* People traveling to or through countries where either faucial or cutaneous diphtheria is common should receive primary immunization if necessary, or a booster dose of Td for those previously immunized.

DIPHYLLOBOTHRIASIS   ICD-9 123.4; ICD-10 B70.0
(Dibothriocephaliasis, Broad or Fish tapeworm infection)

1. Identification—An intestinal tapeworm infection of long duration; symptoms commonly are trivial or absent. A few patients in whom the worms are attached to the jejunum develop vitamin B_{12} deficiency anemia. Massive infections may be associated with diarrhea, obstruction of the bile duct or intestine, and toxic symptoms.

Diagnosis is confirmed by identification of eggs or segments (proglottids) of the worm in feces.

2. Infectious agents—*Diphyllobothrium latum (Dibothriocephalus latus), D. pacificum, D. dendriticum, D. ursi, D. dalliae* and *D. klebanovskii;* cestodes.

3. Occurrence—The disease occurs in lake regions in the Northern Hemisphere, and subarctic, temperate and tropical zones where eating raw or partly cooked freshwater fish is popular. Prevalence increases with age. In North America, endemic foci have been found among Eskimos in Alaska and Canada. Infections in the USA are sporadic and usually come from eating uncooked fish from Alaska or, less commonly, from midwestern or Canadian lakes.

4. Reservoir—Humans; mainly, infected hosts discharging eggs in feces; reservoir hosts other than people include dogs, bears and other fish eating mammals.

5. Mode of transmission—Humans acquire the infection by eating raw or inadequately cooked fish. Eggs in mature segments of the worm are discharged in feces into bodies of fresh water, where they mature, hatch, and the ciliated embryos (coracidium) infect the first intermediate host (copepods of the genera *Cyclops* and *Diaptomus*) and become procercoid larvae. Susceptible species of freshwater fish (pike, perch, turbots, salmon) ingest infected copepods and become second intermediate hosts, in which the worms transform into the plerocercoid (larval) stage, which is infective for people and fish eating mammals, such as the fox, mink, bear, cat, dog, pig, walrus and seal. The egg to egg cycle takes at least 11 weeks.

6. Incubation period—Three to six weeks from ingestion to passage of eggs in the stool.

7. Period of communicability—Not directly transmitted from person to person. Humans and other definitive hosts continue to disseminate eggs into the environment as long as worms remain in the intestine, sometimes for many years.

8. Susceptibility and resistance—People are universally susceptible. No apparent resistance follows infection.

9. **Methods of control—**

A. *Preventive measures:* Thorough heating (at 56°C/133°F for 5 minutes) of freshwater fish, freezing for 24 hours at −18°C (0°F), or irradiation ensures protection.

B. *Control of patient, contacts and the immediate environment:*

1) Report to local health authority: Official report not ordinarily justifiable, Class 5 (see Communicable Disease Reporting). Report is indicated if a commercial source is implicated.
2) Isolation: None.
3) Concurrent disinfection: None; sanitary disposal of feces.
4) Quarantine: None.
5) Immunization of contacts: None.
6) Investigation of contacts and source of infection: Not usually justified.
7) Specific treatment: Praziquantel (Biltricide®) or niclosamide (Niclocide®) is the drug of choice.

C. *Epidemic measures:* None.

D. *Disaster implications:* None.

E. *International measures:* None.

DRACUNCULIASIS ICD-9 125.7; ICD-10 B72
(Guinea worm infection, Dracontiasis)

1. Identification—An infection of the subcutaneous and deeper tissues by a large nematode. A blister appears, usually on a lower extremity (especially the foot) when the gravid 60–100 cm long adult female worm is ready to discharge its larvae. Burning and itching of the skin in the area of the lesion and frequently fever, nausea, vomiting, diarrhea, dyspnea, generalized urticaria and eosinophilia may accompany or precede vesicle formation. After the vesicle ruptures, the worm discharges larvae whenever the infected part is immersed in fresh water. The prognosis is good unless bacterial infection of the lesion occurs; such secondary infections may produce arthritis, synovitis, ankylosis and contractures of the involved limb and may be life threatening.

Diagnosis is made by visual recognition of the adult worm protruding from a skin lesion or by microscopic identification of larvae.

2. Infectious agent—*Dracunculus medinensis,* a nematode.

3. Occurrence—In Africa (16 countries south of the Sahara) and in Asia (India and Yemen), especially in regions with dry climates. Local prevalence varies greatly. In some locales, nearly all inhabitants are infected, in others, few; mainly young adults.

4. Reservoir—Humans; there are no other known animal reservoirs.

5. Mode of transmission—Larvae discharged by the female worm into stagnant fresh water are ingested by minute crustacean copepods (*Cyclops* spp). In about 2 weeks, the larvae develop into the infective stage. People swallow the infected copepods in drinking water from infested step wells and ponds. The larvae are liberated in the stomach, cross the duodenal wall, migrate through the viscera and become adults. The female, after mating, grows and develops to full maturity, then migrates to the subcutaneous tissues (most frequently of the legs).

6. Incubation period—About 12 months.

7. Period of communicability—From rupture of vesicle until larvae have been completely evacuated from the uterus of the gravid worm, usually 2–3 weeks. In water, the larvae are infective for the copepods for about 5 days. After ingestion by copepods, the larvae become infective for people after 12–14 days at temperatures more than 25°C (more than 77°F), and remain infective in the copepods for about 3 weeks, the life span of an infected copepod. Not directly transmitted from person to person.

8. Susceptibility and resistance—Susceptibility is universal. No acquired immunity; multiple and repeated infections may occur in the same person.

9. Methods of control—The provision of safe, filtered drinking water and health education of the populations at risk could lead to eradication of the disease. Foci of disease formerly present in some parts of the Middle East and the Indian subcontinent have been eliminated in this manner.

A. Preventive measures:

1) Provide health education programs in endemic communities to convey three messages: a) that guinea worm infection comes from their drinking water; b) that villagers with blisters or ulcers should not enter any source of drinking water; and c) that drinking water should be filtered through fine mesh cloth (such as nylon gauze with a mesh size of 100 μm) to remove copepods.
2) Provide potable water. Abolish step wells or convert them to draw wells. Construction of wells or rainwater catchments can provide noninfected water.
3) Control copepod populations in ponds, tanks, reservoirs and

step wells by use of the insecticide temefos (Abate®), which is effective and safe.

4) Immunize high risk populations against tetanus.

B. Control of patient, contacts and the immediate environment:

1) Report to local health authority: Case report required wherever the disease occurs, as part of the WHO eradication program, Class 2B (see Communicable Disease Reporting).

2) Isolation: None. Cases are advised not to enter drinking water sources while worm is emerged.

3) Concurrent disinfection: None.

4) Quarantine: None.

5) Immunization of contacts: None.

6) Investigation of contacts and source of infection: Obtain information as to source of drinking water at probable time of infection (about 1 year previously). Search for other cases.

7) Specific treatment: Tetanus toxoid and local treatment with antibiotic ointment and occlusive bandage. Aseptic surgical extraction just prior to worm emergence is effective. Some drugs, such as thiabendazole, albendazole, ivermectin and metronidazole, along with corticosteroids may be of value.

C. Epidemic measures: In hyperendemic situations, field survey to determine prevalence, discover sources of infection and guide control measures as described in 9A, above.

D. Disaster implications: None.

E. International measures: The World Health Assembly adopted a resolution (WHA 44.5, May 1991) to eradicate dracunculiasis by 1995. As of the year 2000, the disease remains endemic in some areas, while in others, eradication has been successful.

EBOLA-MARBURG VIRAL
DISEASES   ICD-9 078.89; ICD-10 A98.3, A98.4
(African hemorrhagic fever, Marburg virus disease, Ebola virus hemorrhagic fever)

1. Identification—Severe acute viral illnesses, usually with sudden onset of fever, malaise, myalgia and headache, followed by pharyngitis, vomiting, diarrhea and maculopapular rash. The accompanying hemorrhagic diathesis is often accompanied by hepatic damage, renal failure, CNS involvement and terminal shock with multiorgan dysfunction. Laboratory findings usually show lymphopenia, severe thrombocytopenia and transaminase elevation (AST greater than ALT), sometimes with hyperamy-lasemia. Approximately 25% of reported primary cases of Marburg virus infection have been fatal; case-fatality rates of Ebola infections in Africa have ranged from 50% to nearly 90%.

Diagnosis is made by ELISA for specific IgG antibody (presence of IgM antibody suggests recent infection); by ELISA antigen detection in blood, serum or organ homogenates; by PCR; by detection of the virus antigen in liver cells by use of monoclonal antibody in an IFA test; or by virus isolation in cell culture or guinea pigs. Virus may sometimes be visualized in liver sections by EM. Postmortem diagnosis through immunohistochemical examination of formalin-fixed skin biopsy specimens is also possible. IFA tests for antibodies have often been misleading, particularly in serosurveys for past infection. Laboratory studies represent an extreme biohazard and should be carried out only where protection against infection of the staff and community is available (BSL-4 containment).

2. Infectious agents—Virions are 80 nm in diameter and 790 nm (Marburg) or 970 nm (Ebola) in length, and are members of the *Filoviridae*. Longer, bizarre virion related structures may be branched or coiled and reach 10 μm in length. The Marburg virus is antigenically distinct from Ebola. Ebola strains from the Democratic Republic of the Congo (formerly Zaire), Ivory Coast, Gabon and Sudan have been associated with human disease. A fourth Ebola strain, Reston, causes fatal hemorrhagic disease in nonhuman primates; few human infections have been documented and those were clinically asymptomatic.

3. Occurrence—Marburg disease has been recognized on six occasions: in 1967, in Germany and Yugoslavia, 31 humans (7 fatalities) were infected following exposure to African green monkeys *(Cercopithecus aethiops)* from Uganda; in 1975, the fatal index case of 3 cases diagnosed in South Africa had originated in Zimbabwe; in 1980, there were 2 confirmed cases in Kenya, 1 fatal; in 1982, 1 case occurred in Zimbabwe; and in 1987, a fatal case occurred in Kenya. In 1999, in the Democratic Republic of the Congo, at least 3 fatal cases of Marburg were confirmed among over 70 suspected cases of viral hemorrhagic fever.

Ebola disease was first recognized in 1976 in the western equatorial province of the Sudan and 500 miles away in Zaire; more than 600 cases were identified in rural hospitals and villages; the case-fatality rate for these nearly simultaneous outbreaks was about 70%. A second outbreak occurred in the same area in Sudan in 1979. A distinct strain was recovered from one person and from chimpanzees in the Ivory Coast in 1994. A major Ebola outbreak in 1995 was centered around Kitwit, Zaire. In 1996–1997 two outbreaks that were recognized in Gabon resulted in 98 recognized cases and 66 deaths. FA antibodies have been found in residents of several other areas of sub-Saharan Africa, but their relation to the highly virulent Ebola virus is unknown.

Ebola related filoviruses have been isolated from cynomolgus monkeys *(Macaca fascicularis)* imported in 1989, 1990 and 1996 to the USA and in 1992 to Italy from the Philippines; many of these monkeys died. Four of five animal handlers with daily exposure to these monkeys in 1989 developed specific antibodies with no antecedent fevers or other illness.

4. Reservoir—Unknown despite extensive studies.

5. Mode of transmission—Person to person transmission occurs by direct contact with infected blood, secretions, organs or semen. Risk is highest during the late stages of illness when the patient is vomiting, having diarrhea, or hemorrhaging. Risk during the incubation period is low. Under natural conditions, airborne transmission among humans has not been documented. Nosocomial infections have been frequent; virtually all Ebola (Zaire) patients who acquired infection from contaminated syringes and needles died. Transmission through semen has occurred 7 weeks after clinical recovery.

6. Incubation period—Three to 9 days with Marburg and 2–21 days in Ebola virus disease.

7. Period of communicability—As long as blood and secretions contain virus. Up to 30% of primary caregivers in Sudan were infected, while most other household contacts remained uninfected. Ebola virus was isolated from the seminal fluid on the 61st, but not on the 76th, day after onset of illness in a laboratory acquired case.

8. Susceptibility and resistance—All ages are susceptible.

9. Methods of control—See control measures for Lassa fever: 9B, C, D and E apply; plus restriction of sexual intercourse for 3 months or until semen can be shown to be free of virus.

ECHINOCOCCOSIS   ICD-9 122; ICD-10 B67

The larval stage (hydatid or cystic) of three species of *Echinococcus* produces disease in humans and other animals; manifestations depend on the infecting species. Cysts usually develop in the liver but are also found in the lungs, kidney, spleen, nervous tissue or bone. They are of three types: 1) unilocular or cystic hydatid disease, 2) multilocular or alveolar hydatid disease, and 3) polycystic hydatid disease.

I. ECHINOCOCCOSIS DUE TO
ECHINOCOCCUS
GRANULOSUS   ICD-9 122.4; ICD-10 B67.0–B67.4
(Cystic or Unilocular echinococcosis, Cystic hydatid disease)

1. Identification—The tapeworm *Echinococcus granulosus* is the most common species of *Echinococcus* and causes cystic hydatid disease, which is infectious by the larval stages of the tapeworm. Hydatid cysts enlarge slowly, and require several years for development. Developed cysts generally are 1-7 cm in diameter, but may exceed 10 cm. Infections may be asymptomatic until cysts cause noticeable mass effect; then, signs and symptoms vary according to location, cyst size and number. Ruptured or leaking cysts can cause severe anaphylactoid reactions and may release protoscolices that can produce secondary echinococcosis. Cysts are typically spherical, thick walled and unilocular and are most frequently found in the liver and lungs, although they may also occur in other organs.

Clinical diagnosis is based on signs and symptoms compatible with a slowly growing tumor, a history of residence in an endemic area, along with association with canines. Differential diagnoses include malignancies, amebic abscesses, congenital cysts and tuberculosis. Radiography, computerized tomography and sonography along with serologic testing are useful for the laboratory diagnosis of human hydatid disease. Definitive diagnosis in seronegative patients, however, requires microscopic identification of specimens obtained at surgery or by percutaneous aspiration; the potential risks of the latter procedure (anaphylaxis, spillage) can be avoided by ultrasound guidance and anthelmintic coverage. Species identification is based on finding thick laminated cyst walls and protoscolices as well as the structure and measurements of protoscolex hooks.

2. Infectious agent—*Echinococcus granulosus,* a small tapeworm of dogs and other canids.

3. Occurrence—The prevalence of this parasite depends on the close association of humans and infected dogs. It occurs on all continents except Antarctica, but is especially common in grazing countries where dogs consume viscera containing cysts. In the USA, the tapeworm has been found in sheep raising regions of Utah, Arizona, New Mexico and California and exists in a sylvatic cycle involving wild ungulates such as moose and caribou in Alaska. Transmission has been completely eliminated in Iceland and greatly reduced in Australia, New Zealand and Cyprus.

4. Reservoir—The domestic dog and other canids are definitive hosts for *E. granulosus;* they may harbor thousands of adult tapeworms in their intestines without signs of infection. Felines and most other carnivores are not suitable hosts for the parasite. Intermediate hosts include herbivores, primarily sheep, cattle, goats, pigs, horses, and other animals.

5. Mode of transmission—Human infection, which often takes place during childhood, occurs directly with hand to mouth transfer of eggs after association with infected dogs or indirectly through contaminated food, water, soil or fomites. In some instances, flies have dispersed eggs after feeding on infected feces.

The adult worms in the small intestines of canines produce eggs containing infective embryos (oncospheres), which are passed in feces; these may survive for several months in pastures or gardens. When ingested by susceptible intermediate hosts, including people, eggs hatch, releasing oncospheres that migrate through the mucosa and are carried by the blood to various organs where they form cysts. Different strains of *E. granulosus* vary in their ability to adapt to various hosts (sheep, cattle, horse, camel, pig, moose) as well as their infectivity to humans.

Canines become infected by eating viscera containing hydatid cysts. Sheep and other intermediate hosts are infected while grazing in areas contaminated with dog feces containing parasite eggs.

6. Incubation period—Variable, from 12 months to many years, depending on the number and location of cysts and how rapidly they grow.

7. Period of communicability—Not directly transmitted from person to person or from one intermediate host to another. Infected dogs begin to pass eggs approximately 7 weeks after infection. Most canine infections resolve spontaneously by 6 months, although adult worms may occasionally survive as long as 2–3 years. Dogs may be infected repeatedly.

8. Susceptibility and resistance—Children are more likely to be exposed to infection because they are more likely to have close contact with infected dogs and are less likely to have adequate hygienic habits. There is no evidence that they are more susceptible to infection than are adults.

9. Methods of control—

  A. Preventive measures:

   1) Educate the public at risk to avoid exposure to dog feces. Handwashing should be emphasized.
   2) Interrupt transmission from intermediate to definitive hosts by preventing dogs' access to uncooked viscera. This includes supervision of livestock slaughtering and safe disposal of infected viscera.
   3) Incinerate or deeply bury infected organs from dead intermediate hosts.
   4) Periodically treat high risk dogs; reduce dog populations to the occupational need for them.
   5) Field and laboratory personnel should observe strict safety precautions to avoid ingestion of tapeworm eggs.

B. *Control of patient, contacts and the immediate environment:*

1) Report to the local health authority: In selected endemic areas; not a reportable disease in most states and countries, Class 3B (see Communicable Disease Reporting).
2) Isolation: None.
3) Concurrent disinfection: None.
4) Quarantine: None.
5) Immunization of contacts: None.
6) Investigation of contacts and source of infection: Examine families and associates for suspicious tumors. Check dogs kept in and about houses for infection. Determine practices leading to infection.
7) Specific treatment: Surgical resection of isolated cysts is the most common treatment; however, mebendazole (Vermox®) and albendazole (Zentel®) have been used successfully and may be the preferred treatment in many cases. If a primary cyst ruptures, praziquantel (Biltricide®), a protoscolicidal agent, reduces the probability of secondary cysts.

C. *Epidemic measures:* In hyperendemic areas, control populations of wild and stray dogs. Treat remaining dogs with praziquantel (Biltricide®). Strictly control slaughtering of livestock.

D. *Disaster implications:* None.

E. *International measures:* Control the movement of dogs from known enzootic areas.

II. ECHINOCOCCOSIS DUE TO *ECHINOCOCCUS MULTILOCULARIS*
ICD-9 122.5, 122.7;
ICD-10 B67.5–B67.7

(Alveolar, echinococcosis or hydatid disease; Multilocular echinococcosis)

1. Identification—This is a highly invasive, destructive disease caused by the larval stage of *E. multilocularis*. Cysts are usually found in the liver, and because growth is not restricted by a thick laminated cyst wall, they continuously expand at the periphery to produce solid, tumor-like masses. Metastases can occur and result in secondary cysts in other organs. Clinical manifestations depend on the size and location of cysts but are often confused with hepatic cirrhosis or carcinoma. The disease is often fatal.

Diagnosis is often based on histopathology, i.e., evidence of the thin host pericyst and multiple microvesicles formed by external proliferation. Humans are an abnormal host, and the cysts rarely produce brood capsules, protoscolices or calcareous corpuscles. Serodiagnosis using purified *E. multilocularis* antigen is highly sensitive and specific.

2. Infectious agent—*Echinococcus multilocularis.*

3. Occurrence—Distribution is limited to areas of the Northern Hemisphere: central Europe, the former Soviet Union, Siberia, northern Japan, Alaska, Canada and rarely the north central USA. The disease is usually diagnosed in adults.

4. Reservoir—The adult tapeworms are restricted largely to wild animals such as foxes, although dogs and cats can be sources of human infection. Intermediate hosts are rodents, including voles, lemmings and mice. *E. multilocularis* is commonly maintained in nature in fox rodent cycles.

5. Mode of transmission—By ingestion of eggs passed in the feces of Canidae and Felidae that have fed on infected rodents. Fecally soiled dog hair, harnesses and environmental fomites also serve as vehicles of infection.

6., 7., 8. and **9. Incubation period, Period of communicability, Susceptibility and resistance** and **Methods of control**—As in section I, *Echinococcus granulosus*, above, except that radical surgical excision is less often successful. For nonresectable cases, continuous treatment with mebendazole or albendazole may prevent progression of the disease.

III. ECHINOCOCCOSIS DUE TO *ECHINOCOCCUS VOGELI*   ICD-9 122.9; ICD-10 B67.9
(Polycystic hydatid disease)

This disease is caused by cysts of *E. vogeli*, that occur in the liver, lungs and other organs. Symptoms vary depending on cyst size and location. This species is distinguished by its rostellar hooks. The polycystic hydatid is unique in that the germinal membrane proliferates externally to form new cysts and internally to form septae that divide the cavity into numerous microcysts. Brood capsules containing many protoscolices develop in the microcysts.

Cases have been identified in Central and South America, mainly in Brazil, Colombia and Ecuador. The principal definitive host is the bush dog; the primary intermediate hosts are pacas, agoutis and spiny rats. Domestic hunting dogs that have fed on the viscera of infected pacas are sources of human infection.

EHRLICHIOSIS ICD-9 083.8; ICD-10 A79.8
(Sennetsu fever, Human ehrlichiosis found in the USA)

1. Identification—Ehrlichiosis is an acute, febrile, bacterial illness caused by a group of small pleomorphic organisms that survive and reproduce in the phagosomes of mononuclear or polymorphonuclear leukocytes of the infected host. The organisms are sometimes observed within these cells.

Sennetsu fever is characterized by sudden onset with fever, chills, general malaise, headache, muscle and joint pain, sore throat and sleeplessness. Generalized lymphadenopathy with tenderness of the enlarged nodes is common. Lymphocytosis with postauricular and posterior cervical lymphadenopathy is similar to that seen in infectious mononucleosis. The disease course is usually benign; fatal cases have not been reported.

Human ehrlichiosis in the USA is a newly recognized disease and is caused by two similar, but distinct, organisms. One type affects primarily mononuclear cells and is known as human monocytic ehrlichiosis (HME). A second type of ehrlichiosis caused by an organism with a predilection for granulocytes is called human granulocytic ehrlichiosis (HGE). The spectrum of disease ranges from subclinical infection or mild illness to a severe, life threatening or fatal disease. Symptoms are usually nonspecific; the most common complaints are fever, headache, anorexia, nausea, myalgia and vomiting. The disease may be confused clinically with Rocky Mountain spotted fever (RMSF) but differs by rarity of a prominent rash. Laboratory findings include leukopenia, thrombocytopenia and elevation of one or more hepatocellular enzymes. In hospitalized cases, the laboratory findings may be only slightly abnormal on admission, and become more abnormal during hospitalization.

Differential diagnosis includes RMSF, Lyme disease, toxic shock syndrome and other multisystem febrile illnesses. The clinical diagnosis of sennetsu fever is confirmed by IF tests by using the etiologic agent isolated in macrophage cultures. Diagnosis is based on clinical and laboratory findings and detection of antibody using organism-specific antigens, and is based on a four-fold rise or fall in titer. Blood smears or buffy coat smears should be examined for the characteristic inclusions (morulae). Other diagnostic techniques include immunohistochemistry, culture and DNA amplification methods (e.g., PCR).

2. Infectious agents—*Ehrlichia sennetsu* is the etiologic agent of sennetsu fever. These organisms are members of the genus *Ehrlichia*, tribe Ehrlichieae and family Rickettsiaceae; until 1984, they were classified as members of the genus *Rickettsia*. The causative agent of HME is *E. chaffeensis*, named after the first human isolate from a patient in Fort Chaffee, Arkansas. The agent of HGE is identical or closely related to *E. phagocytophila* and *E. equi*. A canine ehrlichia (*E. ewingi*), which is commonly found in dogs in Missouri, was identified in 1999 as the cause of a small number of human cases of granulocytic ehrlichiosis.

3. Occurrence— As of 1999, about 1,200 cases of human ehrlichiosis had been recognized in the USA. The majority of HME cases have been diagnosed or reported from southern states whereas the majority of HGE cases have been diagnosed or reported from the upper midwestern and northeastern states. Sennetsu fever appears to be confined to western Japan.

4. Reservoir—Not known for either sennetsu fever or American ehrlichiosis.

5. Mode of transmission—Not known for sennetsu fever, although patients with the disease are frequently reported to have visited rivers or swampy areas near rivers within 3-4 weeks of onset. Ticks, probably *Amblyomma americanum,* are the vectors of HME; most patients report a tick bite or an association with wooded, tick infested areas several weeks prior to onset of illness. *Ixodes scapularis* ticks likely serve as vectors for HGE in the upper Midwest and northeastern USA.

6. Incubation period—For sennetsu fever 14 days; 7-21 days for American ehrlichiosis.

7. Period of communicability—No evidence of transmission from person to person.

8. Susceptibility and resistance—Susceptibility is believed to be general but older or debilated individuals are more likely to suffer a more serious illness. No data are available on protective immunity in humans from infections caused by these organisms.

9. Methods of control—

   A. Preventive measures:

   1) None established for sennetsu fever.
   2) Measures against ticks should be employed (see Lyme disease, 9A) to prevent American ehrlichiosis.

   B. Control of patient, contacts and the immediate environment:

   1) Report to local health authority: Case report required in most states, Class 2B (see Communicable Disease Reporting).
   2) Isolation: None.
   3) Concurrent disinfection: Remove any ticks.
   4), 5) and 6) Quarantine, Immunization of contacts and Investigation of contacts and source of infection: None.
   7) Specific treatment: A tetracycline; chloramphenicol for pregnant women and children under 8 years of age.

C. Epidemic measures: None.

D. Disaster implications: None.

E. International measures: None.

ENCEPHALOPATHY, SUBACUTE
SPONGIFORM   ICD-9 046; ICD-10 A81
(Slow virus infections of the CNS)

A group of subacute degenerative diseases of the brain caused by "unconventional" filterable agents, with very long incubation periods and no demonstrable inflammatory or immune response. The infectious agents are thought by some to be unique proteins replicating by a yet unknown mechanism; if that proves true, then the proposed term "prion" may be an appropriate name for them. Four prion diseases occur in humans (Creutzfeldt-Jakob disease (CJD), Gerstmann-Sträussler-Scheinker syndrome, kuru and fatal familial insomnia) and four in animals (scrapie of sheep and goats, transmissible mink encephalopathy, chronic wasting disease of American mule deer and elk, and bovine spongiform encephalopathy or BSE). During the late 1990s, a new variant of Creutzfeldt-Jakob disease (vCJD) emerged and has been associated with BSE, commonly referred to as "mad cow disease" in the popular press.

I. CREUTZFELDT-JAKOB
DISEASE   ICD-9 046.1; ICD-10 A81.0
(Jakob-Creutzfeldt syndrome, Subacute spongiform encephalopathy)

1. Identification—An insidious onset with confusion, progressive dementia and variable ataxia in patients aged 16 to over 80 years, but almost all (more than 99%) are 35 years of age or older. Later, myoclonic jerks appear, together with a variable spectrum of other neurologic signs. Characteristically, routine laboratory studies of the CSF are normal and there is no fever. Typical periodic high-voltage complexes are common on electroencephalogram (EEG). The disease progresses rapidly; death usually occurs within 3–12 months (median 4 months, mean 7 months). About 5%–10% of cases have a positive family history of presenile dementia, associated with one of several mutations in the gene on chromosome 20 that encodes an amyloidogenic precursor protein (PrP). Pathologic changes are limited to the CNS. One familial subset of this disease, the Gerstmann-Sträussler-Scheinker syndrome (GSS), is characterized neuropathologically by many multicentric plaques. GSS differs from typical Creutzfeldt-Jakob disease (CJD) by the average duration of illness and some symptoms.

CJD must be differentiated from other forms of dementia, especially Alzheimer disease, from other slow infections, from toxic and metabolic encephalopathies and, occasionally, from tumors and other space occupying lesions.

Reports from the UK over the past decade have described thousands of BSE cases in domestic cattle. Concern that BSE might have been transmitted to humans through the consumption of beef products has resulted in a large scale epidemiologic and laboratory study of BSE and its possible relationship to CJD. These studies now suggest that a new form of CJD may also be occurring. This disease, which is designated as new variant Creutzfeld-Jakob disease or vCJD has been described in the UK and other parts of Europe. These two diseases differ in three significant ways. Unlike CJD, vCJD occurs in a younger age group (20-30 years of age). In addition, the characteristic EEG changes seen with CJD are absent in the vCJD. Finally the clinical course of vCJD is typically much longer than CJD (12-15 months versus 3-6 months). In experiments with inbred strains of mice, it has been possible to use brain homogenates of diseased cattle to cause spongiform encephalopathy in the mice. However, this does not necessarily mean that BSE and vCJD are caused by the same agent. Although similarities are clearly apparent, there are sufficient differences to suggest that vCJD may simply be another variant of CJD that has been identified through the intense surveillance studies of humans conducted in the wake of the BSE epizootic in cattle in the UK. Finally, it is also apparent that genetic factors play an important role in the disease, because individuals homozygous for methionine in position 129 of the prion protein (PrP) are known to be at higher risk.

Diagnosis is based on clinical signs and a characteristic periodic EEG. It can be confirmed by histopathologic findings and in research settings by transmission of disease to animals from biopsy specimens. Demonstration of an abnormal amyloid protein in biopsied brain tissue and a pair of abnormal proteins in CSF can verify the diagnosis antemortem; however, the CSF test is not generally available at present.

2. Infectious agent—Many believe CJD is caused by a filterable, self-replicating agent called a prion, transmissible to chimpanzees, monkeys, guinea pigs, mice, hamsters and goats.

3. Occurrence—CJD has been reported from countries all over the world. Average annual mortality rates are 0.5-1/1,000,000 population, with familial clusters reported from Slovakia, Israel and Chile. In the USA, the highest age specific average annual mortality rates (more than 5 cases/1,000,000) occur in the 65-79 year age group. As of mid 1999, over 40 cases of vCJD have been reported, almost all from the UK.

4. Reservoir—Human cases constitute the only known reservoir. There is no documentation of human infection acquired from animals, although this has been hypothesized.

5. Mode of transmission—The mode of transmission for most cases is unknown; de novo spontaneous generation of the self-replicating protein has been hypothesized. Iatrogenic cases have been recognized: these include 1 due to a corneal transplant; 2 to cortical electrodes that had been used on known CJD patients; at least 14 to grafts of human dura mater; and more than 50 to injections of growth or gonadotropic hormones prepared from human pituitary glands. Other patients have had a history of brain surgery within 2 years of onset. Transmission of the possible vCJD causal agent is believed to be through consumption of beef from cattle with BSE.

6. Incubation period—Fifteen months to possibly more than 30 years in the iatrogenic cases. Those with known direct CNS tissue exposures have been associated with incubation periods of less than 10 years. The incubation period is unknown for sporadic cases, but probably as long as in kuru (4 to more than 20 years).

7. Period of communicability—CNS tissues are infectious throughout symptomatic illness. Other tissues and CSF are sometimes infectious. Infectivity during the incubation period is not known, but studies in animals suggest that lymphoid and other organs are probably infectious before signs of illness appear.

8. Susceptibility and resistance—Genetic differences in susceptibility that resemble those of autosomal dominant traits have been shown to explain patterns of disease occurrence in families. Genetic differences in susceptibility to scrapie have been found in animals. Mutations in the "prion protein" gene have been found linked to all forms of familial disease.

9. Methods of control—

 A. ***Preventive measures:*** Great care must be taken to avoid using tissue from infected patients in transplants, EEG electrodes and surgical instruments contaminated by tissue from such patients. Instruments must be sterilized before further use. Transmission of these diseases through the consumption of meat or milk products has not been established. However, concern over this possible route of infection has resulted in a total ban on consumption of beef from cattle herds infected with BSE. Blood transfusions have not been shown to be related to transmission of the agent. Blood donations should not be accepted from individuals at high risk for transmissible spongiform encephalopathies (family history of TSE, previous neurosurgery).

 As a precautionary measure to reduce the theoretical risk of vCJD transmission to blood product recipients, USA and Canadian authorities in August, 1999 requested blood centers to exclude from donating blood potential donors who spent 6 or more cumulative months between Jan 1, 1980 and December 31, 1996 in the UK (England, Scotland, Wales, Northern Ireland, the Isle of Man, and the Channel Islands). Also included in this deferral in the USA were donors who received non-USA licensed bovine insulin or other injectable products made from cattle in BSE endemic countries.

B. Control of patient, contacts and the immediate environment:

1) Report to local health authority: Official case report not ordinarily justifiable, Class 5 (see Communicable Disease Reporting).
2) Isolation: Universal precautions.
3) Concurrent disinfection: Tissues, surgical instruments and all wound drainage should be considered contaminated and must be inactivated. Steam autoclaving is a highly effective method of disinfection (1 hour at 132°C or higher).

   Chemical agents such as 5% sodium hypochlorite and 1N to 2N sodium hydroxide may not be completely effective; after 1 hour, they are best followed by steam autoclaving. Aldehydes are ineffective.
4) Quarantine: None.
5) Immunization of contacts: None.
6) Investigation of contacts and source of infection: A complete medical history, including previous surgical or dental procedures and possible exposure to human hormones or transplanted tissue, as well as a family history of dementia should be obtained.
7) Specific treatment: None.

C., D. and E. Epidemic measures, Disaster implications and International measures: None.

II. KURU   ICD-9 046.0; ICD-10 A81.8

A disease of the CNS manifested by cerebellar ataxia, incoordination, shivering, tremors, rigidity and progressive wasting in patients 4 years of age and older, that occurred exclusively among women and children of the Fore language group in the Papua New Guinea highlands. It is caused by a filterable, self-replicating agent that is transmissible to primates and other animals. Kuru was transmitted by traditional burial practices involving intimate contact with infected tissues and included cannibalism. Formerly very common, kuru now occurs in fewer than 10 patients a year.

ENTEROBIASIS   ICD-9 127.4; ICD-10 B80
(Pinworm infection, Oxyuriasis)

1. Identification—A common intestinal helminthic infection that is often asymptomatic. There may be perianal itching, disturbed sleep, irritability and sometimes secondary infection of the scratched skin. Other clinical manifestations include vulvovaginitis, salpingitis, and pelvic and liver granulomata. Appendicitis and enuresis have been reported as possible associated conditions, but these are rare events.

Diagnosis is made by applying transparent adhesive tape (Scotch tape swab or pinworm paddle) to the perianal region and examining the tape or paddle microscopically for eggs; the material is best obtained in the morning before bathing or defecation. Examination should be repeated three or more times before accepting a negative result. Eggs are sometimes found on microscopic stool and urine examination. Female worms may be found in feces and in the perianal region during rectal or vaginal examinations.

2. Infectious agent—*Enterobius vermicularis,* an intestinal nematode.

3. Occurrence—Worldwide, affecting all socioeconomic classes, with high rates in some areas. It is the most common worm infection in the USA; prevalence is highest in school aged children (in some groups near 50%), followed by preschoolers, and is lowest in adults except for mothers of infected children. Infection often occurs in more than one family member. Prevalence is often high in domiciliary institutions.

4. Reservoir—Humans. Pinworms of other animals are not transmissible to people.

5. Mode of transmission—Direct transfer of infective eggs by hand from anus to mouth of the same or another person, or indirectly through clothing, bedding, food or other articles contaminated with eggs of the parasite. Dustborne infection is possible in heavily contaminated households and institutions. Eggs become infective within a few hours after being deposited at the anus by migrating gravid females; eggs survive less than 2 weeks outside the host. Larvae from ingested eggs hatch in the small intestine; young worms mature in the cecum and upper portions of the colon. Gravid worms usually migrate actively from the rectum and may enter adjacent orifices.

6. Incubation period—The life cycle requires 2–6 weeks to be completed. Symptomatic disease with high worm burdens results from successive reinfections occurring within months after initial exposure.

7. Period of communicability—As long as gravid females are discharging eggs on perianal skin. Eggs remain infective in an indoor environment for about 2 weeks.

8. Susceptibility and resistance—Susceptibility is universal. Differences in frequency and intensity of infection are due primarily to differences in exposure.

9. Methods of control —

    A. Preventive measures:

       1) Educate the public in personal hygiene, particularly the need to wash hands before eating or preparing food. Keep nails short; discourage scratching bare anal area and nail biting.

       2) Remove sources of infection by treatment of cases.

3) Daily morning bathing, with showers (or stand-up baths) preferred to tub baths.
4) Change to clean underclothing, night clothes and bedsheets frquently, preferably after bathing.
5) Clean and vacuum house daily for several days after treatment of cases.
6) Reduce overcrowding in living accommodations.
7) Provide adequate toilets; maintain cleanliness in these facilities.

B. Control of patient, contacts and the immediate environment:

1) Report to local health authority: Official report not ordinarily justifiable, Class 5 (see Communicable Disease Reporting).
2) Isolation: None.
3) Concurrent disinfection: Change bed linen and underwear of infected person daily for several days after treatment, with care to avoid dispersing eggs into the air. Use closed sleeping garments. Eggs on discarded linen are killed by exposure to temperatures of 55°C (131°F) for a few seconds; either boil bed clothing or use a properly functioning household washing machine on the "hot" cycle. Clean and vacuum sleeping and living areas daily for several days after treatment.
4) Quarantine: None.
5) Immunization of contacts: None.
6) Investigation of contacts and source of infection: Examine all members of an affected family or institution.
7) Specific treatment: Pyrantel pamoate (Antiminth®, Combantrin®), mebendazole (Vermox®) or albendazole (Zentel®). Treatment should be repeated after 2 weeks; concurrent treatment of the whole family may be advisable if several members are infected.

C. Epidemic measures: Multiple cases in schools and institutions can best be controlled by systematic treatment of all infected individuals and their household contacts.

D. Disaster implications: None.

E. International measures: None.

ERYTHEMA INFECTIOSUM
HUMAN PARVOVIRUS
INFECTION   ICD-9 057.0; ICD-10 B08.3
(Fifth Disease)

1. Identification—Erythema infectiosum is a mild, usually nonfebrile, viral disease with an erythematous eruption that occurs sporadically or in epidemics, especially among children. Characteristic is a striking erythema of the cheeks (slapped face appearance) frequently associated with a lace-like rash on the trunk and extremities that fades but may recur for 1-3 weeks or longer on exposure to sunlight or heat (e.g., bathing). Mild constitutional symptoms may precede onset of rash. In adults, the rash is often atypical or absent, but arthralgias or arthritis lasting days to months or even years may occur; 25% or more of infections may be asymptomatic. Differentiation from rubella, scarlet fever and erythema multiforme is often necessary.

Severe complications of infection with the causal virus are unusual, but persons with anemia that requires increased red cell production (e.g., sickle cell disease) may develop transient aplastic crisis (TAC), often in the absence of a preceding rash. Intrauterine infection in the first half of pregnancy has resulted in fetal anemia with hydrops fetalis and fetal death in less than 10% of such infections. Immunosuppressed people may develop severe, chronic anemia. A number of other diseases (e.g., rheumatoid arthritis, systemic vasculitis, fulminant hepatitis and myocarditis) have been reported to occur in association with erythema infectiosum, but no causal link has been established.

Diagnosis is usually made on clinical and epidemiologic grounds; it can be confirmed by detection of specific IgM antibodies against parvovirus B19 (B19), or by a rise in B19 IgG antibodies. IgM titers begin to decline 30–60 days after the onset of symptoms. Diagnosis of B19 infection can also be made by detecting viral antigens of DNA. PCR for B19 DNA is the most sensitive of these tests and will often be positive during the first month of an acute infection and in some persons for prolonged periods.

2. Infectious agent—Human parvovirus B19, a 20-25-nm DNA virus belonging to the family Parvoviridae. The virus replicates primarily in erythroid precursor cells.

3. Occurrence—Worldwide. Common in children; both sporadic and epidemic. In the USA, the prevalence of B19 IgG antibodies ranges from 5%-15% in children less than 5 years old to 50%-80% in adults. In temperate zones, epidemics tend to occur in winter and spring, with a periodicity of 3-7 years in a given community.

4. Reservoir—Humans.

5. Mode of transmission—Thought to be primarily through contact with infected respiratory secretions; also, from mother to fetus, and parenterally by transfusion of blood and blood products. B19 is resistant to inactivation by various methods, including heating to 80°C for 72 hours.

6. Incubation period—Variable; 4–20 days to development of rash or symptoms of aplastic crisis.

7. Period of communicability—In people with rash illness alone, greatest before onset of rash and probably not communicable after onset of rash. People with aplastic crisis are communicable up to 1 week after onset of symptoms. Immunosuppressed people with chronic infection and severe anemia may be communicable for months to years.

8. Susceptibility and resistance—Universal susceptibility in persons with the blood group P antigen; protection appears to be conferred with development of B19 antibodies. The receptor for B19 erythroid cells is blood group P antigen. Attack rates among susceptibles can be high: 50% in household contacts, and 10%–60% in the day care or school setting over a 2 to 6 month outbreak period. In the USA, 50%–80% of adults have serologic evidence of past infection depending on age and location.

9. Methods of control—

    A. Preventive measures:

        1) Since the disease is generally benign, prevention should focus on those most likely to develop complications (i.e., those with underlying anemias, immunodeficiencies and non-B19 immune pregnant women). These people may choose to avoid exposure to potentially infectious people in hospital or outbreak settings. Immunoglobulin (IG) has not yet had a trial for efficacy.

        2) Susceptible women who are pregnant or who might become pregnant, and have continued close contact to people with B19 infection (e.g., at school, at home, in health care facilities) should be advised of the potential for acquiring infection and of the potential risk of complications to the fetus. Pregnant women with sick children at home are advised to wash hands frequently and to avoid sharing eating utensils.

        3) Health care workers should be advised of the importance of following good infection control measures. Rare nosocomial outbreaks have been reported.

    B. Control of patient, contacts and the immediate environment:

        1) Report to local health authority: Community wide outbreaks, Class 4 (see Communicable Disease Reporting).

        2) Isolation: Impractical in the community at large. Cases of transient aplastic crisis in the hospital setting should be placed on droplet precautions. Although children with B19 infection

are most communicable before the onset of illness, it may be prudent to exclude them from school or day care attendance while fever is present.

3) Concurrent disinfection: Strict handwashing after patient contact.

4) Quarantine: None.

5) Immunization of contacts: A recombinant B19 capsid vaccine is in the early stages of development.

6) Investigation of contacts and source of infection: Exposed pregnant women should be offered B19 IgG and IgM antibody testing to determine susceptibility and to assist with counseling regarding risks to their fetuses.

7) Specific treatment: Intravenous immunoglobulin (IGIV) has been successfully used to treat chronic anemia in persistent infections, but relapses can occur and require additional IGIV therapy.

C. Epidemic measures: During outbreaks in school or day care settings, those with anemia or immunodeficiencies and pregnant women should be informed of the possible risk of acquiring and transmitting infection.

D. Disaster implications: None.

E. International measures: None.

EXANTHEM SUBITUM   ICD-9 057.8; ICD-10 B08.2
(Sixth disease, Roseola infantum)

1. Identification—Exanthem subitum is an acute, febrile rash illness of viral etiology, that occurs usually in children under 4 years but most common before 2 years of age. It is one manifestation of illnesses caused by human herpesvirus-6B (HHV-6B). A fever, sometimes as high as 41°C (106°F), appears suddenly and lasts 3–5 days. A maculopapular rash on the trunk and later on the remainder of the body ordinarily follows lysis of the fever, and the rash usually fades rapidly. Symptoms are generally mild, but febrile seizures have been reported.

The spectrum of clinical illness in children is now known to include high fever without rash, inflamed tympanic membranes and, rarely, meningoencephalitis, recurrent seizures or fulminant hepatitis. In immunocompetent adults, a mononucleosis-like syndrome has been described, and in immuno-compromised hosts, pneumonitis has been noted. HHV-6 also causes asymptomatic and latent infection. Differentiation of roseola from similar vaccine preventable exanthems (e.g., measles, rubella) is often necessary.

Diagnosis can be confirmed by testing of paired sera for antibodies to HHV-6 by IFA or by isolation of HHV-6. Practical IgM tests are not available; an IgM response is usually not detectable until at least 5 days following the onset of symptoms. Detection of HHV-6 DNA in blood by PCR in the absence of concurrent IgG antibody shows promise as a future practical method for rapid diagnosis.

2. Infectious agent—Human herpesvirus-6 (subfamily, betaherpesvirus, genus *Roseolovirus*) is the most common cause of exanthem subitum. HHV-6 can be divided into HHV-6A and HHV-6B by using monoclonal techniques. Most HHV-6 infections in humans are now known to be caused by HHV-6B. Cases of exanthem subitum due to human herpesvirus 7 also occur.

3. Occurrence—Worldwide. In Japan, the USA, UK and Hong Kong, where the seroepidemiology of HHV-6 has been best described, incidence peaks in 6–12 month olds, with 65%–100% seroprevalence by age 2 years. Seroprevalence in childbearing women ranges from 80%–100% in most of the world, although rates as low as 20% have been observed in Morocco and 49% in Malaysia. Distinct outbreaks of exanthem subitum or HHV-6 are rarely recognized; a seasonal predilection (late winter, early spring) has been described only in Japan.

4. Reservoir—Humans appear to be the main reservoir of infection.

5. Mode of transmission—Not well delineated. In children, the rapid acquisition of early childhood infection that follows the waning of maternal antibodies and the high prevalence of HHV-6 viral DNA in salivary glands of adults suggest that salivary contact with caregivers and parents is the most likely mode of infection. However, in one US study, the age specific infection rate increased when there was more than one sibling in the household, which suggests that children may also be important reservoirs for transmission. Renal and hepatic transplants from HHV-6-infected donors can cause primary infection in seronegative transplant recipients.

6. Incubation period—Ten days, with a usual range of 5–15 days. Onset of illness is usually 2–4 weeks after transplantation in susceptible transplant recipients.

7. Period of communicability—In acute infection, unknown. Following acute infection, the virus may establish latency in lymph nodes, kidney, liver, salivary glands and in monocytes. The duration of potential communicability from these latent infections is unknown but may be lifelong.

8. Susceptibility and resistance—Susceptibility is general. Infection rates in infants less than 6 months of age are low but increase rapidly thereafter, which suggests that temporary protection is conferred by transplacentally acquired maternal antibodies. Second cases of exanthem subitum are rare. Latent infection appears to be established in most persons but is of uncertain clinical significance, notably in persons who are immunosuppressed. Primary disease may be more severe and symptoms last longer in persons who are immunosuppressed.

9. **Methods of control**—Effective measures are not available.

A. *Preventive measures:*

1. There may be a role in the future for avoiding transplantation of organ tissues from HHV-6 seropositive donors to seronegative recipients.

B. *Control of patient, contacts and the immediate environment:*

1. Report to local health authority: Official report not ordinarily justifiable, Class 5 (see Communicable Disease Reporting).
2. Isolation: In hospitals and institutions, patients suspected of having exanthem subitum should be managed under contact isolation precautions and placed in a private room.
3. Concurrent disinfection: None.
4. Quarantine: None.
5. Immunization of contacts: None. Given that sustained immunity against reinfection following primary infections appears to occur, there may be potential for a vaccine in the future.
6. Investigation of contacts and source of infection: None, because of the high prevalence of asymptomatic shedders in the population.
7. Specific treatment: None

C. *Epidemic measures:* None.

D. *Disaster implications:* None.

E. *International measures:* None.

FASCIOLIASIS   ICD-9 121.3; ICD-10 B66.3

1. **Identification**—A disease of the liver caused by a large trematode that is a natural parasite of sheep, cattle and related animals throughout the world. Flukes measuring up to about 3 cm live in the bile ducts; the young stages live in the liver parenchyma and cause tissue damage and enlargement of the liver. During the early period of parenchymal invasion, there

may be right upper quadrant pain, liver function abnormalities and eosinophilia. After migration to the biliary ducts, the flukes may cause biliary colic or obstructive jaundice. Ectopic infection, especially by *Fasciola gigantica,* may produce transient or migrating areas of inflammation in the skin over the trunk or other areas of the body.

Diagnosis is based on finding eggs in feces or in bile aspirated from the duodenum. Serodiagnostic tests, available in some centers, suggest the diagnosis when positive. "Spurious infection" may be diagnosed when nonviable eggs appear in the feces after liver from infected animals has been eaten.

2. Infectious agents—*Fasciola hepatica* and (less commonly) *F. gigantica.*

3. Occurrence—Human infection has been reported in sheep and cattle raising areas of South America, the Caribbean, Europe, Australia, the Middle East and Asia. Sporadic cases are reported in the USA. *F. gigantica* has a restricted distribution in Africa, the western Pacific and Hawaii.

4. Reservoir—Humans are an accidental host. The infection in nature is maintained in a cycle between other animal species, mainly sheep and cattle, and snails of the family Lymnaeidae. Cattle, water buffalo, and other large herbivorous mammals harbor *F. gigantica.*

5. Mode of transmission—Eggs passed in the feces develop in water, and in about 2 weeks a motile ciliated larva (miracidium) hatches. On entering a snail (lymnaeid), this larva develops to produce large numbers of free swimming cercariae that attach to aquatic plants and encyst; these encysted forms (metacercariae) are somewhat resistant to drying. Infection is acquired by eating uncooked aquatic plants (such as watercress) bearing metacercariae. On reaching the intestine, the larvae migrate through the wall into the peritoneal cavity, enter the liver and, after development, enter the bile ducts and begin laying eggs 3–4 months after initial exposure.

6. Incubation period—Variable.

7. Period of communicability—Infection is not transmitted directly from person to person.

8. Susceptibility and resistance—People of all ages are susceptible; infection persists indefinitely.

9. Methods of control —

   A. Preventive measures:

   1) Educate the public in endemic areas to abstain from eating watercress or other aquatic plants of wild or unknown origin, especially from areas where sheep or other animals graze.
   2) Avoid use of sheep feces for fertilizing water plants.

3) Drain the land or use chemical molluscicides to eliminate molluscs where it is technically and economically feasible.

B. Control of patient, contacts and the immediate environment:

1) Report to local health authority: Official report not ordinarily justifiable, Class 5 (see Communicable Disease Reporting).
2) Isolation: None.
3) Concurrent disinfection: None.
4) Quarantine: None.
5) Immunization of contacts: None.
6) Investigation of contacts and source of infection: Identification of the source of infection may be useful in preventing additional infections in the patient or others.
7) Specific treatment: Treatment is generally unsatisfactory. As of late 1999, the recommended treatment of choice is triclabendazole: all requests to CDC for treatment of *Fasciola hepatica* are forwarded to Novartis Pharmaceuticals AG, Basel, Switzerland, suppliers of this drug. Bithionol (Bitin® is no longer in production but available in the USA from CDC for domestic distribution only) was formerly the drug of choice but cure rates with this or praziquantel are inconsistent. During the migratory phase, symptomatic relief may be provided by dehydroemetine, chloroquine or metronidazole.

C. Epidemic measures: Determine source of infection and identify plants and snails involved in transmission. Prevent eating of aquatic plants from contaminated areas.

D. Disaster implications: None.

E. International measures: None.

FASCIOLOPSIASIS   ICD-9 121.4; ICD-10 B66.5

1. Identification—A trematode infection of the small intestine, particularly the duodenum. Symptoms result from local inflammation, ulceration of the intestinal wall and systemic toxic effects. Diarrhea usually alternates with constipation; vomiting and anorexia are frequent. Large numbers of flukes may produce acute intestinal obstruction. Patients may show edema of the face, abdominal wall and legs within 20 days after massive infection; ascites is common. Eosinophilia is usual; secondary anemia is occasional. Death is rare; light infections are usually asymptomatic.

Diagnosis is made by finding the large flukes or characteristic eggs in feces; worms are occasionally vomited.

2. Infectious agent—*Fasciolopsis buski,* a large trematode or fluke reaching lengths up to 7 cm.

3. Occurrence—Widely distributed in rural southeast Asia, especially Thailand, central and south China and parts of India. Prevalence is often high in pig rearing areas.

4. Reservoir—Swine and humans are definitive hosts of adult flukes; dogs less commonly.

5. Mode of transmission—Eggs passed in feces, most often of swine, develop in water within 3-7 weeks under favorable conditions; miracidia hatch and penetrate planorbid snails as intermediate hosts; cercariae develop, are liberated and encyst on aquatic plants to become the infective metacercariae. Human infections result from eating these plants uncooked. In China, the chief sources of infection are the nuts of the red water caltrop, grown in enclosed ponds, and tubers of the so-called water chestnut and water bamboo; infection frequently results when the hull or skin is peeled off with teeth and lips.

6. Incubation period—Eggs appear in the feces about 3 months after infection.

7. Period of communicability—As long as viable eggs are discharged in feces; without treatment, probably for 1 year. Not directly transmitted from person to person.

8. Susceptibility and resistance—Susceptibility is universal. In malnourished individuals, the ill effects are pronounced; number of worms influences severity of disease.

9. Methods of control —

A. *Preventive measures:*

1) Educate the population at risk in endemic areas on the mode of transmission and life cycle of the parasite.
2) Treat night soil to destroy eggs.
3) Bar swine from contaminating areas where water plants are growing; do not feed water plants to pigs.
4) Dry suspected plants, or if plants are to be eaten fresh, dip them in boiling water for a few seconds; both methods kill metacercariae.

B. *Control of patient, contacts and the immediate environment:*

1) Report to local health authority: In selected endemic areas; in most countries, not a reportable disease, Class 3C (see Communicable Disease Reporting).
2) Isolation: None.
3) Concurrent disinfection: Sanitary disposal of feces.

4) Quarantine: None.

5) Immunization of contacts: None.

6) Investigation of contacts and source of infection: In the individual case, of little value. A community problem (see 9C, below).

7) Specific treatment: Praziquantel (Biltricide®) is the drug of choice.

C. Epidemic measures: Identify aquatic plants that harbor encysted metacercariae and are eaten fresh, identify infected snail species living in water with such plants and prevent contamination of water with human and pig feces.

D. Disaster implications: None.

E. International measures: None.

FILARIASIS   ICD-9 125; ICD-10 B74

The term filariasis denotes infection with any of several nematodes belonging to the family Filarioidea. However, as used here, the term refers only to the lymphatic dwelling filariae listed below. For others, refer to the specific disease.

FILARIASIS DUE TO *WUCHERERIA BANCROFTI*   ICD-9 125.0; ICD-10 B74.0
(Bancroftian filariasis)

FILARIASIS DUE TO *BRUGIA MALAYI*   ICD-9 125.1; ICD-10 B74.1
(Malayan filariasis, Brugian filariasis)

FILARIASIS DUE TO *BRUGIA TIMORI*   ICD-9 125.6; ICD-10 B74.2
(Timorean filariasis)

1. Identification—Bancroftian filariasis is an infection with the nematode *Wuchereria bancrofti,* which normally resides in the lymphatics in infected people. Female worms produce microfilariae that reach the bloodstream 6–12 months after infection. Two biologically different forms occur: in one, the microfilariae circulate in the peripheral blood at night (nocturnal periodicity) with greatest concentrations between 10 pm and 2 am; in the other, microfilariae circulate continuously in the peripheral blood, but occur in greater concentration in the daytime (diurnal). The latter form is endemic in the South Pacific and in small rural foci in southeast Asia where the principal vectors are day biting *Aedes* mosquitoes.

The spectrum of clinical manifestations in regions of endemic filariasis includes people who are exposed but remain asymptomatic and parasitologically negative; those who are asymptomatic with microfilaremia; those with acute recurrent filarial fever, lymphadenitis and retrograde lymphangitis who may or may not have microfilaremia; those with chronic signs, including hydrocele, chyluria and elephantiasis of the limbs, breasts and genitalia, who have low-level or undetectable microfilaremia; and those with the tropical pulmonary eosinophilia syndrome, manifested by paroxysmal nocturnal asthma, chronic interstitial lung disease, recurrent low-grade fever, profound eosinophilia and degenerating microfilariae in tissues but not in the bloodstream (occult filariasis).

Brugian filariasis is caused by the nematodes *Brugia malayi* and *B. timori*. The nocturnally periodic form of *B. malayi* occurs in rural populations living in open rice growing areas throughout much of southeast Asia. The subperiodic form infects humans, monkeys and wild and domestic carnivores in the forests of Malaysia and Indonesia. Clinical manifestations are similar to those of Bancroftian filariasis, except that the recurrent acute attacks of filarial fever, adenitis and retrograde lymphangitis are more severe, while chyluria is uncommon and elephantiasis is usually confined to the distal extremities, most frequently to the legs below the knees. Breast lymphedema and hydrocele are rarely, if ever, seen.

Brugia timori **infections** have been described on Timor and other southeastern islands of Indonesia. Clinical manifestations are comparable to those seen in *B. malayi* infections.

Clinical manifestations of filariasis often occur with no demonstrable circulating microfilariae (occult filariasis). In several thousand cases seen in American military personnel during World War II, microfilariae were found in only 10–15 patients despite repeated blood examinations. In some of these cases, infection was manifested by marked eosinophilia often associated with pulmonary symptoms (tropical pulmonary eosinophilia syndrome).

Microfilariae are best detected during periods of maximal microfilaremia. Live microfilariae can be seen under low power in a drop of peripheral blood (finger prick) on a slide or in hemolyzed blood in a counting chamber. Giemsa stained thick and thin smears permit species identification. Microfilariae may be concentrated by filtration through a Nucleopore filter (2–5-μm pore size) in a Swinney adapter and by the Knott technique (centrifugal sedimentation of 2 ml of blood mixed with 10 ml of 2% formalin), or by Quantitative Buffy Coat (QBC) acridine orange/microhematocrit tube technique.

2. Infectious agents—*Wuchereria bancrofti, Brugia malayi* and *B. timori;* long threadlike worms.

3. Occurrence—*W. bancrofti* is endemic in most of the warm humid regions of the world, including Latin America (scattered foci in Brazil, Suriname, Guyana, French Guyana, Haiti, the Dominican Republic and Costa Rica), Africa, Asia and the Pacific islands. It is common in those urban areas where conditions favor breeding of vector mosquitoes. In general, nocturnal periodicity in *Wuchereria* infected areas of the Pacific is found west of 140°E longitude, and diurnal subperiodicity east of 180°E longitude. *B. malayi* is endemic in rural southwest India, southeast Asia, central and northern coastal areas of China and South Korea. *B. timori* occurs on the rural islands of Timor, Flores, Alor and Roti in southeast Indonesia.

4. Reservoir—Humans with microfilariae in the blood for *W. bancrofti,* periodic *B. malayi* and *B. timori.* In Malaysia, southern Thailand, the Philippines and Indonesia, cats, civets *(Viverra tangalunga)* and nonhuman primates serve as reservoirs for subperiodic *B. malayi.*

5. Mode of transmission—By bite of a mosquito harboring infective larvae. *W. bancrofti* is transmitted by many species, the most important being *Culex quinquefasciatus, Anopheles gambiae, An. funestus, Aedes polynesiensis, Ae. scapularis* and *Ae. pseudoscutellaris. B. malayi* is transmitted by various species of *Mansonia, Anopheles* and *Aedes. B. timori* is transmitted by *An. barbirostris.* In the female mosquito, ingested microfilariae penetrate the stomach wall and develop in the thoracic muscles into elongated, infective filariform larvae that migrate to the proboscis. When the mosquito feeds, the larvae emerge and enter the punctured skin following the mosquito bite. They travel via the lymphatics, where they molt twice before becoming adults.

6. Incubation period—While allergic inflammatory manifestations may appear as early as a month after infection, microfilariae may not appear in the blood until 3-6 months in *B. malayi* or 6-12 months in *W. bancrofti* infections.

7. Period of communicability—Not directly transmitted from person to person. Humans may infect mosquitoes when microfilariae are present in the peripheral blood; microfilaremia may persist for 5-10 years or longer after initial infection. The mosquito becomes infective about 12-14 days after an infective blood meal.

8. Susceptibility and resistance—Universal susceptibility to infection is probable; there is considerable geographic difference in the type and severity of disease. Repeated infections occur in endemic regions and lead to the severe manifestations such as elephantiasis.

9. Methods of control —

A. Preventive measures:

1) Educate the inhabitants of endemic areas on the mode of transmission and methods of mosquito control.

2) Identify the vectors by detecting infective larvae in mosquitoes caught on human bait; identify times and places of mosquito biting and locate breeding places. If indoor night biters are responsible, spray inside walls with a residual insecticide, screen houses, or use bed nets (preferably synthetic pyrethroid impregnated) and insect repellents. Eliminate breeding places (e.g., open latrines, old tires, coconut husks) and treat with larvicides. Where *Mansonia* species are vectors, clear ponds of vegetation *(Pistia)* that serve as sources of oxygen for the larvae.

3) Long term control may involve changes in housing construction to include screening, and environmental control to eliminate mosquito breeding sites.

4) Mass treatment with diethylcarbamazine (DEC, Banocide®, Hetrazan®, Notezine®), especially when followed by monthly treatment with a low dose (25–50 mg/kg body weight) of DEC for 1–2 years or the use of DEC-medicated cooking salt (0.2–0.4 mg/g of salt) for 6 months to 2 years, has proven efficacious. However, in some instances, adverse reactions have discouraged community participation, especially where onchocerciasis is endemic (see Onchocerciasis, Mazzotti reaction). Ivermectin and albendazole have also been used; currently, annual single dose treatment with combinations of these drugs is showing promise.

B. Control of patient, contacts and the immediate environment:

1) Report to local health authority: In selected endemic regions; in most countries, not a reportable disease, Class 3C (see Communicable Disease Reporting). Reporting of cases with demonstrated microfilariae provides information on areas of transmission.

2) Isolation: Not practicable. As far as possible, patients with microfilaremia should be protected from mosquitoes to reduce transmission.

3) Concurrent disinfection: None.

4) Quarantine: None.

5) Immunization of contacts: None.

6) Investigation of contacts and source of infection: Only as part of a general community effort (see 9A and 9C).

7) Specific treatment: Diethylcarbamazine (DEC, Banocide®, Hetrazan®, Notezine®) and ivermectin result in rapid disappearance of most or all microfilariae from the blood, but may not destroy all the adult worms. Low level microfilaremia may reappear after treatment. Therefore, treatment must usually be repeated at yearly intervals. Low level microfilaremia can be detected only by concentration techniques. DEC may cause

acute generalized reactions during the first 24 hours of treatment because of death and degeneration of microfilariae; these reactions are often controlled by aspirin, antihistamines or corticosteroids. Localized lymphadenitis and lymphangitis may follow the death of the adult worms. Antibiotics in the early stages of infection may prevent some of the lymphatic sequelae caused by associated bacterial infection.

C. *Epidemic measures:* Vector control is the fundamental measure. In highly endemic areas, it is important to correctly appraise the bionomics of mosquito vectors, prevalence and incidence of disease, and environmental factors responsible for transmission in each locale. Even partial control by antimosquito measures may reduce incidence and restrict the focus. Measurable results are slow because of the long incubation period.

D. *Disaster implications:* None.

E. *International measures:* None.

DIROFILARIASIS   ICD-9 125.6; ICD-10 B74.8
(Zoonotic filariasis)

Certain species of filariae commonly seen in wild or domestic animals occasionally infect humans, but microfilaremia occurs rarely. The genus *Dirofilaria* causes pulmonary and cutaneous disease in humans. *D. immitis,* the dog heartworm, has caused pulmonary disease in the USA (about 50 reported cases) with a few reported infections in Japan, Asia and Australia. Transmission to humans is by mosquito bite. The worm lodges in a pulmonary artery, where it may form the nidus of a thrombus, which leads to vascular occlusion, coagulation, necrosis and fibrosis. Symptoms are chest pain, cough and hemoptysis. Eosinophilia is infrequent. A fibrotic nodule, 1–3 cm in diameter, which most commonly is asymptomatic, is recognizable by x-ray as a "coin lesion."

Cutaneous disease is caused by various species, including *D. tenuis,* a parasite of the raccoon in the USA; *D. ursi,* a parasite of bears in Canada; and adult *D. repens,* a parasite of dogs and cats in Europe, Africa and Asia. The worms develop in or migrate to the conjunctivae and the subcutaneous tissues of the scrotum, breasts, arms and legs, but microfilaremia is rare. Others *(Brugia)* localize in lymph nodes. Diagnosis is usually made by the finding of worms in tissue sections of surgically excised lesions.

OTHER NEMATODES PRODUCING MICROFILARIAE IN HUMANS

Several other nematodes may infect humans and produce microfilariae. These include *Onchocerca volvulus* and *Loa loa*, which cause onchocerciasis and loiasis, respectively (see under each disease listing). Other infections are forms of mansonellosis (ICD-9 125.4 and 125.5; ICD-10 B74.4): *Mansonella perstans* is widely distributed in west Africa and northeastern South America; the adult is found in the body cavities, and the unsheathed microfilariae circulate with no regular periodicity. Infection is usually asymptomatic, but eye infections by immature stages have been reported.

In some countries of west and central Africa, infection with *M. streptocerca* (ICD-9 125.6; ICD-10 B74.4) is common and is suspected of causing cutaneous edema and thickening of the skin, hypopigmented macules, pruritus and papules. Adult worms and unsheathed microfilariae occur in the skin as in onchocerciasis. *M. ozzardi* (ICD-9 125.5; ICD-10 B74.4) occurs from the Yucatan Peninsula in Mexico to northern Argentina and in the West Indies; diagnosis is based on demonstration of the circulating unsheathed nonperiodic microfilariae. Infection is generally asymptomatic but may be associated with allergic manifestations such as articular pain, pruritus, headaches and lymphadenopathy.

Culicoides midges are the main vectors for *M. streptocerca*, *M. ozzardi* and *M. perstans;* in the Caribbean area, *M. ozzardi* is also transmitted by blackflies. *M. rodhaini*, a parasite of chimpanzees, was found in 1.7% of skin snips taken in Gabon.

DEC is effective against *M. streptocerca* and occasionally against *M. perstans* and *M. ozzardi*. Ivermectin is effective against *M. ozzardi*.

FOODBORNE INTOXICATIONS
(Food poisoning)

Foodborne diseases, including foodborne intoxications and foodborne infections, are terms applied to illnesses acquired by consumption of contaminated food; they are frequently and inaccurately referred to as food poisoning. These terms include illnesses caused by chemical contaminants such as heavy metals and many organic compounds; however, the more frequent causes of foodborne illnesses are: (1) toxins elaborated by bacterial growth in the food before consumption (*Clostridium botulinum*, *Staphylococcus aureus*, and *Bacillus cereus*; scombroid fish poisoning, associated not with a specific toxin but with elevated histamine levels) or in the intestines (*Clostridium perfringens*); (2) bacterial, viral, or parasitic infections (brucellosis, *Campylobacter* enteritis, diarrhea caused by *Escherichia coli*, hepatitis A, listeriosis, salmonellosis, shigellosis, toxoplasmosis, viral gastroenteritis, taeniasis, trichinosis, and vibrios); and (3) toxins produced by harmful algal species (ciguatera fish poisoning, paralytic shellfish poisoning, neurotoxic shellfish poisoning, diarrhetic shellfish poisoning, and amnesic shellfish poisoning) or present in specific fish species (puffer fish poisoning).

This chapter deals specifically with toxin related foodborne illnesses (with the exception of botulism). Foodborne illnesses associated with infection by specific agents are covered in specific chapters dealing with these agents.

Foodborne disease outbreaks are recognized by the occurrence of illness within a usually short but variable period of time (from a few hours to a few weeks) after a meal, among individuals who have consumed foods in common. Prompt and thorough laboratory evaluation of cases and implicated foods is essential. Single cases of foodborne disease are difficult to identify unless, as in botulism, there is a distinctive clinical syndrome. Foodborne disease may be one of the most common causes of acute illness; many cases and outbreaks are unrecognized and unreported.

Prevention and control of these diseases, regardless of the specific cause, are based on the same principles: avoidance of food contamination, destruction or denaturation of the contaminants, and prevention of further spread or multiplication of contaminants. Specific problems and appropriate modes of intervention may vary from one country to another and depend on environmental, economic, political, technologic and sociocultural factors. Ultimately, prevention depends on educating food handlers about proper practices in cooking and storage of food and personal hygiene. Toward this end, WHO has developed "Ten Golden Rules for Safe Food Preparation." These are as follows:

1. Choose foods processed for safety.
2. Cook food thoroughly.
3. Eat cooked foods immediately.
4. Store cooked foods carefully.
5. Reheat cooked foods thoroughly.
6. Avoid contact between raw food and cooked food.
7. Wash hands repeatedly.
8. Keep all kitchen surfaces meticulously clean.
9. Protect food from insects, rodents and other animals.
10. Use safe water.

I. STAPHYLOCOCCAL FOOD INTOXICATION ICD-9 005.0; ICD-10 A05.0

1. Identification—An intoxication (not an infection) of abrupt and sometimes violent onset, with severe nausea, cramps, vomiting and prostration, often accompanied by diarrhea, and sometimes with subnormal temperature and lowered blood pressure. Deaths are rare; duration of illness is commonly not more than a day or two, but the intensity of symptoms may require hospitalization and may result in surgical exploration in sporadic cases. Diagnosis is easier when a group of cases is seen with the characteristic acute, predominantly upper GI symptoms and the short interval between eating a common food item and the onset of symptoms.

Differential diagnosis includes other recognized forms of food poisoning as well as chemical poisons.

In the outbreak setting, recovery of large numbers of staphylococci (10^5 organisms or more per gram of food) on routine culture media or detection of enterotoxin from an epidemiologically implicated food item confirms the diagnosis. Absence of staphylococci on culture of a heated food does not rule out the diagnosis; a Gram stain of the food may disclose the organisms that have been heat killed. It may be possible to identify enterotoxin or thermonuclease in the food in the absence of viable organisms. Isolation of organisms of the same phage type from stools or vomitus of two or more ill persons also confirms the diagnosis. Recovery of large numbers of enterotoxin producing staphylococci from stool or vomitus from a single person supports the diagnosis. Phage typing and enterotoxin tests may help epidemiologic investigations but are not routinely available or indicated.

2. Toxic agent—Several enterotoxins of *Staphylococcus aureus,* stable at boiling temperature. Staphylococci multiply in food and produce the toxins.

3. Occurrence—Widespread and relatively frequent; one of the principal acute food intoxications in the USA. About 25% of people are carriers of this pathogen.

4. Reservoir—Humans in most instances; occasionally cows with infected udders, as well as dogs and fowl.

5. Mode of transmission—By ingestion of a food product containing staphylococcal enterotoxin. Foods involved are particularly those that come in contact with food handlers' hands, either without subsequent cooking or with inadequate heating or refrigeration, such as pastries, custards, salad dressings, sandwiches, sliced meat and meat products. Toxin has also developed in inadequately cured ham and salami, and in nonprocessed or inadequately processed cheese. When these foods remain at room temperature for several hours before being eaten, toxin producing staphylococci multiply and elaborate the heat stable toxin.

The organisms may be of human origin from purulent discharges of an infected finger or eye, abscesses, acneiform facial eruptions, nasopharyngeal secretions, or apparently normal skin; or of bovine origin, such as contaminated milk or milk products, especially cheese.

6. Incubation period—Interval between eating food and onset of symptoms is 30 minutes to 8 hours, usually 2–4 hours.

7. Period of communicability—Not applicable.

8. Susceptibility and resistance—Most people are susceptible.

9. **Methods of control—**

 A. *Preventive measures:*

   1) Educate food handlers about: (a) strict food hygiene, sanitation and cleanliness of kitchens, proper temperature control, handwashing, cleaning of fingernails; and (b) the danger of working with exposed skin, nose or eye infections and uncovered wounds.

   2) Reduce food handling time (initial preparation to service) to an absolute minimum, with no more than 4 hours at ambient temperature. Keep perishable foods **hot** (greater than 60°C/140°F) or **cold** (below 10°C /50°F; best is less than 4°C/39°F) in shallow containers and covered, if they are to be stored for more than 2 hours.

   3) Temporarily exclude people with boils, abscesses and other purulent lesions of hands, face or nose from food handling.

 B. *Control of patient, contacts and the immediate environment:*

   1) Report to local health authority: Obligatory report of outbreaks of suspected or confirmed cases, Class 4 (see Communicable Disease Reporting).

   2), 3), 4), 5) and 6) Isolation, Concurrent disinfection, Quarantine, Immunization of contacts and Investigation of contacts and source of infection: Not pertinent. Control is of outbreaks; single cases are rarely identified.

   7) Specific treatment: Fluid replacement when indicated.

 C. *Epidemic measures:*

   1) By quick review of reported cases, determine time and place of exposure and the population at risk; obtain a complete listing of the foods served and embargo, under refrigeration, all foods still available. The prominent clinical features, coupled with an estimate of the incubation period, provide useful leads to the most probable etiologic agent. Collect specimens of feces and vomitus for laboratory examination; alert the laboratory to suspected etiologic agents. Interview a random sample of those exposed. Compare the attack rates for specific food items eaten and not eaten; the implicated food item(s) will usually have the greatest difference in attack rates. Most of the sick will have eaten the contaminated food.

   2) Inquire about the origin of the incriminated food and the manner of its preparation and storage before serving. Look for possible sources of contamination and periods of inadequate refrigeration and heating that would permit growth of staphylococci. Submit any leftover suspected foods promptly for laboratory examination; failure to isolate staphylococci does

not exclude the presence of the heat resistant enterotoxin if the food had been heated.

3) Search for food handlers with skin infections, particularly of the hands. Culture all purulent lesions and collect nasal swabs from all foodhandlers. Antibiograms and/or phage typing of representative strains of enterotoxin producing staphylococci isolated from foods and food handlers and from vomitus or feces of patients may be helpful.

D. **Disaster implications:** A potential hazard in situations involving mass feeding and lack of refrigeration facilities. A particular problem of air travel.

E. **International measures:** WHO Collaborating Centres.

II. *CLOSTRIDIUM PERFRINGENS* FOOD INTOXICATION   ICD-9 005.2; ICD-10 A05.2
(*C. welchii* food poisoning, Enteritis necroticans, Pigbel)

1. Identification—An intestinal disorder characterized by sudden onset of colic followed by diarrhea; nausea is common, but vomiting and fever are usually absent. Generally a mild disease of short duration, 1 day or less, and rarely fatal in healthy people. Outbreaks of severe disease with high case-fatality rates associated with a necrotizing enteritis have been documented in postwar Germany and in Papua New Guinea.

In the outbreak setting, diagnosis is confirmed by demonstration of *Clostridium perfringens* in semiquantitative anaerobic cultures of food (10^5/g or greater) or patients' stool (10^6/g or greater) in addition to clinical and epidemiologic evidence. Detection of enterotoxin in the stool of ill persons also confirms the diagnosis. When serotyping can be performed, the same serotype is usually demonstrated in different specimens; serotyping is done routinely only in Japan and the UK.

2. Infectious agent—Type A strains of *C. perfringens* (*C. welchii*) cause typical food poisoning outbreaks (they also cause gas gangrene); type C strains cause necrotizing enteritis. Disease is produced by toxins elaborated by the organisms.

3. Occurrence—Widespread and relatively frequent in countries with cooking practices that favor multiplication of clostridia to high levels.

4. Reservoir—Soil; also the GI tract of healthy people and animals (cattle, pigs, poultry and fish).

5. Mode of transmission—Ingestion of food that was contaminated by soil or feces and then held under conditions that permit multiplication of the organism. Almost all outbreaks are associated with inadequately heated or reheated meats, usually stews, meat pies, and gravies made of beef, turkey or chicken. Spores survive normal cooking temperatures, germinate and multiply during slow cooling, storage at ambient temperature, and/or inadequate rewarming. Outbreaks are usually traced to food catering firms, restaurants, cafeterias and schools that have inadequate cooling and refrigeration facilities for large-scale service. Heavy bacterial contamination (more than 10^5 organisms per gram of food) is usually required for clinical disease.

6. Incubation period—From 6 to 24 hours, usually 10–12 hours.

7. Period of communicability—Not applicable.

8. Susceptibility and resistance—Most people are probably susceptible. In volunteer studies, no resistance was observed after repeated exposures.

9. Methods of control—

    A. Preventive measures:

      1) Educate food handlers about the risks inherent in large scale cooking, especially of meat dishes. Where possible, encourage serving hot dishes while still hot from initial cooking.

      2) Serve meat dishes hot, as soon as they are cooked, or cool them rapidly in a properly designed chiller and refrigerate until serving time; reheating, if necessary, should be thorough (internal temperature of at least 70°C/158°F, preferably 75°C/167°F or higher) and rapid. Do not partially cook meat and poultry one day and reheat the next, unless it can be stored at a safe temperature. Large cuts of meat should be thoroughly cooked; for more rapid cooling of cooked foods, divide stews and similar dishes prepared in bulk into many shallow containers and place in a rapid chiller.

    B., C. and D. Control of patient, contacts and the immediate environment; Epidemic measures and Disaster implications: See Staphylococcal food intoxication (section I, 9B, 9C and 9D, above).

    E. International measures: None.

III. *BACILLUS CEREUS* FOOD INTOXICATION   ICD-9 005.8; ICD-10 A05.4

1. Identification—An intoxication characterized in some cases by sudden onset of nausea and vomiting, and in others by colic and diarrhea. Illness generally persists no longer than 24 hours and is rarely fatal.

In the outbreak setting, diagnosis is confirmed by performing quantitative cultures with selective media to estimate the number of organisms present in the suspected food (generally more than 10^5 organisms per gram of the incriminated food are required). Diagnosis is also confirmed by isolation of organisms from the stool of two or more ill persons and not from stools of controls. Enterotoxin testing is valuable but may not be widely available.

2. Toxic agent—*Bacillus cereus,* an aerobic spore former. Two enterotoxins have been identified, one (heat stable) causing vomiting, and one (heat labile) causing diarrhea.

3. Occurrence—A well recognized cause of foodborne disease in the world; rarely reported in the USA.

4. Reservoir—A ubiquitous organism in soil and the environment commonly found at low levels in raw, dried and processed foods.

5. Mode of transmission—Ingestion of food that has been kept at ambient temperatures after cooking, permitting multiplication of the organisms. Outbreaks associated with vomiting have been most commonly associated with cooked rice that had subsequently been held at ambient room temperatures before reheating. Various mishandled foods have been implicated in outbreaks associated with diarrhea.

6. Incubation period—From 1 to 6 hours in cases where vomiting is the predominant symptom; from 6 to 24 hours where diarrhea is predominant.

7. Period of communicability—Not communicable from person to person.

8. Susceptibility and resistance—Unknown.

9. Methods of control—

    A. *Preventive measures:* Foods should not remain at ambient temperature after cooking, since the ubiquitous *B. cereus* spores can survive boiling, germinate, and multiply rapidly at room temperature. Refrigerate leftover food promptly; reheat thoroughly and rapidly to avoid multiplication of microorganisms.

    B., C. and D. *Control of patient, contacts and the immediate environment; Epidemic measures* and *Disaster implications:* See Staphylococcal food intoxication (section I, 9B, 9C and 9D, above).

    E. *International measures:* None.

IV. SCOMBROID FISH
   POISONING   ICD-9 988.0; ICD-10 T61.1
(Histamine poisoning)

A syndrome of tingling and burning sensations around the mouth, facial flushing and sweating, nausea and vomiting, headache, palpitations, dizziness and rash that occur within a few hours after eating fish containing high levels of free histamine (more than 20 mg/100 g of fish); this occurs when the fish has undergone bacterial decomposition after capture. Symptoms resolve spontaneously within 12 hours and there are no long-term sequelae.

Occurrence is worldwide; the syndrome was initially associated with fish in the families Scombroidea and Scomberesocidae (tuna, mackerel, skipjack and bonito) which contain high levels of histidine that can be decarboxylated to form histamine by bacteria in the fish. However, nonscombroid fish, such as mahi-mahi (dolphinfish), bluefish and salmon, are commonly associated with illness. Risks appear to be greatest for fish imported from tropical or semitropical areas and fish caught by recreational fishermen, who may lack appropriate storage facilities for large fish. The diagnosis is confirmed by detection of histamine in epidemiologically implicated fish.

Adequate refrigeration or irradiation of caught fish prevents this spoilage. Symptoms usually resolve spontaneously. In severe cases, antihistamines may be effective in relieving symptoms.

While most often associated with fish, any food (such as certain cheeses) that contains the appropriate amino acids and is subjected to certain bacterial contamination and growth may lead to scombroid poisoning when ingested.

V. CIGUATERA FISH
   POISONING   ICD-9 988.0; ICD-10 T61.0

A syndrome of characteristic GI and neurologic symptoms may occur within 1 hour after eating tropical reef fish. GI symptoms (diarrhea, vomiting, abdominal pain) occur first, usually within 24 hours of eating implicated fish. In severe cases, patients may also be hypotensive, with a paradoxical bradycardia. Neurologic symptoms may occur at the same time as the acute symptoms or may follow 1–2 days later; they include pain and weakness in the lower extremities (a very characteristic symptom in the Caribbean) and circumoral and peripheral paresthesias, and may persist for weeks or months.

More bizarre symptoms, such as temperature reversal (ice cream tastes hot, hot coffee seems cold) and "aching teeth," are frequently reported. In very severe cases (particularly in the South Pacific), the neurologic symptoms may progress to coma and respiratory arrest within the first 24 hours of illness. Most patients recover completely within a few weeks, but intermittent recrudescence of symptoms over a period of months to years can occur.

This syndrome is caused by the presence in the fish of toxins elaborated by the dinoflagellate *Gambierdiscus toxicus* and other algae that grow on reefs under the sea. Fish eating the algae become toxic, and the effect is magnified through the food chain so that large predatory fish become the most toxic; this occurs worldwide in tropical areas.

Ciguatera is a significant cause of morbidity in areas in which consumption of reef fish is common—the Caribbean, southern Florida, Hawaii, the South Pacific and Australia. The incidence in the South Pacific has been estimated to be in the range of 500 cases/100,000 population/year, with rates 50 times as high reported for some island groups. In the U.S. Virgin Islands, an incidence rate of 730 cases/100,000 population/year has been reported. More than 400 fish species are said to have the potential for becoming toxic. Worldwide, 50,000 cases of ciguatera occur per year. The diagnosis is confirmed by demonstrating ciguatoxin in epidemiologically implicated fish.

The consumption of large predatory fish should be avoided, especially in the reef area. In areas where assays for toxic fish are available (Hawaii), the risk of toxicity can be reduced by screening all large, "high risk" fish before their consumption. The occurrence of toxic fish is sporadic and not all fish of a given species or from a given locale will be toxic.

Intravenous infusion of mannitol (1 g/kg of a 20% solution, infused over 45 minutes) may have a dramatic effect on acute symptoms of ciguatera fish poisoning, particularly in severe cases; it has the most pronounced effect on neurologic symptoms and may be lifesaving in severe cases that have progressed to coma.

VI. PARALYTIC SHELLFISH POISONING (PSP)   ICD-9 988.0; ICD-10 T61.2

Classic PSP is a syndrome of characteristic symptoms (predominately neurologic) with onset within minutes to several hours after eating bivalve molluscs. Initial symptoms include paresthesias of the mouth and extremities, frequently accompanied by GI symptoms. Symptoms usually resolve within a few days. In severe cases, ataxia, dysphonia, dysphagia and total muscle paralysis with respiratory arrest and death occur. In a retrospective review of PSP outbreaks that occurred in Alaska between 1973 and 1992, 29 (25% of 117 ill persons) required an emergency flight to a hospital, four (3%) required intubation, and one died. Recovery is complete, symptoms usually resolve within hours to days after shellfish ingestion.

This syndrome is caused by the presence in shellfish of saxitoxins produced by *Alexandrium* species and other dinoflagellates. Concentration of these toxins occurs especially during massive algae blooms known as "red tides," but can also occur in the absence of a recognizable algal bloom. PSP is particularly common in shellfish harvested from colder waters above 30°N and below 30°S latitude, but may occur in tropical waters as well. In the USA, PSP is primarily a problem in the New England states, Alaska, California, and Washington. Blooms of the causative *Alexandrium* species occur several times each year, primarily from April through October. Shellfish become toxic and remain toxic for several weeks after the bloom subsides; there are also some shellfish species that remain toxic constantly. Most cases occur in individuals or small groups who gather shellfish for personal consumption. Diagnosis is confirmed by detection of toxin in epidemiologically implicated food. On an experimental basis, it has been possible to demonstrate saxitoxins in serum during acute illness and in urine after acute symptoms resolve.

PSP neurotoxins are heat stable. Surveillance of high risk harvest areas in the USA is routinely conducted by state health departments, by using a standard mouse bioassay; areas are closed to harvesting when toxin levels in shellfish exceed 80 µg/100 g. When toxin levels exceed this value, warnings should be posted in shellfish growing areas, beaches and in the media.

VII. NEUROTOXIC SHELLFISH POISONING   ICD-9 988.0; ICD-10 T61.2

Neurotoxic shellfish poisoning is associated with blooms of *Gymnodinium breve,* which produce brevetoxin. Red tides caused by *G. breve* have occurred along the Florida coast for centuries, with associated fish kills and mortality in seabirds and marine mammals. Symptoms after eating toxic shellfish include circumoral paresthesias and paresthesias of the extremities, dizziness and ataxia, muscle aches, and gastrointestinal symptoms. Symptoms tend to be mild, and resolve quickly and completely. In outbreaks which occurred in 1987 in North Carolina, median duration of illness was 17 hours (range 1–72 hours). Respiratory and eye irritation have also been reported in association with *G. breve* blooms, apparently due to aerosolization of the toxin by wind and wave action.

VIII. DIARRHETIC SHELLFISH POISONING   ICD-9 988.0; ICD-10 T61.2

Illness results from eating mussels, scallops, or clams that have been feeding on *Dinophysis fortii* or *Dinophysis acuminata.* Symptoms include diarrhea, nausea, vomiting, and abdominal pain. Case reports came initially from Japan; however, diarrhetic shellfish poisoning has occurred in France and other parts of Europe, Canada, New Zealand, and South America. There have been no confirmed USA cases, although the causative organisms have been identified in USA coastal waters.

IX. AMNESIC SHELLFISH
POISONING   ICD-9 988.0; ICD-10 T61.2

Amnesic shellfish poisoning results from ingestion of shellfish containing domoic acid, produced by the diatom *Pseudonitzschia pungens*. A series of cases due to this toxin were reported in the Atlantic provinces of Canada in 1987. Symptoms included vomiting, abdominal cramps, diarrhea, headache, and loss of short term memory. On neuropsychological testing several months after the acute intoxication, patients were found to have severe antegrade memory deficits with relative preservation of other cognitive functions; patients also had clinical and electromyographic evidence of pure motor or sensorimotor neuropathy and axonopathy. Neuropathological studies in four patients who died demonstrated neuronal necrosis and loss, predominantly in the hippocampus and amygdala. Canadian authorities now analyze mussels and clams for domoic acid, and close shellfish beds to harvesting when levels exceed 20 µg/g.

In 1991, domoic acid was also identified in razor clams and Dungeness crabs on the Oregon and Washington coast, and it has been found in the marine food web along the Texas coast. While no clear cut human cases of amnesic shellfish poisoning have been identified outside of the original Canadian outbreaks, the clinical significance of ingestion of low levels of domoic acid (as may be occurring in persons eating shellfish and anchovies harvested from these and other areas where *Pseudonitzschia* species are present) is unknown.

X. PUFFER FISH POISONING
(TETRODOTOXIN)   ICD-9 988.0; ICD-10 T61.2

Puffer fish poisoning is characterized by onset of paresthesias, dizziness, GI symptoms and ataxia, which often progresses rapidly to paralysis and death within several hours after eating. The case-fatality rate approaches 60%. The causative toxin is tetrodotoxin, a heat stable, nonprotein neurotoxin concentrated in the skin and viscera of puffer fish, porcupine fish, ocean sunfish, and species of newts and salamanders. More than 6,000 cases have been documented, mostly in Japan. Toxicity can be avoided by not consuming any of the species of fish or amphibians that produce tetrodotoxin.

GASTRITIS CAUSED BY
HELICOBACTER PYLORI   ICD-9 535; ICD-10 K29

1. Identification—A bacterial infection causing chronic gastritis, primarily in the antrum of the stomach, and duodenal ulcer disease.

Eradication of the pathogen is associated with remission of the gastritis and duodenal ulcer disease. Gastric adenocarcinoma and gastric ulcer disease are also epidemiologically associated with *H. pylori* infection.

Diagnosis may be made from a gastric biopsy specimen through the use of culture, histology or the detection of the *H. pylori* urease by using commercially available kits. The organism requires nutrient media for growth, such as Brain-Heart Infusion Agar with added horse blood. Selective media have been developed to prevent contaminating growth when culturing gastric biopsy material. Cultures should be incubated at 37°C (98.6°F) in microaerophilic conditions for 3–5 days. Specific ^{13}C or ^{14}C urea-based breath tests may also be used and are based on the organism's extremely high urease activity. The presence of specific serum antibodies can also be measured, most commonly by ELISA.

2. Infectious agent—*Helicobacter pylori* is a gram-negative, curved, rod-shaped bacillus. Many different *Helicobacter* species have been identified in other animals; *H. cinaedi* and *H. fennelliae* have been associated with diarrhea in homosexual men.

3. Occurrence—*H. pylori* is found worldwide. Only a minority of those infected develop duodenal ulcer disease. Although individuals infected with the organism often have histologic evidence of gastritis, the vast majority are asymptomatic. Cross sectional serologic studies demonstrate increasing prevalence with increasing age. Low socioeconomic status, especially in childhood, is associated with infection. In developing countries, over 75% of adults are affected, with infection occurring predominantly in childhood. Between 20% and 50% of adults from developed countries are infected with *H. pylori*.

4. Reservoir—Humans are the only known reservoir. Most infected persons are asymptomatic, and without treatment infection is often lifelong. Isolation of *H. pylori* from nongastric sites such as oral secretions and stool have been reported but are infrequent.

5. Mode of transmission—The mode(s) of transmission has not been clearly established, but infection is almost certainly a result of ingesting organisms. Transmission is presumed to be either oral-oral and/or fecal-oral. *H. pylori* has been transmitted through incompletely decontaminated gastroscopes and pH electrodes.

6. Incubation period—Data collected from two volunteers who ingested 10^6–10^9 organisms indicated that the onset of gastritis occurred within 5–10 days. No other information about inoculum size or incubation period is available.

7. Period of communicability—Not known. Since infection may be lifelong, those infected are potentially infectious for life. It is not known whether acutely infected patients are more infectious than those with long-standing infection. There is some evidence that persons with low stomach acid may be more infectious.

8. Susceptibility and resistance—All individuals are presumed to be susceptible to infection. Although increasing age and poor socioeconomic conditions are the two most important risk factors for infection, there are scant data on an individual's susceptibility or resistance. It has been postulated that a variety of cofactors are necessary for development of disease. No protective immunity is apparent after infection.

9. Methods of control —

A. *Preventive measures:*

1) Persons living in uncrowded and clean environments are less likely to acquire *H. pylori.*
2) Complete disinfection of gastroscopes, pH electrodes and other instruments entering the stomach.

B. *Control of patient, contacts and the immediate environment:*

1) Report to local health authority: Official report not ordinarily justifiable, Class 5 (see Communicable Disease Reporting).
2) Isolation: None needed.
3) Concurrent disinfection: Of intragastric instruments.
4) Quarantine: Patients infected with *H. pylori* need not be placed in quarantine restrictions.
5) Immunization of contacts: No vaccine is available at present.
6) Investigation of contacts and source of infection: Nonproductive.
7) Specific treatment: Treatment for asymptomatic infection remains controversial. There are a wide variety of treatment regimens available for eradicating infections in individuals with symptoms of disease that are considered attributable to *H. pylori.* The most successful regimens are those that use a combination of antimicrobials for between 2 and 4 weeks. The goal of treatment is eradication rather than temporary clearance. Examples of combination therapy include: a) metronidazole and either amoxycillin or tetracycline, with a bismuth compound such as Pepto-Bismol®; or b) metronidazole and amoxycillin with a proton pump inhibitor such as omeprazole (Prilosec®). Eradication rates of up to 90% have been reported with these regimens. If infection persists, the isolates should be checked for resistance to the antibiotics. Ulcers relapse in those patients in whom eradication was not achieved. In developed countries, reinfection following eradication is infrequent. There are no data on reinfection rates in developing countries.

C. Epidemic measures: None.

D. Disaster implications: None

E. International measures: None.

GASTROENTERITIS, ACUTE VIRAL   ICD-9 008.6; ICD-10 A08

Viral gastroenteritis presents as an endemic or epidemic illness in infants, children and adults. Several viruses (rotaviruses, enteric adenoviruses, astroviruses and caliciviruses including Norwalk-like viruses) infect children in their first years of life and cause a diarrheal illness that may be severe enough to produce dehydration requiring hospitalization for rehydration. Viral agents such as Norwalk-like viruses are also common causes of epidemics of gastroenteritis among children and adults. The epidemiology, natural history and clinical expression of enteric viral infections are best understood for type A rotavirus in infants and Norwalk agent in adults.

I. ROTAVIRAL ENTERITIS   ICD-9 008.61; ICD-10 A08.0
(Sporadic viral gastroenteritis, Severe viral gastroenteritis of infants and children)

1. Identification—A sporadic, seasonal, often severe gastroenteritis of infants and young children, characterized by vomiting, fever and watery diarrhea. Rotaviral enteritis is occasionally associated with severe dehydration and death in young children. Secondary symptomatic cases among adult family contacts can occur, although subclinical infections are more common. Rotavirus infection has occasionally been found in pediatric patients with a variety of clinical manifestations, but the virus is probably coincidental rather than causative in these conditions. Rotavirus is a major cause of nosocomial diarrhea of newborns and infants. Although rotavirus diarrhea is generally more severe than acute diarrhea due to other agents, illness caused by rotavirus is not distinguishable from that caused by other enteric viruses for any individual patient.

Rotavirus can be identified in stool specimens or rectal swabs by EM, ELISA, LA and other immunologic techniques for which commercial kits are available. Evidence of rotavirus infection can be demonstrated by serologic techniques, but diagnosis is usually based on the demonstration of rotavirus antigen in stools. False-positive ELISA reactions are common in newborns; positive reactions require confirmation by an alternative test.

2. Infectious agent—The 70-nm rotavirus belongs to the Reoviridae family. Group A is common, group B is uncommon in infants but has caused large epidemics in adults in China, while group C appears to be uncommon in humans. Groups A, B, C, D, E and F occur in animals. There are 4 major, and at least 10 minor, serotypes of group A human rotavirus, based on antigenic differences in the viral protein 7 (VP7) outer capsid surface protein, the major neutralization antigen. Another outer capsid protein, designated VP4, is associated with virulence and also plays a role in virus neutralization.

3. Occurrence—In both developed and developing countries, rotavirus is associated with about one third of the hospitalized cases of diarrheal illness in infants and young children under 5 years of age. Neonatal rotaviral infections are frequent in certain settings but are usually asymptomatic. Essentially all children are infected by rotavirus in their first 2-3 years of life, with peak incidence of clinical disease in the 6- to 24-month age group. Outbreaks occur among children in day care settings. Rotavirus is more frequently associated with severe diarrhea than other enteric pathogens; in developing countries, it is responsible for an estimated 600,000-870,000 diarrheal deaths each year.

In temperate climates, rotavirus diarrhea occurs in seasonal peaks during cooler months; in tropical climates, cases occur throughout the year, often with a less pronounced peak in the cooler dry months. Infection of adults is usually subclinical, but outbreaks of clinical disease occur in geriatric units. Rotavirus occasionally causes travelers' diarrhea in adults and diarrhea in immunocompromised (including AIDS) patients, parents of children with rotavirus diarrhea and the elderly.

4. Reservoir—Probably humans. The animal viruses do not produce disease in humans; group B and group C rotaviruses identified in humans appear to be quite distinct from those found in animals.

5. Mode of transmission—Probably fecal-oral with possible contact or respiratory spread. Although rotaviruses do not effectively multiply in the respiratory tract, they may be encountered in respiratory secretions. There is some evidence that rotavirus may be present in contaminated water.

6. Incubation period—Approximately 24-72 hours.

7. Period of communicability—During the acute stage of disease, and later while virus shedding continues. Rotavirus is not usually detectable after about the eighth day of infection, although excretion of virus for 30 days or more has been reported in immunocompromised patients. Symptoms last for an average of 4-6 days.

8. Susceptibility and resistance—Susceptibility is greatest between 6 and 24 months of age. By age 3 years, most individuals have acquired rotavirus antibody. Immunocompromised individuals are at particular risk for prolonged rotavirus antigen excretion and intermittent rotavirus diarrhea. Diarrhea is uncommon in infected infants less than 3 months of age.

9. Methods of control—

A. Preventive measures

1) In August 1998, an oral, live, tetravalent, rhesus-based rotavirus vaccine (RRV-TV) was licensed for use among infants in the USA. This vaccine should be administered to infants between the ages of 6 weeks and 1 year. The recommended schedule is a 3-dose series, with doses to be administered at ages 2, 4 and 6 months. The first dose may be administered at ages 6 weeks to 6 months; subsequent doses should be administered with a minimum interval of 3 weeks between any two doses. The first dose should not be administered to children aged greater than or equal to 7 months because of an increased rate of febrile reactions after the first dose among older infants. Second and third doses should be administered before the first birthday. Routine use of this vaccine should prevent most physician visits for rotavirus gastroenteritis and at least 2/3 of hospitalizations and deaths related to rotavirus.

   Intussusception (a bowel obstruction in which one segment of bowel becomes enfolded within another segment) was identified in prelicensure trials as a potential problem associated with RRV-TV. Because of continued reports of intussusception, CDC in July 1999, pending further studies, recommended postponing administration of RRV-TV to children scheduled to receive the vaccine before November 1999; this recommendation includes those who had already begun the RRV-TV series. All cases of intussusception which occur following administration of RRV-TV should be reported to the Vaccine Adverse Events Reporting System (VAERS, 800-822-7967); www.fda.gov/cber/vaers/report.htm). The most current vaccine recommendations will be posted on the CDC immunization website: (http://www.cdc.gov/nip) and also on the CCDM website: (http://www.ccdm.org).

2) The effectiveness of other preventive measures is undetermined. Hygienic measures applicable to diseases transmitted via the fecal-oral route may not be effective in preventing transmission. The virus survives for long periods on hard surfaces, in contaminated water and on hands. It is relatively resistant to commonly used disinfectants but is inactivated by chlorine.

3) In day care, dressing infants with overalls to cover diapers has been demonstrated to decrease transmission of the infection.

4) Prevent exposure of infants and young children to individuals

with acute gastroenteritis in family and institutional (day care or hospital) settings by a high level of sanitary practices; exclusion from day care centers is not necessary.

5) Passive immunization by oral administration of IG has been shown to protect low birthweight neonates and immunocompromised children. Breast feeding does not affect infection rates, but may reduce the severity of the gastroenteritis.

B. Control of patient, contacts and the immediate environment:

1) Report to local health authority: Obligatory report of epidemics; no individual case report, Class 4 (see Comunicable Disease Reporting).

2) Isolation: Enteric precautions, with frequent handwashing by caretakers of infants.

3) Concurrent disinfection: Sanitary disposal of diapers; place overalls over diapers to prevent leakage.

4) Quarantine: None.

5) Immunization of contacts: None.

6) Investigation of contacts and source of infection: Sources of infection should be sought in certain high risk populations and cohorted antigen excreters.

7) Specific treatment: None. Oral rehydration therapy with oral glucose-electrolyte solution is adequate in most cases. Parenteral fluids are needed in cases with vascular collapse or uncontrolled vomiting (see Cholera, 9B7). Antibiotics and antimotility drugs are contraindicated.

C. Epidemic measures: Search for vehicles of transmission and source on epidemiologic bases.

D. Disaster implications: A potential problem with dislocated populations.

E. International measures: WHO Collaborating Centres.

II. EPIDEMIC VIRAL GASTROENTEROPATHY

ICD-9 008.6, 008.8; ICD-10 A08.1

(Norwalk agent disease, Norwalk-like disease, Viral gastroenteritis in adults, Epidemic viral gastroenteritis, Acute infectious nonbacterial gastroenteritis, Viral diarrhea, Epidemic diarrhea and vomiting, Winter vomiting disease, Epidemic nausea and vomiting)

1. Identification—Usually a self-limited, mild to moderate disease that often occurs in outbreaks, with clinical symptoms of nausea, vomiting, diarrhea, abdominal pain, myalgia, headache, malaise, low grade fever or a combination of these symptoms. GI symptoms characteristically last 24-48 hours.

The virus may be identified in stool by direct or immune EM or, for the Norwalk virus, by RIA or by reverse transcription polymerase chain reaction (RT-PCR). Serologic evidence of infection may be demonstrated by IEM or, for the Norwalk virus, by RIA. Diagnosis requires collection of a large volume of stool, with aliquots stored at 4°C (39°F) for EM, and at -20°C (-4°F) for antigen assays. Acute and convalescent sera (3-4-week interval) are essential to link particles observed by EM with disease etiology. RT-PCR seems to be more sensitive than IEM and can be used to examine links among widely scattered clusters of disease.

2. Infectious agents—Norwalk-like viruses are small, 27- to 32-nm, structured RNA viruses classified as caliciviruses; it has been implicated as the most common etiologic agent of the nonbacterial gastroenteritis outbreaks. Several morphologically similar but antigenically distinct viruses have been associated with gastroenteritis outbreaks; these include Hawaii, Taunton, Ditchling or W, Cockle, Parramatta, Oklahoma and Snow Mountain agents.

3. Occurrence—Worldwide and common; most often in outbreaks but also sporadically; all age groups are affected. Outbreaks in the USA are usually associated with consumption of raw shellfish. In one study in the USA, antibodies to Norwalk agent were acquired slowly; by the fifth decade of life, more than 60% of the population had antibodies. In most developing countries studied, antibodies are acquired much earlier. Seroresponse to Norwalk virus was detected in infants and young children in Bangladesh and Finland.

4. Reservoir—Humans are the only known reservoir.

5. Mode of transmission—Probably by the fecal-oral route, although contact or airborne transmission from fomites has been suggested to explain the rapid spread in hospital settings. Several recent outbreaks have strongly suggested primary community foodborne, waterborne and shellfish transmission, with secondary transmission to family members.

6. Incubation period—Usually 24-48 hours; in volunteer studies with Norwalk agent, the range was 10-50 hours.

7. Period of communicability—During acute stage of disease and up to 48 hours after Norwalk diarrhea stops.

8. Susceptibility and resistance—Susceptibility is widespread. Short-term immunity lasting up to 14 weeks has been demonstrated in volunteers after induced Norwalk illness, but long-term immunity was variable; some individuals became ill on rechallenge 27-42 months later. Levels of preexisting serum antibody to Norwalk virus did not correlate with susceptibility or resistance.

9. **Methods of control—**

   A. **Preventive measures:** Use hygienic measures applicable to diseases transmitted via fecal-oral route (see Typhoid fever, 9A). In particular, cooking shellfish and surveillance of shellfish breeding waters can prevent infection from that source.

   B. **Control of patient, contacts and the immediate environment:**

   1) Report to local health authority: Obligatory report of epidemics; no individual case report, Class 4 (see Communicable Disease Reporting).
   2) Isolation: Enteric precautions.
   3) Concurrent disinfection: None.
   4) Quarantine: None.
   5) Immunization of contacts: None.
   6) Investigation of contacts and source of infection: Search for means of spread of infection in outbreak situations.
   7) Specific treatment: Fluid and electrolyte replacement in severe cases (see Cholera, 9B7).

   C. **Epidemic measures:** Search for vehicles of transmission and source; determine course of outbreak to define the epidemiology.

   D. **Disaster implications:** A potential problem.

   E. **International measures:** None.

GIARDIASIS   ICD-9 007.1; ICD-10 A07.1
(*Giardia* enteritis)

   1. **Identification**—A protozoan infection principally of the upper small intestine; while often asymptomatic, it may be associated with a variety of intestinal symptoms, such as chronic diarrhea, steatorrhea, abdominal cramps, bloating, frequent loose and pale greasy stools, fatigue and weight loss. Malabsorption of fats or of fat soluble vitamins may occur. There is usually no extraintestinal invasion, but reactive arthritis may occur and in severe giardiasis, damage to duodenal and jejunal mucosal cells may occur.

   Diagnosis is traditionally made by identification of cysts or trophozoites in feces (to rule out the diagnosis at least three negative test results are needed) or of trophozoites in duodenal fluid (by aspiration or string test) or in mucosa obtained by small intestine biopsy; the latter may be more reliable when results of stool examination are questionable but rarely necessary. Because *Giardia* infection is usually asymptomatic, the presence of *G. lamblia* (either in stool or duodenum) does not necessarily indicate that *Giardia* is the cause of illness. Tests using EIA or direct fluorescent antibody methods for detection of antigen in the stool are commercially available and are generally more sensitive than direct microscopy.

2. Infectious agent—*Giardia lamblia (G. intestinalis, G. duodenalis)*, a flagellate protozoan.

3. Occurrence—Worldwide. Children are infected more frequently than adults. Prevalence is higher in areas of poor sanitation and in institutions with children not toilet trained, including day care centers. The prevalence of stool positivity in different areas may range between 1% and 30%, depending on the community and age group surveyed. Endemic infection in the USA, UK and Mexico most commonly occurs in July–October among children less than 5 years of age and adults 25–39 years old. It is associated with drinking water from unfiltered surface water sources or shallow wells, swimming in bodies of freshwater and having a young family member in day care. Large community outbreaks have occurred from drinking treated but unfiltered water. Smaller outbreaks have resulted from contaminated food, person to person transmission in day care centers and contaminated recreational waters including swimming and wading pools.

4. Reservoir—Humans; possibly beaver and other wild and domestic animals.

5. Mode of transmission—Person to person transmission occurs by hand to mouth transfer of cysts from the feces of an infected individual, especially in institutions and day care centers; this is probably the principal mode of spread. Anal intercourse also facilitates transmission. Localized outbreaks may occur from ingestion of cysts in fecally contaminated drinking and recreational water and less often from fecally contaminated food. Concentrations of chlorine used in routine water treatment do not kill *Giardia* cysts, especially when the water is cold; unfiltered stream and lake waters open to contamination by human and animal feces are a source of infection.

6. Incubation period—Usually 3–25 days or longer; median 7–10 days.

7. Period of communicability—Entire period of infection, often months.

8. Susceptibility and resistance—Asymptomatic carrier rate is high; infection is frequently self-limited. Pathogenicity of *G. lamblia* for humans has been established by clinical studies. Persons with AIDS may have more serious and prolonged infection.

9. Methods of control—

    A. Preventive measures:

        1) Educate families, personnel and inmates of institutions, and especially adult personnel of day care centers, in personal

hygiene and the need for handwashing before handling food, before eating and after toilet use.

2) Filter public water supplies that are exposed to human or animal fecal contamination.

3) Protect public water supplies against contamination with human and animal feces.

4) Dispose of feces in a sanitary manner.

5) Boil emergency water supplies. Less reliable is chemical treatment with hypochlorite or iodine; use 0.1 to 0.2 ml (2 to 4 drops) of household bleach or 0.5 ml of 2% tincture of iodine per liter for 20 minutes (longer if the water is cold or turbid).

B. *Control of patient, contacts and the immediate environment:*

1) Report to local health authority: Case report in selected areas, Class 3B (see Communicable Disease Reporting).

2) Isolation: Enteric precautions.

3) Concurrent disinfection: Of feces and articles soiled therewith. In communities with a modern and adequate sewage disposal system, feces can be discharged directly into sewers without preliminary disinfection. Terminal cleaning.

4) Quarantine: None.

5) Immunization of contacts: None.

6) Investigation of contacts and source of infection: Microscopic examination of feces of household members and other suspected contacts, especially those who are symptomatic.

7) Specific treatment: Metronidazole (Flagyl®) or tinidazole (not licensed in the USA) is the drug of choice. Quinacrine and albendazole are alternatives; furazolidone is available in pediatric suspension for young children and infants, paromomycin can be used during pregnancy. Drug resistance and relapses may occur with any drug.

C. *Epidemic measures:* Institute an epidemiologic investigation of clustered cases in an area or institution to determine source of infection and mode of transmission. A common vehicle, such as water, food or association with a day care center or recreational area, should be sought; institute applicable preventive or control measures. Control of person to person transmission requires special emphasis on personal cleanliness and sanitary disposal of feces.

D. *Disaster implications:* None.

E. *International measures:* None.

GONOCOCCAL INFECTIONS   ICD-9 098; ICD-10 A54

Urethritis, epididymitis, proctitis, cervicitis, Bartholinitis, pelvic inflammatory disease (salpingitis and/or endometritis) and pharyngitis of adults; vulvovaginitis of children; and conjunctivitis of the newborn and adults are localized inflammatory conditions caused by *Neisseria gonorrhoeae*. Gonococcal bacteremia results in the arthritis-dermatitis syndrome, occasionally associated with endocarditis or meningitis. Other complications include perihepatitis and the neonatal amniotic infection syndrome.

Clinically similar infections of the same genital structures may be caused by *Chlamydia trachomatis* and other infectious agents. Simultaneous infections are not uncommon.

I. GONOCOCCAL INFECTION
ICD-9 098.0–098.3; ICD-10 A54.0–A54.2

(Gonorrhea, Gonococcal urethritis, Gonococcal vulvovaginitis, Gonococcal cervicitis, Gonococcal Bartholinitis, Clap, Strain, Gleet, Dose, GC)

1. Identification—A sexually transmitted bacterial disease limited to columnar and transitional epithelium, which differs in males and females in course, severity and ease of recognition. In males, gonococcal infection presents as an acute purulent discharge from the anterior urethra with dysuria within 2-7 days after exposure. Urethritis can be documented by: a) the presence of mucopurulent or purulent discharge; and b) Gram stain of urethral discharge that demonstrates 5 or more WBC per oil immersion field. The Gram stain is highly sensitive and specific for documenting urethritis and the presence of gonococcal infection in symptomatic males. A small percentage of gonococcal infections in males is asymptomatic.

In females infection is followed by the development of mucopurulent cervicitis (MPC) which is often asymptomatic, but some women have abnormal vaginal discharge and vaginal bleeding after intercourse. In about 20% there is also uterine invasion, often at the first, second or later menstrual period, with symptoms of endometritis, salpingitis or pelvic peritonitis, and subsequent risk of infertility and ectopic pregnancy. Prepubescent girls may develop gonococcal vulvovaginitis due to direct genital contact with exudate from infected people during sexual abuse.

In females and homosexual males, pharyngeal and anorectal infections are common and usually asymptomatic, but may cause pruritus, tenesmus and discharge. Conjunctivitis occurs in newborns and rarely in adults; it may cause blindness if not rapidly and adequately treated. Septicemia may occur in 0.5%-1% of all gonococcal infections, with arthritis, skin lesions and (rarely) endocarditis and meningitis. Arthritis can produce permanent joint damage if appropriate antibiotic treatment is delayed. Death is rare except among those with endocarditis.

Nongonococcal urethritis (NGU) and nongonococcal MPC are caused by other sexually transmitted agents and seriously complicate the clinical diagnosis of gonorrhea; frequently the organisms that cause these diseases coexist with gonococcal infections. In many populations, the incidence of NGU exceeds that of gonorrhea. About 30%-40% of NGU in the USA and the UK is caused by *Chlamydia trachomatis* (see Chlamydial infections).

Diagnosis is made by Gram stain of discharges, by bacteriologic culture on selective media (e.g., modified Thayer-Martin agar) or by tests that detect gonococcal nucleic acid. Typical Gram-negative intracellular diplococci can be considered diagnostic in male urethral smears; they are nearly diagnostic when seen in smears from the cervix (specificity is 90%-97%). Culture on selective media followed by presumptive identification based on both macroscopic and microscopic examination and biochemical testing are sensitive and specific, as are nucleic acid detection tests. In cases with potential legal implications, specimens should be cultured and isolates confirmed as *N. gonorrhoeae* by two different methods.

2. Infectious agent—*Neisseria gonorrhoeae,* the gonococcus.

3. Occurrence—Common worldwide, the disease affects both genders, especially sexually active adolescents and younger adults. Prevalence is highest in communities of lower socioeconomic status. In most industrialized countries, the incidence has decreased during the past two decades. In the USA, the incidence of reported cases has declined from a peak of 468/100,000 in 1975 to 122.5/100,000 in 1997. In Canada, incidence has fallen from 216.6/100,000 in 1980 to 18.6/100,000 in 1995. However, the prevalence of resistance to penicillin and tetracycline is widespread, resistance to fluoroquinolones is rare in the US (though common in many parts of the Far East), and resistance to recommended cephalosporins has not been documented.

4. Reservoir—Strictly a human disease.

5. Mode of transmission—By contact with exudates from mucous membranes of infected people, almost always as a result of sexual activity. In children older than 1 year, it is considered an indicator of sexual abuse.

6. Incubation period—Usually 2-7 days, sometimes longer when symptoms occur.

7. Period of communicability—May extend for months in untreated individuals. Effective therapy ends communicability within hours.

8. Susceptibility and resistance—Susceptibility is general. Humoral and secretory antibodies have been demonstrated, but gonococcal strains are antigenically heterogeneous and reinfection is common. Women using an intrauterine contraceptive device have higher risks of salpingitis during the first 3 months after insertion; some people deficient in complement components are uniquely susceptible to bacteremia. Since only columnar and transitional epithelium can be infected by the gonococcus, the vaginal epithelium of adult women (which is covered by stratified squamous epithelium) is resistant to infection, whereas the prepubertal columnar or transitional vaginal epithelium is susceptible.

9. **Methods of control—**

   A. *Preventive measures:*

   1) Same as for syphilis (see Syphilis, 9A), except for measures that apply specifically to gonorrhea, i.e., the use of prophylactic agents in the eyes of the newborn (see section II, 9A2, below) and special attention (presumptive or "epi" treatment) to contacts of infected patients (see 9B6, below).

   2) Prevention is based primarily on safer sexual practices; i.e., mutual monogamy with an noninfected partner, avoiding multiple sexual partners or anonymous and other casual sex, and consistent and correct use of condoms with all partners not known to be free of infection.

   B. *Control of patient, contacts and the immediate environment:*

   1) Report to local health authority: Case report is required in all states and many countries, Class 2B (see Communicable Disease Reporting).

   2) Isolation: Contact isolation for all newborn infants and prepubertal children with gonococcal infection until effective parenteral antimicrobial therapy has been administered for 24 hours. Effective antibiotics in adequate dosage promptly render discharges noninfectious. Patients should refrain from sexual intercourse until antimicrobial therapy is completed, and, to avoid reinfection, abstain from sex with previous sexual partners until they have been treated.

   3) Concurrent disinfection: Care in disposal of discharges from lesions and contaminated articles.

   4) Quarantine: None.

   5) Immunization of contacts: Not available.

   6) Investigation of contacts and source of infection: Interview patients and notify sexual partners. Trained interviewers obtain the best results with uncooperative patients, but clinicians can motivate most patients to help arrange treatment for their partners. Sexual contacts of cases should be examined, tested and treated if their last sexual contact with the case was within 60 days before onset of symptoms or diagnosis in the case. The most recent sexual partner, even if outside these time limits, should be examined, tested and treated. All infants born to infected mothers should be given prophylactic treatment.

   7) Specific treatment: On clinical, laboratory or epidemiologic

grounds (contacts of a diagnosed case), adequate treatment must be given as follows:

For uncomplicated gonococcal infections of the cervix, rectum and urethra in adults, the recommended treatment is cefixime 400 mg orally in a single dose, ceftriaxone 125 mg IM in a single dose, ciprofloxacin 500 mg orally in a single dose or ofloxacin 400 mg orally in a single dose. Patients who can take neither cephalosporins nor quinolones may be treated with spectinomycin 2 gm IM in a single dose. Because of the high probability that patients infected with *N. gonorrhoeae* also have genital infection with *Chlamydia trachomatis,* it is recommended that azithromycin 1g PO in a single dose or doxycycline 100 mg PO twice a day for 7 days be added routinely to the treatment for uncomplicated gonorrhea.

It must be stressed that providing patients under treatment for gonorrhea with a treatment effective against genital chlamydial infection is recommended routinely because chlamydial infection is common among patients diagnosed with gonorrhea. This will also cure incubating syphilis and may inhibit emergence of antimicrobial resistant gonococci.

Gonococcal infections of the pharynx are more difficult to eradicate than infections of the urethra, cervix or rectum. Few regimens can cure such infection more than 90% of the time. Recommended regimens for this infection include ceftriaxone 125 mg IM in a single dose or ciprofloxacin 500 mg orally in a single dose.

Resistance of the gonococcus to common antimicrobials is due to the widespread presence of plasmids which carry genes for resistance. Thus, strains of gonococcus are resistant to penicillin (PPNG), tetracycline (TRNG), and the fluoroquinolones (QRNG). Resistance to third generation and extended spectrum cephalosporins (e.g., ceftriaxone and cefixime) is unknown, and resistance to spectinomycin is rare. Of great importance is resistance to fluoroquinolones (e.g., ciprofloxacin and ofloxacin). Cases of gonorrhea resistant to flouroquinolones are becoming widespread in Asia and have been reported sporadically from many parts of the world, including North America. As of 1997, flouroquinolone resistance was present in about 0.1% of isolates in the USA. Thus, a flouroquinolone regimen can still be used for infections acquired in the USA, but continued surveillance for antimicrobial resistance is essential.

Treatment failure following any of the antigonococcal regimens listed above is rare, and routine culture as a test of cure is unnecessary. If symptoms persist, reinfection is most likely, but specimens should be obtained for culture and antimicrobial susceptibility testing. Retesting of high risk patients after 1-2 months may be advisable to detect late asymptomatic reinfections.

Patients with gonococcal infections are at increased risk of HIV infection and should be offered confidential counseling and testing.

C. Epidemic measures: Intensify routine procedures, especially therapy of contacts on epidemiologic grounds.

D. Disaster implications: None.

E. International measures: See Syphilis, 9E.

II. GONOCOCCAL CONJUNCTIVITIS (NEONATORUM)   ICD-9 098.40; ICD-10 A54.3
(Gonorrheal ophthalmia neonatorum)

1. Identification—Acute redness and swelling of the conjunctiva of one or both eyes, with mucopurulent or purulent discharge in which gonococci are identifiable by microscopic and culture methods. Corneal ulcer, perforation and blindness may occur if specific treatment is not given promptly.

Gonococcal ophthalmia neonatorum is only one of a number of acute inflammatory conditions of the eye or the conjunctiva that occur within the first 3 weeks of life, collectively known as ophthalmia neonatorum. The gonococcus is the most serious, but not the most frequent infectious agent. The most common infectious cause is *Chlamydia trachomatis,* which produces inclusion conjunctivitis that tends to be less acute than gonococcal conjunctivitis and usually appears 5-14 days after birth (see Conjunctivitis, Chlamydial). Any purulent neonatal conjunctivitis should be considered gonococcal until proven otherwise.

2. Infectious agent—*Neisseria gonorrhoeae,* the gonococcus.

3. Occurrence—Varies widely according to the prevalence of maternal infection and the availability of measures to prevent eye infections in the newborn at delivery; infrequent where infant eye prophylaxis is adequate. The disease continues to be an important cause of blindness throughout the world.

4. Reservoir—Infection of the maternal cervix.

5. Mode of transmission—Contact with the infected birth canal during childbirth.

6. Incubation period—Usually 1-5 days.

7. Period of communicability—While discharge persists if untreated; for 24 hours following initiation of specific treatment.

8. Susceptibility and resistance—Susceptibility is general.

9. **Methods of control—**

A. *Preventive measures:*

1) Prevent maternal infection (see section I, 9A, above; and see Syphilis, 9A). Diagnose gonorrhea in pregnant women and treat the woman and her sexual partners. Routine culture of the cervix and rectum for gonococci should be considered during the prenatal period, especially in the third trimester where infection is prevalent.

2) Use an established effective preparation for protection of babies' eyes at birth; instillation of 1% silver nitrate aqueous solution stored in individual wax capsules remains the prophylactic agent most widely used. Erythromycin (0.5%) and tetracycline (1%) ophthalmic ointments are also effective. A study carried out in Kenya found that the incidence of ophthalmia neonatorum in infants treated with a 2.5% ophthalmic solution of povidone-iodine was significantly lower than in those treated with 1% silver nitrate or with 0.5% erythromycin ointment.

B. *Control of patient, contacts and the immediate environment:*

1) Report to local health authority: Case report is required in all states and many countries, Class 2B (see Communicable Disease Reporting).

2) Isolation: Contact isolation for the first 24 hours after administration of effective therapy. Patients should be hospitalized if possible. Bacterial cure after therapy should be confirmed by culture.

3) Concurrent disinfection: Care in disposal of conjunctival discharges and contaminated articles.

4) Quarantine: None.

5) Immunization of contacts: Not applicable; prompt treatment on diagnosis or clinical suspicion of infection.

6) Investigation of contacts and source of infection: Examination and treatment of mothers and their sexual partners.

7) Specific treatment: For gonococcal infections when antibiotic susceptibility is not known, or for penicillin resistant organisms, a single dose of ceftriaxone, 25–50 mg/kg (not to exceed 125 mg) IV or IM, is recommended. Mother and infant should also be treated for chlamydial infection.

C. *Epidemic measures:* None.

D. *Disaster implications:* None.

E. *International measures:* None.

APHA

GRANULOMA INGUINALE   ICD-9 099.2; ICD-10 A.58
(Donovanosis)

1. Identification—A chronic and progressively destructive, but poorly communicable bacterial disease of the skin and mucous membranes of the external genitalia, inguinal and anal regions. An indurated nodule or papule becomes a slowly spreading, nontender, exuberant, granulomatous, ulcerative or cicatricial process. The lesions are characteristically nonfriable, beefy red granulomas that extend peripherally with characteristic rolled edges and eventually form fibrous tissue. Lesions occur most commonly in warm, moist surfaces such as the folds between the thighs, the perianal area, the scrotum, or the vulvar labia and vagina. The genitalia are involved in close to 90% of cases, the inguinal region in close to 10%, the anal region in 5%-10% and distant sites in 1%-5%. If neglected, the process may result in extensive destruction of genital organs and spread by autoinoculation to other parts of the body.

Laboratory diagnosis is based on demonstration of intracytoplasmic rod shaped organisms (Donovan bodies) in Wright or Giemsa-stained smears of granulation tissue or by histologic examination of biopsy specimens; pathognomonic are large infected mononuclear cells filled with deeply staining Donovan bodies. Culture is difficult and unreliable. PCR and serology are available on a research basis. *Haemophilus ducreyi* should be excluded by culture on appropriate selective media.

2. Infectious agent—*Calymmatobacterium granulomatis (Donovania granulomatis)*, a gram-negative bacillus, is the presumed etiologic agent; this is not certain.

3. Occurrence—Rare in industrialized countries (rare in the USA, but cluster outbreaks occasionally occur). Endemic in tropical and subtropical areas, such as: southern India; Papua New Guinea; central and northern Australia; occasionally in Latin America; the Caribbean islands; and central, eastern and southern Africa. It is more frequently seen among males than females and among people of lower socioeconomic status; it may occur in children aged 1-4 years but is predominantly seen at ages 20-40.

4. Reservoir—Humans.

5. Mode of transmission—Presumably by direct contact with lesions during sexual activity, but in various studies only 20%-65% of sexual partners were infected, which suggests some cases are transmitted nonsexually.

6. Incubation period—Unknown; probably between 1 and 16 weeks.

7. Period of communicability—Unknown; probably for the duration of open lesions on the skin or mucous membranes.

8. Susceptibility and resistance—Susceptibility is variable; immunity apparently does not follow attack.

9. Methods of control—

A. *Preventive measures:* Except for those measures applicable only to syphilis, preventive measures are those for Syphilis, 9A. Educational programs in endemic areas should stress the importance of early diagnosis and treatment.

B. *Control of patient, contacts and the immediate environment:*

1) Report to local health authority: A reportable disease in most states and countries, Class 3B (see Communicable Disease Reporting).
2) Isolation: None; avoid close personal contact until lesions are healed.
3) Concurrent disinfection: Care in disposal of discharges from lesions and articles soiled therewith.
4) Quarantine: None.
5) Immunization of contacts: Not applicable; prompt treatment upon recognition or clinical suspicion of infection.
6) Investigation of contacts and source of infection: Examination of sexual contacts.
7) Specific treatment: Erythromycin, TMP-SMX and doxycycline have been reported to be effective but drug resistant strains of the organism occur. Therapy is continued for 3 weeks or until the lesions have resolved; recurrence is not rare but usually responds to a second course of therapy unless malignancy is present. Single dose therapy with ceftriaxone IM or ciprofloxacin PO anecdotally reported to be effective.

C. *Epidemic measures:* Not applicable.

D. *Disaster implications:* None.

E. *International measures:* See Syphilis, 9E.

HANTAVIRAL DISEASES

Hantaviruses infect rodents worldwide; several species have been known for some time to infect humans with varying severity but with their primary effect on the vascular endothelium, which results in increased vascular permeability, hypotensive shock and hemorrhagic manifestations. Many of these agents have been isolated from rodents but are not associated with any human cases. In 1993, an outbreak of disease caused by a previously unrecognized hantavirus occurred in the USA; the principal target organ was not the kidney but the lung. Because they are caused by related etiologic organisms and have similar epidemiologic features and similar pathologic characteristics (a febrile prodrome, thrombocytopenia, leukocytosis and capillary leakage), both syndromes are presented under the rubric of Hantaviral diseases.

I. HEMORRHAGIC FEVER WITH
RENAL SYNDROME   ICD-9 078.6; ICD-10 A98.5
(Epidemic hemorrhagic fever, Korean hemorrhagic fever, Nephropathia epidemica, Hemorrhagic nephrosonephritis, HFRS)

1. Identification—An acute zoonotic viral disease characterized by the abrupt onset of fever, lower back pain, varying degrees of hemorrhagic manifestations and renal involvement. Severe illness is associated with Hantaan virus (primarily in Asia) and Dobrava (in the Balkans). Disease is characterized by five clinical phases which frequently overlap: febrile, hypotensive, oliguric, diuretic and convalescent. High fever, headache, malaise and anorexia, followed by severe abdominal or lower back pain, often accompanied by nausea and vomiting, facial flushing, petechiae and conjunctival injection, characterize the febrile phase which lasts 3–7 days. The hypotensive phase lasts from several hours to 3 days and is characterized by defervescence and abrupt onset of hypotension, which may progress to shock and more apparent hemorrhagic manifestations. Blood pressure returns to normal or is high in the oliguric phase, which lasts 3–7 days; nausea and vomiting may persist, severe hemorrhage may occur and urinary output falls dramatically.

The majority of deaths (the case-fatality rate is variable, but generally ranges from 5%–15%) occur during the hypotensive and oliguric phases. Diuresis heralds the onset of recovery in most cases, with polyuria of 3–6 L per day. Convalescence takes weeks to months.

A less severe illness (case-fatality rate less than 1%) caused by Puumala virus and referred to as nephropathia epidemica is predominant in Europe. Infections caused by Seoul virus, carried by brown or Norway rats, are also clinically milder; severe disease may occur with this virus strain, however. Distinct clinical phases are less obvious with these infections.

Diagnosis is made by demonstration of specific antibodies using ELISA or IFA; most patients have IgM antibodies at the time of hospitalization. The presence of proteinuria, leukocytosis, hemoconcentration, thrombocytopenia and elevated blood urea nitrogen supports the diagnosis. Hantaviruses can be propagated in a limited range of cell cultures and laboratory rats and mice, mainly for research purposes. Leptospirosis and rickettsioses must be considered in the differential diagnosis.

2. Infectious agent—Hantaviruses (a genus of the family Bunyaviridae); 3-segmented RNA viruses with spherical to oval particles, 95–110 nm in diameter. More than 25 antigenically distinguishable viral species exist, each associated primarily with a single rodent species. Hantaan virus is found principally in Asia and less often in Europe, Dobrava (Belgrade) virus in the former Yugoslavia, Puumala virus in Europe and Seoul virus worldwide (see section 4, below).

3. Occurrence—Prior to World War II, Japanese and Soviet authors described HFRS in Manchuria along the Amur River. In 1951, it was recognized in Korea among United Nations troops and since then in both military personnel and civilians. Hantaan virus disease is considered a major public health problem in China and South Korea. The disease is seasonal, with most cases seen in late fall and early winter, and occurs primarily among rural populations. In the Balkans, a severe form of the disease, due to Dobrava virus, affects a few hundred people annually, with mortality rates at least as high as those in Asia. Most cases there are seen during spring and early summer.

Nephropathia epidemica, due to Puumala virus, is found in most European countries, including Russia, west of the Ural mountains, and the Balkans. It is often seen in summer and in the fall and early winter. Seasonal occupational and recreational activities probably influence the risk of exposure, as does the effect of climate cycles and other ecologic factors on rodent population densities. HFRS among medical research personnel and animal handlers in Asia and Europe has been traced to laboratory rats infected with Seoul virus. Seoul virus has been identified in rats captured in major cities worldwide, including Thailand, USA, Brazil and Argentina, but there has been a regular association with human disease only in Asia. With the availability of newer diagnostic techniques, there is an increasing recognition of hantaviruses and hantaviral infections globally.

4. Reservoir—Field rodents (*Apodemus* spp. for Hantaan and Dobrava-Belgrade viruses in Asia and the Balkans; *Clethrionomys* spp. for Puumala in Europe; *Rattus* spp. for Seoul virus worldwide). Humans are an accidental host.

5. Mode of transmission—Aerosol transmission from rodent excreta is presumed (aerosol infectivity has been demonstrated experimentally), though it may not explain all human cases or all forms of transmission between rodents. Virus is present in urine, feces and saliva of persistently infected asymptomatic rodents; the highest virus concentration is found in the lungs. Nosocomial transmission of hantaviruses has been documented but is thought to be extremely rare.

6. Incubation period—As short as a few days, or as long as nearly 2 months, but usually 2–4 weeks.

7. Period of communicability—Not well defiined. Person to person transmission is rare.

8. Susceptibility and resistance—Persons without serologic evidence of past infection appear to be uniformly susceptible. Inapparent infections occur; second attacks have not been documented.

9. Methods of control—

A. *Preventive measures:*

1) Exclude and prevent rodent access to houses and other buildings.
2) Store human and animal food under rodent proof conditions.
3) Disinfect rodent contaminated areas by spraying a disinfectant (such as dilute bleach) solution prior to cleaning. Do not sweep or vacuum rat contaminated areas; use a wet mop or towels moistened with disinfectant. Avoid inhalation of dust by using approved respirators when cleaning previously unoccupied areas.
4) Trap and dispose of rodents using suitable precautions. Live trapping is not recommended.
5) In enzootic areas, minimize exposure to wild rodents and their excreta.
6) Laboratory rodent colonies, particularly *Rattus norvegicus,* should be tested to ensure freedom from asymptomatic hantavirus infection.

B. *Control of patient, contacts and the immediate environment:*

1) Report to local health authority: In selected endemic countries where reporting is required, Class 3A (see Communicable Disease Reporting).
2) Isolation: None.
3) Concurrent disinfection: None.
4) Quarantine: None.
5) Immunization of contacts: None.
6) Investigation of contacts and source of infection: Exterminate rodents in and around the households if feasible.
7) Specific treatment: Bed rest and early hospitalization are critical. Jostling and the effect of lowered atmospheric pressures during airborne evacuation of cases can be deleterious to critically ill hantavirus infected patients. Appropriate and careful attention to fluid management is important to avoid overload and minimize the effects of shock and renal failure. Dialysis is often required. Ribavirin IV as early as possible during the first few days of illness has shown benefit.

C. *Epidemic measures:* Rodent control; surveillance for hantavirus infections in wild rodents. Laboratory associated outbreaks call for evaluation of the associated rodents and, if positive, elimination of the rodents and thorough disinfection.

D. *Disaster implications:* Natural disasters and wars often result in increased numbers of rodents and rodent contact with humans.

E. *International measures:* Control transport of exotic reservoir rodents.

II. HANTAVIRUS PULMONARY
SYNDROME   ICD-9 480.8; ICD-10 J12.8
(Hantavirus adult respiratory distress syndrome, Hantavirus cardiopulmonary syndrome)

1. Identification—An acute zoonotic viral disease characterized by fever, myalgias and GI complaints followed by the abrupt onset of respiratory distress and hypotension. The illness progresses rapidly to severe respiratory failure and shock. An elevated hematocrit, hypoalbuminemia and thrombocytopenia are found in most cases. The crude mortality rate is approximately 40%–50%; it was 43% of the first 217 cases identified. In survivors, the recovery from acute illness is rapid, but full convalescence may require weeks to months. Restoration of normal lung function generally occurs, but pulmonary function abnormalities may persist in some individuals. Renal and hemorrhagic manifestations are usually conspicuously absent except in some severe cases.

Diagnosis is made by the demonstration of specific IgM antibodies by using ELISA, Western blot or strip immunoblot techniques. Most patients have IgM antibodies at the time of hospitalization. PCR analysis of autopsy or biopsy tissues and immunohistochemistry are also established diagnostic techniques in specialized laboratories.

2. Infectious agents—Multiple hantaviruses have been identified in the Americas: Sin Nombre virus is the agent responsible for the 1993 epidemic in southwest USA and most of the other cases identified in North America. Other strains associated with human disease include Black Creek Canal and Bayou viruses (southeastern USA), New York-1 and Monongahela viruses (eastern USA), Andes virus (Argentina, Chile), Laguna Negra virus (Paraguay, Bolivia) and Juquitiba virus (Brazil).

3. Occurrence—The disease was first recognized in the spring and summer of 1993 in the Four Corners area of New Mexico and Arizona, principally among resident Native American populations. Since then, cases have been confirmed in many western states and Canada. Sporadic cases have occurred in eastern regions of the USA. Sporadic cases and several outbreaks have been reported in South American countries (e.g., Argentina, Bolivia, Paraguay, Chile, Brazil). The disease is not restricted to any ethnic group. Incidence appears to coincide with the geographic distribution, population density and proportion of carrier rodents that are infected.

4. Reservoir—The major reservoir of Sin Nombre virus appears to be the deer mouse, *Peromyscus maniculatus*. Antibodies have also been found in other *Peromyscus* species, pack rats, the chipmunk and other rodents. Other hantavirus strains identified thus far have been associated predominantly with other sigmodontine rodent species.

5. Mode of transmission—As with hantavirus caused hemorrhagic fever with renal syndrome, aerosol transmission from rodent excreta is presumed. The natural history of viral infections of host rodents has not been characterized. Indoor exposures in closed, poorly ventilated homes, vehicles and outbuildings with visible rodent infestation are especially prominent.

6. Incubation period—Has not been completely defined but is thought to be approximately 2 weeks with a possibile range of a few days to 6 weeks.

7. Period of communicability— Person to person spread of hantaviruses in the USA has not occurred. However, person to person transmission has been reported during an outbreak in Argentina.

8. Susceptibility and resistance—All persons without prior infection are presumed to be susceptible. No inapparent infections have been documented to date, but milder infections without frank pulmonary edema have been seen. No second cases have been identified, but the protection and duration of immunity conferred by previous infection is unknown.

9. Methods of control—

   A. Preventive measures: See section I, 9A, above.

   B. Control of patient, contacts and the immediate environment:

   1), 2), 3), 4), 5) and 6) Report to local health authority, Isolation, Concurrent disinfection, Quarantine, Immunization of contacts and Investigation of contacts and source of infection— See section I, 9B1 through 9B6, above.
   7) Specific treatment: Provide respiratory intensive care management, carefully avoid overhydration that might lead to exacerbation of pulmonary edema. Use cardiotonic drugs and pressors early under careful monitoring to prevent shock. Strictly avoid hypoxia, particularly if transfer is contemplated. Ribavirin is investigational and of no proven benefit. Extracorporeal membrane oxygenation has been used with some success.

   C. Epidemic measures: Public education regarding rodent avoidance and rodent control in homes is desirable in endemic situations and should be intensified during epidemics. Monitoring of rodent numbers and infection rates is desirable but as yet of unproven value. See section I, 9C, above.

D. Disaster implications: As in section I, 9D, above.

E. International measures: Control transport of exotic reservoir rodents.

HENDRA AND NIPAH VIRAL
DISEASES   ICD-9 078.8; ICD-10 B33.8

1. Identification—These are newly recognized zoonotic viral diseases manifested primarily as encephalitis; they are named for the locations in Australia and Malaysia where the first human isolates were confirmed in 1994 and 1999, respectively. The full course of these diseases are still unknown, but symptoms range in serverity from mild to coma and death and include fever and headaches of varying severity, sore throat, dizziness, drowsiness, and disorientation. Pneumonitis was prominent in the initial Hendra cases, one of which was fatal. Coma usually leads to death in 3–30 days. The case fatality rate for clinical cases is about 50%; subclinical infections may be common.

Serological diagnosis by detection of IgM and IgG by use of an antibody capture ELISA or serum neutralization is available. Diagnosis is confirmed by virus isolation from infected tissues.

2. Infectious agent—Hendra and Nipah viruses are members of the Paramyxoviridae family.

3. Occurrence—Hendra virus caused disease in horses in Queensland, Australia. Three human cases in 1994 and 1995 had close contact with sick horses. Nipah virus affected swine in the pig farming provinces of Perak, Negeri Sembilan, and Selangor in Malaysia. The first human case is believed to have occurred in 1996, although the majority of cases have been identified in late 1998 and early 1999, with 100 confirmed deaths as of mid 1999.

4. Reservoir—Fruit bats for Hendra virus and by analogy, Nipah virus may have a similar reservoir. Hendra virus in horses and Nipah virus in domestic swine cause an acute febrile illness, which may lead to severe respiratory and CNS involvement leading to death. Dogs infected with Nipah virus show a distemper-like manifestation but an epidemiologic role has not been defined. Nipah seropositive horses have been identified, but their role is also undetermined. Nipah serologic testing of cats, goats, cattle, rats, and birds has, as of mid 1999, not been completed.

5. Mode of transmission—Evidence indicates transmission primarily through direct contact with infected horses (Hendra) or swine (Nipah) or contaminated tissues. Oral and nasal routes are suspected in some cases but not confirmed. There is no evidence for person to person transmission.

6. Incubation period—From 4 to 18 days; exceptionally, with Hendra virus, up to 3 months.

7. Period of communicability—unknown

8. Susceptibility and resistance—undetermined

9. Methods of control

    A. Preventive measures: Health education to inform the public about appropriate preventive measures to be taken and the need to avoid fruit bats.

    B. Control of patient, contacts, and the immediate environment:

        1. Report to local authority: Case report should be obligatory wherever these diseases occur; class 2A (see Communicable Disease Reporting).
        2. Isolation: Of infected horses or swine; no evidence for person to person transmission.
        3. Concurrent disinfection: Slaughter infected horses or swine with burial or incineration of carcasses under government supervision.
        4. Quarantine: Restrict movement of horses or pigs from infected farms to other areas.
        5. Immunization of contacts: None.
        6. Investigation of contacts and source of infection: Search for missed cases.
        7. Specific treatment: None.

    C. Epidemic measures:

        1. Proper precautions by animal handlers such as protective clothing, boots, gloves, gowns, goggles and face shields; and washing of hands and body parts with soap before leaving the pig farms.
        2. Slaughter infected horses or swine with burial or incineration of carcasses under government supervision.
        3. Restrict movement of horses or pigs from infected farms to other areas.

D. Disaster implications: None

E. International measures:
Prohibit exportation of horses or pigs and horse/pig products from infected areas.

HEPATITIS, VIRAL ICD-9 070; ICD-10 B15–B19

Several distinct infections are grouped as the viral hepatitides; they are primarily hepatatrophic and have similar clinical presentations, but differ in etiology and in some epidemiologic, immunologic, clinical and pathologic characteristics. Their prevention and control vary greatly. Each will therefore be presented in a separate section.

I. VIRAL HEPATITIS A ICD-9 070.1; ICD-10 B15
(Infectious hepatitis, Epidemic hepatitis, Epidemic jaundice, Catarrhal jaundice, Type A hepatitis, HA)

1. Identification—Onset of illness in adults in nonendemic areas is usually abrupt with fever, malaise, anorexia, nausea and abdominal discomfort, followed within a few days by jaundice. In most developing countries, infection occurs in childhood asymptomatically or with a mild illness. These latter infections may be detectable only through laboratory tests of liver function. The disease varies in clinical severity from a mild illness lasting 1–2 weeks to a severely disabling disease lasting several months. Prolonged, relapsing hepatitis for up to 1 year occurs in 15% of cases; no chronic infection is known to occur. Convalescence is often prolonged. In general, severity of illness increases with age, but complete recovery without sequelae or recurrences is the rule. Reported mortality ranges from 0.1%–0.3%; however, mortality is elevated to 1.8% for adults over 50; persons with chronic liver disease have an elevated risk of death from fulminant hepatitis A. Generally, hepatitis A is considered a disease with a relatively low case-fatality rate.

Diagnosis is established by the demonstration of IgM antibodies against hepatitis A virus (IgM anti-HAV) in the serum of acutely ill or recently ill patients. IgM anti-HAV becomes detectable 5–10 days after exposure. Diagnosis may also be made by a fourfold or greater rise in specific antibodies in paired sera; antibody can be detected by RIA or ELISA. (Assay kits for the detection of IgM and total antibodies to the virus are available commercially.) If laboratory tests are not available, epidemiologic evidence may provide support for the diagnosis.

2. Infectious agent—Hepatitis A virus (HAV), a 27-nm picornavirus (i.e., a positive-strand RNA virus). It has been classified as *Hepatovirus,* a member of the family Picornaviridae.

3. Occurrence—Worldwide, sporadic and epidemic, with a tendency in the past to cyclic recurrences. In developing countries, adults are usually immune and epidemics of HA are uncommon. However, improved sanitation in many parts of the world is leaving many young adults susceptible, and the frequency of outbreaks is increasing. In developed countries, disease transmission is frequent among household and sexual contacts of acute cases, and also occurs sporadically in day care centers with diapered children, among travelers to countries where the disease is endemic, among injecting drug users and among men who have sex with men. Where environmental sanitation is poor, infection is common and occurs at an early age. In the USA, 33% of the general population has serologic evidence of prior HAV infection.

Epidemics often evolve slowly in developed countries, involve wide geographic areas and last many months; common source epidemics may evolve rapidly. In the USA, nationwide epidemic cycles have been observed with peaks in 1961, 1971 and 1989. During some outbreaks, day care center employees or attendees, men with multiple male sex partners and injecting drug users may be at higher risk than the general population. However, in close to half of cases, no source of infection is identified. The disease is most common among school aged children and young adults. In recent years, community wide outbreaks have accounted for most disease transmission, although common source outbreaks due to food contaminated by food handlers and contaminated produce continue to occur. Outbreaks have been reported among susceptible persons working with nonhuman primates raised in the wild.

4. Reservoir—Humans, rarely chimpanzees and certain other nonhuman primates.

5. Mode of transmission—Person to person by the fecal-oral route. The infectious agent is found in feces, reaches peak levels the week or two before onset of symptoms and diminishes rapidly after liver dysfunction or symptoms appear, which is concurrent with the appearance of circulating antibodies to HAV.

Common source outbreaks have been related to contaminated water; food contaminated by infected food handlers, including foods that are not cooked or are handled after cooking; raw or undercooked molluscs harvested from contaminated waters; and contaminated produce such as lettuce and strawberries. A number of outbreaks in the USA and Europe have been associated with injecting and noninjecting drug use. Although rare, instances of transmission by transfusion of blood and clotting factor concentrates obtained from viremic donors during the incubation period have been reported.

6. Incubation period—Fifteen to 50 days, average 28–30 days.

7. Period of communicability—Studies of transmission in humans and epidemiologic evidence indicate that maximum infectivity occurs during the latter half of the incubation period and continues for a few days after onset of jaundice (or during peak aminotransferase activity in anicteric cases). Most cases are probably noninfectious after the first week of jaundice, although prolonged viral excretion (up to 6 months) has been documented in infants and children. Chronic shedding of HAV in feces does not occur.

8. Susceptibility and resistance—Susceptibility is general. Low incidence of manifest disease in infants and preschool children suggests that mild and anicteric infections are common. Homologous immunity after infection probably lasts for life.

9. Methods of control—

 A. Preventive measures:

   1) Educate the public about good sanitation and personal hygiene, with special emphasis on careful handwashing and sanitary disposal of feces.
   2) Provide proper water treatment and distribution systems and sewage disposal.
   3) Two inactivated hepatitis A vaccines are now available in the USA for preexposure immunization of persons 2 years of age and older. These vaccines have been shown to be safe, immunogenic and efficacious in clinical trials. Protection against clinical hepatitis A may begin in some persons as soon as 14–21 days after a single dose of vaccine, and nearly all have protective levels of antibody by 30 days after receiving the first dose of vaccine. A second dose is felt to be necessary for long term protection. The vaccines are not licensed in the USA for persons less than 2 years old; the optimum dose and schedule to overcome interference with passively acquired maternal antibody has not been determined.
   4) In the USA, recommendations for the use of hepatitis A vaccine have been developed and include routine preexposure immunization of the following persons: a) persons at increased risk for HAV infection or its consequences (persons with chronic liver disease or clotting factor disorders, men who have sex with men, injecting drug users, persons traveling to countries where HAV is endemic, persons who work with HAV infected primates or with HAV in research laboratory settings); b) children living in communities that have consistently elevated rates of hepatitis A.

   Close personal contacts (e.g., household, sexual) of hepatitis A patients should be given postexposure prophylaxis with IG within 2 weeks of last exposure. If indicated, hepatitis A vaccine can be given simultaneously at a separate injection site. The efficacy of hepatitis A vaccine alone compared with IG for post exposure prophylaxis has not been determined.

5) Management of day care centers should stress measures to minimize the possibility of fecal-oral transmission, including thorough handwashing after every diaper change and before eating. If one or more hepatitis A cases are associated with a center, or if cases are recognized in two or more households of center attendees, IG should be administered to the staff and attendees. IG administration should be considered for family contacts of children in diapers attending centers where outbreaks occur and cases are recognized in three or more families. If indicated as part of a routine immunization or community wide outbreak control program, hepatitis A immunization of attendees and staff in the involved and also possibly uninvolved centers should also be considered.

6) All travelers to intermediate or highly endemic areas, including Africa, the Middle East, Asia, eastern Europe and Central and South America, should be given IG or hepatitis A vaccine prior to departure. Travelers can be assumed to be protected 4 weeks after receiving the initial vaccine dose. Hepatitis A vaccine is preferred for people who plan to travel repeatedly or reside for long periods in areas of intermediate or high endemicity of HAV infection. If IG is used, IG in a single dose of 0.02 ml/kg, or 2 ml for adults, is recommended for expected exposures of up to 3 months; for more prolonged exposures, 0.06 ml/kg or 5 ml should be given and repeated every 4–6 months if exposure continues.

7) Hepatitis A vaccine should be considered for other populations with increased risk of hepatitis A infection, such as men who have sex with men, injecting drug users and persons who work with HAV-infected primates or with HAV in a research laboratory setting.

8) Oysters, clams and other shellfish from contaminated areas should be heated to a temperature of 85°–90°C (185°–194°F) for 4 minutes or steamed for 90 seconds before eating.

B. *Control of patient, contacts and the immediate environment:*

1) Report to local health authority: Obligatory in all states of the USA and in Canada, although not now required in many countries; Class 2A (see Communicable Disease Reporting).

2) Isolation: For proven hepatitis A, enteric precautions during the first 2 weeks of illness, but no more than 1 week after onset of jaundice; the exception is an outbreak in the neonatal intensive care setting, where prolonged enteric precautions should be considered.

3) Concurrent disinfection: Sanitary disposal of feces, urine and blood.

4) Quarantine: None.

5) Immunization of contacts: Passive immunization with IG (IM), 0.02 ml/kg of body weight, should be given as soon as possible after exposure, but within 2 weeks. Because hepatitis A cannot be reliably diagnosed on clinical presentation alone, serologic confirmation of HAV infection in index patients by IgM anti-HAV testing should be obtained before postexposure treatment of contacts. Persons who have received one dose of hepatitis A vaccine at least 1 month prior to exposure do not need IG.

IG is not indicated for contacts in the usual office, school or factory setting. IG should be administered to previously unimmunized persons in the situations listed below. If indicated, hepatitis A vaccine can be given concurrently at a separate injection site: a) close personal contacts, including household, sexual, drug using and other close personal contacts; b) day care centers if one or more cases of hepatitis A are recognized in children or employees or if cases are recognized in two or more households of center attendees. IG need be given only to classroom contacts of an index case in centers that do not provide care to children in diapers; c) in a common source outbreak, if a food handler is diagnosed with hepatitis A, IG should be administered to other food handlers in the same establishment. IG is usually not offered to patrons; it may be considered if i) the food handlers were involved in the preparations of foods that were not heated; ii) deficiencies in personal hygiene are noted or the food handler has had diarrhea; and iii) the IG can be given within 2 weeks after last exposure.

6) Investigation of contacts and source of infection: Search for missed cases and maintain surveillance of contacts in the patient's household or, in a common source outbreak, people exposed to the same risk.

7) Specific treatment: None.

C. Epidemic measures:

1) Determine mode of transmission by epidemiologic investigation, whether person-to-person or by common vehicle, and identify the population exposed. Eliminate any common sources of infection.

2) Effective use of hepatitis A vaccine in comunity wide outbreak situations is associated with several factors, including identification of an appropriate target group for immunization, initiation of immunization early in the course of the outbreak

and rapid achievement of high (approximately 70% or greater) first-dose vaccine coverage levels. Specific outbreak control measures should be tailored to the characteristics of hepatitis A epidemiology and of the existing hepatitis A immunization program, if any, in the community. Possible strategies include: a) in communities with ongoing programs of routine hepatitis A immunization of young children accelerate immunization of older children who have not previously received vaccine; b) In other outbreak settings, such as day care, hospitals, institutions and schools, routine use of hepatitis A vaccine is not believed to be warranted; and c) target immunization of groups or areas (e.g., age groups, risk groups, census tracts) determined to have the highest disease rates, based on local surveillance and epidemiologic data. However, these immunization programs may reduce disease incidence only in the group(s) targeted for imunization; the effectiveness of this strategy in terminating the outbreak in the entire community has not been determined. Evaluation of effectiveness of this strategy should be part of the outbreak response. Use of IG continues to be the central strategy of outbreak control in these settings. However, if indicated as part of a routine immunization or community wide outbreak control program, concomitant hepatitis A immunization can be considered.

3) Make special efforts to improve sanitary and hygienic practices to eliminate fecal contamination of foods and water.

4) Focal outbreaks in institutions may warrant mass prophylaxis with IG and consideration of hepatitis A vaccine use.

D. Disaster implications: A potential problem in a large collection of people with crowding, inadequate sanitation and water supplies; if cases occur, increased efforts should be exerted to improve sanitation and safety of water supplies. Mass administration of IG is not a substitute for environmental measures.

E. International measures: None.

II. VIRAL HEPATITIS B   ICD-9 070.3; ICD-10 B16
(Type B hepatitis, Serum hepatitis, Homologous serum jaundice, Australia antigen hepatitis, HB)

1. Identification—Only a small proportion of acute hepatitis B virus (HBV) infections may be clinically recognized; less than 10% of children and 30%–50% of adults with acute hepatitis B virus (HBV) infection will have icteric disease. In those with clinical illness, the onset is usually insidious, with anorexia, vague abdominal discomfort, nausea and vomiting, sometimes arthralgias and rash, often progressing to jaundice. Fever may be absent or mild. Severity ranges from inapparent cases detectable only by liver function tests to fulminating, fatal cases of acute hepatic necrosis. The case-fatality rate in hospitalized patients is about 1%; higher in those over 40 years of age. Fulminant HBV infection is also seen in pregnancy and among newborns of infected mothers.

Chronic HBV infection is found in 0.5% of adults in North America and in 0.1%–20% of people from other parts of the world. After acute HBV infection, the risk of developing chronic infection varies inversely with age; chronic HBV infection occurs among about 90% of infants infected at birth, 20%–50% of children infected at 1–5 years of age, and about 1%–10% of persons infected as older children and adults. Chronic HBV infection is also common in persons with immunodeficiency. Persons with chronic infection may or may not have a history of clinical hepatitis. About one third have an elevated aminotransferase; biopsy findings range from normal to chronic active hepatitis, with or without cirrhosis. The prognosis of liver disease in such individuals is variable. An estimated 15%–25% of persons with chronic HBV infection will die prematurely of either cirrhosis or hepatocellular carcinoma. HBV may be the cause of up to 80% of all cases of hepatocellular carcinoma worldwide, second only to tobacco among known human carcinogens.

Diagnosis is confirmed by demonstration in sera of specific antigens and/or antibodies. Three clinically useful antigen-antibody systems have been identified for hepatitis B: 1) hepatitis B surface antigen (HBsAg) and antibody to HBsAg (anti-HBs); 2) hepatitis B core antigen (HBcAg) and antibody to HBcAg (anti-HBc); and 3) hepatitis B *e* antigen (HBeAg) and antibody to HBeAg (anti-HBe). Commercial kits (RIA and ELISA) are available for all markers except HBcAg. HBsAg can be detected in the serum from several weeks before onset of symptoms to days, weeks or months after onset; it persists in chronic infections. Anti-HBc appears at the onset of illness and persists indefinitely. Demonstration of anti-HBc in serum indicates HBV infection, current or past; IgM anti-HBc is present in high titer during acute infection and usually disappears within 6 months, although it can persist in some cases of chronic hepatitis; thus, this test may reliably diagnose acute HBV infection. HBsAg is present in serum during acute infections and persists in chronic infections. The presence of HBsAg indicates that the person is potentially infectious. The presence of HBeAg is associated with relatively high infectivity.

2. **Infectious agent**—The hepatitis B virus (HBV), a hepadnavirus, is a 42-nm partially double-stranded DNA virus composed of a 27-nm nucleocapsid core (HBcAg), surrounded by an outer lipoprotein coat containing the surface antigen (HBsAg). HBsAg is antigenically heterogeneous, with a common antigen designated *a*, and two pairs of mutually exclusive antigens, *d* and *y*, and *w* (including several subdeterminants) and *r*, resulting in 4 major subtypes: *adw, ayw, adr* and *ayr*. The distribution of subtypes varies geographically; because of the common *a* determinant, protection against one subtype appears to confer protection against the

other subtypes, and no differences in clinical features have been related to subtype.

3. Occurrence—Worldwide; endemic with little seasonal variation. WHO estimates that more than 2 billion persons (including 350 million who are chronically infected) have been infected with HBV. Each year about a million persons die as a result of HBV infections and over 4 million new acute clinical cases occur. In countries where HBV is highly endemic (HBsAg prevalence 8% or higher), most infections occur during infancy and early childhood. In countries where HBV is intermediately endemic (HBsAg prevalence ranges from 2%–7%), infections occur commonly in all age groups, although the high rate of chronic infection is primarily maintained by transmission during infancy and early childhood. In countries with low endemicity (HBsAg prevalence less than 2%), most infections occur in young adults, especially among persons who belong to known risk groups. However, even in countries with low HBV endemicity, a high proportion of chronic infections may be acquired during childhood because the development of chronic infection is age dependent. Most of these infections would not be prevented by perinatal hepatitis B prevention programs because they occur among children of HBsAg negative mothers.

In the USA and Canada, serologic evidence of previous infection varies depending on age and socioeconomic class. Overall, 5% of the adult US population has anti-HBc, and 0.5% are HBsAg positive. Exposure to HBV may be common in certain high risk groups, including injecting drug users, heterosexuals with multiple partners, men who have sex with men, household contacts and sex partners of HBV infected persons, health care and public safety workers who have exposure to blood in the workplace, clients and staff in institutions for the developmentally disabled, hemodialysis patients and inmates of correctional facilities.

In the past, recipients of blood products were at high risk. In the many countries in which pretransfusion screening of blood for HBsAg has been required, and where pooled blood clotting factors (especially antihemophilic factor) are processed to destroy the virus, this risk has been virtually eliminated. However, this risk is still present in many developing countries. Contaminated and inadequately sterilized syringes and needles have resulted in outbreaks of hepatitis B among patients in clinics and physicians' offices; this has been a major mode of transmission worldwide. Occasionally, outbreaks have been traced to tattoo parlors and acupuncturists. Rarely, transmission to patients from HBsAg positive health care workers has been documented. A number of outbreaks occurred among patients in dialysis centers in the USA due to failure to adhere to recommended infection control practices for preventing transmission of HBV and other bloodborne pathogens in these settings.

4. Reservoir—Humans. Chimpanzees are susceptible, but an animal reservoir in nature has not been recognized. Closely related hepadnaviruses have been found in woodchucks, ducks and other animals; none cause disease in humans.

5. Mode of transmission—Body substances capable of transmitting HBV include: blood and blood products; saliva; cerebrospinal fluid; peritoneal, pleural, pericardial and synovial fluid; amniotic fluid; semen and vaginal secretions and any other body fluid containing blood; and unfixed tissues and organs. The presence of *e* antigen or viral DNA indicates high virus titer and higher infectivity of these fluids.

Transmission occurs by percutaneous (IV, IM, SC or intradermal) and permucosal exposure to infective body fluids. Because HBV is stable on environmental surfaces for at least 7 days, indirect inoculation of HBV can also occur via inanimate objects. Fecal-oral or vectorborne transmission has not been demonstrated.

Major modes of HBV transmission include sexual or household contact with an infected person, perinatal transmission from mother to infant, injecting drug use and nosocomial exposure. Sexual transmission from infected men to women is about three times more efficient than that from infected women to men. Anal intercourse, insertive and receptive, is associated with an increased risk of infection. Transmission of HBV in households primarily occurs from child to child. Communally used razors and toothbrushes have been implicated as occasional vehicles of HBV transmission in this setting. Perinatal transmission is common, especially when HBV infected mothers are also HBeAg positive. The rate of transmission from HBsAg positive, HBeAg positive mothers is more than 70%, and the rate of transmission from HBsAg positive, HBeAg negative mothers is less than 10%. Transmission associated with injecting drug use can occur though transfer of HBV infected blood by sharing syringes and needles either directly or through contamination of drug preparation equipment. Nosocomial exposures that have resulted in HBV transmission include transfusion of blood or blood products, hemodialysis, acupuncture and needlesticks or other injuries from sharp instruments sustained by hospital personnel. IG, heat treated plasma protein fraction, albumin and fibrinolysin are considered safe.

6. Incubation period—Usually 45-180 days, average 60-90 days. As short as 2 weeks to the appearance of HBsAg, and rarely as long as 6-9 months; the variation is related in part to the amount of virus in the inoculum, the mode of transmission and host factors.

7. Period of communicability—All persons who are HBsAg positive are potentially infectious. Blood from experimentally inoculated volunteers has been shown to be infective many weeks before the onset of first symptoms and to remain infective through the acute clinical course of the disease. The infectivity of chronically infected individuals varies from highly infectious (HBeAg positive) to sparingly infectious (anti-HBe positive).

8. Susceptibility and resistance—Susceptibility is general. Usually the disease is milder and often anicteric in children; in infants it is usually asymptomatic. Protective immunity follows infection if antibody to HBsAg (anti-HBs) develops and HBsAg is negative. Persons with Down syndrome, lymphoproliferative disease, HIV infection and those on hemodialysis appear to be more likely to develop chronic infection.

9. **Methods of control—**

A. *Preventive measures:*

1) Effective hepatitis B vaccines have been available since 1982. Two types of hepatitis B vaccines have been licensed in the USA and Canada. Both have been shown to be safe and highly protective against all subtypes of HBV. The first type is prepared from plasma from HBsAg positive persons; it is no longer produced in the USA but is still used widely elsewhere. The second type is made by recombinant DNA (rDNA) technology; it is produced by using HBsAg synthesized by *Saccharomyces cerevisiae* (common baker's yeast) into which a plasmid containing the gene for HBsAg has been inserted. Combined passive-active immunoprophylaxis with hepatitis B immunoglobulin (HBIG) and vaccine has been shown to stimulate anti-HBs titers comparable to vaccine alone.

a) In all countries, routine infant immunization should be the primary strategy to prevent HBV infection. Immunization of successive infant cohorts should produce a highly immune population sufficient to interrupt transmission. In countries with high endemicity of HBV infection, routine infant immunization will rapidly eliminate transmission because virtually all chronic infections are acquired among young children. In countries with intermediate and low HBV endemicity, immunizing infants alone will not substantially lower disease incidence because most infections occur among adolescents and young adults. In these countries, vaccine strategies for older children, adolescents and adults may be desirable. Strategies to ensure high vaccine coverage of successive age group cohorts are likely to be most effective in eliminating HBV transmission. In addition, immunization strategies can be targeted to high risk groups, which account for most cases among adolescents and adults.

b) Testing to exclude people with preexisting anti-HBs or anti-HBc is not required prior to immunization, but may be desirable as a cost saving method where there is a high level of preexisting infection.

c) Immunity against HBV is believed to persist for at least 15 years after successful immunization.

d) Vaccines licensed in different parts of the world may have varying dosages and schedules; the vaccines currently licensed in the USA are most commonly administered in 3 IM doses: an initial dose with subsequent doses 1 to 2 and 6 to 18 months later; for infants, the first dose is given at birth or at 1–2 months of age. For infants born to HBsAg positive women, the schedule should be birth, 1–2 and 6 months of age. These infants should also receive 0.5 ml of HBIG (see 9B5a, below). The dose of vaccine varies by manufacturer; the package insert should be consulted. In mid 1999, it was announced that very small infants who receive multiple doses of vaccines containing thimerosal could receive more than the recommended limits for mercury exposure based on recently developed guidelines. Reduction or elimination of thimerosal in vaccines as rapidly as possible was encouraged. As of mid 1999, several of the available inactivated vaccines and all live vaccines were thimerosal free. As of mid 1999, only hepatitis B vaccines that were approved for use at birth contained thimerosal. Therefore, it was recommended that hepatitis B immunization be delayed until 2–6 months of age for infants born to hepatitis B surface antigen negative mothers unless hepatitis B vaccines that do not contain thimerosal are available. For infants born to HBsAG positive mothers and mothers who were not screened during pregnancy, the recommendations were unchanged and called for administration of vaccine at birth. Single antigen preservative free hepatitis B vaccine became available in the USA in mid September 1999.

e) Pregnancy is not a contraindication for receiving hepatitis B vaccine.

2) The current hepatitis B prevention strategy in the USA includes the following components: a) screening of all pregnant women for the presence of HBsAg, providing HBIG and hepatitis B vaccine to infants of HBsAg positive mothers, and providing hepatitis B vaccine to susceptible household contacts (see 9B5, below); b) providing routine hepatitis B immunization for all infants; c) providing catch-up immunization to children who are in groups with high rates of chronic HBV infection (Alaskan natives, Pacific Islanders and children of first generation immigrants from countries with a high prevalence of chronic HBV infection); d) catch-up immunization of previously unimmunized children and adolescents, with the highest priority children aged 11–12 years; and e) intensified efforts to immunize adolescents and adults in defined risk groups (see 9A3, next below).

3) Persons at high risk who should routinely receive preexposure hepatitis B immunization include the following: a) sexually active heterosexual men and women, including those who are diagnosed as having recently acquired other STDs, and people who have a history of sexual activity with more than one partner in the previous 6 months; b) men who have sex with men; c) sexual partners and household contacts of HBsAg positive persons; d) inmates of correctional facilities, including juvenile detention facilities, prisons and jails; e) healthcare and public safety workers who perform tasks involving contact with blood or blood contaminated body fluids; f) clients and staff of institutions for the developmentally disabled; g) hemodialysis patients; h) patients with bleeding disorders who receive blood products; and i) international travelers who plan to spend more than 6 months in areas with intermediate to high rates of chronic HBV infection (2% or greater) and who will have close contact with the local population.

4) Adequately sterilize all syringes and needles (including acupuncture needles) and stylets for finger puncture, or preferably use disposable equipment whenever possible. A sterile syringe and needle are essential for each individual receiving skin tests, other parenteral inoculations or venipuncture. Discourage tattooing; enforce aseptic sanitary practices in tattoo parlors.

5) In blood banks, all donated blood should be tested for HBsAg by sensitive tests (RIA or EIA); reject as donors all persons with a history of viral hepatitis, those who have a history of injecting drug use or show evidence of drug addiction or those who have received a blood transfusion or tattoo within the preceding 6 months. Use paid donors only in emergencies.

6) Limit administration of unscreened whole blood or potentially hazardous blood products to those patients in clear and immediate need of such therapeutic measures.

7) Maintain surveillance for all cases of posttransfusion hepatitis, keep a register of all people who donated blood for each case. Notify blood banks of these potential carriers so that future donations may be identified promptly.

8) Medical and dental personnel who are infected with HBV and are HBeAg positive should not perform invasive procedures unless they have sought counsel from an expert review panel and have been advised under what circumstances, if any, they may continue to perform these procedures.

B. Control of patient, contacts and the immediate environment:

1) Report to local health authority: Official report is obligatory in the USA, although not now required in many countries; Class 2A (see Communicable Disease Reporting).

2) Isolation: Universal precautions to prevent exposures to blood and body fluids.

3) Concurrent disinfection: Of equipment contaminated with blood or infectious body fluids.

4) Quarantine: None.

5) Immunization of contacts: Products available for postexposure prophylaxis include HBIG and hepatitis B vaccine. HBIG has high titers of anti-HBs (more than 1:100,000). When indicated, it is important to administer HBIG as soon after exposure as possible.

a) Infants born to HBsAg positive mothers should be given a single dose of HBIG (0.5 ml IM) and vaccine within 12 hours of birth. The first dose of vaccine should be given concurrently with HBIG at birth but at a separate site. The second and third doses of vaccine (without HBIG) are given 1–2 and 6 months later. It is recommended to test the infant for HBsAg and anti-HBs at 9–15 months of age to monitor the success or failure of therapy. Infants who are anti-HBs positive and HBsAg negative are protected and do not need further vaccine doses. Infants found to be anti-HBs negative and HBsAg negative should be reimmunized.

b) After percutaneous (e.g., needle stick) or mucous membrane exposures to blood that contains or might contain HBsAg, a decision to provide postexposure prophylaxis must include consideration of several factors: i) whether the source of the blood is available; ii) the HBsAg status of the source; and iii) the hepatitis B immunization status of the exposed person. For previously unimmunized persons exposed to blood from an HBsAg positive source, a single dose of HBIG (0.06 ml/kg, or 5 ml for adults) should be given as soon as possible, but at least within 24 hours after high risk needle stick exposure, and the hepatitis B vaccine series should be started. If active immunization cannot be given, a second dose of HBIG should be given 1 month after the first. HBIG is not usually given for needle stick exposure to blood that is not known or highly suspected to be positive for HBsAg, since the risk of infection in these instances is small; however, initiation of hepatitis B immunization is recommended if the person had not previously been immunized. For previously immunized persons exposed to an HBsAg positive source, postexposure prophylaxis is not needed for persons who had a protective antibody response to immunization (anti-HBs titer of 10 milli-IUs/ml or greater). For persons whose response to immunization is unknown, hepatitis B vaccine and/or HBIG should be administered.

c) After sexual exposure to a person with acute HBV infection, a single dose of HBIG (0.06 ml/kg) is recommended if it can be given within 14 days of the last sexual contact. For all exposed sexual contacts of persons with acute and chronic HBV infection, vaccine should be administered.

6) Investigation of contacts and source of infection: See 9C, below.

7) Specific treatment: No specific treatment is available for acute hepatitis B. Alpha interferon and lamivudine have been licensed for treatment of chronic hepatitis B in the USA. Candidates for therapy should have liver biopsy evidence of chronic hepatitis B; treatment is most effective in individuals in the high-replicative phase (HBeAg positive) of infection because they are the most likely to be symptomatic, infectious and at greatest risk of long-term sequelae. Studies have shown that alpha interferon is successful in arresting viral replication in about 25%–40% of treated patients. Approximately 10% of patients who respond lose HBsAg 6 months after therapy. Clinical trials of long-term treatment with lamivudine have demonstrated sustained clearance of HBV DNA from serum, followed by improvements in serum aminotransferase levels and histologic improvement.

C. *Epidemic measures:* When two or more cases occur in association with some common exposure, conduct a search for additional cases. Institute strict aseptic techniques. If a plasma derivative such as antihemophilic factor, fibrinogen, pooled plasma or thrombin is implicated, withdraw the lot from use and trace all recipients of the same lot in a search for additional cases.

D. *Disaster implications:* Relaxation of sterilization precautions and emergency use of unscreened blood for transfusions may result in an increased number of cases.

E. *International measures:* None.

III. VIRAL HEPATITIS C   ICD-9 070.5; ICD-10 B17.1
(Parenterally transmitted non-A non-B hepatitis [PT-NANB], Non-B transfusion associated hepatitis, Posttransfusion non-A non-B hepatitis, HCV infection)

1. Identification—Onset is usually insidious, with anorexia, vague abdominal discomfort, nausea and vomiting; progression to jaundice is less frequent than with hepatitis B. Although initial infection may be asymptomatic (more than 90% of cases) or mild, a high percentage (between 50% and 80%) will develop a chronic infection. Of these chronically infected persons, about half will eventually develop cirrhosis or cancer of the liver. Diagnosis depends on detecting antibody to the hepatitis C virus (anti-HCV). As of the late 1990s, the only tests approved in the USA for diagnosis of HCV infection are those that measure anti-HCV. These tests detect anti-HCV in up to 97% of infected patients, but do not distinguish between acute, chronic, or resolved infection. As with any screening test, positive predictive value of EIA for anti-HCV varies depending on prevalence of infection in the population and is low in populations with an HCV prevalence of less than 10%. Supplemental testing with a more specific assay (i.e., recombinant immunoblot assay [RIBATM]) of a specimen with a positive EIA result limits reporting of false-positive results. Supplemental test results might be positive, negative or indeterminate. An anti-HCV positive person is defined as one whose serologic results are EIA test positive and supplemental test positive. Persons with a negative EIA test result or a positive EIA and a negative supplemental test result are considered uninfected, unless other evidence exists to indicate HCV infection (e.g., abnormal ALT levels in immunocompromised persons or persons with no other etiology for their liver disease).

2. Infectious agent—The hepatitis C virus is an enveloped RNA virus classified as a separate genus (*Hepacavirus*) in the Flaviviridae family. At least six different genotypes and greater than 90 subtypes of HCV exist. Evidence is limited regarding differences in clinical features, disease outcome or progression to cirrhosis or hepatocellular carcinoma (HCC) among persons with different genotypes. However, differences do exist in responses to antiviral therapy according to HCV genotypes.

3. Occurrence—Worldwide distribution. HCV prevalence is directly related to the prevalence of persons who routinely share injection equipment and to the prevalence of poor parenteral practices in health care settings. WHO estimated that as of the late 1990s, about 1% of the world's population were infected with HCV. In Europe and North America the prevalence of hepatitis C is between 0.5% and 2.0%; in parts of Africa prevalence is over 4%. There may be close to 1.5 million persons with HCV infections in Europe and close to 4 million in the USA.

4. Reservoir—Humans; virus has been transmitted experimentally to chimpanzees.

5. Mode of transmission—HCV is primarily parenterally transmitted. Sexual transmission has been documented to occur but is far less efficient or frequent than the parenteral route.

6. Incubation period—Ranges from 2 weeks to 6 months; commonly 6-9 weeks. Chronic infection may persist for up to 20 years before the onset of cirrhosis or hepatoma.

7. Period of communicability—From one or more weeks before onset of the first symptoms; may persist in most persons indefinitely. Peaks in virus concentration appear to correlate with peaks in ALT activity.

8. Susceptibility and resistance—Susceptibility is general. The degree of immunity following infection is not known; repeated infections with HCV have been demonstrated in an experimental chimpanzee model.

9. Methods of control —

> **A. Preventive measures:** General control measures against HBV infection apply (see section II, 9A, above). Prophylactic IG is not effective. In blood bank operations, all donors should be routinely screened for anti-HCV. In addition, all donor units with elevated liver enzyme levels and those positive for anti-HBc should continue to be discarded. Routine virus inactivation of plasma derived products, risk reduction counseling for persons uninfected but at high risk (i.e., health care workers) and nosocomial control activities need to be maintained.

> **B. Control of patient, contacts and the immediate environment:** General control measures against HBV apply. Available data suggest that postexposure prophylaxis with IG is not effective in preventing infection. Interferon alpha therapy has been shown to have an overall beneficial effect in about 25% of chronic hepatitis C cases; corticosteroids and acyclovir have not been effective. Studies in patients receiving a combination of ribavirin and interferon have demonstrated a substantial increase in sustained response rates reaching 40%–50%. However, both of these medications have significant side effects that require careful monitoring. Ribavirin is a teratogen; thus pregnancy should be avoided during therapy.

> **C. Epidemic measures:** Same as for hepatitis B.

> **D. Disaster implications:** Same as for hepatitis B.

> **E. International measures:** Ensure adequate virus inactivation for all internationally traded biological products.

IV. DELTA HEPATITIS   ICD-9 070.5; ICD-10 B17.0
(Viral hepatitis D, Hepatitis delta virus, Δ hepatitis, Delta agent hepatitis, Delta associated hepatitis)

1. Identification—Onset is usually abrupt, with signs and symptoms resembling those of hepatitis B; may be severe and is always associated with a coexistent hepatitis B virus infection. Delta hepatitis may be self-limiting or it may progress to chronic hepatitis. Children may have a particularly severe clinical course with usual progression to chronic active hepatitis. Hepatitis delta virus (HDV) and hepatitis B virus (HBV) may coinfect, or delta virus infection may occur in persons with chronic HBV infection. In the latter case, delta hepatitis can be misdiagnosed as an exacerbation of chronic hepatitis B. In several studies throughout Europe and the USA, 25%–50% of fulminant hepatitis cases thought to be caused by HBV were associated with concurrent infection with HDV. The most fulminant disease occurs in superinfections rather than coinfections; a chronic outcome is more commonly associated with superinfection.

Diagnosis is made by detection of total antibody to HDV (anti-HDV) by RIA or EIA. A positive IgM titer indicates ongoing replication; reverse transcription PCR is the most sensitive assay for detecting HDV viremia.

2. Infectious agent—HDV is a 35–37-nm virus-like particle consisting of a coat of HBsAg and a unique internal antigen, the delta antigen. Encapsulated with the delta antigen is the genome, a single-stranded RNA that can have a linear or circular conformation. The RNA does not hybridize with HBV DNA. HDV is unable to infect a cell by itself and requires coinfection with the HBV to undergo a complete replication cycle. Synthesis of HDV, in turn, results in temporary suppression of synthesis of HBV components. HDV is best considered in the new "satellite" family of subvirions, some of which are pathogens of higher plants. Hepatitis D is the only agent in this family that infects animal species. Three genotypes of HDV have been identified: Genotype I is the most prevalent and widespread, Genotype II is represented by two isolates from Japan and Taiwan and Genotype III has been found only in the Amazon basin, where it causes severe fulminant hepatitis with microvesicular steatosis (spongiocytosis).

3. Occurrence—Worldwide, but its prevalence varies widely. An estimated 10 million people are infected with hepatitis D virus and its helper virus HBV. It occurs epidemically or endemically in populations at high risk of HBV infection, such as populations in which hepatitis B is endemic (highest in parts of Russia, Romania, southern Italy, Africa and South America); in hemophiliacs, drug addicts and others who come in frequent contact with blood; in institutions for the developmentally disabled; and, to a lesser extent, in male homosexuals. Severe epidemics have been observed in tropical South America (Brazil, Venezuela, Colombia), in the Central African Republic and among drug addicts in Worcester, Massachusetts (USA).

4. Reservoir—Humans. Virus can be transmitted experimentally to chimpanzees and to woodchucks that are infected with HBV and woodchuck hepatitis virus, respectively.

5. Mode of transmission—Thought to be similar to that of HBV—by exposure to infected blood and serous body fluids, contaminated needles, syringes and plasma derivatives such as antihemophilic factor, and through sexual transmission.

6. Incubation period—Approximately 2–8 weeks.

7. Period of communicability—Blood is potentially infectious during all phases of active delta hepatitis infection. Peak infectivity probably occurs just prior to onset of acute illness, when particles containing the delta antigen are readily detected in the blood. Following onset, viremia probably falls rapidly to low or undetectable levels. HDV has been transmitted to chimpanzees from the blood of chronically infected patients in which particles containing delta antigen could not be detected.

8. Susceptibility and resistance—All people susceptible to HBV infection or who have chronic HBV can be infected with HDV. Severe disease can occur even in children.

9. Methods of control—

  A. *Preventive measures:* For people susceptible to HBV infection, same as for hepatitis B, above. Prevention of HBV infection with hepatitis B vaccine prevents infection with HDV. Among persons with chronic HBV, the only effective measure is avoidance of exposure to any potential source of HDV. HBIG, IG and hepatitis B vaccine do not protect persons with chronic HBV from infection by HDV. Studies reported from Taiwan suggest that measures which decrease sexual exposure and needle sharing have been associated with a decline in the incidence of HDV infection.

  B., C., D. and E. *Control of patient, contacts and the immediate environment; Epidemic measures; Disaster implications* and *International measures:* Same as for hepatitis B, above.

V. VIRAL HEPATITIS E ICD-9 070.5; ICD-10 B17.2
(Enterically transmitted non-A non-B hepatitis [ET-NANB], Epidemic non-A non-B hepatitis, Fecal-oral non-A non-B hepatitis)

1. Identification—The clinical course is similar to that of hepatitis A; there is no evidence of a chronic form. The case-fatality rate is similar to that of hepatitis A except in pregnant women, where the rate may reach 20% among those infected during the third trimester of pregnancy. Epidemic and sporadic cases have been described.

Diagnosis depends on clinical and epidemiologic features and exclusion of other etiologies of hepatitis, especially hepatitis A, by serologic means. Serologic tests have been developed for antibody to HEV, but are not commercially available in the USA. However, several diagnostic tests are available in research laboratories, which include: enzyme immunoassays and Western blot assays to detect IgM and IgG anti-HEV in serum; polymerase chain reaction tests to detect HEV RNA in serum and stool, and immunofluorescent antibody blocking assays to detect antibody to HEV antigen in serum and liver.

2. Infectious agent—The hepatitis E virus (HEV), a spherical, nonenveloped, single-stranded RNA virus that is approximately 32 to 34 nm in diameter. HEV has been provisionally classified in the Caliciviridae family.

However, the organization of the HEV genome is substantially different from other caliciviruses, and HEV may eventually be classified in a separate family.

3. Occurrence—HEV is the major etiologic agent of enterically transmitted non-A, non-B hepatitis throughout the world. Outbreaks of hepatitis E and sporadic cases have occurred over a wide geographic area, primarily in countries with inadequate environmental sanitation. Outbreaks often occur as waterborne epidemics, but sporadic cases and epidemics not clearly related to water have been reported. The highest rates of clinically evident disease have been in young to middle aged adults; lower disease rates in younger age groups may be the result of anicteric and/or subclinical HEV infection. In the USA and most other industrialized countries, hepatitis E cases have been documented only among travelers returning from HEV endemic areas. Outbreaks have been identified in India, Myanmar (Burma), Iran, Bangladesh, Ethiopia, Nepal, Pakistan, central Asian Republics of the former Soviet Union, Algeria, Libya, Somalia, Mexico, Indonesia and China. A large waterborne outbreak consisting of 3,682 cases occurred in 1993 in Uttar Pradesh.

4. Reservoir—Recent studies suggest a reservoir may exist in domestic animals, including swine; however, this has not been proved. HEV is transmissible to chimpanzees, cynomolgus macaques, tamarins and pigs.

5. Mode of transmission—HEV is transmitted primarily by the fecal-oral route; fecally contaminated drinking water is the most commonly documented vehicle of transmission. Transmission probably also occurs from person to person by the fecal-oral route, though secondary household cases are not common during outbreaks. Recent studies have suggested that hepatitis E may in fact be a zoonotic infection with coincident areas of high human infection.

6. Incubation period—The range is 15 to 64 days; the mean incubation period has varied from 26 to 42 days in different epidemics.

7. Period of communicability—Not known. However, HEV has been detected in stools 14 days after the onset of jaundice and approximately 4 weeks after oral ingestion of contaminated food or water and persists for about 2 weeks.

8. Susceptibility and resistance—Susceptibility is unknown. More than 50% of HEV infections may be anicteric; the expression of icterus appears to increase with increasing age. Women in the third trimester of pregnancy are especially susceptible to fulminant disease. The occurrence of major epidemics among young adults in geographic regions where other enteric viruses are highly endemic and most of the population acquires infection in infancy remains unexplained.

9. Methods of control—

A. Preventive measures: Provide educational programs to stress sanitary disposal of feces and careful handwashing after defecation and before handling food; follow basic measures to prevent fecal-oral transmission, as listed under Typhoid fever, 9A. It is unlikely that IG prepared from the serum of donors in the USA or Europe will protect against hepatitis E.

B. Control of patient, contacts and the immediate environment:

1), 2) and 3) Report to local health authority, Isolation and Concurrent disinfection: Same as for hepatitis A, above.

4) Quarantine: None.

5) Immunization of contacts: No products are available to prevent hepatitis E. IG prepared from plasma collected in non-HEV endemic areas is not effective in preventing clinical disease during hepatitis E outbreaks, and the efficacy of IG prepared from plasma collected in HEV endemic areas is unclear. In studies conducted with prototype vaccines in animals, vaccine induced antibody attenuated HEV infection but did not prevent virus excretion in stools.

6) Investigation of contacts and source of infection: Same as for hepatitis A, above.

7) Specific treatment: None.

C. Epidemic measures: Determine mode of transmission by epidemiologic investigation; investigate water supply and identify the population at increased risk of infection. Make special efforts to improve sanitary and hygienic practices in order to eliminate fecal contamination of foods and water.

D. Disaster implications: A potential problem where there is mass crowding and inadequate sanitation and water supplies. If cases occur, increased effort should be exerted to improve sanitation and the safety of water supplies.

E. International measures: None.

HERPES SIMPLEX   ICD-9 054; ICD-10 B00
ANOGENITAL HERPESVIRAL
INFECTIONS   ICD-10 A60
(Alphaherpesviral disease, Herpesvirus hominis, Human herpesviruses 1 and 2)

1. Identification—Herpes simplex is a viral infection characterized by a localized primary lesion, latency and a tendency to localized recurrence. The two etiologic agents—herpes simplex virus (HSV) types 1 and

2—generally produce distinct clinical syndromes, depending on the portal of entry. Either may infect the genital tract or oral mucosa.

The primary infection with HSV 1 may be mild and inapparent and occur in early childhood. In approximately 10% of primary infections, overt disease may appear as an illness of varying severity, marked by fever and malaise lasting a week or more; it may be associated with gingivostomatitis accompanied by vesicular lesions in the oropharynx, severe keratoconjunctivitis, a generalized cutaneous eruption complicating chronic eczema, meningoencephalitis or some of the fatal generalized infections in newborn infants (congenital herpes simplex, ICD-9 771.2, ICD-10 P35.2). HSV 1 causes about 2% of acute pharyngotonsillitis, usually as a primary infection.

Reactivation of latent infection commonly results in herpes labialis (fever blisters or cold sores) manifested by superficial clear vesicles on an erythematous base, usually on the face or lips, which crust and heal within a few days. Reactivation is precipitated by various forms of trauma, fever, physiologic changes or intercurrent disease, and may also involve other body tissues; it occurs in the presence of circulating antibodies, which are seldom elevated by reactivation. Severe and extensive spread of infection may occur in those who are immunosuppressed.

CNS involvement may appear in association with either a primary infection or a recrudescence. HSV 1 is a common cause of meningoencephalitis. Fever, headache, leukocytosis, meningeal irritation, drowsiness, confusion, stupor, coma and focal neurologic signs may occur and are frequently referable to one or the other temporal region. The condition may be confused with a variety of other intracranial lesions including brain abscess and tuberculous meningitis. Because antiviral therapy may reduce the high mortality, PCR for DNA of herpes virus in the CSF or biopsy of cerebral tissue should be considered early in clinically suspected cases to establish the diagnosis.

Genital herpes, usually caused by HSV 2, occurs mainly in adults and is sexually transmitted. Primary and recurrent infections occur, with or without symptoms. In women, the principal sites of primary disease are the cervix and the vulva; recurrent disease generally involves the vulva, perineal skin, legs and buttocks. In men, lesions appear on the glans penis or prepuce, and in the anus and rectum of those engaging in anal sex. Other genital or perineal sites, as well as the mouth, may be involved in either gender, depending on sexual practices. HSV 2 has been associated with aseptic meningitis and radiculitis rather than meningoencephalitis.

Neonatal infections can be divided into three clinical presentations: disseminated infections involving particularly the liver, encephalitis and infection limited to the skin, eyes or mouth. The first two forms are often lethal. Infections are most frequently due to HSV 2, but HSV 1 is also common. Risk to the infant depends on two important maternal factors: stage of pregnancy at which the mother excretes HSV, and whether the infection is primary or secondary. Only excretion at the time of delivery is dangerous to the newborn, with the rare exception of intrauterine infections. Primary infection in the mother raises the risk of infection from 3% to over 30%, presumably because maternal immunity confers a degree of protection.

Diagnosis is suggested by characteristic cytologic changes (multinucleated giant cells with intranuclear inclusions in tissue scrapings or biopsy), but is confirmed by direct FA tests or isolation of the virus from oral or genital lesions or from a brain biopsy in cases of encephalitis or by demonstration of HSV DNA in lesion or spinal fluid by PCR. Diagnosis of primary infection can be confirmed by a fourfold rise in titer in paired sera in various serologic tests; the presence of herpes specific IgM is suggestive but not conclusive evidence of primary infection. Reliable techniques to differentiate type 1 from type 2 antibody are now available in diagnostic laboratories; virus isolates can be distinguished readily from one another by DNA analysis. Type specific serologic tests are not yet widely available.

2. Infectious agent—Herpes simplex virus in the virus family Herpesviridae, subfamily Alphaherpesvirinae. HSV types 1 and 2 can be differentiated immunologically (especially when highly specific or monoclonal antibodies are used) and differ with respect to their growth patterns in cell culture, embryonated eggs and experimental animals.

3. Occurrence—Worldwide; 50%-90% of adults possess circulating antibodies against HSV 1; initial infection with HSV 1 usually occurs before the 5th year of life, but more primary infections in adults are now being reported. HSV 2 infection usually begins with sexual activity and is rare before adolescence, except in sexually abused children. HSV 2 antibody is found in about 20%-30% of American adults. The prevalence is greater (up to 60%) in lower socioeconomic groups and persons with multiple sexual partners.

4. Reservoir—Humans.

5. Mode of transmission—Contact with HSV 1 virus in the saliva of carriers is probably the most important mode of spread. Infection on the hands of health care personnel (e.g., dentists) from patients shedding HSV results in herpetic whitlow. Transmission of HSV 2 is usually by sexual contact. Both types 1 and 2 may be transmitted to various sites by oral-genital, oral-anal or anal-genital contact. Transmission to the neonate usually occurs via the infected birth canal, but less commonly occurs in utero or postpartum.

6. Incubation period—From 2-12 days.

7. Period of communicability—HSV can be isolated for 2 weeks and occasionally up to 7 weeks after primary stomatitis or primary genital lesions. Both primary and recurrent infections may be asymptomatic. After either, HSV may be shed intermittently from mucosal sites for years and possibly lifelong, in the presence or absence of clinical manifestations. In recurrent lesions, infectivity is shorter than after primary infection, and usually the virus cannot be recovered after 5 days.

8. Susceptibility and resistance—Humans are probably universally susceptible.

9. Methods of control—

A. Preventive measures:

1) Health education and personal hygiene directed toward minimizing the transfer of infectious material.
2) Avoid contaminating the skin of eczematous patients with infectious material.
3) Health care personnel should wear gloves when in direct contact with potentially infectious lesions.
4) Cesarean section is advised before the membranes rupture when primary genital herpes infections occur in late pregnancy because of the risk of highly fatal neonatal infection (30-50%). Use of scalp electrodes is contraindicated. The risk of fatal neonatal infection after recurrent infection is much lower (3-5%), and cesarean section is advisable only when active lesions are present at delivery.
5) Use of latex condoms in sexual practice may decrease the risk of infection; no antiviral agent has yet been proved to be practical in prophylaxis of primary infection, although acyclovir may be used prophylactically to reduce the incidence of recurrences and of herpes infections in immunodeficient patients.

B. Control of patient, contacts and the immediate environment:

1) Report to local health authority: Official case report in adults not ordinarily justifiable, but some states have reporting requirements for genital herpes, Class 5; neonatal infections reportable in some states, Class 3B (see Communicable Disease Reporting).
2) Isolation: Contact isolation for neonatal and disseminated or primary severe lesions; for recurrent lesions, drainage and secretion precautions. Patients with herpetic lesions should have no contact with newborns, children with eczema or burns or immunosuppressed patients.
3) Concurrent disinfection: None.
4) Quarantine: None.
5) Immunization of contacts: None.
6) Investigation of contacts and source of infection: Seldom of practical value.

7) Specific treatment: The acute manifestations of herpetic keratitis and early dendritic ulcers may be treated with trifluridine or adenine arabinoside (vidarabine, Vira-A® or Ara-A®) as an ophthalmic ointment or solution. Corticosteroids should never be used for ocular involvement unless administered by an experienced ophthalmologist. Acyclovir IV is of value in herpes simplex encephalitis, but may not prevent residual neurologic problems. Acyclovir (Zovirax®) used orally, intravenously or topically has been shown to reduce shedding of virus, diminish pain and accelerate healing time in primary genital and recurrent herpes, rectal herpes and herpetic whitlow. The oral preparation is most convenient to use and may benefit patients with extensive recurrent infections as well. However, mutant strains of herpes virus resistant to acyclovir have been reported. Valacyclovir and famciclovir are recently licensed congeners of acyclovir that have equivalent efficacy. Prophylactic daily administration of these drugs can reduce the frequency of HSV recurrences in adults. Neonatal infections should be treated with intravenous acyclovir.

C. *Epidemic measures:* Not applicable.

D. *Disaster implications:* None.

E. *International measures:* None.

MENINGOENCEPHALITIS DUE TO CERCOPITHECINE HERPES VIRUS 1   ICD-9 054.3; ICD-10 B00.4
(B-virus, Simian B disease)

While HSV 1 (occasionally, type 2) can cause meningoencephalitis, the picture is distinctly different with B-virus infection, a CNS disease caused by cercopithecine herpesvirus 1, a virus closely related to HSV. This virus causes an ascending encephalomyelitis seen in veterinarians, laboratory workers and other individuals having close contact with Eastern Hemisphere monkeys or monkey cell cultures. After an incubation period of 3 days to 3 weeks, there is an acute febrile onset with headache, often local vesicular lesions, lymphocytic pleocytosis and variable neurologic patterns, ending in death in over 70% of cases, 1 day to 3 weeks after onset of symptoms. The occasional recoveries have been associated with considerable residual disability, but a few recent cases, treated with acyclovir, have recovered completely. The virus causes a natural infection of monkeys analogous to HSV infection in humans; 30%–80% of rhesus monkeys are seropositive. During periods of stress (shipping and handling), they have high rates of viral shedding. Human illness is extremely rare but highly fatal; it is acquired by the bite of apparently normal monkeys, or by exposure of naked skin or mucous membrane to infected saliva or monkey cell cultures. Prevention depends on proper use of protective gauntlets and care to minimize exposure to monkeys. All bite or scratch wounds incurred from macaques or from cages that might be contaminated with macaque secretions and result in bleeding should be immediately and thoroughly scrubbed and cleaned with soap and water. Prophylactic treatment with an antiviral agent such as acyclovir may be considered when an animal handler sustains a deep, penetrating wound that cannot be adequately cleaned; the B-virus status of the monkey should be determined. The appearance of any skin lesions or neurologic symptoms, such as itching, pain, or numbness near the site of the wound calls for expert medical consultation for diagnosis and possible treatment.

HISTOPLASMOSIS ICD-9 115; ICD-10 B39

Two clinically different mycoses have been designated as histoplasmosis because the pathogens that cause them cannot be distinguished morphologically when growing on culture media as molds. Detailed information will be given for the infection caused by *Histoplasma capsulatum* var. *capsulatum,* followed by a brief summary of histoplasmosis caused by *H. capsulatum* var. *duboisii.*

I. INFECTION BY *HISTOPLASMA CAPSULATUM* ICD-9 115.0; ICD-10 B39.4
(Histoplasmosis capsulati, Histoplasmosis due to *H. capsulatum* var. *capsulatum*, American histoplasmosis)

1. Identification—A systemic mycosis of varying severity, with the primary lesion usually in the lungs. While infection is common, overt clinical disease is not. Five clinical forms are recognized.

1) Asymptomatic with only hypersensitivity to histoplasmin.

2) Acute benign respiratory, which varies from a mild respiratory illness to temporary incapacity with general malaise, fever, chills, headache, myalgia, chest pains and a nonproductive cough; occasional erythema multiforme and erythema nodosum. Multiple, small scattered calcifications in the lung, hilar lymph nodes and spleen may be late findings.

3) Acute disseminated histoplasmosis with debilitating fever, GI symptoms, evidence of bone marrow suppression, hepatosplenomegaly, lymphadenopathy and a rapid course, most frequent in infants and young children and immunocompromised patients including those with AIDS. Without therapy, this form of the disease is usually fatal.

4) Chronic disseminated disease with low-grade intermittent fever, weight loss, weakness, hepatosplenomegaly, mild hematologic abnormali-

ties and focal disease (e.g., endocarditis, meningitis, mucosal ulcers of mouth, larynx, stomach or bowel and Addison's disease). This form has a subacute course with progression over 10-11 months and is usually fatal unless treated.

5) Chronic pulmonary, which clinically and radiologically resembles chronic pulmonary tuberculosis with cavitation; occurs most often in middle aged and elderly men with underlying emphysema and progresses over months or years, with periods of quiescence and sometimes spontaneous cure.

Clinical diagnosis is confirmed by culture or by visualizing the fungus in Giemsa or Wright stained smears of ulcer exudates, bone marrow, sputum or blood; special stains are necessary to demonstrate the fungus in biopsies of ulcers, liver, lymph nodes or lung. The histoplasmin skin test is helpful in epidemiologic studies but not in diagnosis. Among the available serologic tests, the immunodiffusion test is the most specific and reliable. A rise in CF titers in paired sera may be encountered early in acute infection and is suggestive evidence of active disease; however, recent positive skin tests with histoplasmin can raise the titer against the mycelial form, and the serologic tests can cross react with other mycoses. False negative tests are common enough so that negative serologic tests do not exclude the diagnosis. Detection of antigen in serum or urine is useful in making the diagnosis and following the results of therapy in disseminated histoplasmosis.

2. Infectious agent—*Histoplasma capsulatum* var. *capsulatum (Ajellomyces capsulatus),* a dimorphic fungus growing as a mold in soil and as a yeast in animal and human hosts.

3. Occurrence—Infections commonly occur in specific geographic foci over wide areas of the Americas, Africa, eastern Asia and Australia; rare in Europe. Histoplasmin hypersensitivity, indicating antecedent infection, sometimes is present in as much as 80% of a population in parts of eastern and central USA. Clinical disease is far less frequent, and severe progressive disease is rare. Prevalence increases from childhood to 15 years of age; differences by gender are usually not observed except that the chronic pulmonary form is more common in males. Outbreaks have occurred in endemic areas in families, students and workers with exposure to bird, chicken or bat droppings or recently disturbed contaminated soil. Histoplasmosis also occurs in dogs, cats, cattle, horses, rats, skunks, opossums, foxes and other animals, often with a clinical picture comparable to the disease in humans.

4. Reservoir—Soil with high organic content and undisturbed bird droppings, in particular that around and in old chicken houses, in caves harboring bats and around starling, blackbird and pigeon roosts.

5. Mode of transmission—Growth of the fungus in soil produces microconidia and tuberculate macroconidia; infection results from inhalation of airborne conidia. Person to person transmission can occur only if infected tissue is inoculated into a healthy person.

6. Incubation period—Symptoms appear within 3-17 days after exposure but may be shorter with heavy exposure; commonly 10 days.

7. Period of communicability—Not transmitted from person to person.

8. Susceptibility and resistance—Susceptibility is general. Inapparent infections are extremely common in endemic areas and usually result in increased resistance to infection. May be an opportunistic infection in those with compromised immunity.

9. Methods of control—

    A. Preventive measures: Minimize exposure to dust in a contaminated environment, such as chicken coops and their surrounding soil. Spray with water or oil to reduce dust; use protective masks.

    B. Control of patient, contacts and the immediate environment:

        1) Report to local health authority: In selected endemic areas (USA); in many countries, not a reportable disease, Class 3B (see Communicable Disease Reporting).
        2) Isolation: None.
        3) Concurrent disinfection: Of sputum and articles soiled therewith. Terminal cleaning.
        4) Quarantine: None.
        5) Immunization of contacts: None.
        6) Investigation of contacts and source of infection: Household and occupational contacts for evidence of infection from a common environmental source.
        7) Specific treatment: Oral ketoconazole is approved for treatment of immunocompetent patients. Oral itraconazole is also approved for pulmonary and disseminated histoplasmosis in non-HIV infected individuals. Neither should be used in patients with CNS involvement. For other patients with disseminated histoplasmosis, amphotericin B (Fungizone®) IV is the drug of choice. Itraconazole is effective chronic suppressive therapy in AIDS patients previously treated with amphotericin B.

    C. Epidemic measures: Occurrence of grouped cases of acute pulmonary disease in or outside of an endemic area, particularly with history of exposure to dust within a closed space as within caves or construction sites, should arouse suspicion of histoplasmosis. Suspected sites such as attics, basements, caves or construction sites with large amounts of bird droppings or bat guano should be investigated.

D. Disaster implications: None. Possible hazard if large groups, especially from nonendemic areas, are forced to move through or live in areas where the mold is prevalent.

E. International measures: None.

II. HISTOPLASMOSIS DUBOISII   ICD-9 115.1; ICD-10 B39.5
(Histoplasmosis due to *H. capsulatum* var. *duboisii*, African histoplasmosis)

This usually presents as a subacute granuloma of the skin or bone. Infection, though usually localized, may be disseminated in the skin, subcutaneous tissue, lymph nodes, bones, joints, lungs and abdominal viscera. Disease is more common in males and may occur at any age, but especially in the second decade of life. Thus far, the disease has been recognized only in Africa and Madagascar. Diagnosis is made by culture and by demonstrating the yeast cells of *H. capsulatum* var. *duboisii* in tissue by smear or biopsy. These cells are much larger than the yeast cells of *H. capsulatum* var. *capsulatum*. The true prevalence of *H. duboisii*, its reservoir, mode of transmission and incubation period are unknown. It is not communicable from person to person. Treatment is probably the same as for American histoplasmosis.

HOOKWORM DISEASE   ICD-9 126; ICD-10 B76
(Ancylostomiasis, Uncinariasis, Necatoriasis)

1. Identification—A common chronic parasitic infection with a variety of symptoms, usually in proportion to the degree of anemia. In heavy infections, the bloodletting activity of the nematode leads to iron deficiency and hypochromic, microcytic anemia, the major cause of disability. Children with heavy, long term infection may have hypoproteinemia and may be retarded in mental and physical development. Occasionally, severe acute pulmonary and GI reactions follow exposure to infective larvae. Death is infrequent and usually can be attributed to other infections. Light hookworm infections generally produce few or no clinical effects.

Infection is confirmed by finding hookworm eggs in feces; stool examination may be negative early in the course of the infection until the worms mature. Species differentiation requires microscopic examination of larvae cultured from the feces, or examination of adult worms expelled by purgation following a vermifuge. Differentiation of the species can be made by using PCR-RFLP techniques.

2. Infectious agents—*Necator americanus, Ancylostoma duodenale, A. ceylanicum* and *A. caninum.*

3. Occurrence—Widely endemic in tropical and subtropical countries where sanitary disposal of human feces is not practiced and soil, moisture and temperature conditions favor development of infective larvae. May also occur in temperate climates under similar environmental conditions (e.g., in mines). Both *Necator* and *Ancylostoma* occur in many parts of Asia (particularly in southeast Asia), the South Pacific and east Africa. *N. americanus* is the prevailing species throughout southeast Asia, most of tropical Africa and America; *A. duodenale* prevails in North Africa, including the Nile Valley, in northern India, in northern parts of the Far East and in the Andean areas of South America. *A. ceylanicum* occurs in southeast Asia but is less common than either *N. americanus* or *A. duodenale. A. caninum* has been described in Australia as a cause of eosinophilic enteritis syndrome.

4. Reservoir—Humans for *N. americanus* and *A. duodenale;* cats and dogs for *A. ceylanicum* and *A. caninum.*

5. Mode of transmission—Eggs in feces are deposited on the ground and hatch; under favorable conditions of moisture, temperature and soil type, larvae develop to the third stage, becoming infective in 7–10 days. Human infection occurs when the infective larvae penetrate the skin, usually of the foot; in so doing, they produce a characteristic dermatitis (ground itch). The larvae of *A. caninum* die within the skin, having produced cutaneous larva migrans. The larvae of *Necator* and other *Ancylostoma* normally enter the skin and pass via lymphatics and bloodstream to the lungs, enter the alveoli, migrate up the trachea to the pharynx, are swallowed and reach the small intestine where they attach to the intestinal wall, develop to maturity in 6–7 weeks (3–4 weeks in the case of *A. ceylanicum*) and typically produce thousands of eggs per day. Infection with *Ancylostoma* may also be acquired by ingesting infective larvae; possible vertical transmission has been reported.

6. Incubation period—Symptoms may develop after a few weeks to many months, depending on intensity of infection and iron intake of the host. Pulmonary infiltration, cough and tracheitis may occur during the lung migration phase of infection, particularly in *Necator* infections. After entering the body, *A. duodenale* may become dormant for about 8 months, after which development resumes, with a patent (stools containing eggs) infection a month later.

7. Period of communicability—Not transmitted from person to person, but infected people can contaminate soil for several years in the absence of treatment. Under favorable conditions, larvae remain infective in soil for several weeks.

8. Susceptibility and resistance—Universal; there is no evidence that immunity develops with infection.

9. Methods of control—

A. *Preventive measures:*

1) Educate the public to the dangers of soil contamination by human, cat or dog feces, and in preventive measures, including wearing shoes in endemic areas.
2) Prevent soil contamination by installation of sanitary disposal systems for human feces, especially sanitary privies in rural areas. Night soil and sewage effluents are hazardous, especially where they are used as fertilizer.
3) Examine and treat people migrating from endemic to receptive nonendemic areas, especially those who work barefooted in mines, construct dams or work in the agricultural sector.

B. *Control of patient, contacts and the immediate environment:*

1) Report to local health authority: Official report not ordinarily justifiable, Class 5 (see Communicable Disease Reporting).
2) Isolation: None.
3) Concurrent disinfection: Sanitary disposal of feces to prevent contamination of soil.
4) Quarantine: None.
5) Immunization of contacts: None.
6) Investigation of contacts and source of infection: Each infected contact and carrier is a potential or actual indirect spreader of infection.
7) Specific treatment: Single dose treatment with mebendazole (Vermox®), albendazole (Zentel®), levamisole (Ketrax®) or pyrantel pamoate (Antiminth®) is recommended; adverse reactions are infrequent. Follow-up stool examination is indicated after 2 weeks, and therapy should be repeated if a heavy worm burden persists. Iron supplementation will correct the anemia and should be used in conjunction with worm therapy. Transfusion may be necessary for severe anemia. As a general rule, pregnant women should not be treated in the first trimester unless there are specific indications to do so.

C. *Epidemic measures:* Survey for prevalence in highly endemic areas and provide periodic mass treatment. Provide health educa-

tion in environmental sanitation and personal hygiene, and provide facilities for excreta disposal.

D. Disaster implications: None.

E. International measures: None.

HYMENOLEPIASIS   ICD-9 123.6; ICD-10 B71.0
I. HYMENOLEPIASIS DUE TO
   HYMENOLEPIS NANA
(Dwarf tapeworm infection)

1. Identification—An intestinal infection with very small tapeworms; light infections are usually asymptomatic. Massive numbers of the worms may cause enteritis with or without diarrhea, abdominal pain and other vague symptoms such as pallor, loss of weight and weakness.

Diagnosis is made by the microscopy identification of eggs in feces.

2. Infectious agent—*Hymenolepis nana* (dwarf tapeworm), the only human tapeworm without an obligatory intermediate host.

3. Occurrence—Cosmopolitan; more common in warm than cold, and in dry than wet climates. Dwarf tapeworm is the most common human tapeworm in the USA and Latin America; it is common in Australia, Mediterranean countries, the Near East and India.

4. Reservoir—Humans; possibly mice.

5. Mode of transmission—Eggs of *H. nana* are infective when passed in the feces. Infection is acquired through ingestion of eggs in contaminated food or water; directly from fecally contaminated fingers (i.e., autoinfection or person to person transmission); or by ingestion of insects bearing larvae that have developed from eggs ingested by the insect. When *H. nana* eggs are ingested, they hatch in the intestine, liberating oncospheres that enter mucosal villi and develop into cysticercoids; these rupture into the lumen and grow into adult tapeworms. Some *H. nana* eggs are immediately infectious when released from the proglottids in the human gut, so autoinfections or person to person transmission can occur. If *H. nana* eggs are ingested by mealworms, larval fleas, beetles or other insects, they may develop into cysticercoids that are infective to humans and rodents when ingested.

6. Incubation period—Onset of symptoms is variable; the development of mature worms requires about 2 weeks.

7. Period of communicability—As long as eggs are passed in the feces. *H. nana* infections may persist for several years.

8. Susceptibility and resistance—Universal; infection produces resistance to reinfection. Children are more susceptible than adults; intensive infection occurs in immunodeficient and malnourished children.

9. Methods of control—

A. Preventive measures:

1) Educate the public in personal hygiene and sanitary disposal of feces.
2) Provide and maintain clean toilet facilities.
3) Protect food and water from contamination with human and rodent feces.
4) Treat to remove sources of infection.
5) Eliminate rodents from the home environment.

B. Control of patient, contacts and the immediate environment:

1) Report to local health authority: Official report not ordinarily justifiable, Class 5 (see Communicable Disease Reporting).
2) Isolation: None.
3) Concurrent disinfection: Sanitary disposal of feces.
4) Quarantine: None.
5) Immunization of contacts: Not applicable.
6) Investigation of contacts and source of infection: Fecal examination of family or institution members.
7) Specific treatment: Praziquantel (Biltricide®) or niclosamide (Yomesan®, Niclocide®) is effective.

C. Epidemic measures: Outbreaks in schools and institutions can be controlled best by treatment of infected individuals and by special attention to personal and group hygiene.

D. Disaster implications: None.

E. International measures: None.

II. HYMENOLEPIASIS DUE TO *HYMENOLEPIS DIMINUTA*   ICD-9 123.6; ICD-10 B71.0
(Rat tapeworm infection, Hymenolepiasis diminuta)

The rat tapeworm, *H. diminuta,* occurs accidentally in humans, usually in young children. The eggs passed in rodent feces are ingested by insects such as flea larvae, grain beetles and cockroaches in which cysticercoids develop in the hemocele. The mature tapeworm develops in rats, mice or other rodents when the insect is ingested. People are rare accidental hosts, usually of a single or few tapeworms; human infections are rarely symptomatic. Definitive diagnosis is based on finding characteristic eggs in the feces; treatment as for *H. nana*.

III. DIPYLIDIASIS ICD-9 123.8; ICD-10 B71.1
(Dog tapeworm infection)

Toddler aged children are occasionally infected with the dog tapeworm *(Dipylidium caninum)*, the adult of which is found worldwide in dogs and cats. It rarely if ever produces symptoms in the child but is distressful to the parent who sees motile, seed-like proglottids (tapeworm segments) at the anus or on the surface of the stool. Infection is acquired when the child ingests fleas that, in their larval stage, have eaten eggs from proglottids. In 3-4 weeks the tapeworm becomes mature. Infection is prevented by keeping dogs and cats free of fleas and worms; niclosamide or praziquantel is effective for treatment.

INFLUENZA ICD-9 487; ICD-10 J10, 11

1. Identification—An acute viral disease of the respiratory tract characterized by fever, headache, myalgia, prostration, coryza, sore throat and cough. Cough is often severe and protracted, but other manifestations are usually self-limited, with recovery in 2-7 days. Recognition is commonly by epidemiologic characteristics; sporadic cases can be identified only by laboratory procedures. Influenza in individuals may be indistinguishable from disease caused by other respiratory viruses. The clinical picture may range from the common cold, croup, bronchiolitis, viral pneumonia and undifferentiated acute respiratory disease. GI tract manifestations (nausea, vomiting, diarrhea) are uncommon, but may accompany the respiratory phase in children, and have been reported in up to 25% of children in school outbreaks of influenza B and A (H1N1).

Influenza derives its importance from the rapidity with which epidemics evolve, the widespread morbidity and the seriousness of complications, notably viral and bacterial pneumonias. During major epidemics, severe illness and death occur, primarily among the elderly and those debilitated by chronic cardiac, pulmonary, renal or metabolic disease, anemia or immunosuppression. The proportion of total deaths associated with pneumonia and influenza in excess of the proportion expected for the time of year (excess mortality) varies from epidemic to epidemic and depends on the prevalent virus type. From 1972-73 through 1994-95, an estimated more than 20,000 influenza associated deaths occurred during each of 11 different US epidemics, and more than 40,000 influenza associated deaths occurred during 6 of those 11 epidemics. In all 11 epidemics, 80%–90% of deaths occurred in persons more than 65 years of age. However, in the 1918 pandemic, the highest mortality rates were among young adults. Reye syndrome, involving the CNS and liver, is a rare complication in children who have ingested salicylates; it occurs mainly in children with influenza B disease and less frequently with influenza A.

During the early febrile stage of disease, laboratory confirmation is made by isolation of influenza viruses from pharyngeal or nasal secretions or washings in cell culture or embryonated eggs, by direct identification of viral antigens in nasopharyngeal cells and fluids by FA test or ELISA, or by amplification of viral RNA. Infection may also be confirmed by demonstration of a specific serologic response between acute and convalescent sera.

2. **Infectious agents**—Three types of influenza virus are recognized: A, B and C. Type A includes three subtypes (H1N1, H2N2 and H3N2) that have been associated with widespread epidemics and pandemics; type B has been infrequently associated with regional or widespread epidemics; type C has been associated with sporadic cases and minor localized outbreaks. Virus type is determined by the antigenic properties of the two relatively stable internal structural proteins, the nucleoprotein and the matrix protein.

Influenza A subtypes are classified by the antigenic properties of the surface glycoproteins, the hemagglutinin (H) and the neuraminidase (N). Frequent mutation of the genes encoding the surface glycoproteins of influenza A and influenza B viruses results in emergence of variants that are described by the geographic site of isolation, the culture number and the year of isolation. Examples of prototype strains with these designations include A/Beijing/262/95 (H1N1), A/Japan/305/57 (H2N2), A/Sydney/5/97 (H3N2) and B/Yamanashi/166/98.

Emergence of completely new subtypes (antigenic shift) occurs at irregular intervals and only with type A viruses; they are responsible for pandemics and result from the unpredictable recombination of human and swine or avian antigens. The relatively minor antigenic changes (antigenic drift) of A and B viruses responsible for frequent epidemics and regional outbreaks occur constantly and necessitate annual reformulation of influenza vaccine.

3. **Occurrence**—In pandemics, epidemics, localized outbreaks and as sporadic cases. During the past 100+ years, pandemics occurred in 1889, 1918, 1957 and 1968. Clinical attack rates during epidemics range from 10% to 20% in the general community to more than 50% in closed populations such as boarding schools or nursing homes. Epidemics of influenza occur in the USA almost every year; they may be caused primarily by Type A viruses, occasionally by influenza B viruses or by both. In temperate zones, epidemics tend to occur in winter; in the tropics, they often occur in the rainy season, but outbreaks or sporadic cases may occur in any month.

Influenza viral infections with different antigenic subtypes also occur naturally in swine, horses, mink and seals, and in many domestic and wild avian species in many parts of the world. Interspecies transmission and reassortment of influenza A viruses have been reported to occur between swine, humans and wild and domestic fowl. The human influenza viruses responsible for the 1918, 1957 and 1968 pandemics contained gene segments closely related to those of avian influenza viruses.

4. Reservoir—Humans are the primary reservoir for human infections; however, mammalian reservoirs such as swine and birds are likely sources of new human subtypes thought to emerge through genetic reassortment. New subtypes of a virulent virus strain with new surface antigens cause pandemic influenza by spreading through an essentially nonimmune population.

5. Mode of transmission—Airborne spread predominates among crowded populations in enclosed spaces, such as school buses; transmission may also occur by direct contact, since the influenza virus may persist for hours, particularly in the cold and in low humidity.

6. Incubation period—Short, usually 1–3 days.

7. Period of communicability—Probably 3–5 days from clinical onset in adults; up to 7 days in young children.

8. Susceptibility and resistance—When a new subtype appears, all children and adults are equally susceptible, except for those who have lived through earlier epidemics caused by the same or an antigenically similar subtype. Infection produces immunity to the specific infecting virus, but the duration and breadth of immunity depend on the degree of antigenic drift and the number of previous infections. Vaccines produce serologic responses specific for the included viruses and elicit booster responses to related strains with which the individual has had prior experience.

Age specific attack rates during an epidemic reflect persisting immunity from past experience with strains related to the epidemic subtype, so that the incidence of infection is often highest in school aged children. Thus, with the H1N1 epidemics that occurred after 1977, the incidence of disease was greatest among those born after 1957; most people born before this time had partial immunity from infection with antigenically similar H1N1 viruses that circulated between 1918 and 1957.

9. Methods of control—Detailed recommendations for the prevention and control of influenza are issued annually by CDC and WHO.

A. Preventive measures:

1) Educate the public and health care personnel in basic personal hygiene, especially the danger of unprotected coughs and sneezes, and hand to mucous membrane transmission.

2) Immunization with available inactivated virus vaccines may provide 70%–80% protection against infection in healthy young adults when the vaccine antigen closely matches the circulating strains of virus. In the elderly, immunization may be less effective in preventing illness, but it may reduce the severity of disease and the incidence of complications by 50%–60% and death by approximately 80%. Hospitalization of those 65 years of age or older for pneumonia and influenza in the USA over the period 1989–92 was reduced an estimated 30%–50% by immunization. Influenza immunization should be coupled with immunization against pneumococcal pneumonia (q.v.).

A single dose suffices for those with prior exposure to influenza A and B viruses; 2 doses of vaccine 1 month apart are required for persons who have no previous immunization history. Routine immunization programs should be directed primarily at those at greatest risk of serious complications or death (see Identification, above) and those who might spread infection to them (health care personnel and household contacts of high risk people). Immunization of children on long term aspirin therapy is also recommended to prevent development of Reye syndrome after influenza infection. Intranasally administered, cold adapted live attenuated trivalent influenza vaccines are in the final stages of clinical efficacy testing in children and adults and are expected to become generally available in the new millennium.

Immunization should also be considered for those engaged in essential community services and is recommended for military personnel. However, any individual may benefit from immunization.

The vaccine should be given each year **before** influenza is expected in the community (November to March in the USA). For those living or traveling outside the USA, timing of immunization should be based on the different seasonal patterns of influenza in different parts of the world (April to September in the Southern Hemisphere and tropics). Biannual recommendations for vaccine components are based on the viral strains currently circulating as determined by international surveillance.

Contraindications: Allergic hypersensitivity to egg protein or other vaccine components is a contraindication. During the swine influenza vaccine program in 1976, an increased risk of developing Guillain-Barré syndrome (GBS) within 6 weeks after vaccination was reported in the USA. Subsequent vaccines produced from other virus strains have not been clearly associated with an increased risk of GBS.

3) Amantadine hydrochloride (Symmetrel®, Symadine®) or riman-

tadine hydrochloride (Flumadine®) is effective in the chemo-prophylaxis of influenza A, but not influenza type B. Amantadine is associated with CNS side effects in 5%–10% of recipients; these may be more severe in the elderly or those with impaired kidney function. For this reason, persons with underlying renal disease should receive reduced dosages that reflect the degree of renal impairment. Rimantadine is reported to cause fewer CNS side effects. The use of these drugs should be considered in nonimmunized persons or groups at high risk of complications, such as residents of institutions or nursing homes for the elderly, when an appropriate vaccine is not available or as a supplement to vaccine when immediate maximal protection is desired against influenza A infection. The drug should be continued throughout the epidemic; it will not interfere with the response to influenza vaccine. Inhibitors of influenza neuraminidase have been shown to be safe and partially effective for both prophylaxis and treatment of influenza A and B. These new drugs were initially licensed for use in Australia and Sweden, and were licensed in mid 1999 in the USA. Neuraminidase inhibitors are expected to be widely marketed in the new millennium.

B. *Control of patient, contacts and the immediate environment:*

1) Report to local health authority: Reporting outbreaks or laboratory confirmed cases assists disease surveillance. Report identity of the infectious agent as determined by laboratory examination if possible, Class 1A (see Communicable Disease Reporting).

2) Isolation: Impractical under most circumstances because of the delay in diagnosis, unless rapid, direct viral tests are available. In epidemics, due to increased patient load, it would be desirable to isolate patients (especially infants and young children) believed to have influenza by placing them in the same room (cohorting) during the initial 5–7 days of illness.

3) Concurrent disinfection: None.

4) Quarantine: None.

5) Protection of contacts: A specific role has been shown for antiviral chemoprophylaxis with amantadine or rimantadine against type A strains (see 9A3, above).

6) Investigation of contacts and source of infection: Of no practical value.

7) Specific treatment: Amantadine or rimantadine started within 48 hours of onset of influenza A illness and given for approximately 3–5 days reduces symptoms and virus titers in the respiratory secretions. Dosages are 5 mg/kg/day in 2 divided doses for those 1–9 years of age, and 100 mg twice a

day for those more than 9 years (if weight is less than 45 kg, use 5 mg/kg/day in 2 doses) for 2-5 days. Doses should be reduced for those 65 years of age and older or with decreased hepatic and renal function. Newly developed neuraminidase inhibitors may also be considered for the treatment of influenza A and B, but they became available in the USA only with the 1999/2000 influenza season.

During treatment with either drug, drug resistant viruses may emerge late in the course of treatment and may be transmitted to others; therefore, cohorting people on antiviral therapy should be considered, especially in closed populations with many high risk individuals. Patients should be watched for development of bacterial complications, and only then should antibiotics be administered. Because of the association with Reye syndrome, salicylates should be avoided in children.

C. Epidemic measures:

1) The severe and often disruptive effects of epidemic influenza on community activities may be reduced in part by effective health planning and education, particularly locally organized immunization programs for high risk patients and their care providers. Surveillance by health authorities of the extent and progress of outbreaks and the reporting of findings to the community are important.

2) Closure of individual schools has not proven to be an effective control measure; it has generally been applied too late and only because of high absenteeism of students and staff.

3) Hospital administrators should anticipate the increased demand for medical care during epidemic periods; there may also be excessive absenteeism of health care personnel as a result of influenza. To prevent this, health care personnel should be immunized annually or use antiviral drugs during influenza A epidemics.

4) Maintain adequate supplies of antiviral drugs to treat high risk patients and essential personnel in the event of the emergence of a new pandemic strain for which no suitable vaccine is available in time for the first wave.

D. Disaster implications: Aggregations of people in emergency shelters will favor outbreaks of disease if the virus is introduced.

E. International measures: A Disease under Surveillance by WHO. The following are recommended:

1) Report epidemics within a country to WHO.

2) Identify the causative virus in reports, and submit prototype strains to one of the four WHO Centres for Reference and

Research on Influenza (Atlanta, London, Tokyo and Melbourne). Throat secretion specimens, nasopharyngeal aspirates and paired blood samples may be sent to any WHO recognized national influenza center.

3) Conduct epidemiologic studies and promptly identify viruses to the national health agencies.

4) Ensure sufficient commercial and/or governmental facilities to provide rapid production of adequate quantities of vaccine and antiviral drugs, and maintain programs for vaccine and antiviral drug administration to high risk people and essential personnel.

KAWASAKI SYNDROME   ICD-9 446.1; ICD-10 M303
(Kawasaki disease, Mucocutaneous lymph node syndrome, Acute febrile mucocutaneous lymph node syndrome)

1. Identification—An acute febrile, self-limited, systemic vasculitis of early childhood, presumably of infectious or toxic origin. Clinically characterized by a high, spiking fever (mean duration 12 days), unresponsive to antibiotics, associated with pronounced irritability and mood change; usually solitary, frequently unilateral nonsuppurative cervical adenopathy; bilateral nonexudative bulbar conjunctival injection; an enanthem consisting of a "strawberry tongue," injected oropharynx or dry fissured or erythematous lips; limb changes consisting of edema, erythema or periungual or generalized desquamation; and a generalized polymorphous erythematous exanthem that can be truncal or perineal and can range from a morbilliform maculopapular rash to an urticarial rash to a vasculitic exanthem.

Typically there are three phases: 1) an acute febrile phase of about 10 days characterized by high, spiking fever, rash, adenopathy, peripheral erythema or edema, conjunctivitis and enanthem; 2) a subacute phase lasting about 2 weeks characterized by thrombocytosis, desquamation, and resolution of fever; and 3) a lengthy convalescent phase during which clinical signs fade.

The case-fatality rate is between 0.1% and 1.0%; half of the deaths occur within 2 months of illness.

There is no pathognomonic laboratory test for Kawasaki syndrome (KS), but an elevated ESR, C-reactive protein and platelet counts above 450,000/mm³ (SI units 450×10^9/L) are common laboratory features. Diagnosis is based on the presence of fever lasting more than 5 days, exclusion of other causes and at least four of the following: 1) bilateral conjunctival injection;

2) injected or fissured lips, or injected pharynx, or "strawberry tongue"; 3) erythema of palms or soles, or edema of the hands or feet, or generalized or periungual desquamation; 4) rash; and 5) cervical lymphadenopathy (at least 1 node equal to or greater than 1.5 cm). The criterion for fever more than 5 days is waived if intravenous immune globulin (IVIG) therapy is administered within 5 days of onset while the patient is still febrile. Atypical KS may be diagnosed with fewer than five of the diagnostic criteria in the presence of documented coronary artery aneurysm.

2. Infectious agent—Unknown. Currently, the cause is postulated to be a superantigen bacterial toxin secreted by *Staphylococcus aureus* or group A streptococci, but this has not been confirmed or generally accepted.

3. Occurrence—Worldwide, although most cases (more than 100,000) have been reported from Japan, where nationwide epidemics have been documented. In the USA, the estimated number of new cases each year is approximately 2,000. Approximately 80% of cases are diagnosed in children less than 5 years old, with a peak incidence in those 1–2 years old, more in boys than in girls. Cases are more frequent in the winter and spring. Outbreaks have been reported in various cities and states throughout the USA. In Japan, where the disease has been tracked since 1970, peak incidence occurred in 1984-85. Since then, the incidence rate has been steady, with an incidence of 108 per 100,000 hospitalized children in 1996.

4. Reservoir—Unknown, perhaps humans.

5. Mode of transmission—Unknown; no firm evidence of person to person transmission, even within families. Seasonal variation, limitation to the pediatric age group and outbreak occurrence in communities is consistent with an infectious etiology.

6. Incubation period—Unknown.

7. Period of communicability—Unknown.

8. Susceptibility and resistance—Children, especially those of Asian ancestry, are most likely to develop KS, but given the relatively low number of these individuals in the USA, the majority of cases are reported among African American and Caucasian children. Recurrences are very infrequently reported.

9. Methods of control—

A. Preventive measures: Unknown.

B. Control of patient, contacts and the immediate environment:

1) Report to local health authority: Voluntary reporting in the USA to the Kawasaki Surveillance System, Centers for Disease

Control and Prevention (CDC 55.54 Rev. 1-91) through local and state health departments. Clusters and epidemics should be reported immediately, Class 5 (see Communicable Disease Reporting).

2) Isolation: None.

3) Concurrent disinfection: None.

4) Quarantine: None.

5) Immunization of contacts: Not applicable.

6) Investigation of contacts: Not profitable except in outbreaks and clusters.

7) Specific treatment: High-dose IVIG, preferably as a single dose, within 10 days of onset of fever can reduce fever, inflammatory signs and aneurysm formation and should be considered even if the duration of fever is greater than 10 days. About 10% of patients may not respond and may require retreatment. High dose aspirin is recommended during the acute phase, followed by low doses for at least 2 months. Measles and/or Varicella vaccine should usually be deferred following receipt of IVIG.

C. Epidemic measures: Outbreaks and clusters should be investigated to elucidate etiology and risk factors.

D. Disaster implications: None.

E. International measures: None.

LASSA FEVER   ICD-9 078.8; ICD-10 A96.2

1. Identification—An acute viral illness of 1–4 weeks duration. Onset is gradual, with malaise, fever, headache, sore throat, cough, nausea, vomiting, diarrhea, myalgia and chest and abdominal pain; fever is persistent or spikes intermittently. Inflammation and exudation of the pharynx and conjunctivae are commonly observed. About 80% of human infections are mild or asymptomatic; the remaining cases have a severe multisystem disease. In severe cases, hypotension or shock, pleural effusion, hemorrhage, seizures, encephalopathy and edema of the face and neck are frequent. Albuminuria and hemoconcentration are common. Early lymphopenia may be followed by late neutrophilia. Platelet counts are only moderately depressed, but platelet function is abnormal. Disease is more severe in pregnancy, and fetal loss occurs in more than 80% of cases. Transient alopecia and ataxia may occur in convalescence, and 8th cranial nerve deafness occurs in 25% of patients; only half recover some function after 1–3 months. Though only about 1% of infected persons die, the case-fatality rate is about 15% among hospitalized cases; higher rates may be observed in epidemics. Women in the third trimester of pregnancy and fetuses fare poorly. AST levels more than 150 and high viremia indicate poor prognosis. Inapparent infections, diagnosed serologically, are common in endemic areas.

Diagnosis is made by IgM antibody capture and antigen detection by ELISA or by PCR; by isolation of virus from blood, urine or throat washings; and IgG seroconversion by ELISA or IFA. Laboratory specimens may be biohazardous and must be handled with extreme care that includes BSL-4 containment, if available. Heating serum at 60°C (140°F) for 1 hour will largely inactivate the virus, and the serum can then be used to measure heat stable substances such as electrolytes, BUN or creatinine.

2. Infectious agent—Lassa virus, an arenavirus, serologically related to lymphocytic choriomeningitis, Machupo, Junín, Guanarito and Sabiá viruses.

3. Occurrence—Endemic in Sierra Leone, Liberia, Guinea and regions of Nigeria. Cases have also been reported from the Central African Republic. Serologic evidence of human infection has also been recognized in the Congo, Mali and Senegal. Serologically related viruses of lesser virulence for laboratory hosts from Mozambique and Zimbabwe have not yet been associated with human infection or disease.

4. Reservoir—Wild rodents; in west Africa, the multimammate mouse of the *Mastomys* species complex.

5. Mode of transmission—Primarily through aerosol or direct contact with excreta of infected rodents deposited on surfaces such as floors and beds or in food and water. Laboratory infections occur, especially in the hospital environment, direct contact with blood through inoculation with contaminated needles and pharyngeal secretions or urine of a patient. Infection can also be spread from person to person by sexual contact.

6. Incubation period—Commonly 6–21 days.

7. Period of communicability—Person to person spread may occur during the acute febrile phase when virus is present in the throat. Virus may be excreted in urine of patients for 3–9 weeks from onset of illness.

8. Susceptibility and resistance—All ages are susceptible; the duration of immunity following infection is unknown.

9. Methods of control —

   A. Preventive measures: Specific rodent control.

   B. Control of patient, contacts and the immediate environment:

   1) Report to local health authority: Individual cases should be reported, Class 2A (see Communicable Disease Reporting).

2) Isolation: Institute immediate strict barrier isolation in a private hospital room away from traffic patterns. Entry of nonessential staff and visitors should be restricted. Because of the low incidence of nosocomial infections reported from African hospitals, transfer to special isolation units is not considered necessary; however, nosocomial transmission has occurred, and strict procedures for isolation of body fluids and excreta should be maintained. A negative pressure room and respiratory protection is desirable. Male patients should refrain from unprotected sexual activity until the semen has been shown to be free of virus or for 3 months. To reduce exposure to infectious materials, laboratory tests should be kept to the minimum necessary for proper diagnosis and patient care. Technicians should be alerted to the nature of the specimens and supervised to ensure that appropriate specimen inactivation/isolation procedures are followed. Dead bodies should not be embalmed but rather sealed in leakproof material and cremated or buried promptly in a sealed casket.

3) Concurrent disinfection: Patient's excreta, sputum, blood and all objects with which the patient has had contact, including laboratory equipment used to carry out tests on blood, should be disinfected with 0.5% sodium hypochlorite solution or 0.5% phenol with detergent, and, as far as possible, appropriate heating methods, such as autoclaving, incineration or boiling. Laboratory tests should be carried out in special high containment facilities; if there is no such facility, tests should be kept to a minimum and specimens handled by experienced technicians using all available precautions such as gloves and biological safety cabinets. When appropriate, serum may be heat inactivated at 60°C (140°F) for 1 hour. Thorough terminal disinfection with 0.5% sodium hypochlorite solution or a phenolic compound is adequate; formaldehyde fumigation can be considered.

4) Quarantine: Only surveillance is recommended for close contacts (see 9B6, below).

5) Immunization of contacts: None.

6) Investigation of contacts and source of infection: Identify all close contacts (people living with, caring for, testing laboratory specimens from or having noncasual contact with the patient) in the 3 weeks after the onset of illness. Establish close surveillance of contacts as follows: body temperature checks at least 2 times daily for at least 3 weeks after last exposure. In case of temperature greater than 38.3°C (101°F), hospitalize immediately in strict isolation facilities. Determine patient's place of residence during 3 weeks prior to onset, and search for unreported or undiagnosed cases.

7) Specific treatment: Ribavirin (Virazole®), most effective within the first 6 days of illness, should be given IV, 30 mg/kg initially, followed by 15 mg/kg every 6 hours for 4 days and 8 mg/kg every 8 hours for 6 additional days.

C. Epidemic measures: Not determined.

D. Disaster implications: *Mastomys* may become more numerous in homes and food storage areas and increase the risk of human exposures.

E. International measures: Notification of source country and to receiving countries of possible exposures by infected travelers.

LEGIONELLOSIS   ICD-9 482.8; ICD-10 A48.1
(Legionnaires' disease; Legionnaires' pneumonia)
NONPNEUMONIC LEGIONELLOSIS   ICD-10 A48.2
(Pontiac fever)

1. Identification—An acute bacterial disease with two currently recognized, distinct clinical and epidemiologic manifestations: Legionnaires' disease (ICD-10 A48.1) and Pontiac fever (ICD-10 A48.2). Both are characterized initially by anorexia, malaise, myalgia and headache. Within a day, there is usually a rapidly rising fever associated with chills. Temperatures commonly reach 39°C-40.5°C (102°F-105°F). A nonproductive cough, abdominal pain and diarrhea are common. In Legionnaires' disease, a chest radiograph may show patchy or focal areas of consolidation that may progress to bilateral involvement and ultimately to respiratory failure; the case-fatality rate has been as high as 39% in hospitalized cases of Legionnaires' disease; it is generally higher in those with compromised immunity.

Pontiac fever is not associated with pneumonia or death; patients recover spontaneously in 2-5 days without treatment; this clinical syndrome may represent reaction to inhaled antigen rather than bacterial invasion.

Diagnosis depends on isolation of the causative organism on special media, its demonstration by direct IF stain of involved tissue or respiratory secretions, or detection of antigens of *Legionella pneumophila* serogroup 1 in urine by RIA or by a fourfold or greater rise in IFA titer between an acute phase serum and one drawn 3-6 weeks later.

2. Infectious agent—*Legionellae* are poorly staining, Gram-negative bacilli that require cysteine and other nutrients to grow in vitro. Eighteen serogroups of *L. pneumophila* are currently recognized; however, *L. pneumophila* serogroup 1 is most commonly associated with disease. Related organisms, including *L. micdadei, L. bozemanii, L. longbeachae* and *L. dumoffii,* have been isolated, predominantly from immunosuppressed patients with pneumonia. In all, 35 species of *Legionella* with at least 45 serogroups are currently recognized.

3. Occurrence—Legionellosis is neither new nor localized. The earliest documented case occurred in 1947; the earliest documented outbreak in 1957 in Minnesota. Since then, the disease has been identified throughout North America, as well as in Australia, Africa, South America and Europe. Although cases occur throughout the year, both sporadic cases and outbreaks are recognized more commonly in summer and autumn. Serologic surveys suggest a prevalence of antibodies to *L. pneumophila* serogroup 1 at a titer of 1:128 or greater in 1%–20% of the general population in the few locations studied. The proportion of cases of community acquired pneumonias that are due to *Legionella* ranges between 0.5% and 5.0%.

Outbreaks of legionellosis usually occur with low attack rates (0.1%–5%) in the population at risk. Epidemic Pontiac fever has had a high attack rate (about 95%) in several outbreaks.

4. Reservoir—Probably primarily aqueous. Hot water systems (showers), air conditioning cooling towers, evaporative condensers, humidifiers, whirlpool spas, respiratory therapy devices and decorative fountains have been implicated epidemiologically; the organism has been isolated from water in these, as well as from hot and cold water taps and showers, hot tubs and from creeks and ponds and the soil from their banks. The organism survives for months in tap and distilled water. An association of Legionnaires' disease with soil disturbances or excavation has not been clearly established.

5. Mode of transmission—Epidemiologic evidence supports airborne transmission; other modes are possible, including aspiration of water.

6. Incubation period—Legionnaires' disease 2–10 days, most often 5–6 days; Pontiac fever 5–66 hours, most often 24–48 hours.

7. Period of communicability—Person to person transmission has not been documented.

8. Susceptibility and resistance—Illness occurs most frequently with increasing age (most cases are at least 50 years of age), especially in patients who smoke and in those with diabetes mellitus, chronic lung disease, renal disease or malignancy; and in the immunocompromised, particularly those who are receiving corticosteroids or who have had an organ transplant. The male:female ratio is about 2.5:1. The disease is extremely rare in those under 20 years of age. Several outbreaks have occurred among hospitalized patients.

9. **Methods of control—**

A. *Preventive measures:* Cooling towers should be drained when not in use, and they should be mechanically cleaned periodically to remove scale and sediment. Appropriate biocides should be used to limit the growth of slime forming organisms. Tap water should not be used in respiratory therapy devices. Cost-effective preventive guidelines for domestic water systems have not been established; maintaining hot water system temperatures at 50°C (122°F) or higher may reduce the risk of transmission.

B. *Control of patient, contacts and the immediate environment:*

1) Report to local health authority: In selected areas (USA); in many countries, not a reportable disease, Class 3B (see Communicable Disease Reporting).
2) Isolation: None.
3) Concurrent disinfection: None.
4) Quarantine: None.
5) Immunization of contacts: None.
6) Investigation of contacts and source of infection: Search (households, business) for additional cases due to infection from a common environmental source. Initiate an investigation for a hospital source should a single confirmed nosocomial case be identified.
7) Specific treatment: Erythromycin appears to be the agent of choice; the newer macrolides, clarithromycin and azithromycin, may be effective. Rifampin may be a valuable adjunct but should not be used alone. Experience with fluoroquinolones is encouraging but limited. Penicillin, the cephalosporins and the aminoglycosides are ineffective.

C. *Epidemic measures:* Search for common exposures among cases and possible environmental sources of infection. Decontamination of implicated sources by chlorination and/or superheating water supplies has been effective.

D. *Disaster implications:* None known.

E. *International measures:* None.

LEISHMANIASIS   ICD-9 085; ICD-10 B55
I. CUTANEOUS AND MUCOSAL
   LEISHMANIASIS   ICD-9 085.1–085.5;
                                                   ICD-10 B55.1, B55.2
(Aleppo evil, Baghdad or Delhi boil, Oriental sore; in the Americas,
Espundia, Uta, Chiclero ulcer)

1. Identification—A polymorphic protozoan disease of skin and mucous membranes caused by a number of species of the genus *Leishmania*. These protozoa exist as obligate intracellular parasites in humans and other mammalian hosts. The disease starts with a papule that enlarges and typically becomes an indolent ulcer. Lesions may be single or multiple, occasionally nonulcerative and diffuse. Lesions may heal spontaneously within weeks to months, or last for a year or more. In some individuals, certain parasite strains (mainly from the Western Hemisphere) can disseminate to cause mucosal lesions (espundia), even years after the primary cutaneous lesion has healed. These sequelae involve nasopharyngeal tissues, are characterized by progressive tissue destruction and often scanty presence of parasites and can be severely disfiguring. Recurrence of cutaneous lesions after apparent cure may occur as ulcers, papules or nodules at or near the healed original ulcer.

Diagnosis is made by microscopic identification of the nonmotile, intracellular form (amastigote) in stained specimens from lesions, and by culture of the motile, extracellular form (promastigote) on suitable media. An intradermal (Montenegro) test with antigen derived from the promastigotes (not available in the USA) generally is positive in established disease; it is not helpful with very early lesions or anergic disease. Serologic (IFA or ELISA) testing can be done, but antibody levels typically are low or undetectable, so this may not be helpful in diagnosis (except for mucosal leishmaniasis). Species identification requires testing for biological (development in sand flies, culture media and animals), immunologic (monoclonal antibodies), molecular (DNA techniques) and biochemical (isoenzyme analysis) criteria.

2. Infectious agents—Eastern Hemisphere: *Leishmania tropica, L. major, L. aethiopica*. Western Hemisphere: *L. braziliensis* and *L. mexicana* complexes of species. Members of the *L. braziliensis* complex are more likely to produce mucosal lesions; *L. tropica* is the usual cause of the "leishmaniasis recidivans" cutaneous lesions. Members of the *L. donovani* complex usually cause visceral disease in the Eastern Hemisphere; in the Western Hemisphere the responsible organism is *L. chagasi*. Both may cause cutaneous leishmaniasis without concomitant visceral involvement, as well as post-kala-azar dermal leishmaniasis.

3. Occurrence—Pakistan, India and recently China, the Middle East, including Iran and Afghanistan; southern regions of the former Soviet Union, the Mediterranean littoral; the sub-Saharan African savanna and

Sudan, the highlands of Ethiopia, Kenya and Namibia; south central Texas, Mexico (especially Yucatan), all of Central America, the Dominican Republic and every country of South America except Chile and Uruguay. A nonulcerative, keloid-like form has been observed with increasing frequency in Central America, especially Honduras, where it is called atypical cutaneous leishmaniasis. There are increasing numbers of cases of diffuse leishmaniasis in Mexico and the Dominican Republic. In some areas in the Eastern Hemisphere, urban population groups, including children, may be at risk. In the Western Hemisphere, disease is usually restricted to occupational groups, such as those involved in work in forested areas; to those whose homes are in or next to a forest; and to visitors to such areas from nonendemic countries. Generally more common in rural than urban areas.

4. Reservoir—Locally variable; humans, wild rodents, hydraxes, edentates (sloths), marsupials and carnivores (Canidae), often including domestic dogs; unknown hosts in many areas.

5. Mode of transmission—From the zoonotic reservoir host through the bite of infective female phlebotomines (sand flies). After feeding on an infected mammalian host, motile promastigotes develop and multiply in the sand fly gut; in 8–20 days, infective parasites develop, which are injected during biting. In humans and other mammals, the organisms are taken up by macrophages and transform into amastigote forms, which multiply within the macrophages until the cells rupture and enable spread to other macrophages. Transmission from person to person and by blood transfusion and sexual contact has been reported, but is rare.

6. Incubation period—At least a week, up to many months.

7. Period of communicability—Not typically transmitted from person to person, but infectious to sand flies as long as parasites remain in lesions; in untreated cases, usually a few months to 2 years. Eventual spontaneous healing occurs in most cases. A small proportion of patients infected with *L. amazonensis* or *L. aethiopica* may develop diffuse cutaneous lesions that are rich in parasites and do not heal spontaneously. Infections with parasites of the *L. braziliensis* complex can heal spontaneously, but a small proportion are followed, months or years later, by metastatic mucosal lesions.

8. Susceptibility and resistance—Susceptibility is probably general. Lifelong immunity may be present after lesions due to *L. tropica* or *L. major* heal but may not protect against other leishmanial species. Factors responsible for late mutilating disease, such as espundia, are unknown; occult infections may be activated years after the primary infection. The most important factor in immunity is development of an adequate cell mediated response.

9. **Methods of control—**

A. ***Preventive measures:*** Control measures vary from area to area, depending on the habits of the mammalian hosts and the phlebotomine vectors. Where these habits are known, applicable control measures may be carried out. These include the following:

1) Detect cases systematically and treat rapidly. This applies to all forms of leishmaniasis and is one of the important measures to prevent development of destructive mucosal lesions in the Western Hemisphere and "recidivans forms" in the Eastern Hemisphere, particularly in those situations where the reservoir is largely or solely in people.

2) Apply insecticides with residual action periodically. Phlebotomine sand flies have a relatively short flight range and are highly susceptible to control by systematic spraying with residual insecticides. Spraying should cover exteriors and interiors of doorways and other openings if transmission occurs in dwellings. Possible breeding places of Eastern Hemisphere sand flies, such as stone walls, animal houses and rubbish heaps, should be sprayed.

Exclude vectors by screening, this requires a fine mesh screen (10–12 holes per linear cm or 25–30 holes per linear inch, an aperture size not more than 0.89 mm or 0.035 inches). Insecticide impregnated bed nets are currently under trial.

3) Eliminate rubbish heaps and other breeding places for Eastern Hemisphere phlebotomines.

4) Destroy gerbils (and their burrows) implicated as reservoirs in local areas by deep ploughing and removal of chenopods. Dog control in specific areas.

5) In the Western Hemisphere, avoid sand fly infested and thickly forested areas, particularly after sundown; use insect repellents and protective clothing if exposure to sand flies is unavoidable.

6) Apply appropriate environmental management and forest clearance.

B. ***Control of patient, contacts and the immediate environment:***

1) Report to local health authority: Official report not ordinarily justifiable, Class 5 (see Communicable Disease Reporting).

2) Isolation: None. Only of theoretical value.

3) Concurrent disinfection: None.

4) Quarantine: None.

5) Immunization of contacts: None.

6) Investigation of contacts and source of infection: Determine

local transmission cycle and interrupt it in most practical fashion.

7) Specific treatment: Mainly pentavalent antimonials, either sodium stibogluconate (Pentostam®), which is available in the USA from CDC, Atlanta or meglumine antimonate (Glucantime®), which is used in South America and some other areas. Pentamidine is used as a second line drug for cutaneous leishmaniasis. The imidazoles, ketoconazole and itraconazole, may have moderate antileishmanial activity against some leishmanial species. Amphotericin B (Fungizone®) may be required in South American mucosal disease if it does not respond to antimonial therapy. While spontaneous healing of simple cutaneous lesions occurs, infections acquired in geographic regions where mucosal disease has been reported should be treated promptly.

C. *Epidemic measures:* In areas of high incidence, use intensive efforts to control the disease by provision of diagnostic facilities and appropriate measures directed against phlebotomine flies and the mammalian reservoir hosts.

D. *Disaster implications:* None.

E. *International measures:* WHO Collaborating Centres.

II. VISCERAL LEISHMANIASIS ICD-9 085.0; ICD-10 B55.0
(Kala-azar)

1. **Identification**—A chronic systemic disease caused by intracellular protozoa of the genus *Leishmania*. The disease is characterized by fever, hepatosplenomegaly, lymphadenopathy, anemia, leukopenia, thrombocytopenia and progressive emaciation and weakness. Untreated clinically evident disease is usually fatal. Fever is of gradual or sudden onset, persistent and irregular, often with two daily peaks, with alternating periods of apyrexia and low-grade fever. Post-kala-azar dermal lesions may occur after apparent cure of systemic disease.

Diagnosis is made preferably by culture of the organism from a biopsy specimen or aspirated material, or by demonstration of intracellular amastigotes (Leishman-Donovan bodies) in stained smears from bone marrow, spleen, liver, lymph node or blood. The PCR technique can detect one leishmanial infected macrophage in 8 ml of peripheral blood (see section I, above).

2. **Infectious agents**—Typically, but not exclusively, *Leishmania donovani, L. infantum, L. tropica* and *L. chagasi.*

3. Occurrence—A rural disease of some tropical and subtropical areas, occurring in foci in India, Bangladesh, Pakistan, China, southern regions of the former Soviet Union, the Middle East including Turkey, the Mediterranean basin, Mexico, Central and South America (mostly in Brazil), and in Sudan, Kenya, Ethiopia and sub-Saharan savanna parts of Africa. In many affected areas, the disease occurs commonly as scattered cases among infants, children and adolescents but occasionally in epidemic waves. Incidence is modified by the use of antimalarial insecticides. Where dog populations have been drastically reduced, human disease has also been reduced.

4. Reservoir—Known or presumed reservoirs include humans, wild Canidae and domestic dogs. Humans are the only known reservoir in India, Nepal and Bangladesh.

5. Mode of transmission—Through bite of infected phlebotomine sand flies. (See section I, 5, above.)

6. Incubation period—Generally 2–6 months; range is 10 days to years.

7. Period of communicability—Not usually transmitted from person to person, but infectious to sand flies as long as parasites persist in the circulating blood or skin of the mammalian reservoir host. Infectivity for phlebotomines may persist even after clinical recovery of human patients.

8. Susceptibility and resistance—Susceptibility is general. Kala-azar apparently induces lasting homologous immunity. Considerable evidence indicates that inapparent and subclinical infections are common and that malnutrition predisposes to clinical disease and activation of inapparent infections. Manifest disease occurs among AIDS patients, presumably as reactivation of latent infections.

9. Methods of control—

A. *Preventive measures:* See section I, 9A, above. In selected areas, eliminate domestic canine reservoir.

B. *Control of patient, contacts and the immediate environment:*

1) Report to local health authority: In selected leishmaniasis-endemic areas, Class 3B (see Communicable Disease Reporting).
2) Isolation: Blood and body fluid precautions.
3) Concurrent disinfection: None.
4) Quarantine: None.
5) Immunization of contacts: None.
6) Investigation of contacts and source of infection: Ordinarily none.

7) Specific treatment: Sodium stibogluconate (Pentostam®), available from CDC, Atlanta, and meglumine antimonate (Glucantime®) are effective. Cases that do not respond to antimony may be treated with amphotericin B or pentamidine; these are not used routinely because of toxicity. In some regions, such as Kenya and India, the disease is less responsive to treatment than in Mediterranean countries and may require longer courses of therapy than are typically used.

C. *Epidemic measures:* Effective control must include an understanding of the local ecology and transmission cycle, followed by adoption of practical measures to stop transmission.

D. *Disaster implications:* None.

E. *International measures:* Institute coordinated programs of control among neighboring countries where the disease is endemic. WHO Collaborating Centres.

LEPROSY
(Hansen's disease)

ICD-9 030; ICD-10 A30

1. Identification—A chronic bacterial disease of the skin, peripheral nerves and (in lepromatous patients) the upper airway. The manifestations of the disease vary in a continuous spectrum between the two polar forms, lepromatous and tuberculoid leprosy. In lepromatous leprosy, nodules, papules, macules and diffuse infiltrations are bilaterally symmetrical and usually numerous and extensive; involvement of the nasal mucosa may lead to crusting, obstructed breathing and epistaxis; ocular involvement leads to iritis and keratitis.

In tuberculoid leprosy, skin lesions are single or few, sharply demarcated, anesthetic or hypesthetic, and bilaterally asymmetrical; peripheral nerve involvement tends to be severe. Borderline leprosy has features of both polar forms and is more labile, with a tendency to shift toward the lepromatous form in the untreated patient, and toward the tuberculoid form in the treated patient. An early form of the disease, indeterminate leprosy, is manifested by a hypopigmented macule with ill defined borders and, if untreated, may progress to tuberculoid, borderline or lepromatous disease. The clinical manifestations can include "reactions" of leprosy, i.e., acute adverse episodes, which are termed erythema nodosum leprosum in lepromatous patients and reversal reactions in borderline leprosy.

Clinical diagnosis is based on complete skin examination. Search for signs of peripheral nerve involvement (hypesthesia, anesthesia, paralysis, muscle wasting or trophic ulcers) with bilateral palpation of peripheral nerves (ulnar nerve at the elbow, peroneal nerve at the head of the fibula and the great auricular nerve) for enlargement and tenderness. Test skin lesions for sensation (light touch, pinprick, temperature discrimination).

Differential diagnosis includes many infiltrative skin diseases, including lymphomas, lupus erythematosus, psoriasis, scleroderma and neurofibromatosis. Diffuse cutaneous leishmaniasis, some mycoses, myxedema and pachydermoperiostosis may resemble lepromatous leprosy, but acid-fast bacilli are not present. Several skin conditions, such as vitiligo, tinea versicolor, pityriasis alba, nutritional dyschromia, nevus and scars may resemble tuberculoid leprosy.

The diagnosis in lepromatous leprosy (the multibacillary form) is strongly supported by demonstration of acid-fast bacilli in skin smears made by the scraped incision method; in tuberculoid disease (the paucibacillary form), the bacilli may be so few that they are not demonstrable. Whenever possible, a skin biopsy confined to the affected area should be sent to a pathologist experienced in leprosy diagnosis. Nerve involvement with acid-fast bacilli is pathognomonic of leprosy.

2. Infectious agent—*Mycobacterium leprae*. The organism has not been grown in bacteriologic media or cell cultures. It can be grown in mouse foot pads to 10^6/g of tissue; in disseminated infections of the nine-banded armadillo, it grows to 10^9–10^{10}/g.

3. Occurrence—The world prevalence in 1997 was estimated by WHO to be 1.15 million cases. Prevalence rates of more than 5/1,000 are common in the rural tropics and subtropics; socioeconomic conditions may be more important than climate itself. The chief endemic areas are in south and southeast Asia, including the Philippines, Indonesia, Papua New Guinea, some Pacific islands, India, Bangladesh, Myanmar (Burma) and Indonesia; tropical Africa; and some areas of Latin America. Reported rates in the Americas range from less than 0.1 to 14/10,000.

Newly recognized cases in the USA are diagnosed principally in California, Florida, Hawaii, Louisiana, Texas and New York City, and in Puerto Rico. Most of these cases are in immigrants and refugees whose disease was acquired in their native countries; however, the disease remains endemic in California, Hawaii, Louisiana, Texas and Puerto Rico.

4. Reservoir—Humans are the only reservoir of proven significance. Feral armadillos in Louisiana and Texas have been found naturally afflicted with a disease identical to experimental leprosy in this animal, and there have been reports suggesting that disease in armadillos has been naturally transmitted to humans. Naturally acquired leprosy has been observed in a mangabey monkey and in a chimpanzee captured in Nigeria and Sierra Leone, respectively.

5. Mode of transmission—Although the exact mode of transmission is not clearly established, household and prolonged close contact appear to be important. Millions of bacilli are liberated daily in the nasal discharges of untreated lepromatous patients, and bacilli have been shown to remain viable for at least 7 days in dried nasal secretions. Cutaneous ulcers in lepromatous patients may also shed large numbers of bacilli. The organisms probably gain entrance through the upper respiratory tract and possibly through broken skin. In cases in children under 1 year of age, transmission is presumed to be transplacental.

6. Incubation period—The range is from 9 months to 20 years, the average is probably 4 years for tuberculoid leprosy and twice that for lepromatous leprosy. The disease is rarely seen in children under age 3; however, more than 50 cases have been identified in children less than 1 year of age, the youngest was 2.5 months.

7. Period of communicability—Clinical and laboratory evidence suggests that infectiousness is lost in most instances within 3 months of continuous and regular treatment with dapsone (DDS) or clofazimine, or within 3 days of treatment with rifampin.

8. Susceptibility and resistance—The persistence and form of leprosy depend on the ability to develop effective cell mediated immunity. The lepromin test is an intradermal injection of autoclaved *M. leprae;* the presence or absence of induration at 28 days is called the Mitsuda reaction. The reaction is negative in lepromatous leprosy and positive in tuberculoid disease and in a proportion of normal adults. Because the test has only very limited value for diagnosistic classification and as a marker of protective immunity, the WHO Expert Committee on Leprosy recommends the use of lepromin be restricted to research purposes.

The rate of positive tests in the general population increases with age. In addition, the high prevalence of *M. leprae* specific lymphocyte transformation and antibodies specific for *M. leprae* among close contacts of leprosy patients suggests that infection is frequent yet clinical disease occurs in only a small proportion of such close contacts.

9. Methods of control—The availability of drugs effective in treatment and in rapid elimination of infectiousness, such as rifampin, has changed the management of the patient with leprosy from, societal isolation with attendant despair to one of ambulatory treatment. Hospitalization is reserved only for managing reactions, surgical correction of deformities and treatment of ulcers resulting from anesthesia of the extremities.

A. Preventive measures:

1) Health education should stress the availability of effective multidrug therapy, the absence of infectivity of patients under continuous treatment and the prevention of physical and social disabilities.

2) Detect cases, particularly infectious multibacillary cases, early

and administer multidrug therapy on a regular outpatient basis whenever possible.

3) In field trials in Uganda, India, Malawi, Myanmar and Papua New Guinea, prophylactic *Bacillus Calmette-Guérin* (BCG) apparently effected a considerable reduction in the incidence of tuberculoid leprosy among contacts. A study in India indicated significant protection against leprosy but not against tuberculosis; studies in Myanmar and India showed less protection than in Uganda. Chemoprophylaxis studies suggest that approximately 50% protection against disease can be achieved with dapsone or acedapsone, but this is not recommended unless closely supervised. The addition of killed *M. leprae* does not seem to improve the protection achieved by BCG immunization.

B. Control of patient, contacts and the immediate environment:

1) Report to local health authority: Case report obligatory in many states (USA) and countries and desirable in all, Class 2B (see Communicable Disease Reporting).

2) Isolation: None for cases of tuberculoid leprosy; contact isolation for cases of lepromatous leprosy until multidrug therapy has been established. Hospitalization is often indicated during treatment of reactions. No special procedures are required when cases are hospitalized, but in a general hospital, a separate room may be desirable for aesthetic or social reasons. No restrictions in employment or attendance at school are indicated for patients whose disease is regarded as noninfectious.

3) Concurrent disinfection: Of nasal discharges of infectious patients. Terminal cleaning.

4) Quarantine: None.

5) Immunization of contacts: Not routinely practiced (see 9A3, above).

6) Investigation of contacts and source of infection: The initial examination is more productive, but periodic examination of household and other close contacts is recommended at 12-month intervals for at least 5 years after last contact with an infectious case.

7) Specific treatment: With the widespread prevalence of dapsone resistance and the emergence of resistance to rifampin, combined chemotherapy regimens are essential. The minimal regimen recommended by WHO for multibacillary leprosy is rifampin, 600 mg once monthly; dapsone (DDS), 100 mg/day; and clofazimine, 300 mg once monthly and 50 mg/day. The monthly rifampin and clofazimine are administered under supervision. The WHO Expert Committee on Leprosy has

determined that the minimum duration of therapy for multibacillary leprosy can be shortened to 12 months from the previously recommended 24 months. Treatment should be continued longer, as necessary, until skin smears are negative. For early paucibacillary (tuberculoid) leprosy, or patients with a single skin lesion, a single dose of multidrug therapy (600 mg rifampin, 400 mg ofloxacin and 100 mg minocyclone) is sufficient. In paucibacillary leprosy patients with more than one skin lesion, the recommended regimen (600 mg rifampin once a month (supervised) and 100 mg dapsone daily) should be given for 6 months. Patients under treatment should be monitored for drug side effects, for leprosy reactions and for development of trophic ulcers. Some complications may need to be treated in a referral center.

C. Epidemic measures: Not applicable.

D. Disaster implications: Any interruption of treatment schedules is serious. During wars, diagnosis and treatment of leprosy patients has often been neglected.

E. International measures: International controls should be limited to untreated infectious cases. WHO Collaborating Centres.

LEPTOSPIROSIS   ICD-9 100; ICD-10 A27
(Weil disease, Canicola fever, Hemorrhagic jaundice, Mud fever, Swineherd disease)

   1. Identification—A group of zoonotic bacterial diseases with protean manifestations. Common features are fever with sudden onset, headache, chills, severe myalgia (calves and thighs) and conjunctival suffusion. Other manifestations that may be present are diphasic fever, meningitis, rash (palatal exanthem), hemolytic anemia, hemorrhage into skin and mucous membranes, hepatorenal failure, jaundice, mental confusion and depression, myocarditis and pulmonary involvement with or without hemoptysis. In areas of endemic leptospirosis, a majority of infections are clinically inapparent or too mild to be diagnosed definitively.

Cases are often misdiagnosed as meningitis, encephalitis or influenza; serologic evidence of leptospiral infection is found among 10% of cases with otherwise undiagnosed meningitis and encephalitis. Clinical illness lasts from a few days to 3 weeks or longer. Generally, there are two phases in the illness; the leptospiremic or febrile stage, followed by the convalescent or immune phase. Recovery of untreated cases can take several months. Infections may be asymptomatic; severity varies with the infecting serovar. Case-fatality rate is low but increases with advancing age and may reach 20% or more in patients with jaundice and kidney damage who have not been treated with renal dialysis; deaths are due predominantly to hepatorenal failure, vascular abnormalities with hemorrhage, adult respiratory distress syndrome or cardiac arrhythmias due to myocarditis.

Different types of leptospires tend to occur in different locales, so serologic tests should utilize a panel of locally occurring leptospires. Difficulties in diagnosis have compromised disease control in a number of settings and resulted in increased severity and elevated mortality. Diagnosis is confirmed by rising titers in specific serologic tests, such as the microscopic agglutination test, and by isolation of leptospires from blood (first 7 days) or CSF (days 4–10) during the acute illness, and from urine after the 10th day, by using special media. Inoculation of young guinea pigs, hamsters or gerbils is often positive. IF and ELISA techniques are used for detection of leptospires in clinical and autopsy specimens.

2. **Infectious agent**—Leptospires, members of the order Spirochaetales. Pathogenic leptospires belong to the species *Leptospira interrogans,* which is subdivided into serovars. More than 200 serovars have been identified, and these fall into about 23 serogroups based on serologic relatedness. Important changes in leptospiral nomenclature are being made, based on DNA relatedness. Commonly identified serovars in the USA are *icterohaemorrhagiae, canicola, autumnalis, hebdomidis, australis* and *pomona.* In the UK, New Zealand and Australia, *L. interrogans* serovar *hardjo* infection in humans is the most common among those in close contact with infected livestock.

3. **Occurrence**—Worldwide; in urban and rural, developed and developing areas, except for polar regions. The disease it is an occupational hazard for rice and sugarcane fieldworkers, farmers, sewer workers, miners, veterinarians, animal husbandrymen, dairymen, abattoir workers, fish workers and military troops; outbreaks occur among those exposed to fresh river, stream, canal and lake water contaminated by urine of domestic and wild animals, and to urine and tissues of infected animals. The disease is a recreational hazard to bathers, campers and sportsmen in infected areas, and predominantly a disease of males, related to occupation. It appears to be increasing among urban children. A major outbreak in Nicaragua in 1995 caused extensive mortality. In 1997 and 1998 outbreaks were reported in India, Singapore, Thailand and Kazakhstan.

4. **Reservoir**—Wild and domestic animals; serovars vary with the animal affected. Notable are rats *(icterohemorrhagiae)*, swine *(pomona)*, cattle *(hardjo)*, dogs *(canicola)* and raccoons *(autumnalis)*. In the USA, swine appear to be the reservoir hosts of *bratislava;* in Europe, also badgers. Alternative animal hosts with usually shorter carrier states abound and include feral rodents, deer, squirrels, foxes, skunks, raccoons, opossums and marine mammals (sea lions). Serovars infecting reptiles and

amphibians (frogs) have not been shown to infect humans but have been suspected in Barbados and Trinidad. In carrier animals, an asymptomatic infection occurs in the renal tubules, with leptospiruria persisting for long periods or, especially in reservoir species, for life.

5. Mode of transmission—Contact of the skin, especially if abraded, or of mucous membranes with water, moist soil or vegetation, especially sugarcane contaminated with urine of infected animals, as in swimming, accidental immersion or occupational abrasion; direct contact with urine or tissues of infected animals; occasionally through ingestion of food contaminated with urine of infected rats; and occasionally by inhalation of droplet aerosols of contaminated fluids.

6. Incubation period—Usually 10 days, with a range of 4–19 days.

7. Period of communicability—Direct transmission from person to person is rare. Leptospires may be excreted in the urine, usually for 1 month, but leptospiruria has been observed in humans and in animals for as long as 11 months after the acute illness.

8. Susceptibility and resistance—Susceptibility of humans is general; immunity to the specific serovar follows infection or (occasionally) immunization, but this may not protect against infection with a different serovar.

9. Methods of control—

    A. Preventive measures:

      1) Educate the public on modes of transmission, to avoid swimming or wading in potentially contaminated waters and to use proper protection when work requires such exposure.

      2) Protect workers in hazardous occupations by providing boots, gloves and aprons.

      3) Recognize potentially contaminated waters and soil and drain such waters when possible.

      4) Control rodents in human habitations, especially rural and recreational. Burn sugarcane fields before harvest.

      5) Segregate infected domestic animals; prevent contamination of human living, working and recreational areas by urine of infected animals.

      6) Immunization of farm and pet animals prevents illness, but not necessarily infection and renal shedding. The vaccine must contain the dominant local strains.

      7) Immunization of people has been carried out against occupational exposures to specific serovars in Japan, China, Italy, Spain, France and Israel.

      8) Doxycycline has been shown in Panama to be effective in preventing leptospirosis in exposed military personnel when

administered in an oral dose of 200 mg once weekly during periods of high exposure.

B. Control of patient, contacts and the immediate environment:

1) Report to local health authority: Obligatory case report in many states (USA) and countries, Class 2B (see Communicable Disease Reporting).
2) Isolation: Blood and body fluid precautions.
3) Concurrent disinfection: Articles soiled with urine.
4) Quarantine: None.
5) Immunization of contacts: None.
6) Investigation of contacts and source of infection: Search for exposure to infected animals and potentially contaminated waters.
7) Specific treatment: Penicillins, cephalosporins, lincomycin and erythromycin are inhibitory in vitro. Doxycycline and penicillin G have been shown to be effective in double blind placebo controlled trials; penicillin G and amoxicillin were effective as late as 7 days into an illness. Prompt specific treatment, as early in the illness as possible, is essential.

C. Epidemic measures: Search for source of infection, such as a contaminated swimming pool or other water source; eliminate the contamination or prohibit use. Investigate industrial and occupational sources, including direct animal contact.

D. Disaster implications: A potential problem following flooding of certain areas with a high water table.

E. International measures: WHO Collaborating Centres.

LISTERIOSIS   ICD-9 027.0; ICD-10 A32

1. Identification—A bacterial disease usually manifested as meningoencephalitis and/or septicemia in newborns and adults; manifestations in pregnant women are fever and abortion. Those at highest risk are neonates, the elderly, immunocompromised individuals and pregnant women. The onset of meningoencephalitis (which is rare in pregnant women) can be sudden, with fever, intense headache, nausea, vomiting and signs of meningeal irritation, or may be subacute, particularly in an immunocompromised or elderly host. Delirium and coma may appear early; occasionally there is collapse and shock. Endocarditis, granulomatous lesions in the liver and other organs, localized internal or external abscesses, and pustular or papular cutaneous lesions may occur on rare occasion.

The normal host who acquires infection may exhibit only an acute, mild, febrile illness, but, in pregnant women infection can be transmitted to the fetus. Infants may be stillborn, born with septicemia, or develop meningitis in the neonatal period even though the mother may be asymptomatic at delivery. The postpartum course of the mother is usually uneventful, but the case-fatality rate is 30% in newborn infants and approaches 50% when onset occurs in the first 4 days. In a recent epidemic, the overall case-fatality rate among nonpregnant adults was 35%: 11% in those less than 40 years old and 63% in those more than 60 years of age.

Diagnosis is confirmed by isolation of the infectious agent from CSF, blood, amniotic fluid, placenta, meconium, lochia, gastric washings and other sites of infection. *Listeria monocytogenes* can be isolated readily from normally sterile sites on routine media, but care must be taken to distinguish this organism from other gram-positive rods, particularly diphtheroids. Isolations from contaminated specimens are more frequent with improved selective enrichment media. Microscopic examination of CSF or meconium permits presumptive diagnosis; serologic tests are unreliable.

2. Infectious agent—*Listeria monocytogenes,* a gram-positive rod shaped bacterium; human infections are usually caused by serovars 1/2a, 1/2b and 4b.

3. Occurrence—An uncommonly diagnosed infection; in the USA, the incidence of illness severe enough to require hospitalization is about 1/200,000 population. Typically, it occurs sporadically; however, several outbreaks that occurred in all seasons were recognized in recent years. About 30% of clinical cases occur within the first three weeks of life; in nonpregnant adults, infection occurs mainly after age 40. Nosocomial acquisition has been reported. Asymptomatic infections probably occur at all ages, although these are of importance only during pregnancy. Abortion can occur at any point in pregnancy but it usually occurs in the second half; perinatal infection is acquired during the last trimester.

4. Reservoir—The principal reservoir of the organism is in soil, forage, water, mud and silage. The seasonal use of silage as fodder is frequently followed by an increased incidence of listeriosis in animals. Other reservoirs include infected domestic and wild mammals, fowl and people. Asymptomatic fecal carriage is common in humans (up to 10%) and has been much higher in abattoir workers and laboratory workers who work with *Listeria monocytogenes* cultures. Soft cheeses may support the growth of *Listeria* during ripening and have caused outbreaks. Unlike most other foodborne pathogens, *Listeria* tends to multiply in refrigerated foods that are contaminated.

5. Mode of transmission—Outbreaks of listeriosis have been reported in association with ingestion of raw or contaminated milk, soft cheeses, vegetables, and ready-to-eat meats, such as pâté. A substantial proportion of sporadic cases of listeriosis result from foodborne transmission. Papular lesions on hands and arms may occur from direct contact with infectious material.

In neonatal infections, the organism can be transmitted from mother to fetus in utero or during passage through the infected birth canal. There are rare reports of nursery outbreaks attributed to contaminated equipment or materials.

6. Incubation period—Variable; outbreak cases have occurred 3-70 days following a single exposure to an implicated product. Median incubation is estimated to be 3 weeks.

7. Period of communicability—Mothers of infected newborn infants can shed the infectious agent in vaginal discharges and urine for 7-10 days after delivery, rarely longer. However, infected individuals can shed the organisms in their stools for several months.

8. Susceptibility and resistance—Fetuses and newborn infants are highly susceptible. Children and young adults generally are resistant, adults less so after age 40, especially the immunocompromised and the elderly. Disease is usually superimposed on other debilitating illnesses such as cancer, organ transplantation, diabetes and AIDS. There is little evidence of acquired immunity, even after prolonged severe infection.

9. Methods of control—

A. *Preventive measures:*

1) Pregnant women and immunocompromised individuals should avoid soft cheeses such as Brie, Camembert, and Mexican style cheeses. They should cook, until steaming hot, leftover foods or foods such as hot dogs. They should avoid deli meats and eat only properly cooked meats and pasteurized dairy products. They should also avoid contact with potentially infective materials, such as aborted animal fetuses on farms.

2) Ensure safety of foods of animal origin. Pasteurize all dairy products where possible. Irradiate soft cheeses after ripening or monitor nonpasteurized dairy products, such as soft cheeses, by culturing for *Listeria.*

3) Processed foods that are found to be contaminated by *Listeria monocytogenes* (e.g., during routine bacteriologic surveillance) should be recalled.

4) Thoroughly wash raw vegetables before eating.

5) Thoroughly cook raw food from animal sources such as beef, pork, or poultry.

6) Wash hands, knives, and cutting boards after handling uncooked foods.

7) Avoid the use of untreated manure on vegetable crops.

8) Veterinarians and farmers should take proper precautions in handling aborted fetuses and sick or dead animals, especially sheep that died of encephalitis.

B. Control of patient, contacts and the immediate environment:

1) Report to local health authority: Obligatory case report required in many states (USA) and some countries, Class 2B; in others, report of clusters of cases required, Class 4 (see Communicable Disease Reporting).

2) Isolation: Enteric precautions.

3) Concurrent disinfection: None.

4) Quarantine: None.

5) Immunization of contacts: None.

6) Investigation of contacts and source of infection: Case surveillance data should be analyzed frequently for possible clusters; all suspected clusters should be investigated for common-source exposures.

7) Specific treatment: Penicillin or ampicillin alone or together with aminoglycosides. For penicillin-allergic patients, TMP-SMX or erythromycin is preferred. Cephalosporins, including third generation cephalosporins, are not effective in the treatment of clinical listeriosis. Tetracycline resistance has been observed. A gram-stained smear of meconium from clinically suspected newborn infants should be examined for short gram-positive rods resembling *L. monocytogenes.* If positive, prophylactic antibiotics should be administered as a precaution.

C. Epidemic measures: Investigate outbreaks to identify a common source of infection, and prevent further exposure to that source.

D. Disaster implications: None.

E. International measures: None.

LOIASIS   ICD-9 125.2; ICD-10 B74.3
(Loa loa infection, Eyeworm disease of Africa, Calabar swelling)

1. Identification—A chronic filarial disease characterized by migration of the adult worm through subcutaneous or deeper tissues of the body, causing transient swellings several centimeters in diameter, located on any part of the body. These swellings may be preceded by localized pain accompanied by pruritus. Pruritus localized on arms, thorax, face and shoulders is a major symptom. Local names include "fugitive swelling" and "Calabar swelling." Migration under the bulbar conjunctivae may be accompanied by pain and edema. Allergic reactions with giant urticaria and fever may occur occasionally.

Infections with other filariae, such as *Wuchereria bancrofti, Onchocerca volvulus, Mansonella (Dipetalonema) perstans* and *M. streptocerca* (which are common in areas where *Loa loa* is endemic) should be considered in the differential diagnosis.

Larvae (microfilariae) are present in peripheral blood during the daytime and can be demonstrated in stained thick blood smears, stained sediment of laked blood or by membrane filtration. Eosinophilia is frequent. Loa loa specific DNA can be detected in the blood from occult infected individuals. A travel history is essential for diagnosis.

2. Infectious agent—*Loa loa*, a filarial nematode.

3. Occurrence—Widely distributed in the African rain forest, especially in central Africa. In the Congo River basin, up to 90% of indigenous inhabitants of some villages are infected.

4. Reservoir—Humans.

5. Mode of transmission—Transmitted by a deer fly of the genus *Chrysops. Chrysops dimidiata, C. silacea* and other species ingest blood containing microfilariae; the larvae develop to their infectious stage within 10–12 days in the fly. They then migrate to the proboscis and are transferred to a human host by the bite of the infective fly.

6. Incubation period—Symptoms usually do not appear until several years after infection but may occur as early as 4 months. Microfilariae may appear in the peripheral blood as early as 6 months after infection.

7. Period of communicability—The adult worm may persist in humans, shedding microfilariae into the blood for as long as 17 years; in the fly, "communicability" is from 10–12 days after its infection until all infective larvae have been released, or until the fly dies.

8. Susceptibility and resistance—Susceptibility is universal; repeated infections occur and immunity, if present, has not been demonstrated.

9. Methods of control—

    A. Preventive measures:

        1) Measures directed against the fly larvae are effective but have not proven practical because the moist, muddy breeding areas are usually too extensive.

        2) Diethyltoluamide (Deet®, Autan®) or dimethyl phthalate applied to exposed skin are effective fly repellents.

3) Wear protective clothing (long sleeves and trousers), screen houses.

4) For temporary residents of endemic areas whose risk of exposure is high or prolonged, a weekly dose of diethylcarbamazine (300 mg) is prophylactic.

B. Control of patient, contacts and the immediate environment:

1) Report to local health authority: Official report not ordinarily required, Class 5 (see Communicable Disease Reporting).

2) Isolation: As far as possible, patients with microfilaremia should be protected from *Chrysops* bites to reduce transmission.

3) Concurrent disinfection: None.

4) Quarantine: None.

5) Immunization of contacts: None.

6) Investigation of contacts and source of infection: None; a community problem.

7) Specific treatment: Diethylcarbamazine (DEC, Banocide®, Hetrazan®, Notezine®) causes disappearance of microfilariae and may kill the adult worm with resulting cure. During therapy, however, hypersensitivity reactions (sometimes severe) are common but controllable with steroids and/or antihistamines. When microfilaremia is heavy (greater than 2,000/ml blood), there is a risk of meningoencephalitis, and the advantages of treatment must be weighed against the risk of life threatening encephalopathy; thus, treatment with DEC must be individualized and undertaken under close medical supervision. Ivermectin (Mectizan®) treatment also results in a reduction of microfilaremia, and the adverse reactions may be milder than with DEC. Albendazole also causes a slow decrease in microfilaremia and probably kills adult worms. Surgical removal of the migrating adult worm under the bulbar conjunctivae is indicated when feasible. Loa loa encephalopathy has been reported following ivermectin treatment for onchocerciasis.

C. Epidemic measures: Not applicable.

D. Disaster implications: None.

E. International measures: None.

LYME DISEASE

ICD-9 104.8, 088.81;
ICD-10 A69.2, L90.4

(Lyme borreliosis, Tickborne meningopolyneuritis)

1. Identification—This tickborne, spirochetal, zoonotic disease is characterized by a distinctive skin lesion, systemic symptoms and neurologic, rheumatologic and cardiac involvement that occur in varying combinations over a period of months to years. The early symptoms are intermittent and changing. The illness typically begins in the summer, and the first manifestation in about 90% of patients appears as a red macule or papule that expands slowly in an annular manner, often with central clearing. This distinctive skin lesion is called "erythema migrans" (EM; formerly "erythema chronicum migrans"). EM may be single or multiple. To be considered significant for case surveillance purposes, the EM lesion must reach 5 cm in diameter. With or without EM, early systemic manifestations may include malaise, fatigue, fever, headache, stiff neck, myalgia, migratory arthralgias and/or lymphadenopathy, all of which may last several weeks or more in untreated patients.

Within weeks to months after onset of the EM lesion, neurologic abnormalities such as aseptic meningitis and cranial neuritis—including facial palsy, chorea, cerebellar ataxia, motor or sensory radiculoneuritis, myelitis and encephalitis—may develop; symptoms fluctuate, may last for months and may become chronic. Cardiac abnormalities (including atrioventricular block and rarely, acute myopericarditis or cardiomegaly) may occur within a few weeks after onset of EM. Weeks to years after onset (mean, 6 months), intermittent episodes of swelling and pain in large joints, especially the knees, may develop and recur for several years; chronic arthritis may occasionally result. Similarly, sometimes following long periods of latent infection, chronic neurologic manifestations may develop and include encephalopathy, polyneuropathy or leukoencephalitis; the CSF often shows lymphocytic pleocytosis and elevated protein levels, while the electromyogram is usually abnormal.

Diagnosis is currently based on clinical findings supported by serologic tests performed in two stages, by IFA, ELISA, then Western immunoblot. Serologic tests, which are poorly standardized, must be interpreted with caution. They are insensitive during the first several weeks of infection and may remain negative in people treated early with antibiotics. An ELISA for IgM antibodies that uses a recombinant outer surface protein C (rOspC) has been shown to be more sensitive for early diagnosis than either whole cell ELISA or immunoblot assay. Test sensitivity increases when patients progress to later stages of the disease, but a small proportion of chronic Lyme disease patients may remain seronegative. Cross-reacting IFA and ELISA antibodies may cause false positive reactions in patients with syphilis, relapsing fever, leptospirosis, HIV infection, Rocky Mountain spotted fever, infectious mononucleosis, lupus or rheumatoid arthritis. The specificity of serologic testing is enhanced by immunoblot testing of all specimens that are positive or equivocal on IFA or ELISA. The etiologic agent, *Borrelia burgdorferi*, grows at 33°C (91.4°F) in the Barbour, Stoenner, Kelly (BSK) medium; other species causing Lyme-like disease may not grow well in this medium. Isolation from blood and tissue biopsies is difficult, but biopsies of the EM lesions may yield the organism in 80% or more of cases. By PCR, *B. burgdorferi* genetic material has been detected in synovial fluid, CSF, skin and other tissues, blood and urine; however, the usefulness of PCR in the routine management of Lyme disease patients has yet to be verified.

2. Infectious agents—The causative spirochete of North American Lyme disease, *B. burgdorferi*, was identified in 1982. Three genomic groups of *B. burgdorferi* sensu lato have now been identified in Europe; they have been named *B. burgdorferi* sensu stricto, *B. garinii* and *B. afzelii*.

3. Occurrence—In the USA, endemic foci exist along the Atlantic coast and are concentrated between Massachusetts and Maryland; in the upper midwest, an expanding focus is currently concentrated in Wisconsin and Minnesota; and in the west, in some areas of California and Oregon. Currently, increasing recognition of the disease is redefining endemic areas; cases have been reported from 47 states and from Ontario and British Columbia, Canada. Elsewhere, it has been found in Europe, the former Soviet Union, China and Japan.

Initial infection occurs primarily during summer, with a peak in June and July, but may occur throughout the year, depending on the seasonal abundance of the tick in different geographic areas. The distribution of the majority of cases coincides with the distribution of *Ixodes scapularis* (formerly called *I. dammini*) ticks in the eastern and midwestern USA, *I. pacificus* in western USA, *I. ricinus* in Europe and *I. persulcatus* in Asia. Dogs, cattle and horses develop systemic disease that may include the articular and cardiac manifestations seen in human patients. The explosive repopulation of white-tailed deer in the eastern USA by white-tailed deer has been linked to the spread of Lyme disease in this region.

4. Reservoir—Certain ixodid ticks through transstadial transmission. Wild rodents, especially *Peromyscus* spp. in the northeastern and midwestern USA and *Neotoma* spp. in the western USA maintain the enzootic transmission cycle. Deer serve as important maintenance mammalian hosts for vector tick species. Larval and nymphal ticks feed on small mammals, and adult ticks feed primarily on deer. The majority of Lyme disease cases result from bites by infected nymphs.

5. Mode of transmission—Tickborne; in experimental animals, transmission by *I. scapularis* and *I. pacificus* usually does not occur until the tick has been attached for 24 hours or more; this may also be true in humans.

6. Incubation period—For EM, from 3 to 32 days (mean 7 to 10 days) after tick exposure; however, the early stages of the illness may be inapparent, and the patient may present with later manifestations.

7. Period of communicability—No evidence of natural transmission from person to person. There are rare case reports of congenital transmission, but epidemiologic studies have not shown a link between maternal Lyme disease and adverse outcomes of pregnancy.

8. Susceptibility and resistance—All persons are probably susceptible. Reinfection has occurred in those treated with antibiotics for early disease.

9. Methods of control—

   A. Preventive measures:

   1) Educate the public about the mode of tick transmission and the means for personal protection.
   2) Avoid tick infested areas when feasible. To minimize exposure, wear light colored clothing that covers legs and arms so that ticks may be more easily seen; tuck pants into socks and apply tick repellent such as diethyltoluamide (Deet®, Autan®) to the skin or permethrin (a repellent and contact acaricide) to pant legs and sleeves.
   3) If working or playing in an infested area, search the total body area daily, do not neglect haired areas, and remove ticks promptly; these ticks may be very small. Remove any attached ticks by using gentle, steady traction with forceps (tweezers) applied close to the skin to avoid leaving mouth parts in the skin; protect hands with gloves, cloth or tissue when removing ticks from humans or animals. Following removal, cleanse the attachment site with soap and water.
   4) Measures designed to reduce tick populations on residential properties are available (host management, habitat modification, chemical control), but are generally impractical on a large-scale basis.
   5) During the late 1990s, two Lyme disease vaccines were developed that use recombinant *B. burgdorferi* lipidated outer-surface protein A (rOspA) as immunogen. As of late 1999, one of these vaccines was licensed by the FDA for persons aged 15–70 years in the USA. This vaccine is administered on a 3 dose schedule of 0, 1, and 12 months and was found to be safe (does not cause chronic arthritis) and is 76% effective in preventing overt Lyme disease after three doses. Information regarding vaccine safety and efficacy beyond the transmission season immediately after the third dose is not available. Thus, as of late 1999, the duration of protective immunity and need for booster doses beyond the third dose was unknown.
      a) Vaccine induced anti-rOspA antibodies routinely cause false positive ELISA results for Lyme disease. However,

experienced laboratory workers, through careful interpretation of the results of Western blot assay, can usually discriminate between *B. burgdorferi* infection and previous rOspA immunization, because anti-OspA antibodies do not develop after natural infection.

b) Lyme disease vaccine does not protect all recipients against infection with *B. burgdorferi* and offers no protection against other tickborne diseases. Decisions regarding the use of vaccine should be based on individual assessment of the risk of exposure to infected ticks and on careful consideration of the relative risks and benefits of the vaccine compared with other protective measures that include early diagnosis and treatment of Lyme disease.

c) Risk assessment should include consideration of the geographic distribution of Lyme disease. The areas of highest risk in the USA are concentrated within some northeastern and north central states. However, the risk for Lyme disease differs not only between regions, states and counties within states, but even within counties and townships. Detailed information about the distribution of Lyme disease risk within specific areas is best obtained from state and local public health authorities.

d) In areas of moderate to high risk, immunization should be considered for persons aged 15–70 years who engage in activities (e.g., recreational, property maintenance, occupational or leisure) that result in frequent or prolonged exposure to tick infested habitats. Lyme disease vaccine may be considered for persons aged 15–70 years who are exposed to tick infested habitats but whose exposure is neither frequent nor prolonged. The benefit of Lyme disease vaccine beyond that provided by basic personal protection and early diagnosis and treatment of infection is uncertain. Lyme disease vaccine is not recommended for persons who have minimal or no exposure to tick infested habitats.

B. *Control of patient, contacts and the immediate environment:*

1) Report to local health authority: Case report obligatory in all states (USA) and some countries, Class 3B (see Communicable Disease Reporting).
2) Isolation: None.
3) Concurrent disinfection: Carefully remove all ticks from patients.
4) Quarantine: None.
5) Immunization of contacts: None applicable.
6) Investigation of contacts and source of infection: Studies to

determine source of infection are indicated when cases occur outside a recognized endemic focus.

7) Specific treatment: For adults, the EM stage can usually be treated effectively with doxycycline (100 mg twice daily) or amoxicillin (500 mg 3–4 times daily). For localized EM, 2 weeks of therapy is usually sufficient; for early disseminated infection, 3–4 weeks of therapy should be given. Children less than 9 years of age can be treated with amoxicillin, 50 mg/kg/day in divided doses, for the same period of time as adults. Cefuroxime axetil or erythromycin can be used in those who are allergic to penicillin or who cannot take tetracyclines. Lyme arthritis can usually be treated successfully with a 4-week course of the oral agents. However, objective neurologic abnormalities, with the possible exception of facial palsy alone, are best treated with IV ceftriaxone, 2 g once daily, or IV penicillin, 20 m.u. in 6 divided doses, for 3–4 weeks. Treatment failures may occasionally occur with any of these regimens and retreatment may be necessary.

C. Epidemic measures: In hyperendemic areas, particular attention should be paid to identification of the tick species involved and the areas infested, and to recommendations in 9A1 through 9A3, above.

D. Disaster implications: None.

E. International measures: WHO Collaborating Centres.

LYMPHOCYTIC CHORIOMENINGITIS ICD-9 049.0; ICD-10 A87.2
(LCM, Benign [or serous] lymphocytic meningitis)

1. **Identification**—A viral infection of animals, especially mice, transmissible to humans, with a marked diversity of clinical manifestations. At times, there may be influenza-like symptoms, with myalgia, retroorbital headache, leukopenia and thrombocytopenia, followed by complete recovery; in some cases, the illness may begin with meningeal or meningoencephalomyelitic symptoms, or they may appear after a brief remission. Orchitis, parotitis, arthritis, myocarditis and rash occur occasionally. The acute course is usually short, very rarely fatal, and even with extremely severe manifestations (e.g., coma with meningoencephalitis), prognosis for recovery without sequelae is usually good, although convalescence with fatigue and vasomotor instability may be prolonged. The CSF in

cases with neurologic involvement typically shows a lymphocytic pleocytosis and, at times, a low glucose level. The primary pathologic finding in the rare human fatality is diffuse meningoencephalitis. A few fatal cases of hemorrhagic fever-like disease have been reported. Transplacental infection of the fetus that leads to hydrocephalus and chorioretinitis occurs and should be tested for in such cases.

Laboratory diagnostic methods include isolation of virus from blood or CSF early in the course of the illness by intracerebral inoculation of LCM-free 3 to 5 week old mice or cell cultures. Presence of specific IgM in serum or CSF by IgM capture ELISA or rising titers of antibodies by IFA in paired sera are considered diagnostic. LCM requires differentiation from other aseptic meningitides and viral encephalitides.

2. Infectious agent—Lymphocytic choriomeningitis virus, an arenavirus, serologically related to Lassa, Machupo, Junin, Guaranito and Sabia viruses.

3. Occurrence—Not uncommon in Europe and the Americas; underdiagnosed. Loci of infection among feral mice often persist over long periods and results in sporadic clinical disease. Outbreaks have occurred from exposure to pet hamsters and laboratory animals. Nude mice, now extensively used in many research laboratories, are susceptible to infection and may be prolific chronic excreters of virus.

4. Reservoir—The infected house mouse, *Mus musculus,* is the natural reservoir; infected females transmit infection to the offspring, which become asymptomatic persistent viral shedders. Infection also occurs in mouse and hamster colonies and in transplantable tumor lines.

5. Mode of transmission—Virus is excreted in urine, saliva and feces of infected animals, usually mice. Transmission to humans is probably through oral or respiratory contact with virus contaminated excreta, food or dust, or by contamination of skin lesions or cuts. Handling articles contaminated by naturally infected mice may place individuals at a high risk of infection.

6. Incubation period—Probably 8-13 days; 15-21 days until meningeal symptoms appear.

7. Period of communicability—Transmission from person to person has not been demonstrated and is unlikely.

8. Susceptibility and resistance—Recovery from the disease probably indicates immunity of long duration. Cell mediated mechanisms are important, and antibodies may play a secondary role.

9. Methods of control—

   A. Preventive measures: Provide a clean home and place of work; eliminate mice and dispose of diseased animals. Keep foods in closed containers. Virologic surveillance of commercial rodent breeding establishments, especially those producing hamsters and mice, is helpful. Ensure that laboratory mice are not infected and that personnel handling mice follow established procedures to prevent transmission from infected animals.

B. *Control of patient, contacts and the immediate environment:*

1) Report to local health authority: Reportable in selected endemic areas, Class 3C (see Communicable Disease Reporting).
2) Isolation: None.
3) Concurrent disinfection: Of discharges from the nose and throat, urine, feces and articles soiled therewith during acute febrile period. Terminal cleaning.
4) Quarantine: None.
5) Immunization of contacts: None.
6) Investigation of contacts and source of infection: Search home and place of employment for presence of house mice or rodent pets.
7) Specific treatment: None.

C. *Epidemic measures:* Not applicable.

D. *Disaster implications:* None.

E. *International measures:* None.

LYMPHOGRANULOMA
VENEREUM   ICD-9 099.1; ICD-10 A55
(Lymphogranuloma inguinale, Climatic or tropical bubo, LGV)

1. Identification—A sexually acquired chlamydial infection beginning with a small, painless, evanescent erosion, papule, nodule or herpetiform lesion on the penis or vulva, frequently unnoticed. Regional lymph nodes undergo suppuration followed by extension of the inflammatory process to the adjacent tissues. In the male, inguinal buboes are seen that may become adherent to the skin, fluctuate and result in sinus formation. In the female, inguinal nodes are less frequently affected and involvement is mainly of the pelvic nodes with extension to the rectum and rectovaginal septum, the result is proctitis, stricture of the rectum and fistulae. Proctitis may result from rectal intercourse; LGV is a fairly common cause of severe proctitis in homosexual men. Elephantiasis of the genitalia may occur in either gender. Fever, chills, headache, joint pains and anorexia are usually present. The disease course is often long and the disability great, but generally not fatal. Generalized sepsis with arthritis and meningitis is a rare occurrence.

Diagnosis is made by demonstration of chlamydial organisms by IF, EIA, DNA probe, PCR, culture of bubo aspirate or by specific micro-IF serologic test. CF testing is of diagnostic value if there is a fourfold rise or a single titer of 1:64 or greater. A negative CF test rules out the diagnosis.

2. Infectious agent—*Chlamydia trachomatis,* immunotypes L-1, L-2 and L-3; related to the organisms of trachoma and oculogenital chlamydial infections.

3. Occurrence—Worldwide, especially in tropical and subtropical areas; more common than ordinarily believed. Endemic in parts of Asia and Africa, particularly among lower socioeconomic classes. Age incidence corresponds with sexual activity. The disease is less commonly diagnosed in women, probably due to frequency of asymptomatic infections; however, gender differences are not pronounced in countries with high endemicity. All races are affected. In temperate climates, it is seen predominantly among male homosexuals.

4. Reservoir—Humans; often asymptomatic (particularly in females).

5. Mode of transmission—Direct contact with open lesions of infected people, usually during sexual intercourse.

6. Incubation period—Variable, with a range of 3-30 days for a primary lesion; if a bubo is the first manifestation, 10-30 days to several months.

7. Period of communicability—Variable, from weeks to years during presence of active lesions.

8. Susceptibility and resistance—Susceptibility is general; status of natural or acquired resistance is unclear.

9. Methods of control—

   A. *Preventive measures:* Except for measures that are specific for syphilis, preventive measures are those for sexually transmitted diseases. See Syphilis, 9A, and Granuloma inguinale, 9A.

   B. *Control of patient, contacts and the immediate environment:*

   1) Report to local health authority: A reportable disease in selected endemic areas; not a reportable disease in most countries, Class 3B (see Communicable Disease Reporting).
   2) Isolation: None. Refrain from sexual contact until all lesions are healed.
   3) Concurrent disinfection: None; care in disposal of discharges from lesions and of articles soiled therewith.

4) Quarantine: None.

5) Immunization of contacts: Not applicable; prompt treatment on recognition or clinical suspicion of infection.

6) Investigation of contacts and source of infection: Search for infected sexual contacts of patient. Recent contacts of confirmed active cases should receive specific therapy.

7) Specific treatment: Tetracycline and doxycycline are effective for all stages, including buboes and ulcerative lesions; administer orally for at least 2 weeks. Erythromycin or sulfonamides may be used when tetracycline is contraindicated. Do not incise buboes; drain by aspiration through healthy tissue.

C. Epidemic measures: Not applicable.

D. Disaster implications: None.

E. International measures: See Syphilis, 9E.

MALARIA ICD-9 084; ICD-10 B50–B54

1. Identification—A parasitic disease; infections with the four human malarias can present sufficiently similar symptoms to make species differentiation generally impossible without laboratory studies. Furthermore, the fever pattern of the first few days of infection resembles that seen in early stages of many other illnesses (bacterial, viral and parasitic). Even the demonstration of parasites, particularly in highly malarious areas, does not necessarily mean that malaria is the patient's sole illness (e.g., early yellow fever, Lassa fever, typhoid fever). The most serious malarial infection, **falciparum malaria** (malignant tertian, ICD-9 084.0, ICD-10 B50) may present a quite varied clinical picture, including fever, chills, sweats, cough, diarrhea, respiratory distress and headache, and may progress to icterus, coagulation defects, shock, renal and liver failure, acute encephalopathy, pulmonary and cerebral edema, coma and death. It is a possible cause of coma and other CNS symptoms, such as disorientation and delirium, in any nonimmune person recently returned from a tropical area. Prompt treatment is essential, even in mild cases, since irreversible complications may appear suddenly; case-fatality rates among untreated children and nonimmune adults can be 10%–40% or higher.

The other human malarias, **vivax** (benign tertian, ICD-9 084.1, ICD-10 B51), **malariae** (quartan, ICD-9 084.2, ICD-10 B52) and **ovale** (ICD-9 084.3, ICD-10 B53), generally are not life-threatening. Illness may begin with indefinite malaise and a slowly rising fever of several days' duration, followed by a shaking chill and rapidly rising temperature, usually accompanied by headache and nausea, and ending with profuse sweating. After an interval free of fever, the cycle of chills, fever and sweating is repeated, either daily, every other day or every third day. Duration of an untreated primary attack varies from a week to a month or longer. True relapses following periods with no parasitemia (seen with vivax and ovale infections) may occur at irregular intervals for up to 5 years. Malariae infections may persist for life with or without recurrent febrile episodes.

Persons who are partially immune or who have been taking prophylactic drugs may show an atypical clinical picture and a prolonged incubation period.

Laboratory confirmation of the diagnosis is made by demonstration of malaria parasites in blood films. Repeated microscopic examinations every 12–24 hours may be necessary because the density of *Plasmodium falciparum* parasites in the peripheral blood varies and parasites are often not demonstrable in films from patients recently or actively under treatment. Several tests are under study. The most promising are dipsticks that detect circulating plasmodial antigens in the bloodstream. While licensed abroad, none were, as of late 1999, licensed in the USA. Diagnosis by PCR is the most sensitive method available, but is a specialized assay not generally available in diagnostic laboratories. Antibodies, demonstrable by IFA or other tests, may appear after the first week of infection but may persist for years, indicating past malarial experience; thus antibody determinations are not helpful for diagnosis of current illness.

2. Infectious agents—*Plasmodium vivax, P. malariae, P. falciparum* and *P. ovale;* sporozoan parasites. Mixed infections are not infrequent in endemic areas.

3. Occurrence—Endemic malaria no longer occurs in many temperate-zone countries and in some areas of subtropical countries, but is still a major cause of ill health in many tropical and subtropical areas; high transmission areas are found on the fringes of forests in South America (e.g., Brazil), southeast Asia (e.g., Thailand and Indonesia) and throughout sub-Saharan Africa. Ovale malaria occurs mainly in sub-Saharan Africa where vivax malaria is much less frequent.

P. falciparum, refractory to cure with the 4 aminoquinolines (such as chloroquine) and other antimalarial drugs (such as sulfa-pyrimethamine combinations and mefloquine) occurs in the tropical portions of both hemispheres, particularly in the Amazon region and parts of Thailand and Cambodia. *P. vivax* refractory to treatment with chloroquine is present in Papua New Guinea and is prevalent in Irian Jaya (Indonesia) and has been reported from Sumatra (Indonesia), the Solomon Islands, and Guyana. The hepatic stages of some *P. vivax* strains may also be relatively resistant to treatment with primaquine. In the USA, a few episodes of locally acquired malaria have occurred since the mid-1980s. Current information on foci of drug-resistant malaria is published annually by WHO and can also be obtained from the Malaria Section, CDC, Atlanta or by consulting the CDC's travel web site: http://www.cdc.gov/travel.

4. Reservoir—Humans are the only important reservoir of human malaria. Nonhuman primates are naturally infected by many malarial species, including *P. knowlesi, P. cynomolgi, P. brazilianum, P. inui, P. schwetzi* and *P. simium,* which can infect humans experimentally, but natural transmission to humans is rare.

5. Mode of transmission—By the bite of an infective female *Anopheles* mosquito. Most species feed at dusk and during early night hours; some important vectors have biting peaks around midnight or the early hours of the morning. When a female *Anopheles* mosquito ingests blood containing the sexual stages of the parasite (gametocytes), male and female gametes unite to form the ookinete in the mosquito stomach which then penetrates the stomach wall to form a cyst on the outer surface in which thousands of sporozoites develop; this requires 8-35 days, depending on the species of parasite and the temperature to which the vector is exposed. These sporozoites migrate to various organs of the infected mosquito, and some that reach the salivary glands mature and are infective when injected into a person as the insect takes the next blood meal.

In the susceptible host, the sporozoites enter liver hepatocytes and develop into exoerythrocytic schizonts. The hepatocytes rupture and asexual parasites (tissue merozoites) reach the bloodstream through the hepatic sinusoids and invade the erythrocytes to grow and multiply cyclically. Most will develop into asexual forms, from trophozoites to mature blood schizonts that rupture the erythrocyte within 48-72 hours, to release 8-30 (depending on the species) free erythrocytic merozoites that invade other erythrocytes. Clinical symptoms are produced at the time of each cycle, by the rupture of large numbers of erythrocytic schizonts. Within infected erythrocytes, some of the merozoites may develop into the male (microgametocyte) or the female (macrogametocyte), the sexual forms.

The period between the infective bite and the detection of the parasite in a thick blood smear is the "prepatent period," which is generally 6-12 days with *P. falciparum,* 8-12 days with *P. vivax* and *P. ovale,* and 12-16 days with *P. malariae* (but may be shorter or longer). Delayed primary attacks of some *P. vivax* strains may occur 6-12 months after exposure. Gametocytes usually appear in the blood stream within 3 days of parasitemia with *P. vivax* and *P. ovale,* and after 10-14 days with *P. falciparum.* Some exoerythrocytic forms of *P. vivax* and *P. ovale* exist as dormant forms (hypnozoites) that remain in hepatocytes to mature months or years later and produce relapses. This phenomenon does not occur in falciparum or malariae malaria, and reappearance of these forms of the disease is the result of inadequate treatment or of infection with drug-resistant strains. With *P. malariae,* low levels of erythrocytic parasites may persist for many years, to multiply at some future time to a level that may result again in clinical illness. Malaria may also be transmitted by injection or transfusion of blood from infected persons or by use of contaminated needles and syringes, as by injecting drug users. Congenital transmission occurs rarely, but stillbirth from infected mothers is more frequent.

6. Incubation periods—The time between the infective bite and the appearance of clinical symptoms is approximately 7-14 days for *P. falciparum*, 8-14 days for *P. vivax* and *P. ovale*, and 7-30 days for *P. malariae*. With some strains of *P. vivax*, mostly from temperate areas, there may be a protracted incubation period of 8-10 months. With infection by blood transfusion, incubation periods depend on the number of parasites infused and are usually short, but may range up to about 2 months. Suboptimal drug suppression, such as from prophylaxis, may result in a prolonged incubation period.

7. Period of communicability—For infectivity of mosquitoes, as long as infective gametocytes are present in the blood of patients; this varies with species and strain of parasite and with response to therapy. Untreated or insufficiently treated patients may be a source of mosquito infection for more than 3 years in malariae, 1-2 years in vivax, and generally not more than 1 year in falciparum malaria; the mosquito remains infective for life. Transmission by transfusion may occur as long as asexual forms remain in the circulating blood; with *P. malariae* this can continue for 40 years or longer. Stored blood can remain infective for at least a month.

8. Susceptibility and resistance—Susceptibility is universal except in humans with specific genetic traits. Tolerance or refractoriness to clinical disease is present in adults in highly endemic communities where exposure to infective anophelines is continuous over many years. Most black Africans show a natural resistance to infection with *P. vivax*, which is associated with the absence of Duffy factor on their erythrocytes. Persons with sickle cell trait have relatively low parasitemia when infected with *P. falciparum*, and therefore are relatively protected from severe disease.

9. Methods of control—

A. Preventive measures:
I Community based measures

  1) Encourage source reduction and control of larval stages by sanitary improvements that will result in permanent elimination or reduction of anopheline mosquito breeding habitats close to human population settlements. Methods to eliminate unusable impounded water (filling in and draining) and to increase the speed that water flows in natural or artificial channels (rectification and clearing of path and margins) are very effective adjunct measures for permanent malaria control. Use of chemical and biological control methods on useful impounded water requires more recurrent cost and efforts than the maintenance required for permanent elimination of

breeding sites, but is another important adjunct to malaria control at the local level of transmission.

2) Any large scale use of residual insecticides against adult anopheline vectors should be preceded by a careful appraisal of the transmission characteristics in the problem area. Even in those transmission foci characterized by mosquitoes that tend to rest and feed indoors (endophilic and endophagic vectors), the sole application of residual insecticides on the inside walls of dwellings may not necessarily result in permanent malaria control. Residual insecticide on the inside walls of dwellings and on other surfaces will generally be ineffective where the vector has developed resistance to these insecticides or the vectors do not enter houses.

3) Other important considerations of an integrated control plan should include:

a) Access to health care services for early diagnosis and prompt treatment.

b) Intersectoral epidemiologic monitoring of human population movement patterns (migration and circulation): these are the source of introduction and spread of *Plasmodium* spp. into areas ecologically prone to transmission.

c) Massive public information measures directed to those exposed to risk on how best to protect themselves, their families and their community.

d) Prompt and effective treatment of acute and chronic cases is an important measure of malaria control. Moreover, the mortality from all *P. falciparum* infections is strongly associated with delayed diagnosis and delay in receiving effective treatment.

e) Blood donors should be questioned for a history of malaria or a history of travel to, or residence in a malarious area. In most nonendemic areas, travelers who have not taken antimalarial drugs and have been free of symptoms may donate 6 months (in the USA, this period is 1 year) after return from an endemic area. For long term (more than 6 months) visitors to malarious areas who have been on antimalarials and have not had malaria, or for persons who have immigrated or are visiting from an endemic area, they may be accepted as donors 3 years after cessation of prophylactic antimalarial drugs and departure from the endemic area, if they have remained asymptomatic. A period of more than 6 months is considered residence in a malarious area, and the donor should be evaluated as an immigrant from that area. An immigrant or visitor from an area where malariae malaria is or had been endemic may be a source of transfusion induced infection for many years. Such areas include but are not limited to malaria endemic countries of the Americas, tropical Africa, Papua New Guinea, south and southeast Asia and even countries of the Mediterranean region of Europe, where malariae transmission no longer occurs.

II Personal protective measures

Because of the resurgence of malaria during the past decade, the following guidelines on prevention, especially prophylaxis and treatment are presented in detail. Travelers to malarious areas need to realize that: protection from biting mosquitoes continues to be of paramount importance; no antimalarial prophylactic regimen gives complete protection; prophylaxis with antimalarial drugs should not automatically be prescribed for all travelers to malarious areas; and ''standby'' or emergency self-treatment is recommended when a febrile illness occurs in a falciparum malaria area where professional medical care is not readily available.

1) Measures to reduce the risk of mosquito bites include:
   a) Avoid going out between dusk and dawn when anopheline mosquitoes commonly bite. Wear long sleeved clothing and long trousers when going out at night, and avoid dark colors which attract mosquitoes.
   b) Apply insect repellent to exposed skin; choose one containing either N, N-diethyl-m-toluamide (Deet®) or dimethyl phthalate. The manufacturers' recommendations for use must not be exceeded, particularly with small children.
   c) Stay in a well-constructed and well-maintained building in the most developed part of town.
   d) Use screens over doors and windows; if no screens are available, close windows and doors at night.
   e) If accommodation allows entry of mosquitoes, use a mosquito net over the bed, with edges tucked in under the mattress, and ensure that the net is not torn and that there are no mosquitoes inside it; increased protection may be obtained by impregnating the net with synthetic pyrethroid insecticides.
   f) Use antimosquito sprays or insecticide dispensers (mains or battery operated) that contain tablets impregnated with pyrethroids, or burn pyrethroids, or pyrethroid mosquito coils in bedrooms at night.
2) People who are or will be exposed to mosquitoes in malarious areas should be given the following information:
   a) The risk of malaria infection varies among countries and within different areas of each country. See country list in WHO's annual publication *International Travel and Health*, ISBN-9241580208.

    b) Pregnant women and young children when exposed and infected are highly susceptible to development of severe and complicated malaria (see below).

    c) Malaria can kill if treatment is delayed. Medical help must be sought promptly if malaria is suspected; a blood sample should be examined for malaria parasites on more than one occasion and a few hours apart.

    d) Symptoms of malaria may be mild; malaria should be suspected if, 1 week after entry into a transmission area, an individual suffers any fever, malaise with or without headache, backache, muscular aching and/or weakness, vomiting, diarrhea and cough. Prompt medical advice must be sought.

3) Pregnant women and parents of young children should be advised of the following:

    a) Malaria in a pregnant woman increases the risk of maternal death, miscarriage, stillbirth and neonatal death.

    b) A malarious area should not be visited unless absolutely necessary.

    c) Extra diligence is needed in using measures to protect against mosquito bites.

    d) Chloroquine (5.0 mg/kg/week—the equivalent of 8.0 mg of diphosphate salt/kg/week; 6.8 mg of sulphate salt/kg/week and 6.1 of hydrochloride salt/kg/week) and proguanil (3.0 mg/kg/day—the equivalent of 3.4 mg of hydrochloride salt/kg/day) should be taken for prophylaxis (proguanil is not available in the USA). In areas with chloroquine-resistant *P. falciparum,* chloroquine and proguanil should be taken during the first 3 months of pregnancy; mefloquine prophylaxis (5.0 mg/kg/week—the equivalent of 5.48 mg of hydrochloride salt/kg/week) may be considered; start from the fourth month of pregnancy.

    e) Doxycycline prophylaxis should not be taken.

    f) Medical help should be sought immediately if malaria is suspected; emergency "standby" treatment should be taken only if no medical help is immediately available. Medical help must still be sought as soon as possible after standby treatment (see 9AII4 and 9AII5c below).

    g) Malaria prophylaxis is important for the protection of young children. Chloroquine (5 mg/kg/week) plus proguanil (3 mg/kg/day) may be given safely to infants (proguanil is not available in the USA).

    h) Mefloquine prophylaxis (5 mg/kg/week) may be taken by women of childbearing age, but pregnancy should be avoided for 3 months after stopping the drug. Cumulative evidence from women inadvertently given mefloquine chemoprophylaxis during pregnancy and from clinical trials has not shown embryotoxic or teratogenic effects. Mefloquine may therefore be given during the second and third trimesters. Data concerning use during the first trimester are limited, but in situations of inadvertent pregnancy, prophylaxis with mefloquine is not considered an indication for pregnancy termination.

i) Doxycycline prophylaxis (1.5 mg dihydrochloride salt/kg/day) may be taken by women of childbearing age, but pregnancy should be avoided for about 1 week after stopping the drug.

j) If pregnancy occurs during antimalarial prophylaxis (except with chloroquine plus proguanil), information about congenital risks should be sought from the drug manufacturer by the woman's doctor.

4) Standby treatment: The most important factors that determine the survival of patients with falciparum malaria are early diagnosis and immediate treatment. Most nonimmune individuals exposed to or infected with malaria should be able to obtain prompt medical attention when malaria is suspected. However, a minority will be exposed to a high risk of infection, and will be at least 12–24 hours away from competent medical attention. In such cases, WHO recommends that prescribers issue antimalarial drugs to be carried by the persons who may be in such exposed situations for self-administration. Persons prescribed such standby treatment should be given precise instructions on the recognition of symptoms, the complete treatment regimen to be taken, possible side effects and the action to be taken in the event of drug failure. Moreover, they should be made aware that self-treatment is a temporary measure and medical advice is still to be sought as soon as possible.

5) Prophylaxis: Nonimmune individuals who will be exposed to mosquitoes in malarious areas must make use of the protective measures against mosquito bites and could also benefit from the use of suppressive drugs for chemoprophylaxis. The possible side effects of long term (up to 3 to 5 months) use of the drug or drug combination recommended for use in any particular area should be weighed against the actual likelihood of being bitten by an infected mosquito. There may be no risk of exposure to those visitors or residents in most urban areas in many malarious countries, including southeast Asia and South America, so suppressive drugs may not be indicated. In some urban centers, notably in Indian subcontinent countries, there may be a risk of exposure to malaria. If there is any risk, all protective measures should be used. The geographic distribution and specific drug sensitivities of malaria parasites can change rapidly: the most recent information about drug

patterns must be sought before prescribing chemoprophylaxis.

a) For suppression of malaria in nonimmune individuals temporarily residing in or traveling through endemic areas where, as of late 1999, the plasmodia are chloroquine sensitive (Central America west of the Panama Canal, the island of Hispaniola—Haiti and Dominican Republic—and malarious areas of the Middle East, and mainland China): chloroquine (Aralen, 5 mg base/kg body weight, 300 mg base or 500 mg chloroquine phosphate for the average adult) once weekly, or hydroxychloroquine (plaquenil, 5 mg base/kg body weight to the adult dose of 310 mg base or 400 mg salt) is recommended. Pregnancy is not a contraindication. The drug must be continued on the same schedule for 4 weeks after leaving endemic areas. Minor side effects may occur at prophylactic doses, which may be alleviated by taking the drug with meals, or changing to hydroxychloroquine. Psoriasis may be exacerbated particularly in Africans and African Americans; chloroquine may interfere with the immune response to intradermal rabies vaccine.

b) For suppressive malaria drug therapy for travelers who will be exposed to chloroquine resistant *P. falciparum* infection (southeast Asia, sub-Saharan Africa, rain forest areas of South America, and western Pacific Islands), mefloquine alone (5 mg/kg/week) is recommended. Suppressive drug treatment should be continued weekly, starting 1–2 weeks before travel and continued weekly during travel or residence in malarious area and for 4 weeks after the return to nonmalarious areas. Mefloquine is contraindicated only in those with a known hypersensitivity to it. It is not recommended for women in the first trimester of pregnancy unless exposure to chloroquine-resistant *P. falciparum* is unavoidable (see 9AII3h above). Suppressive drug treatment should not be continued for more than 12 to 20 weeks, with the same drug. For those with prolonged residence in high risk areas, the seasonality of transmission and improved protective measures against mosquito bites should be weighed against the long term risk of drug reactions.

As of late 1999, mefloquine is not recommended for individuals with underlying cardiac arrhythmias, or individuals with a recent history of epilepsy, or severe psychiatric disorders. For those who are unable to take mefloquine and for those going to malaria endemic areas of Thailand (forested rural areas principally along the borders with Cambodia and Myanmar), doxycycline alone, 100 mg once daily, is an alternative regimen. Doxycycline may cause diarrhea, candida vaginitis and photosensitivity. It should not be given to pregnant women and children less than 8 years old. Doxycycline prophylaxis can begin 1-2 days prior to travel to malarious areas and should be continued daily during travel and for 4 weeks after leaving the malarious area.

Long-term travelers at risk of infection by chloroquine-resistant *P. falciparum* strains for whom mefloquine or doxycycline is not recommended should take once weekly chloroquine alone. Limited data indicate that weekly chloroquine together with daily proguanil (paludrine, 200 mg) is more effective than chloroquine alone in Africa, but it cannot be expected to prevent most cases; in Asia and Oceania, proguanil adds no benefit to chloroquine alone (proguanil is not available in the USA). Travelers in this category should carry a treatment dose of a locally effective antimalarial or Fansidar® (sulfadoxine 500 mg/pyrimethamine 25 mg) unless they have a history of sulfonamide intolerance. In the event of a febrile illness when professional medical care is not readily available, they should take the complete antimalarial dosage (Fansidar®—adult dose 3 tablets) and obtain medical consultation as soon as possible. **It must be emphasized that such presumptive self-treatment is only a temporary measure and that prompt medical evaluation is imperative.**

In areas of chloroquine resistance to both *P. vivax* and *P. falciparum,* an alternative prophylactic regimen for adults who do not have glucose-6-phosphate dehydrogenase (G-6-PD) deficiency and women who are not pregnant and not nursing, was proposed based on clinical studies reported during the late 1990s. This regimen consists of primaquine only at 0.5 mg base/kg/day, beginning on the first day of exposure and continued for 1 week after leaving the risk area. Compliance with this regimen achieved a protective efficacy of close to 95% for *P. falciparum* and about 85%–90% for *P. vivax* in the South Pacific and South America. The most common side effect was epigastric or abdominal pain and vomiting in less than 10% of recipients. Longer term exposure, up to 50 weeks of daily administration of primaquine, showed a slight increase of methahemoglobin level to 5.8%, which declined by half within a week after ending primaquine administration.

c) These chemosuppressive drugs do not eliminate intrahepatic parasites, so that clinical relapses of vivax or ovale malaria may occur after the drug is discontinued. Primaquine, 0.3 mg base/kg/day for 14 days (15 mg base or 26.3

mg of primaquine phosphate for the average adult) is often effective and may be given after leaving endemic areas, concurrently with or following the suppressive drug. However, it can produce hemolysis in those with G-6-PD deficiency. The decision to administer primaquine is made on an individual basis, after consideration of the potential risk of adverse reactions, and is generally indicated only for persons who have had prolonged exposure, e.g., missionaries, Peace Corps volunteers, and some military personnel. Larger daily doses (30 mg base) are generally required for most southeast Asian, southwest Pacific, and some South American strains.

Alternatively, primaquine, 0.75 mg base/kg, may be given once weekly for 8 doses (45 mg base or 79 mg primaquine phosphate for the average adult) after leaving endemic areas. Prior to primaquine administration, the patient should be tested for G-6-PD deficiency. Primaquine should not be administered during pregnancy; chloroquine should be continued weekly for the duration of the pregnancy.

B. Control of patient, contacts and the immediate environment:

1) Report to local health authority: Obligatory case report as a Disease under Surveillance by WHO, Class 1A (see Communicable Disease Reporting) in nonendemic areas, preferably limited to smear confirmed cases (USA); Class 3C is the more practical procedure in endemic areas.
2) Isolation: For hospitalized patients, blood precautions. Patients should be in mosquito proof areas from dusk to dawn.
3) Concurrent disinfection: None.
4) Quarantine: None.
5) Immunization of contacts: Not applicable.
6) Investigation of contacts and source of infection: Determine history of previous infection or of possible exposure. If a history of needle sharing is obtained from the patient, investigate and treat all persons who shared the equipment. In transfusion-induced malaria, all donors must be located and their blood examined for malaria parasites and for antimalarial antibodies; parasite positive donors should receive treatment.
7) Specific treatment for all forms of malaria:
    a) The treatment of malaria due to infection with chloroquine sensitive *P. falciparum, P. vivax, P. malariae* and *P. ovale* is the oral administration of a total of 25 mg of chloroquine base/kg administered over a 3-day period: 15 mg/kg the first day (10 mg/kg initially and 5 mg/kg 6 hours later; 600 and 300 mg doses for the average adult); 5 mg/kg the second day; and 5 mg/kg the third day. *P. vivax* acquired in

Oceania may be resistant to chloroquine, in which case treatment should be repeated or a single dose of mefloquine, 25 mg/kg may be given.

b) For emergency treatment of adults with severe or complicated infections or for people unable to retain orally administered medication, quinine dihydrochloride, 20 mg base/kg, diluted in 500 ml of normal saline, glucose or plasma, may be administered by slow IV (over 2-4 hours); repeated in 8 hours at a lower dose (10 mg/kg) if needed, and then the lower dose is given every 8 hours until it can be supplanted by oral quinine. The pediatric dosage is the same. If there is improvement within 48 hours and drug levels cannot be monitored, each dose should be reduced by 30%; hypoglycemia is a common side effect.

In the USA, parenteral quinine is not available but parenteral quinidine can be substituted and is equally effective in treatment of severe malaria. A loading dose of 10 mg quinidine gluconate base/kg body weight is administered by slow IV infusion over 1-2 hours, followed by a constant IV infusion of 0.02 mg base/kg/minute, preferably controlled by a constant-infusion pump, monitoring of cardiac function, and fluid balance through a central venous catheter; the quinidine infusion should be temporarily slowed or stopped for a QT interval greater than 0.6 seconds, an increase in the QRS complex by more than 50%, or hypotension unresponsive to fluid challenges. The infusion may continue for a maximum of 72 hours. All parenteral drugs should be discontinued as soon as oral drug administration can be initiated.

In extremely severe falciparum infections, particularly those with altered mental status or with a parasitemia approaching or exceeding 10%, exchange transfusion should be considered. When infections, especially severe cases, were acquired in areas where quinine resistance occurs (as of late 1999 in Thai border areas), use artemether IM (3.2 mg/kg the first day, followed by 1.6 mg/kg/day); or artesunate IV or IM (2 mg/kg on the first day, followed by 1 mg/kg/day). In hyperparasitemic cases, artesunate 1 mg/kg may be given 4-6 hours after the first dose: to limit potential neurotoxicity, it should be given for no more than 5-7 days or until the patient can take an effective antimalarial drug, such as mefloquine, 25 mg/kg, by mouth. These drugs, which are not available in the USA, are used only in combination with other antimalarials.

c) For *P. falciparum* infections acquired in areas where

chloroquine-resistant strains are present, administer quinine, 30 mg/kg/day divided into 3 doses, for 3–7 days. (For severe infections, administer IV quinine as described above.) Along with quinine, administer doxycycline (2 mg/kg twice a day, maximal 100 mg/dose) or tetracycline (20 mg/kg dose, maximal 250 mg/ day) given in 4 doses daily, for 7 days. Quinine may be discontinued after 3 days, except for infections acquired in Thailand and the Amazon Basin, in which case the quinine should be continued for all 7 days. Mefloquine (15–25 mg/kg) is effective for treatment of chloroquine resistant *P. falciparum* from most parts of the world, but is poorly effective on its own for *P. falciparum* in Thailand and neighboring countries. Failures have also been reported from Brazil. Every effort should be made to determine the therapeutic course producing the best results in the area where the disease was contracted, since drug resistance patterns may vary in time and locale.

d) For *P. vivax* infections acquired in Papua New Guinea or Irian Jaya, Indonesia, mefloquine should be used for treatment (15 mg/kg in a single dose). Halofantrine is a possible alternative drug; consult package insert.

e) For prevention of relapses in mosquito acquired *P. vivax* and *P. ovale* infections, administer primaquine, as described in 9A5c, above, on completion of the treatment of an acute attack. It is desirable to test all patients (especially Africans, African Americans, Asians and Mediterraneans) for G-6-PD deficiency to prevent drug induced hemolysis. Many, particularly Africans and African Americans, are able to tolerate the hemolysis, but consideration may have to be given to immediate discontinuance of primaquine: However, the induced problem must be balanced against the possible recurrence of malaria. Primaquine is not required in nonmosquito transmitted disease (e.g., transfusion), since no liver phase occurs.

C. *Epidemic measures:* Determine the nature and extent of the epidemic situation. Intensify case detection as well as control measures directed against adult and larval stages of the important vectors: eliminate breeding places; treat acute cases; use personal protection and suppressive drugs. Mass treatment may be considered.

D. *Disaster implications:* Throughout history the malarias have been a concomitant or the result of wars and social upheavals. Any abnormal climatic or edaphic change that increases the availability of mosquito breeding sites in endemic areas can lead to an increase in malaria.

E. *International measures:*

1) Important international measures include the following:
   a) Disinsectization of aircraft before boarding passengers or in transit by using a residual spray application of a type of insecticide to which the vectors are susceptible;
   b) Disinsectization of aircraft, ships and other vehicles on arrival if the health authority at the place of arrival has reason to suspect importation of malaria vectors;
   c) Enforcing and maintaining rigid antimosquito sanitation within the mosquito flight range of all ports and airports.
2) In special circumstances, administer antimalarial drugs to potentially infected migrants, refugees, seasonal workers and persons taking part in periodic mass movement into an area or country where malaria has been eliminated. Primaquine, 30–45 mg base (0.5–0.75 mg/kg), given as a single dose, renders the gametocytes of falciparum malaria noninfectious.
3) Malaria is a Disease under Surveillance by WHO, as its control is considered an essential element of the world strategy for primary health care. National health administrations are expected to notify WHO twice a year of the following:
   a) those areas originally malarious with no present risk of infection;
   b) those malaria cases imported into areas free of disease but with continuing potential for risk of transmission;
   c) those areas with chloroquine resistant strains of parasites; and
   d) those international ports and airports free of malaria.
4) WHO Collaborating Centres.

MALIGNANT NEOPLASMS ASSOCIATED WITH INFECTIOUS AGENTS

Infectious agents are risk factors for a number of malignancies. Several parasites, the bacterium *Helicobacter pylori* and several viruses have been implicated in the pathogenesis of various human malignancies, either directly or indirectly. These malignancies usually represent the late outcome of the infection. Cofactors, both external (environmental) and internal (genetic and physiologic at the immunologic and molecular levels), play important roles in each of these malignancies. The infectious agent is neither a necessary nor sufficient cause of all cases of agent-related malignancy; other causes are involved in some and cofactors are almost always involved.

Most of the infectious agents implicated in the etiology of tumors are viruses. A common feature of most virus-related cancers is the persistence of the virus following infection early in life or the presence of immunosuppression: this leads to integration and development of cancer, usually in a single cell clone (monoclonal tumor). Both DNA and RNA viruses are involved.

The four strongest DNA virus candidates as agents directly or indirectly involved in the pathogenesis of human malignancies are: (1) hepatitis B virus (HBV); (2) Epstein-Barr virus (EBV); (3) human papillomaviruses (HPV, mainly types 16 and 18); and (4) human herpesvirus-8 (HHV-8), also called Kaposi's sarcoma associated virus (KSHV). The first three of these viruses are ubiquitous throughout the world and produce much more inapparent than apparent infection; most result in a latent virus state that is subject to reactivation. Monoclonality of the tumor cells and integration of the virus into the tumor cell indicate a causal association. The associated malignancies are relatively rare events that occur in special host and geographic settings.

Among the RNA viruses, the retroviruses—which include human T-cell lymphotropic virus (HTLV-1) and human immunodeficiency virus (HIV)—are associated with human T-cell leukemia/lymphoma. In contrast to oncogenic DNA viruses, these viruses are less ubiquitous and are more localized geographically. These viruses are strongly implicated in the causation of specific malignancies by serologic, virologic and epidemiologic evidence.

I. HEPATOCELLULAR
CARCINOMA   ICD-9 155.0; ICD-10 C22.0
(HCC, Primary liver cancer, Primary hepatocellular carcinoma)

Chronic infection with hepatitis B or C is an important risk factor for primary hepatocellular cancer (PHC or HCC). Prospective studies in Taiwan have shown a hundred fold higher risk of HCC in persons chronically infected with HBV than in noncarriers. Many patients go through stages of chronic hepatitis and cirrhosis before development of the tumor.

Periodic screening of hepatitis B virus (HBV) carriers for alpha-fetoprotein, a serologic marker associated with HCC, and screening with ultrasound can, in some cases, detect the tumor at an early, resectable stage.

HCC is among the most common malignant neoplasms in many parts of Asia and Africa; it occurs with highest frequency in areas with high prevalence of HBV carriers. These areas include most of Asia, Africa and the South Pacific. Rates are intermediate on the Indian subcontinent and in the Middle East and are relatively low in North America and Western Europe. Hepatitis C virus (HCV) infection has been shown in case-control studies to be strongly associated with HCC among patients with and without HBV infections; in addition there is laboratory evidence for transforming properties of HCV. HCV infection may be the dominant cause of HCC in Japan.

See Viral hepatitis B for methods of control. Development of the tumor can be prevented by administration of hepatitis B (HB) vaccine alone or HB vaccine plus hepatitis B immune globulin (HBIG) to all newborns. Immunization interrupts transmission of HBV infection from mother to infant. WHO recommends that all countries integrate HB vaccine into routine childhood immunization schedules. Many countries, including the USA, are implementing this recommendation, which should eventually lead to elimination of HBV and control of HCC caused by HBV. HCC cases should be reported to a tumor registry. No vaccine is available for HCV infection but testing the blood supply for HCV antibody will prevent its transmission by transfusion.

II. BURKITT LYMPHOMA   ICD-9 200.2; ICD-10 C83.7
(BL, African Burkitt lymphoma, Endemic Burkitt lymphoma, Burkitt tumor)

Burkitt lymphoma (BL) is a monoclonal tumor of B cells. It occurs worldwide but is hyperendemic in highly malarious areas, such as tropical Africa and lowland Papua New Guinea, which have heavy rainfall (usually more than 40 inches/year) and are below 3,000 feet elevation. In African children, jaw involvement is common. The tumor may also develop as a rare event in immunosuppressed patients (organ transplant patients, those with familial and X-linked immunodeficiency, and more commonly in AIDS—about 25%–30% of these are EBV related). The tumors may be monoclonal, polyclonal or mixed; not all are Burkitt-type, but all are acute lymphoblastic sarcomas.

Epstein-Barr virus (EBV), a herpesvirus responsible for infectious mononucleosis plays an important pathogenic role in about 97% of BL cases in Africa and Papua New Guinea, where EBV infection occurs in infancy, and malaria, which appears to be a cofactor, is holoendemic. EBV is also associated with BL in about 30% of cases in low BL-endemic and nonmalarious areas (American BL). The estimated range of tumor development is 2–12 years from primary EBV infection but is much shorter in AIDS patients in whom an EBV related lymphoma (often CNS) develops. EBV infection is strongly implicated in the causation of African BL by serologic, virologic, and epidemiologic evidence. Prevention of EBV infection early in life and control of malaria (see Malaria, section 9) might reduce tumor incidence in Africa and Papua New Guinea. Subunit vaccines against EBV are in the trial stage. Chemotherapy of the tumor is usually effective after the tumor develops. Cases should be reported to a tumor registry.

III. NASOPHARYNGEAL
CARCINOMA   ICD-9 147.9; ICD-10 C11

Nasopharyngeal carcinoma (NPC) is a malignant tumor of the epithelial cells of the nasopharynx that usually occurs in adults aged 20–40 years. There is an approximate tenfold higher incidence among groups of

Chinese from southern China and Taiwan; incidence remains high even in those who have moved elsewhere (including the USA), when compared with the general population. However, the risk decreases in subsequent generations after emigration from Asia.

IgA antibody to the EBV viral capsid antigen in both serum and nasopharyngeal secretions is a characteristic feature of the disease and has been used in China as a screening test for the tumor. Its appearance may precede the clinical appearance of NPC by several years, and its reappearance after treatment heralds recurrence.

The serologic and virologic evidence relating EBV to NPC is similar to that for African BL (high EBV antibody titers, genome in tumor cells), and this relationship has been found without respect to the geographic origin of the patient. The tumor occurs throughout the world, but is highest in southern China, southeast Asia, north and east Africa and the Arctic. Males outnumber females by about 2:1. Chinese with HLA-2 and SIN-2 antigen profiles have an approximately fivefold higher risk.

EBV infection occurs early in life in settings where NPC is most common, yet the tumor does not appear until age 20–40, which suggests the occurrence of some secondary, reactivating factor, with epithelial invasion later in life. Repeated respiratory infections or chemical irritants, such as nitrosamines in dried foods, may play a role. The higher frequency of the tumor in persons of southern Chinese origin, without respect to later residence, and the association with certain HLA haplotypes suggest a genetic susceptibility. A lower incidence among those who have migrated to the USA and elsewhere suggests that environmental factor(s) may be associated cofactors, such as the nitrosamines present in smoked fish and other foods.

Early detection in highly endemic areas by screening for EBV IgA antibodies to viral capsid antigen permits early treatment. A subunit vaccine against EBV infection is under study. Chemotherapy after early recognition is the only specific therapy. Cases should be reported to a tumor registry.

IV. MALIGNANCIES POSSIBLY RELATED TO EBV

A. HODGKIN'S DISEASE   ICD-9 201; ICD-10 C81

Hodgkin's disease (HD) is a tumor of the lymphatic system that occurs in four histologic subtypes—nodular sclerosis, lymphocyte predominance, mixed cellularity and lymphocyte depletion. The histologic picture is characterized by the presence of a highly specific, but nonpathognomonic cell, the Reed-Sternberg cell (RSC), also seen in cases of infectious mononucleosis (IM).

The cause of HD is not certain, but laboratory and epidemiologic evidence implicates EBV in at least half of the cases. HD is more common in developed countries, but of relatively low age adjusted incidence. It is more common in higher socioeconomic settings, in smaller families, and in Caucasians compared with African Americans.

Cases that develop after IM, which has a peak in the USA at about age 17–19, occur some 10 years later, but cases in older adults, if EBV related, are probably the result of virus reactivation in the presence of a deteriorating immune system. The high frequency of EBV found in HD diagnosed in AIDS patients and the relatively short incubation period appear to be related to the severe immunodeficiency due to HIV infection, but whether the presence of EBV in the tumor cell is cause or effect is not known.

Among AIDS patients, particularly those infected by IV drug use, a significantly higher proportion of HD cases are EBV associated. Cases should be reported to a tumor registry.

B. NON-HODGKIN'S LYMPHOMAS
ICD-10 B21.2, C83.0, C83.8, C83.9, C85

The incidence of lymphomas in AIDS patients is about 50–100 times that of the general population. While a substantial number of these cases are related to EBV, the virus most associated with non-Hodgkin's lymphoma (NHL) tumors, such as high grade and CNS lymphomas, is HIV. Since 1980, NHL has shown a dramatic increase in young, single white men with AIDS. About 4% of AIDS patients present with lymphoma, and perhaps 30% will eventually develop one if survival is sufficiently long. Whether EBV is a causal factor in these EBV associated lymphomas in AIDS patients, or simply enters the tumor cell after it has been formed is not clear, but accumulating evidence points to the former possibility.

A marked increase in NHL not explained by the increase in AIDS patients has been noted in recent years. The disease commonly occurs in the presence of other forms of immunodeficiency, such as that seen in posttransplant patients, those given immunosuppressive drugs and persons with inherited forms of immunodeficiency. There are few epidemiologic clues to the risk factors responsible. Altered antibody patterns to EBV characteristic of those seen in immunodeficiency states are seen in many cases of NHL and these changes have been shown to precede the development of NHL. Molecular techniques have shown the EBV genome to be present in some 10%–15% of tumor cells in the spontaneous form of NHL. Cases should be reported to a tumor registry.

V. KAPOSI'S SARCOMA
ICD-9 173.0–173.9; ICD-10 C46.0–46.9

(Idiopathic multiple pigmented hemorrhagic sarcoma)

Kaposi's sarcoma (KS) is a vascular neoplastic disorder that involves spindle cell proliferation. It is characterized by red-purple or blue-brown macules, plaques, and nodules of the skin and other organs. The skin lesions may be firm or compressible, solitary or legion. KS, first described in 1872, was considered a rare tumor of unknown etiology before its frequent diagnosis in AIDS patients.

There are four distinct epidemiologic forms of KS. The classical form occurs in older males of mainly Mediterranean or eastern European Jewish backgrounds. A second endemic form, found in parts of equatorial Africa, occurs in all age groups; neither of these two forms has a known precipitating environmental factor nor is either associated with immune deficiency. In contrast, the remaining two types of KS—those associated with recipients of organ transplants who undergo immunosuppressive treatment and with individuals infected with HIV-1—are accompanied by immune impairment. In all forms, males are predominantly afflicted. The epidemic form of KS presents the most aggressive clinical course and is seen almost exclusively in HIV infected individuals. Despite differences in clinical manifestations and HIV-1 serostatus, it is more appropriate to consider all forms of KS as one entity given the identical immunohistochemical features of the characteristic spindle cell of the tumor.

It is now believed that Kaposi's sarcoma associated herpesvirus (KSHV), also called human herpesvirus 8 (HHV-8), is the etiologic agent of KS. This herpesvirus, discovered in 1994, is a novel human *Gammaherpesvirus* that is related to an oncogenic herpesvirus of monkeys, *Herpesvirus saimiri*. Evidence of viral infection is found in virtually all cases of KS and several lines of evidence point to a key etiologic role in this disease. KSVH infection precedes clinical KS, is highly associated with increased KS risk in all populations thus far studied, and targets the endothelial (spindle) cell thought to be the prime determinant of KS tumorigenesis. KSHV has also been shown to induce transformation of primary endothelial cells.

Seroepidemiologic analysis suggests that KSHV has a more limited distribution than any of the other seven human herpesviruses. In North America, seroprevalence ranges from 0%–1% in blood donors to about 35% in HIV infected individuals and up to 100% in KS patients with AIDS. In contrast, in Milan, Italy where KS is endemic, blood donors have a 4% seropositivity rate. Data suggest even higher KSHV rates are present in Central Africa—58% of persons aged 14–84 were KSHV positive in one study while seroprevalence increased linearly with age and seroprevalence was similar in men and women.

Serologic analyses also suggest that infection occurs primarily in sexually active people, particularly homosexual men. Support for sexual transmission comes from the striking differences in KS risk for AIDS patients who acquire HIV via sexual transmission and those whose HIV infections derive from blood product exposure: the proportion of hemophiliac and transfusion related AIDS patients who develop KS are in the range of 1%–3%. Evidence for other routes of transmission come from infants born to HIV-1 positive women who developed KS at a very young age. In Africa, the high seroprevalence among adolescents and the relatively linear increase in prevalence with age suggest that nonsexual modes of transmission for KSHV may be important.

There is no known cure for Kaposi's sarcoma, although partial and complete remissions have been noted. Cases should be reported to a tumor registry.

VI. LYMPHATIC TISSUE, MALIGNANCY

ICD-9 202; ICD-10 C84.1, C84.5, C91.4, C91.5

(Adult T-cell leukemia [ATL], T-cell lymphosarcoma [TLCL], peripheral T-cell lymphoma [Sézary disease], Hairy cell leukemia)

Adult T-cell leukemia (ATL), a leukemia/lymphoma of T-cell origin commonly seen in Japan, is identical to T-cell lymphoma sarcoma-cell leukemia (TLCL) seen less commonly in the Caribbean, the Pacific coast of South America, equatorial Africa, and southern USA. These malignancies involve adults primarily and are associated with human T-cell lymphotrophic virus (HTLV-1), a member of the family of retroviruses. Infection early in life, primarily through breast milk, leads to tumor development in the adult with a peak at about age 50. This suggests the risk of ATL is lower should infection occur later in life through transfer of blood or blood products, IV drug use, or sexual activity. The same virus also causes tropical spastic paraparesis (TSP; also called HTLV-1-associated myelopathy [HAM] in Japan). Adult Japanese and Caribbean blacks are at highest risk.

HTLV-1 is strongly implicated in the causation of leukemia/lymphoma by serologic, virologic and epidemiologic evidence. In general, control measures are similar to those for prevention of AIDS (see AIDS, section 9). Effectiveness of screening donor blood for antibodies against HTLV-1 and 2 has yet to be demonstrated. In the USA, transmission from blood donors is a rare event because of the very low prevalence of the virus in the general population, but screening donor units for the virus is now a standard procedure. Cases should be reported to a tumor registry.

VII. CERVICAL CANCER

ICD-9 180; ICD-10 C53

(Carcinoma of the uterine cervix)

Cervical cancer is the sixth most common cancer worldwide and the highest among women in many economically developing areas. It occurs in westernized countries; incidence is higher in women who have a history of early and frequent intercourse with multiple sex partners and who are of lower socioeconomic status. Three quarters of all patients are in developing countries.

Human papillomavirus (HPV) has been strongly implicated in the etiology of cervical cancer. While HPV is usually the cause of benign warts and verrucae (see Warts, Viral), evidence of HPV types 16 and 18 has been found in tumor tissue from cervical neoplasia, with the genome demonstrated inside the cells in 80%–90% of the neoplasias. Cases should be reported to a tumor registry.

APHA

MEASLES   ICD-9 055; ICD-10 B05
(Rubeola, Hard measles, Red measles, Morbilli)

1. Identification—An acute, highly communicable viral disease with prodromal fever, conjunctivitis, coryza, cough and small spots with white or bluish white centers on an erythematous base on the buccal mucosa (Koplik spots). A characteristic red blotchy rash appears on the third to seventh day; the rash begins on the face, then becomes generalized, lasts 4-7 days, and sometimes ends in brawny desquamation. Leukopenia is common. The disease is more severe in infants and adults than in children. Complications may result from viral replication or bacterial superinfection, and include otitis media, pneumonia, laryngotracheobronchitis (croup), diarrhea and encephalitis.

In the USA, during the 1990s, death from measles occurred at a rate of about 2-3/1,000 cases; deaths occur mainly in children under 5 years of age, primarily from pneumonia and occasionally from encephalitis. Measles is a more severe disease in the very young and in malnourished children, in whom it may be associated with hemorrhagic rash, protein losing enteropathy, otitis media, oral sores, dehydration, diarrhea, blindness and severe skin infections. Children with clinical or subclinical vitamin A deficiency are at particularly high risk. The case-fatality rates in developing countries are estimated to be 3%-5%, but are commonly 10%-30% in some localities. Acute and delayed mortality in infants and children have been documented. In children who are borderline nourished, measles often precipitates acute kwashiorkor and exacerbates vitamin A deficiency, that may lead to blindness. Subacute sclerosing panencephalitis (SSPE) develops very rarely (about 1/100,000) several years after infection; over 50% of SSPE cases have had measles diagnosed in the first 2 years of life.

Diagnosis is usually made on clinical and epidemiologic grounds although laboratory confirmation is preferred. The detection of measles specific IgM antibodies which are present by 3-4 days after rash onset, or a significant rise in antibody concentrations between acute and convalescent sera confirms the diagnosis of measles. Techniques used less commonly include identification of viral antigen in nasopharyngeal mucosal swab by use of FA techniques, or by virus isolation in cell culture from blood or nasopharyngeal swab collected before the fourth day of rash, or urine specimens taken before the eighth day of rash.

2. Infectious agent—Measles virus, a member of the genus *Morbillivirus* of the family Paramyxoviridae.

3. Occurrence—Prior to widespread immunization, measles was common in childhood, so that more than 90% of people had been infected by age 20; few went through life without an attack. Measles was endemic in large metropolitan communities, and attained epidemic proportion about every second or third year. In smaller communities and areas, outbreaks tended to be more widely spaced and somewhat more severe. With longer intervals between outbreaks, as in the Arctic and some islands, measles outbreaks often involved a large proportion of the population with a high case-fatality rate. With effective childhood immunization programs, measles cases in the USA, Canada and other countries (e.g., Finland, the Czech Republic) have dropped by 99% and generally occur in young unimmunized children or older children, adolescents or young adults who have received only one dose of vaccine.

In the USA, there was a marked increase in measles incidence during 1989-1991. The majority of cases occurred in unimmunized children, including those under 15 months of age. Also, sustained outbreaks occurred in school populations among the 2%-5% who failed to seroconvert after 1 dose of vaccine. Similar outbreaks have occurred in Canada prior to the adoption of a 2 dose immunization schedule. Since 2 dose immunization schedules have been adopted, measles incidence has declined to record low levels and recent data indicate interuption of endogenous transmission in the USA. In Latin America, programs to administer supplemental doses of measles vaccine in regional National Immunization Day campaigns have resulted in the near elimination of measles from most countries. In 1994, the countries of the Western Hemisphere agreed to set a target of complete elimination of measles transmission by the end of the year 2005. In temperate climates, measles occurs primarily in the late winter and early spring. In tropical climates, measles occurs primarily in the dry season.

4. **Reservoir**—Humans.

5. **Mode of transmission**—Airborne by droplet spread, direct contact with nasal or throat secretions of infected persons, and, less commonly, by articles freshly soiled with nose and throat secretions. Measles is one of the most highly communicable infectious diseases.

6. **Incubation period**—About 10 days, but may be 7 to 18 days from exposure to onset of fever, usually 14 days until rash appears; rarely as long as 19-21 days. IG given for passive protection later than the third day of the incubation period, may extend the incubation period.

7. **Period of communicability**—From 1 day before the beginning of the prodromal period (usually about 4 days before rash onset) to 4 days after appearance of the rash; minimal after the second day of rash. The vaccine virus has not been shown to be communicable.

8. **Susceptibility and resistance**—All persons who have not had the disease or who have not been successfully immunized are susceptible. Acquired immunity after illness is permanent. Infants born to mothers who have had the disease are protected against disease for approximately the first 6-9 months or more, depending on the amount of residual maternal antibody at the time of pregnancy and the rate of antibody degradation. Maternal antibody interferes with response to vaccine. Immunization at

12-15 months induces immunity in 94%–98% of recipients; reimmunization increases immunity levels to about 99%. Children born to mothers with vaccine induced immunity receive less passive antibody, and these infants may become susceptible to measles and require measles immunization at an earlier age than is usually recommended.

9. **Methods of control—**

A. *Preventive measures:*

1) Public education by health departments and private physicians should encourage measles immunization for all susceptible infants, children, adolescents and young adults born in 1957 or later. Those for whom vaccine is contraindicated, and unimmunized persons identified more than 72 hours after exposure to measles in families or institutions may be partially or completely protected by IG given within 6 days after exposure.

2) Immunization: Live attenuated measles vaccine is the agent of choice and is indicated for all persons not immune to measles, unless specifically contraindicated (see 9A2c, below). A single injection of live measles vaccine, which is usually combined with other live vaccines (mumps, rubella), can be administered concurrently with other inactivated vaccines or toxoids; it should induce active immunity in 94–98% of susceptible individuals, possibly for life, by producing a mild or inapparent, noncommunicable infection. A second dose of measles vaccine may increase immunity levels to as high as 99%.

   About 5%–15% of nonimmune vaccinees may develop malaise and fever to 39.4°C (103°F) within 5-12 days postimmunization which lasts 1-2 days, but with little disability. Rash, coryza, mild cough and Koplik spots may occasionally occur. Febrile seizures occur infrequently and without sequelae; the highest incidence is in children with a previous history or a close family history (parents or siblings) of seizures. Encephalitis and encephalopathy have been reported following measles immunization (less than one case per million doses distributed).

   To reduce the number of vaccine failures, the current recommendation in the USA is a routine 2 dose measles vaccine schedule, with the initial dose administered at 12-15 months of age or as soon as possible thereafter. The second dose should be given at school entry (4-6 years of age), but can be administered as early as 4 weeks after the first dose in settings where the risk of exposure to measles is high. Both doses should generally be given as combined measles, mumps and rubella vaccine (MMR).

   Routine immunization with MMR at 12 months of age is

particularly important in areas where measles cases occur. During community outbreaks, the recommended age for immunization using monovalent measles vaccine can be lowered to 6-11 months. A second dose of measles vaccine is then given at 12-15 months and a third dose at school entry.

Studies in Africa and Latin America indicate that the optimal age for immunization in developing countries depends on the persistence of maternal antibodies in the infant and the increased risk of exposure to measles at a younger age. In most settings, WHO recommends measles immunization at 9 months of age. In Latin America, PAHO now recommends routine immunization at 12 months of age and periodic supplemental National Immunization Day campaigns to prevent outbreaks.

a) Vaccine shipment and storage: Immunization may not produce protection if the vaccine has been improperly handled or stored. Prior to reconstitution, freeze-dried measles vaccine is relatively stable and can be stored in a freezer or at refrigerator temperatures (2°-8°C; 35.6°-46.4°F) with safety for a year or more. Reconstituted vaccine should be kept at refrigerator temperatures and discarded after 8 hours. Both freeze-dried and reconstituted vaccine should be protected from prolonged exposure to ultraviolet light, which may inactivate the virus.

b) Reimmunizations: In the USA, in addition to routine reimmunization of children entering school, reimmunization should be required of persons entering high school, educational institutions beyond high school, or entering medical care facilities, unless they have a documented history of measles, serologic evidence of measles immunity, or have received 2 doses of measles containing vaccines. In those who received only inactivated measles vaccine, reimmunization may produce more severe reactions, such as local edema and induration, lymphadenopathy and fever, but will protect against the atypical measles syndrome.

c) Contraindications to the use of live virus vaccines:

i) Patients with primary immune deficiency diseases affecting T-cell function or acquired immune deficiency due to leukemia, lymphoma or generalized malignancy, or therapy with corticosteroids, irradiation, alkylating drugs or antimetabolites, should not receive live virus vaccines. Infection with HIV is not an absolute contraindication. In the USA, immunization with MMR can be considered for asymptomatic HIV infected persons without evidence of severe immunosuppression. WHO recommends measles immunization of all infants and children regardless of HIV status because of the greater risk of severe measles in such persons.

ii) Patients with severe acute illness with or without fever should have immunization deferred until they have recovered from the acute phase of their illness; minor febrile illnesses, such as diarrhea or upper respiratory infections, are not a contraindication.

iii) Persons with anaphylactic hypersensitivity to a previous dose of measles vaccine, gelatin or neomycin should not receive measles vaccine. Egg allergy, even if anaphylactic, is no longer considered a contraindication.

iv) Pregnancy. Purely on theoretical grounds, vaccine should not be given to pregnant women; others should be advised of the theoretical risk of fetal damage if they become pregnant within 1 month after receipt of monovalent measles vaccine or 3 months after receipt of MMR vaccine.

v) Vaccine should be given at least 14 days before IG or blood transfusion. IG or blood products can interfere with the response to measles vaccine for varying periods depending on the dose of IG. The usual dose administered for hepatitis A prevention can interfere for 3 months; very large doses of intravenous IG can interfere for up to 11 months.

3) The requirement for measles immunization for school attendance—from day care centers through college—is an important and effective means of measles control in the USA and some provinces of Canada. Since sustained outbreaks have occurred in schools with immunization rates more than 95%, even higher levels of immunity are needed to prevent outbreaks from occurring. This may be achieved by routine reimmunization as a school entry requirement.

B. Control of patient, contacts and the immediate environment:

1) Report to local health authority: Obligatory case report in most states (USA) and in many countries, Class 2A (see Communicable Disease Reporting). Early reporting (within 24 hours) provides opportunity for better outbreak control.

2) Isolation: Impractical in the community at large; children with measles should be kept out of school for 4 days after appearance of the rash. In hospitals, respiratory isolation from onset of catarrhal stage of the prodromal period through fourth day of rash reduces the exposure of other patients at high risk.

3) Concurrent disinfection: None.

4) Quarantine: Usually impractical. Quarantine of institutions, wards or dormitories can sometimes be of value; strict segregation of infants if measles occurs in an institution.

5) Immunization of contacts: Live virus vaccine, if given within 72 hours of exposure, may provide protection. IG may be used within 6 days of exposure for susceptible household or other

contacts for whom risk of complications is very high (particularly contacts under 1 year of age, pregnant women or immunocompromised persons), or for whom measles vaccine is contraindicated. The dose is 0.25 ml/kg (0.11 ml/lb) up to a maximum of 15 ml. For immunocompromised persons, 0.5 ml/kg is given, up to a maximum of 15 ml. Live measles vaccine should be given 5–6 months later to those for whom vaccine is not contraindicated.

6) Investigation of contacts and source of infection: A search for and immunization of exposed susceptible contacts should be carried out to limit the spread of disease. Carriers are unknown.

7) Specific treatment: None.

C. Epidemic measures:

1) Prompt reporting (within 24 hours) of suspected cases and comprehensive immunization programs for all susceptibles are needed to limit spread. In day care, school and college outbreaks in the USA, all persons without documentation of 2 doses of live virus vaccine at least 1 month apart on or after the first birthday should be immunized unless they have documentation of prior physician diagnosed measles or laboratory evidence of immunity.

2) In institutional outbreaks, new admissions should receive vaccine or IG.

3) In many less developed countries, measles has a relatively high case-fatality rate. If vaccine is available, prompt use at the beginning of an epidemic is essential to limit spread; if vaccine supply is limited, priority should be given to young children for whom the risk is greatest.

D. Disaster implications: Introduction of measles into refugee populations with a high proportion of susceptibles can result in devastating epidemics with high fatality rates.

E. International measures: None.

MELIOIDOSIS   ICD-9 025; ICD-10 A24
(Whitmore disease)

1. Identification—An uncommon bacterial infection with a range of clinical manifestations, from no disease or asymptomatic pulmonary consolidation to necrotizing pneumonia and/or a rapidly fatal septicemia.

It may simulate typhoid fever or, more commonly, tuberculosis; the clinical picture may include pulmonary cavitation, empyema, chronic abscesses and osteomyelitis.

Diagnosis depends on isolation of the causative agent; a rising antibody titer in serologic tests is confirmatory. The possibility of melioidosis should be kept in mind in any unexplained suppurative disease, especially cavitating pulmonary disease, in a patient living in or returned from southeast Asia and other endemic areas; disease may become manifest as long as 25 years after exposure.

2. Infectious agent—*Pseudomonas pseudomallei,* the Whitmore bacillus.

3. Occurrence—Clinical disease is uncommon, it generally occurrs in individuals whose abraded, lacerated or burned skin has had intimate contact with contaminated soil and surface water. It may appear as a complication of an overt wound or may follow aspiration of water. Cases have been recorded in, but probably are not restricted to, southeast Asia (Myanmar, Thailand, Malaysia, Indonesia and Vietnam), the Philippines, Iran, Turkey, northeastern Australia, Papua New Guinea, Guam, Burkina Faso (Upper Volta), Ivory Coast, Sri Lanka, Madagascar, Brazil, Ecuador, Panama, Mexico, Haiti, El Salvador, Puerto Rico and Aruba. In certain of these areas, 5%–20% of agricultural workers have demonstrable antibodies but no history of overt disease; in Thailand it is considered to be a disease of rice farmers.

4. Reservoir—The organism is saprophytic in certain soils and waters. Various animals, including sheep, goats, horses, swine, monkeys and rodents (and a variety of animals and birds in zoological gardens) can become infected. There is no evidence that they are important reservoirs, except that they transfer the agent to new foci.

5. Mode of transmission—Usually by contact with contaminated soil or water through overt or inapparent skin wounds, by aspiration or ingestion of contaminated water or by inhalation of dust from soil.

6. Incubation period—Can be as short as 2 days. However, years may elapse between the presumed exposure and the appearance of clinical disease.

7. Period of communicability—Person to person transmission has not been proven; it has been reported only following sexual contact with an individual with prostatic infection. Laboratory acquired infections are uncommon but do occur, especially if procedures produce aerosols.

8. Susceptibility and resistance—Disease in humans is uncommon even among people in endemic areas who have close contact with soil or water containing the infectious agent. Many chronically infected, asymptomatic patients develop clinical disease following severe injuries or burns or disease may be due to the presence of an underlying predisposing condition such as diabetes or renal failure. These conditions may precipitate disease or recrudescence of disease in asymptomatic infected individuals.

9. Methods of control—

A. Preventive measures:

1) Persons with debilitating disease, including diabetes, and those with traumatic wounds should avoid exposure to soil or water, such as rice paddies, in endemic areas.

2) In endemic areas, skin lacerations, abrasions or burns that have been contaminated with soil or surface water should be immediately and thoroughly cleaned.

B. Control of patient, contacts and the immediate environment:

1) Report to local health authority: No official report, Class 5 (see Communicable Disease Reporting).

2) Isolation: Respiratory and sinus drainage precautions.

3) Concurrent disinfection: Safe disposal of sputum and wound discharges.

4) Quarantine: None.

5) Immunization of contacts: None.

6) Investigation of contacts and source of infection: Human carriers are not known.

7) Specific treatment: The most effective agent is TMP-SMX. A favorable outcome may be expected in most subacute and chronic cases. For cases with acute sepsis, some recommend ceftazidime plus TMP-SMX plus gentamicin. In a study in Thailand, relapses were significantly less frequent after therapy with ceftazidime or an oral multidrug combination of chloramphenicol, doxycycline and TMP-SMX. The best treatment for severe septicemic cases was found to be IV ceftazidime, with amoxicillin/clavulanate as an alternative.

C. Epidemic measures: Not applicable to humans; a sporadic disease.

D. Disaster implications: None.

E. International measures: None. Introduction should be considered when animals are moved to areas where the disease is unknown.

GLANDERS   ICD-9 024; ICD-10 A24.0

Glanders is a highly communicable disease of horses, mules and donkeys; it has disappeared from most areas of the world, although enzootic foci are believed to exist in Asia and some eastern Mediterranean countries. Clinical glanders no longer occurs in the Western Hemisphere. Human infection has occurred rarely and sporadically and almost exclusively in those whose occupations involve contact with animals or work in laboratories (e.g., veterinarians, equine butchers and pathologists). Infection with the etiologic organism, *Pseudomonas mallei (Actinobacillus mallei),* the glanders bacillus, cannot be differentiated serologically from *P. pseudomallei;* specific diagnosis can be made only by characterization of the isolated organism. Prevention depends on control of glanders in the equine species and care in handling causative organisms. Treatment is the same as for melioidosis.

MENINGITIS
I. VIRAL MENINGITIS   ICD-9 047.9; ICD-10 A87
(Aseptic meningitis, Serous meningitis, Nonbacterial or Abacterial meningitis)
(Nonpyogenic meningitis: ICD-9 322.0; ICD-10 G03.0)

1. Identification—A relatively common but rarely serious clinical syndrome with multiple viral etiologies, characterized by sudden onset of febrile illness with signs and symptoms of meningeal involvement. CSF findings are pleocytosis (usually mononuclear but may be polymorphonuclear in early stages), increased protein, normal sugar and absence of bacteria. A rash resembling rubella characterizes certain types caused by echoviruses and coxsackieviruses; vesicular and petechial rashes may also occur. Active illness seldom exceeds 10 days. Transient paresis and encephalitic manifestations may occur; paralysis is unusual. Residual signs that last a year or more may include weakness, muscle spasm, insomnia and personality changes. Recovery is usually complete. GI and respiratory symptoms may be associated with enterovirus infection.

Various diseases caused by nonviral agents may mimic aseptic meningitis: these include inadequately treated pyogenic meningitis, tuberculous and cryptococcal meningitis, meningitis caused by other fungi, cerebrovascular syphilis and lymphogranuloma venereum. Postinfectious and postvaccinal reactions require differentiation, these include sequelae to measles, mumps, varicella and immunization against rabies and smallpox; these syndromes are usually encephalitic in type. Leptospirosis, listeriosis, syphilis, lymphocytic choriomeningitis, viral hepatitis, infectious mononucleosis, influenza and other diseases may produce the same clinical syndrome, and these are discussed in individual chapters.

Under optimal conditions, specific identification can be made in about half the cases by using serologic and isolation techniques. Viral agents may be isolated in early stages from throat washings and stool, occasionally from CSF and blood, and by cell culture techniques and animal inoculation.

2. Infectious agents—A wide variety of infectious agents, many of which are associated with other specific diseases. Many viruses are capable of producing meningeal features. Half or more of the cases have no etiology demonstrated. In epidemic periods, mumps may be responsible for more than 25% of cases of established etiology in nonimmunized populations. In the USA, enteroviruses (picornaviruses) cause most cases of known etiology. Coxsackievirus group B, types 1–6, cause roughly one third; and echovirus, types 2, 5, 6, 7, 9 (most), 10, 11, 14, 18 and 30, about one half. Coxsackievirus group A (types 2, 3, 4, 7, 9 and 10), arboviruses, measles, herpes simplex and varicella viruses, lymphocytic choriomeningitis virus, adenovirus and others are responsible for sporadic cases. The incidence of specific types varies with geographic location and time. *Leptospira* may be responsible for up to 20% of cases of aseptic meningitis in various areas of the world (see Leptospirosis).

3. Occurrence—Worldwide, as epidemics and sporadic cases. Actual incidence is unknown. Seasonal increases in late summer and early autumn are due mainly to arboviruses and enteroviruses, while late winter outbreaks may be due primarily to mumps.

4., 5., 6., 7. and **8. Reservoir, Mode of transmission, Incubation period, Period of communicability** and **Susceptibility and resistance**—Vary with the specific infectious agent (refer to specific disease chapters).

9. Methods of control—

    A. Preventive measures: Depend on etiology (see specific disease).

    B. Control of patient, contacts and the immediate environment:

        1) Report to local health authority: In selected endemic areas; in many countries and states (USA), not a reportable disease, Class 3B (see Communicable Disease Reporting). If confirmed by laboratory means, specify the infectious agent; otherwise, report as cause undetermined.

        2) Isolation: Specific diagnosis depends on laboratory data not usually available until after recovery. Therefore, enteric precautions are indicated for 7 days after onset of illness unless a nonenteroviral diagnosis is established.

        3) Concurrent disinfection: No special precautions are needed beyond routine sanitary practices.

        4) Quarantine: None.

        5) Immunization of contacts: See specific disease.

        6) Investigation of contacts and source of infection: Not usually indicated.

        7) Specific treatment: None for the usual causative viral agents.

    C. Epidemic measures: See specific disease.

D. Disaster implications: None.

E. International measures: WHO Collaborating Centres.

II. BACTERIAL MENINGITIS   ICD-9 320; ICD-10 G00

The reported incidence of bacterial meningitis more than 10 years after licensure of the first vaccine against *Haemophilus influenzae* serotype b (Hib) is 2.2/100,000/year in the USA, and about one third of cases are in children under 5. Any agent may cause infection at any age, but, as of the late 1990s, the most common agents are *Neisseria meningitidis* and *Streptococcus pneumoniae.* Meningococcal disease occurs sporadically and in epidemics; in many parts of the world, it is the leading cause of bacterial meningitis. Meningitis due to Hib, previously one of the most common causes of bacterial meningitis, has largely been eliminated in the USA. The less common bacterial causes of meningitis, such as staphylococci, enteric bacteria, group B streptococci and *Listeria*, occur in persons with specific susceptibilities (such as neonates and patients with impaired immunity) or as the consequence of head trauma.

II.A. MENINGOCOCCAL
INFECTION   ICD-9 136; ICD-10 A39
(Cerebrospinal fever)
MENINGOCOCCAL
MENINGITIS   ICD-9 036.0; ICD-10 A39.0
(Meningococcemia, not meningitis: ICD-10 A39.2–A39.4)

1. Identification—An acute bacterial disease, characterized by sudden onset of fever, intense headache, nausea and often vomiting, stiff neck and, frequently, a petechial rash with pink macules or, very rarely, vesicles. Delirium and coma often appear; occasional fulminant cases exhibit sudden prostration, ecchymoses and shock at onset. Formerly, case-fatality rates exceeded 50%, but with early diagnosis, modern therapy and supportive measures, the case-fatality rate is between 5% and 15%.

Up to 5%–10% of populations in countries with endemic disease may be asymptomatic carriers with the nasopharynx colonized with *Neisseria meningitidis.* A small minority of persons who become colonized will progress to invasive disease, characterized by one or more clinical syndromes including bacteremia, sepsis, meningitis or pneumonia. Many patients with sepsis develop a petechial rash, sometimes with joint involvement. Meningococcemia may occur without extension to the meninges and should be suspected in cases of unexplained acute febrile illness associated with petechial rash and leukocytosis. In fulminating meningococcemia, the death rate remains high despite prompt antibacterial treatment.

Diagnosis is confirmed by the recovery of meningococci from the CSF or blood. In culture negative cases, the diagnosis may be supported by identification of group specific meningococcal polysaccharides in CSF by LA, CIE and coagglutination techniques, or meningococcal DNA in CSF or plasma by PCR. Microscopic examination of Gram-stained smears from petechiae may reveal organisms.

2. **Infectious agent**—*N. meningitidis,* the meningococcus. Group A organisms have caused the major epidemics in the USA (none since 1945) and elsewhere; groups B, C and Y are, as of the late 1990s, responsible for most cases in the USA. Certain genotypes have been associated with outbreaks of disease. Additional serogroups have been recognized as pathogens (e.g., groups W-135, X and Z). Organisms belonging to some of these serogroups may be less virulent, but fatal infections and secondary cases have occurred with all. Outbreaks of *N. meningitidis* are usually caused by closely related strains. Subtyping of isolates by use of methods such as multilocus enzyme electrophoresis or pulsed-field gel electrophoresis of enzyme-restricted DNA fragments, may allow identification of an "outbreak strain" and aid in better defining the extent of an outbreak.

3. **Occurrence**—Meningococcal infections are ubiquitous, but the incidence of meningococcal disease peaks in late winter to early spring. Meningococcal disease, while primarily a disease of very small children, occurs commonly in children and young adults; in many countries in males more than females, and more commonly among newly aggregated adults under crowded living conditions such as in barracks and institutions. An area of high incidence has existed for many years in the sub-Saharan region of mid-Africa, where the disease is usually caused by group A organisms. In 1996, the largest recorded epidemic of meningococcal disease occurred in west Africa, with close to 150,000 cases reported in Burkina Faso, Chad, Mali, Niger and Nigeria. Over the past 10 years, there have also been group A epidemics in Nepal and India, as well as in Ethiopia, Sudan and other African countries. During the 1980s and 1990s, group B has emerged as the most common cause of disease in Europe and most of the Americas. Epidemics, characterized by a 5-10 fold increase in incidence have been reported from many countries in Europe, Central and South America and most recently in New Zealand and the US Pacific northwest. Community outbreaks of group C disease have been observed with increasing frequency in the USA and Canada since 1990. These outbreaks have particularly affected school and college aged persons, and transmission has occasionally occurred among persons congregating in bars or nightclubs. During the late 1990s, group Y disease has become as common as groups B and C in many parts of the USA. Circulation of new strains of meningococci is usually characterized by an increase in the average age of persons reported with meningococcal disease.

4. **Reservoir**—Humans.

5. **Mode of transmission**—By direct contact, including respiratory

droplets from nose and throat of infected people; infection usually causes only a subclinical mucosal infection; invasion sufficient to cause systemic disease is comparatively rare. Carrier prevalence of 25% or greater may exist without cases of meningitis. During epidemics, over half the men in a military unit may be healthy carriers of pathogenic meningococci. Fomite transmission is insignificant.

6. Incubation period—Varies from 2 to 10 days, commonly 3–4 days.

7. Period of communicability—Until meningococci are no longer present in discharges from nose and mouth. Meningococci usually disappear from the nasopharynx within 24 hours after institution of treatment with antimicrobial agents to which the organisms are sensitive and which attain substantial concentrations in oropharyngeal secretions. Penicillin will temporarily suppress the organisms, but it does not usually eradicate them from the oronasopharynx.

8. Susceptibility and resistance—Susceptibility to the clinical disease is low and decreases with age; a high ratio of carriers to cases prevails. Those who are deficient in certain complement components are especially prone to recurrent disease. Splenectomized persons are susceptible to bacteremic illness. Group specific immunity of unknown duration follows even subclinical infections.

9. Methods of control—

A. Preventive measures:

1) Educate the public on the need to reduce direct contact and exposure to droplet infection.
2) Reduce overcrowding in living quarters and workplaces, such as barracks, schools, camps and ships.
3) Vaccines containing groups A, C, Y and W-135 meningococcal polysaccharides have been licensed in the USA and other countries for use in adults and older children; currently only the quadrivalent vaccine is available in the USA. Meningococcal vaccine is effective in adults and has been given to military recruits in the USA since 1971; it has also been used to control community and college outbreaks of group C disease during the 1990s. It should be given to certain high risk groups over 2 years of age who are especially susceptible to serious meningococcal infections, including asplenic patients, persons with terminal complement deficiencies and laboratory personnel who are exposed routinely to *N. meningitidis* in solutions that may be aerosolized. Unfortunately, the C component is poorly immunogenic and ineffective in children under 2 years of age. Serogroup A vaccine is probably effective in younger children; however, for those 3 months to 2 years of age, 2 doses are given 3 months apart instead of the single dose given to those

over 2 years of age. The duration of protection is limited, particularly in children less than 5 years of age. Routine immunization of civilians in the USA is not recommended. Immunization will reduce the risk to travelers who plan to have prolonged contact with the local populace in countries experiencing epidemic meningococcal group A or C disease. Reimmunization may be considered within 3-5 years if indications for receipt of vaccine still exist. No vaccine effective against group B meningococci is currently licensed in the USA, although several have been developed and demonstrated to have some efficacy in older children and adults. Conjugate vaccines against serogroups A and C are in clinical trials, but their efficacy, as of late 1999, has not been evaluated. For infants and young children, conjugate serogroup A, C, Y, and W135 meningococcal vaccines have been developed through methods similar to those used for *Haemophilus influenzae* type b conjugate vaccines. These vaccines are expected to be used routinely in the United Kingdom starting around the year 2000 and should become become available in the USA within 2-4 years thereafter.

B. Control of patient, contacts and the immediate environment:

1) Report to local health authority: Obligatory case report in most states (USA) and countries, Class 2A (see Communicable Disease Reporting).

2) Isolation: Respiratory isolation for 24 hours after start of chemotherapy.

3) Concurrent disinfection: Of discharges from the nose and throat and articles soiled therewith. Terminal cleaning.

4) Quarantine: None.

5) Protection of contacts: Close surveillance of household, daycare, and other intimate contacts for early signs of illness, especially fever, to initiate appropriate therapy without delay; prophylactic administration of an effective chemotherapeutic agent to intimate contacts (household contacts, military personnel sharing the same sleeping space and people socially close enough to have shared eating utensils, e.g., close friends at school but not the whole class). Younger children in day care centers are exceptions and, even if not close friends, all should be given prophylaxis after an index case is identified. The prophylactic antibiotic agent of choice is rifampin administered twice daily for 2 days: adults 600 mg per dose; children over 1 month old, 10 mg/kg; and for those less than 1 month old, 5 mg/kg. Rifampin should be avoided by pregnant women. Rifampin may reduce the effectiveness of oral contraceptives.

For adults, ceftriaxone, 250 mg IM, given in a single dose, is effective; 125 mg IM for children under 15 years of age. Ciprofloxacin, 500 mg PO, may be given as a single dose to adults. If the organisms have been shown to be sensitive to sulfadiazine, it may be given to adults and older children at a dosage of 1.0 g every 12 hours for 4 doses; for infants and children, the dosage is 125–150 mg/kg/day divided into 4 equal doses, on each of 2 consecutive days. As of 1993, sulfadiazine is no longer manufactured in the USA, and assistance may be needed from CDC to obtain this drug. Health care personnel are rarely at risk even when caring for infected patients; only intimate exposure to nasopharyngeal secretions (e.g., as in mouth to mouth resuscitation) warrants prophylaxis. There would be insufficient time for immunization of close household contacts to be of any value.

6) Investigation of contacts and source of infection: Throat or nasopharyngeal cultures are of no value in deciding who should receive prophylaxis since carriage is variable and there is no consistent relationship between that found in the normal population and in an epidemic.

7) Specific treatment: Penicillin given parenterally in adequate doses is the drug of choice for proven meningococcal disease; ampicillin and chloramphenicol are also effective. However, strains resistant to penicillin have been reported in multiple countries, including Spain, England and the USA; strains resistant to chloramphenicol have been reported in Vietnam and France. Treatment should begin immediately when the presumptive clinical diagnosis is made, even before meningococci have been identified. In children, until the specific etiologic agent has been identified, the therapy must be effective against *Haemophilus influenzae* type b (Hib) as well as *Streptococcus pneumoniae*. While ampicillin is the drug of choice for both as long as the organisms are ampicillin sensitive, it should be combined with a third generation cephalosporin, or chloramphenicol or vancomycin should be substituted in the many places where ampicillin resistant *H. influenzae* b or penicillin-resistant *S. pneumoniae* strains are known to occur. Patients with meningococcal or Hib disease should be given rifampin prior to discharge from the hospital if neither a third generation cephalosporin nor ciprofloxacin was given as treatment to ensure elimination of the organism.

C. Epidemic measures:

1) When an outbreak occurs, major emphasis must be placed on careful surveillance, early diagnosis and immediate treatment of suspected cases. A high index of suspicion is invaluable.

2) Separate individuals, and ventilate living and sleeping quarters of all people who are exposed to infection because of crowding or congested living conditions (e.g., soldiers, miners and prisoners).

3) Mass chemoprophylaxis is usually not effective in controlling outbreaks. However, in outbreaks involving small populations (e.g., a single school), administration of chemoprophylaxis to all persons within the population may be considered, especially if the outbreak is caused by a serogroup not included in the available vaccine. If undertaken, it should be administered to all members of the community at the same time. All intimate contacts should still be considered for prophylaxis, regardless of whether the entire small population is treated (see 9B5, above).

4) The use of vaccine in all age groups affected should be strongly considered if an outbreak occurs in a large institutional or community setting in which the cases are due to groups A, C, W-135 or Y (see 9A3, above). Meningococcal vaccine has been very effective in halting epidemics due to A and C serogroups. The following may help in deciding whether to immunize persons at risk during possible group C outbreaks: a) determine the epidemiology of the outbreak to find the least common age and social denominator (e.g., a school, day care setting, organization, night club, town) among affected persons; b) calculate attack rates with the outbreak strain among the population at risk; and c) subtype *N. meningitidis* isolates, if available, from cases of disease, using molecular typing methods. If at least 3 cases of group C disease with the same subtype have occurred during a 3 month period, new cases are still occurring and the attack rate exceeds 10 group C cases per 100,000 in the population at risk, then immunization of those in the group at risk should be considered.

D. Disaster implications: Epidemics may develop in situations of forced crowding.

E. International measures: WHO Collaborating Centres. While not covered by *International Health Regulations,* a valid certificate of immunization against meningococcal meningitis may be required by some countries, as by Saudi Arabia for religious visitors.

II.B. *HAEMOPHILUS* MENINGITIS ICD-9 320.0; ICD-10 G00.0
(Meningitis due to *Haemophilus influenzae*)

1. Identification—In the era before widespread use of *Haemophilus* b conjugate vaccines, this was the most common bacterial meningitis in children aged 2 months to 5 years in the USA. It is usually associated with a bacteremia. The onset can be subacute but is usually sudden; symptoms include fever, vomiting, lethargy and meningeal irritation, with bulging fontanelle in infants or stiff neck and back in older children. Progressive stupor or coma is common. Occasionally, there is a low grade fever for several days, with more subtle CNS symptoms.

Diagnosis may be made by isolation of organisms from blood or CSF. Specific capsular polysaccharide may be identified by CIE or LA techniques.

2. Infectious agent—Most commonly *H. influenzae* serotype b (Hib). This organism may also cause epiglottitis, pneumonia, septic arthritis, cellulitis, pericarditis, empyema and osteomyelitis. Other serotypes rarely cause meningitis.

3. Occurrence—Worldwide; most prevalent among children aged 2 months to 3 years; unusual over the age of 5 years. In developing countries, peak incidence is in children less than 6 months of age; in the USA, in children 6-12 months of age. In the prevaccine era in the USA, about 12,000 cases of Hib meningitis occurred among children less than 5 years compared with about 25 reported cases in 1998. As of the late 1990s, with widespread vaccine use in early childhood, Hib meningitis has virtually disappeared; more cases now occur in adults than in young children. Secondary cases may occur in families and day care centers.

4. Reservoir—Humans.

5. Mode of transmission—By droplet infection and discharges from nose and throat during the infectious period. The portal of entry is most commonly the nasopharynx.

6. Incubation period—Unknown; probably short, 2-4 days.

7. Period of communicability—As long as organisms are present, which may be for a prolonged period even without nasal discharge. Noncommunicable within 24-48 hours after starting effective antibiotic therapy.

8. Susceptibility and resistance—Susceptibility is assumed to be universal. Immunity is associated with the presence of circulating bactericidal and/or anticapsular antibody, acquired transplacentally, from prior infection or from immunization.

9. Methods of control—

   A. Preventive measures:

   1) Routine childhood immunization. Several protein polysaccharide conjugate vaccines have been shown to prevent meningitis in children more than 2 months of age and are licensed in the USA both individually and combined with other vaccines.

Immunization is recommended starting at 2 months of age, followed by additional doses after 2 months; dosages vary with the vaccine in use. All vaccines require boosters at 12–15 months of age. Immunization is not routinely recommended for children more than 5 years of age.

2) Monitor for cases occurring in susceptible population settings, such as day care centers and large foster homes.

3) Educate parents about the risk of secondary cases in siblings less than 4 years old and the need for prompt evaluation and treatment if fever or stiff neck develops.

B. *Control of patient, contacts and the immediate environment:*

1) Report to local health authority: In selected endemic areas (USA), Class 3B (see Communicable Disease Reporting).

2) Isolation: Respiratory isolation for 24 hours after start of chemotherapy.

3) Concurrent disinfection: None.

4) Quarantine: None.

5) Protection of contacts: Rifampin prophylaxis (orally once daily for 4 days in a 20 mg/kg dose, maximal dose 600 mg/day) for all household contacts (including adults) in households where there are one or more infants (other than the index case) less than 12 months of age or with a child 1–3 years of age who is inadequately immunized. When two or more cases of invasive disease have occurred within 60 days and unimmunized or incompletely immunized children attend the child care facility, administration of rifampin to all attendees and supervisory personnel is indicated. When a single case has occurred, the use of rifampin prophylaxis is controversial.

6) Investigation of contacts and source of infection: Observe contacts under 6 years old, and especially infants including those in household, day care centers and nurseries for signs of illness, especially fever.

7) Specific treatment: Ampicillin has been the drug of choice (parenteral 200–400 mg/kg/day). However, since about 30% of strains are now resistant due to beta-lactamase production, ceftriaxone, cefotaxime or chloramphenicol is recommended concurrently or singly until antibiotic sensitivities are known. The patient should be given rifampin prior to discharge from the hospital to assure elimination of the organism.

C. *Epidemic measures:* Not applicable.

D. *Disaster implications:* None.

E. *International measures:* None.

II.C. PNEUMOCOCCAL
MENINGITIS   ICD-9 320.1; ICD-10 G00.1

Pneumococcal meningitis has a high case-fatality rate. It can be fulminant and occurs with bacteremia but not necessarily with any other focus, although there may be otitis media or mastoiditis. The onset is usually sudden with high fever, lethargy or coma and signs of meningeal irritation. It is a sporadic disease in young infants, the elderly and in certain high risk groups, including asplenic and hypogammaglobulinemic patients. Basilar fracture causing persistent communication with the nasopharynx is a recognized predisposing factor. (See Pneumonia, pneumococcal.)

II.D. NEONATAL
MENINGITIS   ICD-9 320.8, 771.8;
ICD-10 P37.8, P35–P37, G00, G03

Infants with neonatal meningitis develop lethargy, seizures, apneic episodes, poor feeding, hypothermia or hyperthermia and sometimes respiratory distress, usually in their first week of life. The WBC count may be elevated or depressed. Culture of the CSF yields group B streptococci, *Listeria monocytogenes* (see Listeriosis), *E. coli* K-1 or other organisms acquired from the birth canal. Infants 2 weeks to 2 months of age may develop similar symptoms, with recovery from the CSF of group B streptococci or organisms of the *Klebsiella-Enterobacter-Serratia* group, acquired from the nursery environment. The meningitis in both groups is associated with septicemia. Treatment is with ampicillin, plus a third-generation cephalosporin or aminoglycoside, until the etiologic organism has been identified and its antibiotic susceptibilities determined.

MOLLUSCUM
CONTAGIOSUM   ICD-9 078.0; ICD-10 B08.1

1. Identification—A viral disease of the skin that results in a smooth-surfaced, firm and spherical papule with umbilication of the vertex. The lesions may be flesh colored, white, translucent or yellow. Most molluscum papules are 2–5 mm in diameter, but giant-cell molluscum papules (greater than 15 mm in diameter) are occasionally seen. Lesions in adults are most often on the lower abdominal wall, pubis, genitalia or inner thighs; lesions on children are most often on the face, trunk and proximal extremities. Lesions tend to disseminate in patients with HIV infection. Occasionally the lesions itch and a linear orientation is seen, which suggests autoinoculation by scratching. Also, in some patients, 50-100 lesions may become confluent and form a single plaque.

Without treatment, molluscum contagiosum persists for 6 months to 2 years. Any one lesion has a life span of 2-3 months. Lesions may resolve spontaneously or as a result of the inflammatory response following trauma or secondary bacterial infection. Treatment (i.e., mechanically removing the molluscum lesions) may shorten the course of the illness.

Diagnosis can be made clinically when multiple lesions are present. For confirmation, the core can be expressed onto a glass slide and examined by ordinary light microscopy for classic basophilic, Feulgen-positive, intracytoplasmic inclusions, the "molluscum bodies" or "Henderson-Paterson bodies." Histology can confirm the diagnosis.

2. Infectious agent—Member of Poxviridae family, genus *Molluscipoxvirus;* the genus comprises at least two species differentiated by DNA endonuclease cleavage maps. Virus has not been grown in cell culture.

3. Occurrence—Worldwide. Serologic tests are not well standardized. Inspection of the skin is the only screening technique available. Therefore, epidemiologic studies of the disease have been limited. Population surveys have been conducted only in Papua New Guinea and Fiji, where the peak disease incidence occurs in childhood.

4. Reservoir—Humans.

5. Mode of transmission—Usually by direct contact. Transmission is both sexual and nonsexual, the latter includes spread via fomites. Autoinoculation is also suspected.

6. Incubation period—For experimental inoculation, 19-50 days; clinical reports, 7 days to 6 months.

7. Period of communicability—Unknown, but probably as long as lesions persist.

8. Susceptibility and resistance—Any age may be affected; more often seen in children. Disease is more common in patients with AIDS, in whom lesions may disseminate.

9. Methods of control—

    A. Preventive measures: Avoid contact with affected patients.

    B. Control of patient, contacts and the immediate environment:

        1) Report to local health authority: Official report not ordinarily justifiable, Class 5 (see Communicable Disease Reporting).

        2) Isolation: Generally not indicated. Infected children with visible lesions should be excluded from close contact sports such as wrestling.

3) Concurrent disinfection: None.
4) Quarantine: None.
5) Immunization of contacts: None.
6) Investigation of contacts and source of infection: Examine sexual partners where applicable.
7) Specific treatment: Indicated to minimize risk of transmission. Curettage with local anesthesia or topical application of cantharidin or peeling agents (salicylic or lactic acid). Freezing with liquid nitrogen has some advocates.

C. Epidemic measures: Suspend direct contact activities.

D. Disaster implications: None.

E. International measures: None.

MONONUCLEOSIS, INFECTIOUS   ICD-9 075; ICD-10 B27

(Gammaherpesviral mononucleosis, Mononucleosis due to Epstein-Barr virus, Glandular fever, Monocytic angina)

1. Identification—An acute viral syndrome characterized clinically by fever, sore throat (often with exudative pharyngotonsillitis), lymphadenopathy (especially posterior cervical) and splenomegaly; characterized hematologically by mononucleosis and lymphocytosis of 50% or greater, including 10% or more atypical cells; and characterized serologically by the presence of heterophile and Epstein-Barr virus (EBV) antibodies. Recovery usually occurs in a few weeks, but a very small proportion of individuals can take months to regain their former level of energy. There is no evidence that this is due to abnormal persistence of the infection in a chronic form.

In young children the disease is generally mild and more difficult to recognize. Jaundice occurs in about 4% of infected young adults, although 95% will have abnormal liver function tests; splenomegaly occurs in 50%. Duration is from 1 to several weeks; the disease is rarely fatal. The disease is more severe in older adults.

The causal agent, EBV, is also closely associated with the pathogenesis of several lymphomas and nasopharyngeal cancer. (see Malignant Neoplasms Associated with Infectious Agents). Fatal immunoproliferative disorders involving a polyclonal expansion of EBV infected B-lymphocytes may occur in persons with an X-linked recessive immunoproliferative disorder; they can also occur in persons with acquired immune defects, including AIDS patients, transplant recipients and persons with other medical conditions requiring long-term immunosuppressive therapy.

About 10%–15% of infectious mononucleosis cases are heterophile negative. A heterophile-negative form of a syndrome resembling infectious mononucleosis is due to cytomegalovirus and accounts for 5%–7% of the "mono syndrome" (see Cytomegalovirus Infections); other rare causes are toxoplasmosis (q.v.) and herpesvirus type 6 (see Exanthem Subitum following Rubella). A mono-like illness may occur early in HIV infected patients. Differentiation depends on laboratory results that include the EBV IgM test; only EBV elicits the "true" heterophile antibody. EBV accounts for over 80% of both heterophile positive and heterophile negative cases of the "mono" syndrome.

Laboratory diagnosis is based on the finding of a lymphocytosis exceeding 50% (including 10% or more abnormal forms), abnormalities in liver function tests (AST) or an elevated heterophile antibody titer after absorption of the serum with guinea pig kidney. The most sensitive and commercially available test is the absorbed horse-RBC test; the most specific of the common tests is the beef-cell hemolysin test; and the most frequently used procedure is a commercial, qualitative slide agglutination assay. Very young children may not show an elevation of the heterophile titer, and heterophile negative and clinically atypical forms rarely occur in the elderly. If available, the IFA test for IgM and IgA antibody specific for viral capsid antigen (VCA) or antibody against "early antigen" of the causal virus is very helpful in diagnosis of heterophile negative cases; antibody specific for the EBV nuclear antigen (EBNA) is usually absent during the acute phase of illness. Therefore, a positive anti-VCA titer and a negative anti-EBNA titer are characteristic diagnostic responses of an early primary EBV infection.

2. Infectious agent—Epstein-Barr virus, human (gamma) herpesvirus 4, is closely related to other herpesviruses morphologically, but distinct serologically; it infects and transforms B-lymphocytes.

3. Occurrence—Worldwide. Infection is common and widespread in early childhood in developing countries and in socioeconomically depressed population groups, where it is usually mild or asymptomatic. Typical infectious mononucleosis occurs primarily in developed countries, where the age of infection is delayed until older childhood and young adulthood, so that it is most commonly recognized in high school and college students. About 50% of those infected will develop clinical infectious mono; the others are mostly asymptomatic.

4. Reservoir—Humans.

5. Mode of transmission—Person to person spread by the oropharyngeal route, via saliva. Young children may be infected by saliva on the hands of nurses and other attendants and on toys, or by prechewing of baby food by the mother, a practice in some developing countries. Kissing facilitates spread among young adults. Spread may also occur via blood transfusion to susceptible recipients, but ensuing clinical disease is uncommon. Reactivated EBV may play a role in the interstitial pneumonia of HIV infected infants and in hairy leukoplakia and B-cell tumors in HIV infected adults.

6. Incubation period—From 4 to 6 weeks.

7. Period of communicability—Prolonged; pharyngeal excretion may persist in cell free form for a year or more after infection; 15%–20% or more of EBV antibody positive healthy adults are long-term oropharyngeal carriers.

8. Susceptibility and resistance—Susceptibility is general. Infection confers a high degree of resistance; immunity from unrecognized childhood infection may account for low rates of clinical disease in lower socioeconomic groups. Reactivation of EBV may occur in immunodeficient individuals and result in elevated antibody titers to EBV but not heterophile antibody, and possibly to the development of lymphomas.

9. Methods of control—

A. *Preventive measures:* Undetermined. Use hygienic measures including handwashing to avoid salivary contamination from infected individuals; avoid drinking beverages from a common container to minimize contact with saliva.

B. *Control of patient, contacts and the immediate environment:*

1) Report to local health authority: Official report not ordinarily justifiable, Class 5 (see Communicable Disease Reporting).
2) Isolation: None.
3) Concurrent disinfection: Of articles soiled with nose and throat discharges.
4) Quarantine: None.
5) Immunization of contacts: None.
6) Investigation of contacts and source of infection: For the individual case, of little value.
7) Specific treatment: None. Nonsteroidal anti-inflammatory drugs, or steroids given in small doses in decreasing amounts over about a week are of value in severe toxic cases and in patients with severe oropharyngeal involvement and airway encroachment.

C. *Epidemic measures:* None.

D. *Disaster implications:* None.

E. *International measures:* None.

MUMPS
ICD-9 072; ICD-10 B26
(Infectious parotitis)

1. Identification—An acute viral disease characterized by fever, swelling and tenderness of one or more salivary glands, usually the parotid and sometimes the sublingual or submaxillary glands. Orchitis, most commonly unilateral, occurs in 20%–30% of postpubertal males, and mastitis occurs in up to 31% of females older than 15 years; sterility is an extremely rare sequel. As many as 40%–50% of mumps infections have been associated with respiratory symptoms, particularly in children less than 5 years. Not all cases of parotitis are caused by mumps infection; however, other parotitis causing agents do not produce parotitis on an epidemic scale. Mumps can cause sensorineural hearing loss in children, at an incidence of 5 per 100,000 cases. Encephalitis is rare (1–2/10,000 cases); pancreatitis, usually mild, occurs in 4% of cases but a suggested association with diabetes remains unproven.

Permanent sequelae such as paralysis, seizures and hydrocephalus are rare, as are deaths due to mumps. Mumps infection during the first trimester of pregnancy may increase the rate of spontaneous abortion, but there is no firm evidence that mumps during pregnancy causes congenital malformations.

Acute mumps infection can be confirmed by a significant rise in IgG antibody titer in acute and convalescent sera, by the presence of mumps specific IgM or by positive mumps viral cultures. Serologic tests used to confirm acute or recent mumps infection include enzyme-linked immunosorbant assay, hemmagglutination inhibition and complement fixation. Mumps immunity can be documented by the presence of IgG mumps specific antibodies by EIA, IFA or neutralization. Virus may be isolated from the buccal mucosa from 7 days before until 9 days after salivary enlargement and from urine from 6 days before to 15 days after the onset of parotitis.

2. Infectious agent—Mumps virus, a member of the family Paramyxoviridae, genus *Paramyxovirus,* is antigenically related to the parainfluenza viruses.

3. Occurrence—Mumps is recognized less regularly than other common communicable diseases of childhood, such as measles and chickenpox, although serologic studies show that 85% or more of people have had mumps infection by adult life in the absence of immunization. About 1/3 of exposed susceptible people have inapparent infections; most infections in children less than 2 years of age are subclinical. Winter and spring are seasons of greatest incidence.

In the USA, the incidence of mumps has declined dramatically since the wide use of mumps vaccine began after its licensure in 1967. This decline has occurred in all age groups, but with effective pediatric and preschool immunization programs, the greatest risk of infection has shifted toward older children, adolescents and young adults. While mumps outbreaks in the 1980s were attributed to failure to immunize susceptible individuals, more recent outbreaks have occurred among highly immunized populations. During the 1990s, the annual incidence of mumps declined steadily. In 1997, fewer than 700 cases of mumps were reported in the USA.

4. Reservoir—Humans.

5. Mode of transmission—Airborne transmission or by droplet spread and by direct contact with the saliva of an infected person.

6. Incubation period—About 15-18 days (range, 14-25).

7. Period of communicability—Virus has been isolated from saliva from 6-7 days before overt parotitis to 9 days after onset of illness. Maximum infectiousness occurs between 2 days before to 4 days after onset of illness. Inapparent infections can be communicable.

8. Susceptibility and resistance—Immunity is generally lifelong and develops after either inapparent or clinical infections. Most adults, particularly those born before 1957, are likely to have been infected naturally and may be considered to be immune, even if they did not have recognized disease. The demonstration of mumps IgG antibody by serologic assays is acceptable evidence of mumps immunity.

9. Methods of control—

A. Preventive measures:

1) Public education by health care providers should encourage mumps immunization for all susceptible individuals over 1 year of age who were born in 1957 or later.

2) A live attenuated mumps virus vaccine (Jeryl Lynn strain) was introduced in the USA in 1967 and is available either as a single vaccine or in combination with rubella and measles live virus vaccines (MMR). The reported incidence of adverse reactions depends on the strain of mumps virus used. In controlled trials, the incidence of fever in vaccines was similar to that in placebo recipients. Parotitis, usually unilateral, has been reported in 1% of recipients about 2 weeks after immunization with the vaccine used in the USA. Other reactions, including aseptic meningitis, encephalitis and thrombocytopenia, have been reported rarely.

Immunization of people already immune, either by wild or vaccine virus infection, is not associated with increased risk of adverse reactions. More than 95% of recipients develop immunity that is long-lasting and may be lifelong. Vaccine may be administered any time after 1 year of age, preferably as MMR at 12-15 months of age.

Present recommendations in the USA for 2-dose immunization with MMR will protect against mumps. The first dose of MMR is recommended at 12 months of age with a second dose recommended at 4-6 years. However, in an accelerated MMR schedule, or a catch-up opportunity, the second dose may be given as soon as 1 month (28 days) after the first dose. Special effort should be made to immunize before puberty all persons with no definite history of mumps or mumps immunization.

Vaccine is contraindicated in the immunosuppressed; however, treatment with a low dose of steroid (less than 2 mg/kg/day), steroids given on alternate days, topical steroid use or aerosolized steroid preparations are not contraindications to mumps vaccine. Pregnant females or females trying to get pregnant in the next 3 months should not receive mumps vaccine for theoretical reasons, although no evidence exists that mumps vaccine causes fetal damage. See Measles or Rubella for vaccine storage and transport and for greater detail on contraindications.

B. *Control of patient, contacts and the immediate environment:*

1) Report to local health authority: Selectively reportable, Class 3B (see Communicable Disease Reporting).
2) Isolation: Respiratory isolation and private room for 9 days from onset of swelling; less if swelling has subsided. Exclusion from school or workplace until 9 days after onset of parotitis if susceptible contacts (those not immunized) are present.
3) Concurrent disinfection: Of articles soiled with nose and throat secretions.
4) Quarantine: Exclusion of susceptibles from school or the workplace from the 12th through the 25th day after exposure if other susceptibles are present.
5) Immunization of contacts: Although immunization after exposure to natural mumps may not prevent disease in contacts, those who do not develop disease would be protected against infection from subsequent exposures. IG is not effective and not recommended.
6) Investigation of contacts and source of infection: Susceptible contacts should be immunized.
7) Specific treatment: None.

C. *Epidemic measures:* Immunize susceptibles, especially those at risk of exposure; serologic screening to identify susceptibles is impractical and unnecessary, since there is no risk in immunizing those who are already immune.

D. *Disaster implications:* None.

E. *International measures:* None.

MYALGIA, EPIDEMIC   ICD-9 074.1; ICD-10 B33.0
(Epidemic pleurodynia, Bornholm disease, Devil's grippe)

1. Identification—An acute viral disease characterized by paroxysmal spasmodic pain localized in the chest or abdomen, which may be intensified by movement, usually accompanied by fever and frequently by headache. The pain tends to be more abdominal than thoracic in infants and young children, while the reverse applies to older children and adults. Most patients recover within 1 week of onset, but relapses do occur; no fatalities have been reported. Localized epidemics are characteristic. It is important to differentiate from more serious medical or surgical conditions.

Complications occur relatively infrequently and include orchitis, pericarditis, pneumonia and aseptic meningitis. During outbreaks of epidemic myalgia, cases of group B coxsackievirus myocarditis of the newborn have been reported; while myocarditis in adults is a rare complication, the possibility should always be considered.

Diagnosis is suggested by multiple family members with similar symptoms; the diagnosis is confirmed by a significant rise in antibody titer against specific etiologic agents in acute and convalescent sera, or by isolation of the virus in cell culture or neonatal mice from throat secretions or feces of patients.

2. Infectious agents—Group B coxsackievirus types 1-3, 5 and 6, and echoviruses 1 and 6 are associated with the illness. Many group A and B coxsackieviruses and echoviruses have been reported in sporadic cases.

3. Occurrence—An uncommon disease, occurring in summer and early autumn; usually seen in children and young adults, aged 5-15, but all ages may be affected. Multiple cases in a household can occur frequently. Outbreaks have been reported in Europe, Australia, New Zealand and North America.

4. Reservoir—Humans.

5. Mode of transmission—Directly by fecal oral or respiratory droplet contact with an infected person, or indirectly by contact with articles freshly soiled with feces or throat discharges of an infected person who may or may not have symptoms. Group B coxsackieviruses have been found in sewage and flies, though the relationship to transmission of human infection is not clear.

6. Incubation period—Usually 3-5 days.

7. Period of communicability—Apparently during the acute stage of disease; stools may contain virus for several weeks.

8. Susceptibility and resistance—Susceptibility is probably general; type specific immunity presumably results from infection.

9. **Methods of control—**

   A. *Preventive measures:* None.

   B. *Control of patient, contacts and the immediate environment:*

   1) Report to local health authority: Obligatory report of epidemics, Class 4 (see Communicable Disease Reporting).
   2) Isolation: Ordinarily limited to enteric precautions. Because of the possibility of serious illness in the newborn, if a patient in a maternity unit or nursery develops an illness suggestive of enterovirus infection, precautions should be instituted at once. Similarly, individuals (including medical personnel) with suspected enterovirus infections should be excluded from visiting maternity and nursery units and from contact with infants and women near term.
   3) Concurrent disinfection: Prompt and safe disposal of respiratory discharges and feces; wash or dispose of articles soiled therewith. Careful attention should be given to prompt, thorough handwashing when handling discharges, feces and articles soiled therewith.
   4) Quarantine: None.
   5) Immunization of contacts: None.
   6) Investigation of contacts and source of infection: Of no practical value.
   7) Specific treatment: None.

   C. *Epidemic measures:* General notice to physicians of the presence of an epidemic and the necessity for differentiation of cases from more serious medical or surgical emergencies.

   D. *Disaster implications:* None.

   E. *International measures:* None.

MYCETOMA	ICD-9 039; ICD-10 B47
ACTINOMYCETOMA	ICD-9 039; ICD-10 B47.1
EUMYCETOMA	ICD-9 117.4; ICD-10 B47.0

(Maduromycosis, Madura foot)

1. **Identification**—A clinical syndrome caused by a variety of aerobic actinomycetes (bacteria) and eumycetes (fungi), characterized by swelling and suppuration of subcutaneous tissues and formation of sinus tracts with visible granules in the pus draining from the sinus tracts. Lesions are usually

on the foot or lower leg, sometimes on the hand, shoulders and back, and rarely at other sites.

Mycetoma may be difficult to distinguish from chronic osteomyelitis and botryomycosis, the latter being a clinically and pathologically similar entity caused by a variety of bacteria, including staphylococci and gram-negative bacteria.

Specific diagnosis depends on visualizing the granules in fresh preparations or histopathologic slides and isolation of the causative actinomycete or fungus in culture.

2. Infectious agents—Eumycetoma is caused by *Madurella mycetomatis, M. grisea, Pseudallescheria (Petriellidium) boydii, Scedosporium (Monosporium) apiospermum, Exophiala (Phialophora) jeanselmei, Acremonium (Cephalosporium) recifei, A. falciforme, Leptosphaeria senegalensis, Neotestudina rosatii, Pyrenochaeta romeroi* or several other species. Actinomycetoma is caused by *Nocardia brasiliensis, N. asteroides, N. otitidiscaviarum, Actinomadura madurae, A. pelletieri, Nocardiopsis dassonvillei* or *Streptomyces somaliensis.*

3. Occurrence—Rare in continental USA; common in Mexico, northern Africa, southern Asia and other tropical and subtropical areas, especially where people go barefoot (e.g., Sudan).

4. Reservoir—Soil and decaying vegetation.

5. Mode of transmission—Subcutaneous implantation of conidia or hyphal elements from a saprophytic source by penetrating wounds (thorns, splinters).

6. Incubation period—Usually months.

7. Period of communicability—Not transmitted from person to person.

8. Susceptibility and resistance—While etiologic agents are widespread in nature, clinical infection is rare, which suggests intrinsic resistance.

9. Methods of control—

  A. *Preventive measures:* Protect against puncture wounds by wearing shoes and protective clothing.

  B. *Control of patient, contacts and the immediate environment:*

    1) Report to local health authority: Official report not ordinarily justifiable, Class 5 (see Communicable Disease Reporting).
    2) Isolation: None.
    3) Concurrent disinfection: None. Ordinary cleanliness.
    4) Quarantine: None.

5) Immunization of contacts: None.

6) Investigation of contacts and source of infection: Not indicated.

7) Specific treatment: Some patients with eumycetoma may benefit from itraconazole or ketoconazole; some cases of actinomycetoma from clindamycin, TMP-SMX or long acting sulfonamides. Unlike actinomycosis, penicillin is usually not useful. Resection of small lesions may be helpful, while amputation may be required for an extremity with advanced lesions.

C. Epidemic measures: Not applicable, a sporadic disease.

D. Disaster implications: None.

E. International measures: WHO Collaborating Centres.

NAEGLERIASIS AND ACANTHAMEBIASIS
(Primary amebic meningoencephalitis)

ICD-9 136.2;
ICD-10 B60.2, B60.1

1. Identification—In naegleriasis, a free-living ameboflagellate invades the brain and meninges via the nasal mucosa and olfactory nerve; it causes a typical syndrome of fulminating pyogenic meningoencephalitis (primary amebic meningoencephalitis [PAM]) with sore throat, severe frontal headache, occasional olfactory hallucinations, nausea, vomiting, high fever, nuchal rigidity and somnolence, and death within 10 days, usually on the fifth or sixth day. The disease occurs mainly in active immunocompetent young people of both genders.

In contrast, several species of *Acanthamoeba* and *Balamuthia mandrillaris* (leptomyxid amebae) can invade the brain and meninges of immunocompromised individuals, probably secondary to entry through a skin lesion and without involvement of the nasal and olfactory tissues; this causes a granulomatous disease (granulomatous amebic encephalitis [GAE]) characterized by insidious onset and a course lasting from 8 days to several months.

In acanthamebiasis, in addition to causing GAE, species of *Acanthamoeba (A. polyphaga, A. castellanii)* have been associated with chronic granulomatous lesions of the skin, with or without secondary invasion of the CNS. Infections of the eye (Conjunctivitis due to *Acanthamoeba*, ICD-10 H13.1) and of the cornea (Keratoconjunctivitis due to *Acanthamoeba*, ICD-10 H19.2) have resulted in blindness.

Diagnosis of suspected PAM or GAE is made by microscopic examination of wet mount preparations of fresh CSF in which motile amebae may be seen and in stained smears of the CSF. In suspected *Acanthamoeba* infections, diagnosis is made by microscopic examination of scrapings, swabs or aspirates of the eye and skin lesions; or by culture on nonnutrient agar seeded with *Escherichia coli, Klebsiella aerogenes* or other suitable *Enterobacter* species. *Balamuthia* require mammalian cell cultures for isolation. The trophozoites of *Naegleria* may become flagellated after a few hours in water. The pathogenic *N. fowleri, Acanthamoeba* species and *Balamuthia* can be differentiated from each other morphologically and through immunologic testing. Amebae have been misidentified as macrophages and have been mistaken for *Entamoeba histolytica* when microscopic diagnoses are made under low magnification.

2. Infectious agents—*Naegleria fowleri,* several species of *Acanthamoeba (A. culbertsoni, A. polyphaga, A. castellanii, A. astronyxis)* and *Balamuthia mandrillaris.*

3. Occurrence—The organisms are distributed globally in the environment. More than 160 cases of PAM in healthy people, over 100 cases of GAE in immunoincompetent patients (including several with AIDS) and over 1,000 cases of keratitis, primarily in contact lens wearers, have been diagnosed in many countries on all continents.

4. Reservoir—*Acanthamoeba* and *Naegleria* are free living in aquatic and soil habitats. Little is known about the reservoir of *Balamuthia.*

5. Mode of transmission—*Naegleria* infection is acquired by exposure of the nasal passages to contaminated water, most commonly by diving or swimming in fresh water, especially somewhat stagnant ponds or lakes in areas of warm climate or during late summer; or in thermal springs or in bodies of water warmed by the effluent of industrial plants; or in hot tubs, spas or inadequately maintained public swimming pools. The *Naegleria* trophozoites colonize the nasal tissues, then invade the brain and meninges by extension along the olfactory nerves.

Acanthamoeba and *Balamuthia* trophozoites reach the CNS by hematogenous spread, probably from a skin lesion or other site of primary colonization, frequently in chronically ill or immunosuppressed patients with no history of swimming or known source of infection. Eye infections have occurred primarily in soft contact lens wearers; homemade saline used as a cleaning or wetting solution and exposure to spas or hot tubs have been implicated as sources of corneal infection.

6. Incubation period—From 3 to 7 days in documented cases of *Naegleria* infection; usually much longer in infection with *Acanthamoeba* and *Balamuthia.*

7. Period of communicability—No person to person transmission has been observed.

8. Susceptibility and resistance—Unknown. Apparently healthy individuals develop *Naegleria* infection; immunosuppressed individuals have increased susceptibility to infection with *Acanthamoeba* and probably *Balamuthia*. *Naegleria* and *Balamuthia* have not been found in asymptomatic individuals; *Acanthamoeba* has been found in the respiratory tract of healthy people.

9. **Methods of control —**

   A. *Preventive measures:*

   1) Educate the public to the dangers of swimming in lakes and ponds where infection is known or presumed to have been acquired, and of allowing such water to be forced into the nose by diving or underwater swimming.
   2) Protect the nasopharynx from exposure to water likely to contain *N. fowleri*. In practice, this is difficult to accomplish since the amebae may occur in a wide variety of aquatic bodies, including swimming pools.
   3) Swimming pools containing residual free chlorine of 1–2 ppm are considered safe. No infection is known to have been acquired in a standard chlorinated swimming pool in the USA.
   4) Soft contact lens wearers should not wear the lenses while swimming or in hot tubs, and should strictly follow the wear and care procedures recommended by lens manufacturers and health care professionals.

   B. *Control of patient, contacts and the immediate environment:*

   1) Report to local health authority: Not reportable in most countries, Class 3B (see Communicable Disease Reporting).
   2) Isolation: None.
   3) Concurrent disinfection: None.
   4) Quarantine: None.
   5) Immunization of contacts: Not applicable.
   6) Investigation of contacts and source of infection: A history of swimming or introducing water into the nose within the week prior to onset of symptoms may suggest the source of *Naegleria* infection.
   7) Specific treatment: *N. fowleri* is sensitive to amphotericin B (Fungizone®); recovery has followed intravenous and intrathecal administration of amphotericin B and miconazole in conjunction with oral rifampin. Despite sensitivity of the organisms to antibiotics in laboratory studies, recoveries have been rare. For eye infections, no reliable treatment has been reported, but topical propamidine isethionate (Brolene®) has been reported to be effective in several cases; clotrimazole, miconazole and pimaricin have been used in small numbers of patients with some response.

C. Epidemic measures: Multiple cases may occur following exposure to an apparent source of infection. Any grouping of cases warrants prompt epidemiologic investigation and the prohibition of swimming in implicated waters.

D. Disaster implications: None.

E. International measures: None.

NOCARDIOSIS   ICD-9 039.9; ICD-10 A43

1. Identification—A chronic bacterial disease usually originating in the lungs, which may spread via the blood to produce abscesses of the brain, subcutaneous tissue and other organs; the case-fatality rate is high in cases with other than subcutaneous involvement. The frequent isolation of *Nocardia asteroides* from patients with other chronic pulmonary diseases may represent cases of endobronchial colonization. The etiologic agent may also cause cutaneous and/or lymphocutaneous disease of the extremities and actinomycotic mycetomas (see Mycetoma, Actinomycetoma, Eumycetoma).

Microscopic examination of stained smears of sputum, pus or CSF may reveal gram-positive, weakly acid-fast, branched filaments; culture confirmation is desirable but difficult from most sources. Biopsy or autopsy establishes involvement in causing disease.

2. Infectious agents—*Nocardia asteroides* complex (includes *N. asteroides sensu strictu, N. farcinica* and *N. nova*), *N. brasiliensis, N. transvalensis* and *N. otitidiscaviarum;* aerobic actinomycetes.

3. Occurrence—An occasional sporadic disease in people and animals in all parts of the world. No evidence of age, gender or racial differences.

4. Reservoir—Found worldwide as a soil saprophyte.

5. Mode of transmission—*Nocardia* species are presumed to enter the body principally by inhalation of contaminated dust. Inoculation or soil contamination of a wound may result in cutaneous infection.

6. Incubation period—Uncertain; probably a few days to a few weeks.

7. Period of communicability—Not directly transmitted from humans or animals to humans.

8. Susceptibility and resistance—Unknown. Endogenous or iatrogenic adrenal hypercorticism, and probably pulmonary alveolar proteinosis predispose to infection. *Nocardia* species may cause opportunistic infection in patients with compromised immunity.

9. Methods of control—

A. Preventive measures: None.

B. Control of patient, contacts and the immediate environment:

1) Report to local health authority: Official report not ordinarily justifiable, Class 5 (see Communicable Disease Reporting).
2) Isolation: None.
3) Concurrent disinfection: Of discharges and contaminated dressings.
4) Quarantine: None.
5) Immunization of contacts: None.
6) Investigation of contacts and source of infection: Not indicated.
7) Specific treatment: TMP-SMX, sulfisoxazole or sulfadiazine is effective in systemic infections if given early and for prolonged periods. Minocycline may be tried in sulfa-allergic patients who do not have brain abscess. Amikacin, imipenem or high dose ampicillin has been added to sulfonamides in patients failing to respond. Surgical drainage of abscesses may be needed in addition to antibiotic therapy.

C. Epidemic measures: Not applicable, a sporadic disease.

D. Disaster implications: None.

E. International measures: None.

ONCHOCERCIASIS
(River blindness)

ICD-9 125.3; ICD-10 B73

1. Identification—A chronic, nonfatal filarial disease with fibrous nodules in subcutaneous tissues, particularly of the head and shoulders (America) or pelvic girdle and lower extremities (Africa). The adult worms are found in these nodules, which occur superficially and also in deep-seated bundles lying against the periosteum of bones or near joints. The female worm discharges microfilariae that migrate through the skin, often causing an intense pruritic rash when they die, chronic dermatitis-altered pigmentation, edema and atrophy of the skin. Pigment changes, particularly of the lower limbs, gives the condition known as "leopard skin," while loss of skin elasticity and lymphadenitis may result in "hanging groin." Microfilariae frequently reach the eye, where their invasion and subsequent death causes visual disturbance and blindness. Microfilariae may be found in organs and tissues other than skin and eye, but the clinical significance of this is not yet clear; in heavy infections they may also be found in the blood, tears, sputum and urine.

Laboratory diagnosis is made by microscopic examination of fresh superficial skin biopsy incubated in water or saline with observation of microfilariae; by evidence of microfilariae in urine; or by excising nodules and finding adult worms. Differentiation of the microfilariae from those of other filarial diseases is required where these are also endemic. Other diagnostic clues include evidence of ocular manifestations, slit-lamp observations of microfilariae in the cornea, anterior chamber or vitreous body. In low density infections, where microfilariae are not found in the skin and are not present in the eyes, the Mazzotti reaction (which may be dangerous in heavily infected individuals) may be used. Oral administration of 25 mg of diethylcarbamazine citrate, or topical application of the drug, produces characteristic pruritus. This test has been abandoned in many countries. PCR on material obtained from skin scratches can be used to detect parasite DNA.

2. Infectious agent—*Onchocerca volvulus,* a filarial worm belonging to the class Nematoda.

3. Occurrence—Geographic distribution in the Western Hemisphere is limited to Guatemala (principally on the western slope of the Continental Divide); southern Mexico (states of Chiapas and Oaxaca); foci in northern and southern Venezuela; and small areas in Colombia, Ecuador, Brazil (states of Amazonas and Goiás). In sub-Saharan Africa, the disease occurs in an area extending from Senegal to Ethiopia down to Angola in the west and Malawi in the east; also in Yemen. In some endemic areas in west Africa, until recent years, a high percentage of the population was infected, and visual impairment and blindness were serious problems. People abandoned the valleys and migrated to safer higher ground, where the soil was far less fertile. The disease thus had grave socioeconomic consequences. This problem has now been largely overcome through the activities of the Onchocerciasis Control Programme in west Africa.

4. Reservoir—Humans. The disease can be transmitted experimentally to chimpanzees and has been found rarely in nature in gorillas. Other *Onchocerca* species found in animals cannot infect humans but may occur together with *O. volvulus* in the insect vector.

5. Mode of transmission—Only by the bite of infected female black flies of the genus *Simulium:* in Central America, mainly *S. ochraceum;* in South America, *S. metallicum* complex, *S. sanguineum/amazonicum* complex, *S. quadrivittatum* and other species; in Africa, *S. damnosum* complex and *S. neavei* complex, as well as *S. albivirgulatum* in Zaire. Microfilariae, ingested by a black fly feeding on an infected person, penetrate thoracic muscles of the fly, develop into infective larvae, migrate to the cephalic capsule and are liberated on the skin and enter the bite wound during a subsequent blood meal.

6. Incubation period—Microfilariae are found in the skin usually only after 1 year or more from the time of the infective bite; in Guatemala they have been found in children as young as 6 months of age. In Africa, vectors could be infective 7 days after a blood meal; in Guatemala the extrinsic incubation period is measurably longer (up to 14 days) because of lower temperatures.

7. Period of communicability—People can infect flies as long as living microfilariae occur in their skin, i.e., for 10-15 years after last exposure to *Simulium* bites if untreated. The disease is not directly transmitted from person to person.

8. Susceptibility and resistance—Susceptibility is probably universal. Reinfection of infected people may occur; severity of disease depends on cumulative effects of the repeated infections.

9. Methods of control—

A. Preventive measures:

1) Avoid bites of *Simulium* flies by wearing protective clothing and headgear as much as possible or by use of an insect repellent such as diethyltoluamide (Deet®).

2) Identify the vector species and their breeding sites; control the larvae (which usually develop in rapidly running streams and in artificial waterways) by use of biodegradable insecticides such as temefos (Abate®) at low concentrations, spraying 0.05 mg/L for 10 minutes weekly in the wet season and 0.1 mg/L for 10 minutes weekly in the dry season. *B.t.* H-14, a biological insecticide formulated as an aqueous suspension, can be used at a dose 2.5 times higher than temefos. In contrast to temefos, resistance is unlikely to develop against *B.t.* H-14, which has a much shorter carry and therefore needs numerous application points along the river. Aerial spraying may be used to ensure coverage of breeding places in large scale control operations such as in Africa. Because of the mountainous terrain, such procedures generally are not feasible in the Americas. Elimination of *S. neavei* (which develop on crabs) has been effective by use of insecticides.

3) Provide facilities for diagnosis and treatment.

B. Control of patient, contacts and the immediate environment:

1) Report to local health authority: Official report not ordinarily justifiable, Class 5 (see Communicable Disease Reporting).

2) Isolation: None.

3) Concurrent disinfection: None.
4) Quarantine: None.
5) Immunization of contacts: None.
6) Investigation of contacts and source of infection: A community problem.
7) Specific treatment: Ivermectin (Mectizan®) is being provided for treatment of onchocerciasis in humans by Merck and Company. Given in a single oral dose of 150 µg/kg, with annual retreatment, this drug reduces the microfilarial load and morbidity; it kills microfilariae and also blocks release of microfilariae from the uterus of the adult worm and effectively suppresses the number of microfilariae in the skin and eyes over a period of 6–12 months.

Research is under way to develop safe and effective drugs that would sterilize or kill the adult worm; some of these are undergoing clinical trials. Albendazole has been reported to interfere with embryogenesis.

While diethylcarbamazine citrate (DEC, Banocide®, Hetrazan®, Notezine®) is effective against microfilariae, it may cause severe adverse reactions that only partially respond to corticosteroids. It is no longer recommended for treatment of onchocerciasis. Ivermectin should be used in conjunction with suramin for full treatment of selected patients. Suramin (Bayer 205, Naphuride®, Antrypol®), which is available in the USA from CDC, Atlanta, kills the adult worms and leads to gradual disappearance of microfilariae. Nephrotoxicity and other undesirable reactions may occur, so the use of suramin requires close medical supervision. Neither drug is suited for mass treatment because of the possible serious side effects.

In Central America, where nodules commonly occur on the head, their excision is often carried out, as this may reduce symptoms and prevent blindness.

C. *Epidemic measures:* In areas of high prevalence, make concerted effort to reduce incidence, taking measures listed under 9A, above.

D. *Disaster implications:* None.

E. *International measures:* The Onchocerciasis Control Programme (OCP), a coordinated program in west Africa sponsored by the World Bank, UNDP, FAO and WHO, covers the area in 11 countries where primarily the savanna ("blinding") form of the infection is endemic. Control has been based mainly on anti-black fly measures, with insecticides applied systematically to breeding sites in the rivers of the area. Ivermectin is now being distributed to communities on an ever increasing scale as a replacement for larvicides. However, in the northwestern part of the western extension of the OCP area, ivermectin is the sole control measure. The Onchocerciasis Elimination Program for the Americas is a multinational multiagency effort to eliminate, by the year 2000, blindness and skin sequelae from the most endemic foci in the Americas. The program is based on sustained yearly or twice yearly administration of ivermectin, together with improved health education and community participation.

ORF VIRUS DISEASE   ICD-9 051.2; ICD-10 B08.0
(Contagious pustular dermatitis, Human orf, Ecthyma contagiosum)

1. Identification—A proliferative cutaneous viral disease transmissible to humans by contact with infected sheep and goats, and occasionally wild ungulates (deer, reindeer). The lesion in the human, usually solitary and located on hands, arms or face, is a red to violet vesiculonodule, maculopapule or pustule, that progresses to a weeping nodule with central umbilication. There may be several lesions, each measuring up to 3 cm in diameter, which last 3–6 weeks. With secondary bacterial infection, lesions may become pustular. Regional adenitis occurs in a minority of cases. A maculopapular rash may occur on the trunk. Erythema multiforme and erythema multiforme bullosum are rare complications. Disseminated disease and serious ocular damage have been reported. The disease has been confused with cutaneous anthrax and malignancy.

Diagnosis is made by a history of contact with sheep, goats or wild ungulates, and in particular, their young; by EM demonstration of ovoid parapoxvirions in the lesion; by negative conventional bacteriology; by growth of the virus in cell cultures of ovine, bovine or primate origin; or by positive results of serologic tests.

2. Infectious agent—Orf virus, a DNA virus belonging to the genus *Parapoxvirus* of Poxviruses (family Poxviridae). The causative agent is closely related to other parapoxviruses that can be transmitted to humans as occupational diseases—milkers' nodule virus of dairy cattle and bovine papular stomatitis virus of beef cattle. Contagious ecthyma parapoxvirus of domesticated camels may infect people on rare occasion.

3. Occurrence—Probably worldwide among farm workers. It is a common infection among shepherds, veterinarians and abattoir workers in areas producing sheep and goats and is an important occupational disease in New Zealand.

4. Reservoir—Probably in various ungulates (e.g., sheep, goats, reindeer and musk oxen). The virus is very resistant to physical factors, except UV light, and may persist for months in soil and on animal skin and hair.

5. Mode of transmission—By direct contact with the mucous membranes of infected animals, with lesions on udders of nursing dams, or through intermediate passive transfer from apparently normal animals contaminated by contact, knives, shears, stall manger and sides, trucks and clothing. Person to person transmission is rare. Human infection may follow production and administration of vaccines to animals.

6. Incubation period—Generally 3–6 days.

7. Period of communicability—Unknown. Human lesions show a decrease in the number of virus particles as the disease progresses.

8. Susceptibility and resistance—Susceptibility is probably universal; recovery produces variable levels of immunity.

9. Methods of control —

 A. ***Preventive measures:*** Good personal hygiene and washing the exposed area with soap and water. Domestic and wild ungulates should be considered a potential source of infection. Ensure general cleanliness of animal housing areas. The efficacy and safety of *Parapoxvirus* vaccines in animals has not been fully determined.

 B. ***Control of patient, contacts and the immediate environment:***

 1) Report to local health authority: Not required, but desirable when a human case occurs in areas not previously known to have the infection, Class 5 (see Communicable Disease Reporting).
 2) Isolation: None.
 3) Concurrent disinfection: Boil, autoclave or incinerate dressings.
 4) Quarantine: None.
 5) Immunization of contacts: None.
 6) Investigation of contacts and source of infection: Important to secure history of contact.
 7) Specific treatment: None.

 C. ***Epidemic measures:*** None.

 D. ***Disaster implications:*** None.

 E. ***International measures:*** None for humans.

PARACOCCIDIOIDOMYCOSIS
ICD-9 116.1;
ICD-10 B41

(South American blastomycosis, Paracoccidioidal granuloma)

1. Identification—A serious and at times fatal chronic (also known as adult type) mycosis characterized by patchy pulmonary infiltrates and/or ulcerative lesions of the mucosa (oral, nasal, GI) and of the skin. Lymphadenopathy is frequent. In disseminated cases all viscera may be affected; adrenal glands are especially susceptible. The juvenile (acute) form, which is less common, is characterized by reticuloendothelial system involvement and bone marrow dysfunction.

Keloidal blastomycosis (Lobo disease), a disease with only skin involvement, formerly confused with paracoccidioidomycosis, is caused by *Loboa loboi*, a fungus known only in its tissue form and not yet grown in culture.

Diagnosis is confirmed histologically or by culture of the infectious agent. Serologic techniques are useful in diagnosis.

2. Infectious agent—*Paracoccidioides brasiliensis,* a dimorphic fungus.

3. Occurrence—Endemic in the tropical and subtropical regions of South America and, to a lesser extent, of Central America and Mexico. Workers in contact with soil, such as farmers, laborers and construction workers, are especially at risk. Highest incidence is in adults aged 30–50 years; much more common in males than in females.

4. Reservoir—Presumably soil or fungus laden dust.

5. Mode of transmission—Presumably acquired through inhalation of contaminated soil or dust.

6. Incubation period—Highly variable, from 1 month to many years.

7. Period of communicability—Direct transmission of clinical disease from person to person is not known.

8. Susceptibility and resistance—Unknown.

9. Methods of control—

    A. Preventive measures: None.

    B. Control of patient, contacts and the immediate environment:

        1) Report to local health authority: Official report not ordinarily justifiable, Class 5 (see Communicable Disease Reporting).
        2) Isolation: None.
        3) Concurrent disinfection: Of discharges and contaminated articles. Terminal cleaning.
        4) Quarantine: None.
        5) Immunization of contacts: None.

6) Investigation of contacts and source of infection: Not indicated.
7) Specific treatment: Itraconazole appears to be the drug of choice for all but patients ill enough to require hospitalization, who should receive amphotericin B (Fungizone®) IV followed by prolonged therapy with itraconazole. Sulfonamides are cheaper but less effective than azoles.

C. Epidemic measures: Not applicable, a sporadic disease.

D. Disaster implications: None.

E. International measures: None.

PARAGONIMIASIS   ICD-9 121.2; ICD-10 B66.4
(Pulmonary distomiasis, Lung fluke disease)

1. Identification—This is a trematode disease that most frequently involves the lungs. Symptoms include cough, hemoptysis and pleuritic chest pain. X-ray findings may include diffuse and/or segmental infiltrates, nodules, cavities, ring cysts and/or pleural effusions. Extrapulmonary disease is not uncommon, with flukes found in such sites as the CNS, subcutaneous tissues, intestinal wall, peritoneal cavity, liver, lymph nodes and genitourinary tract. Infection usually lasts for years, and the infected person may appear well. In Asian immigrants, the disease may be mistaken for tuberculosis on chest x-rays.

The sputum generally contains orange-brown flecks, sometimes diffusely distributed, in which masses of eggs are seen microscopically and establish the diagnosis. However, acid-fast staining for tuberculosis destroys the eggs and precludes diagnosis. Eggs are also swallowed, especially by children, and may be found in feces by some concentration techniques. A highly sensitive and specific immunoblot serologic test is available at CDC, Atlanta.

2. Infectious agents—*Paragonimus westermani, P. skrjabini* and other species in Asia; *P. africanus* and *P. uterobilateralis* in Africa; *P. mexicanus (P. peruvianus)* and other species in the Americas; and *P. kellicotti* in the USA and Canada.

3. Occurrence—The disease has been reported in the Far East, southwest Asia, India, Africa and the Americas. China is now the major endemic country, where 20 million people are estimated to be infected; Laos, Manipur province of India and Myanmar (Burma) probably follow China. The disease has been nearly eliminated in Japan, while fewer than 1,000 people are infected in Korea. Of the Latin American countries,

Ecuador is the most affected, with about 500,000 estimated to be infected; cases have also occurred in Brazil, Colombia, Peru, Venezuela, Costa Rica and Mexico. The disease is less common in the USA and Canada.

4. Reservoir—Humans, dogs, cats, pigs and wild carnivores are definitive hosts and act as reservoirs.

5. Mode of transmission—Infection occurs when the raw, salted, marinated or partially cooked flesh of freshwater crabs, such as *Eriocheir* and *Potamon,* or of crayfish, such as *Cambaroides,* containing infective larvae (metacercariae), are eaten. The larvae excyst in the duodenum, penetrate the intestinal wall, migrate through the tissues, become encapsulated (usually in the lungs) and develop into egg producing adults. Eggs are expectorated in sputum and, when this is swallowed, are passed in the feces, gain access to freshwater and embryonate in 2-4 weeks. Larvae (miracidia) hatch, penetrate suitable freshwater snails *(Semisulcospira, Thiara, Aroapyrgus* or other genera) and undergo a cycle of development of approximately 2 months. Larvae (cercariae) emerge from the snails and penetrate and encyst in freshwater crabs and crayfish. Pickling of these crustaceans in wine, brine or vinegar, a common practice in Asia, does not kill the encysted larvae. Many infections occur in tourists sampling "native" or exotic foods.

6. Incubation period—Flukes mature and begin to lay eggs approximately 6-10 weeks after a person ingests the infective larvae. The interval until symptoms appear is long, variable, poorly defined, and depends on the organ invaded and the number of worms involved.

7. Period of communicability—Eggs may be discharged by those infected for up to 20 years; duration of infection in mollusk and crustacean hosts is not well defined. Not directly transmitted from person to person.

8. Susceptibility and resistance—Susceptibility is general.

9. Methods of control—

A. Preventive measures:

1) Educate the public in endemic areas about the life cycle of the parasite.
2) Stress thorough cooking of crustaceans.
3) Dispose of sputum and feces in a sanitary manner.
4) Control snails by molluscicides where feasible.

B. Control of patient, contacts and the immediate environment:

1) Report to local health authority: Official report not ordinarily justifiable, Class 5 (see Communicable Disease Reporting).
2) Isolation: None.

3) Concurrent disinfection: Of sputum and feces.
4) Quarantine: None.
5) Immunization of contacts: None.
6) Investigation of contacts and source of infection: None.
7) Specific treatment: Praziquantel (Biltricide®), triclabendazole and bithionol (Bitin®). The latter drug is no longer in production but is available in the USA from CDC for domestic distribution only.

C. Epidemic measures: In an endemic area, occurrence of small clusters of cases, or even sporadic infections, is an important signal for examination of local waters for infected snails, crabs and crayfish, and determination of reservoir mammalian hosts to establish appropriate controls.

D. Disaster implications: None.

E. International measures: WHO Collaborating Centres.

PEDICULOSIS AND PHTHIRIASIS   ICD-9 132; ICD-10 B85

1. Identification—Infestation by head lice *(Pediculus humanus capitis)* occurs on the hair, eyebrows and eyelashes; infestation by body lice *(P. h. corporis)* is of the clothing, especially along the seams of inner surfaces. Crab lice *(Phthirus pubis)* infestation is usually of the pubic area; they may also infest facial hair (including eyelashes in cases of heavy infestation), axillae and body surfaces. Infestations may result in severe itching and excoriation of the scalp or body. Secondary infection may occur with ensuing regional lymphadenitis (especially cervical).

2. Infesting agents—*P. h. capitis,* the head louse; *P. h. corporis,* the body louse; and *Phthirus pubis,* the crab louse; adult lice, nymphs and nits (egg cases) infest people. Lice are host specific and those of lower animals do not infest people, although they may be present transiently. Both sexes feed on blood.

The body louse is the species involved in outbreaks of epidemic typhus caused by *Rickettsia prowazeki*, trench fever caused by *R. quintana* and epidemic relapsing fever caused by *Borrelia recurrentis*.

3. Occurrence—Worldwide. Outbreaks of head lice are common among children in schools and institutions everywhere. Body lice are still prevalent among populations with poor personal hygiene, especially in cold climates where heavy clothing is worn and bathing is infrequent or when people cannot change their clothes (refugees).

4. **Reservoir**—Humans.

5. **Mode of transmission**—For head and body lice, direct contact with an infested person and objects used by them; for body lice, indirect contact with the personal belongings of infested persons, especially shared clothing and headgear. Head and body lice can survive for only a week without a food source. Crab lice are most frequently transmitted through sexual contact. Lice leave a febrile host; fever and overcrowding increase transfer from person to person.

6. **Incubation period**—The life cycle is composed of three stages: eggs, nymphs and adults. The most suitable temperature for the life cycle is 32°C (89.6°F). Eggs of head lice do not hatch at temperatures less than 22°C (71.6°F). Under optimal conditions, the eggs of lice hatch in 7-10 days. The nymphal stages last about 7-13 days depending on temperatures. The egg to egg cycle averages about 3 weeks. The average life cycle of the body or head louse extends over a period of 18 days and that of the crab louse, 15 days.

7. **Period of communicability**—As long as lice or eggs remain alive on the infested person or on fomites. The adult's life span is approximately 1 month. Lice eggs ("nits") remain viable on clothing for 1 month. Body and head lice survive for a week without food (implies off the host), crab lice only 2 days. Nymphs survive 24 hours without food.

8. **Susceptibility and resistance**—Any person may become louse infested under suitable conditions of exposure. Repeated infestations may result in dermal hypersensitivity.

9. **Methods of control**—

   A. *Preventive measures:*

      1) Educate the public on the value of destroying eggs and lice by early detection, safe and thorough treatment of the hair, laundering clothing and bedding in hot water (55°C or 131°F for 20 min), dry cleaning or setting dryers at hot cycle.
      2) Avoid physical contact with infested individuals and their belongings, especially clothing and bedding.
      3) Perform regular, direct inspection of children in a group setting for head lice and, when indicated, of body and clothing for body lice.
      4) In high risk situations, use appropriate repellents on hair, skin and clothing.

   B. *Control of patient, contacts and the immediate environment:*

      1) Report to local health authority: Official report not ordinarily justifiable; school authorities should be informed, Class 5 (see Communicable Disease Reporting).

2) Isolation: For body lice, contact isolation if possible until 24 hours after application of an effective insecticide.

3) Concurrent disinfection: Clothing, bedding and fomites should be treated by laundering in hot water, dry cleaning or applying an effective chemical insecticide (see 9B7, below).

4) Quarantine: None.

5) Immunization of contacts: Does not apply.

6) Investigation of contacts and source of infestation: Examination of household and close personal contacts, and treatment of those infested.

7) Specific treatment: For head and pubic lice: 1% permethrin (a synthetic pyrethroid) cream rinse (NIX®), pyrethrins synergized with piperonyl butoxide (A-200 Pyrinate®, RID® and XXX®, Pronto, R & C commercial products containing pyrethrins with piperonyl butoxide), carbaryl, benzyl benzoate; and 1% gamma benzene hexachloride lotions (Lindane, Kwell®; not recommended for infants, young children and pregnant or lactating women). None of these is 100% effective, so retreatment may be necessary after an interval of 7–10 days if eggs survive.

For body lice: Clothing and bedding should be washed using the hot water cycle of an automatic washing machine or dusted with pediculicides using power dusters, hand dusters or 2-ounce sifter cans. Dusts recommended by WHO include 1% malathion, 0.5% permethrin, 2% Abate® (temefos), 5% iodofenphos, 1% propoxur, 5% carbaryl, 10% DDT or 1% gamma benzene hexachloride or lindane (resistance is widespread to DDT and lindane).

C. *Epidemic measures:* Mass treatment as recommended in 9B7, above, using insecticides known from careful monitoring to be effective against prevalent strains of lice. In typhus epidemics, individuals may protect themselves by wearing silk or plastic clothing tightly fastened around wrists, ankles and neck, and by impregnating their clothes with repellents.

D. *Disaster implications:* Diseases for which body and head lice are vectors are particularly prone to occur at times of social upheaval (see Typhus fever, section I, Epidemic louseborne).

E. *International measures:* None.

APHA

PERTUSSIS   ICD-9 033.0; ICD-10 A37.0
PARAPERTUSSIS   ICD-9 033.1; ICD-10 A37.1
(Whooping Cough)

1. **Identification**—An acute bacterial disease involving the respiratory tract. The initial catarrhal stage has an insidious onset with an irritating cough that gradually becomes paroxysmal, usually within 1-2 weeks, and lasts for 1-2 months or longer. Paroxysms are characterized by repeated violent coughs; each series of paroxysms has many coughs without intervening inhalation and can be followed by a characteristic crowing or high-pitched inspiratory whoop. Paroxysms frequently end with the expulsion of clear, tenacious mucus, often followed by vomiting. Infants less than 6 months old, adolescents and adults often do not have the typical whoop or cough paroxysm.

The number of fatalities in the USA is low; approximately 80% of deaths are among children under 1 year of age, and 70% are under 6 months. The case-fatality rate is less than 1% in infants under 6 months of age in the USA. Morbidity is slightly higher in adult females than males. In nonimmunized populations, especially those with underlying malnutrition and multiple enteric and respiratory infections, pertussis is among the most lethal diseases of infants and young children. Pneumonia is the most common cause of death; fatal encephalopathy, probably hypoxic, and inanition from repeated vomiting occasionally occur.

In recent years in the USA, pertussis has been recognized with increasing frequency in adolescents and young adults, whose symptoms varied in severity from a mild, atypical respiratory illness to the full-blown syndrome. Many of these cases occur in previously immunized persons and indicate waning immunity following immunization.

Parapertussis is a similar but usually milder disease. It usually occurs in school age children and is relatively infrequent. Differentiation between *Bordetella parapertussis* and *B. pertussis* is based on culture, biochemical and immunologic differences. A similar acute clinical syndrome has been reported in association with viruses, especially adenoviruses; however, the duration of cough is usually less than 28 days.

Diagnosis is based on the recovery of the etiologic organism from nasopharyngeal specimens obtained during the catarrhal and early paroxysmal stages on appropriate culture media. DFA staining of nasopharyngeal secretions can provide rapid presumptive diagnosis but requires an experienced laboratory technician; false positive and false negative results can occur. PCR and serologic tests for diagnosis of pertussis have not been standardized. These methods are best used as presumptive assays in conjunction with culture.

2. **Infectious agents**—*B. pertussis,* the pertussis bacillus; *B. parapertussis* causes parapertussis.

3. **Occurrence**—An endemic disease common to children (especially young children) everywhere, regardless of ethnicity, climate or geographic

location. Outbreaks occur periodically. A marked decline has occurred in incidence and mortality rates during the past four decades, chiefly in communities with active immunization programs and where good nutrition and medical care are available. From 1980 to 1989, an average of 2,800 cases was reported annually in the USA, but the number of cases increased in 1995-98, to an average of 6,500. With higher immunization levels in Latin America, reported cases declined from 120,000 in 1980 to 40,000 in 1990. Incidence rates have increased in countries where antipertussis immunization rates have fallen (e.g., England, Japan in the early 1980s and Sweden).

4. Reservoir—Humans are believed to be the only host.

5. Mode of transmission—Primarily by direct contact with discharges from respiratory mucous membranes of infected persons by the airborne route, probably by droplets. Frequently brought home by an older sibling and sometimes by a parent.

6. Incubation period—Commonly 7-20 days.

7. Period of communicability—Highly communicable in the early catarrhal stage before the paroxysmal cough stage. Thereafter, communicability gradually decreases and becomes negligible in about 3 weeks for nonhousehold contacts, despite persisting spasmodic cough with whoop. For control purposes, the communicable stage extends from the early catarrhal stage to 3 weeks after onset of typical paroxysms in patients not treated with antibiotics. When treated with erythromycin, the period of infectiousness usually is 5 days or less after onset of therapy.

8. Susceptibility and resistance—Susceptibility of nonimmunized individuals is universal. Transplacental immunity in infants has not been demonstrated. It is predominantly a childhood disease; incidence rates of reported (i.e., recognized) disease are highest in children under 5 years of age. Milder and missed atypical cases occur in all age groups. One attack usually confers prolonged immunity, although second attacks (some of which may be due to *B. parapertussis*) can occasionally occur. Cases in previously immunized adolescents and adults in the USA occur because of waning immunity and are an increasing source of infection for nonimmunized young children.

9. Methods of control—

A. Preventive measures:

1) Educate the public, particularly parents of infants, about the dangers of whooping cough and on the advantages of initiating immunization at 2 months of age and adhering to the immunization schedule. This continues to be important because of the wide publicity given the relatively rare adverse reactions.

2) Active primary immunization against *B. pertussis* infection is recommended with 3 doses of a vaccine consisting of a suspension of killed bacteria, usually in combination with diphtheria and tetanus toxoids adsorbed on aluminum salts (Diphtheria and Tetanus Toxoids and Pertussis Vaccine Adsorbed USP, DTP). Acellular preparations (DTaP) that contain two or more protective antigens of *B. pertussis* are used in the USA for the primary (3 doses) series and booster doses. Nonadsorbed ("plain") preparations (not available except in Michigan) have no advantage, either for primary or booster immunization. In the USA, DTaP is recommended to be given at 2, 4 and 6 months of age; booster doses are recommended at 15–18 months of age and at school entry. Vaccines containing pertussis are not recommended after the 7th birthday. Some countries recommend different ages of administration and/or number of doses (e.g., most developing countries give DTP vaccine at 6, 10 and 14 weeks of age).

DTaP/DTP can be given simultaneously with oral poliovirus vaccine (OPV), inactivated poliovirus vaccine (IPV), *Haemophilus influenzae* type b (Hib), hepatitis B vaccine and measles, mumps and rubella vaccines (MMR) at different sites. Combination vaccines containing DTaP/DTP and Hib are available in the USA.

In the USA, a family history of convulsive seizures is not considered a contraindication to pertussis vaccine; antipyretics may prevent febrile seizure. Immunization with DTaP or DTP should be delayed if the child has an intercurrent febrile infection; however, a mild illness, with or without fever, is not a contraindication. In young infants with suspected evolving and progressive neurologic disease, immunization may be delayed for some months to permit the diagnosis to be established and to avoid possible confusion about the cause of symptoms. In some cases of progressive neurologic illness the child should receive DT rather than DTaP/DTP vaccine. Stable neurologic disorders, such as well-controlled seizures, are not a contraindication.

In general, pertussis vaccine is not given to persons 7 years of age or older, since reactions to the vaccine may be increased in older children and adults. Those who experience severe reactions such as convulsions, persistent or unusually severe screaming, collapse or temperature greater than 40.5°C (greater than 105°F) may not be given further doses of a vaccine containing pertussis if the risks outweigh the benefits. In circumstances in which further pertussis immunization is indicated (e.g., during an outbreak of pertussis), DTaP should be used. An anaphylactic reaction or acute encephalopathy within 48–72 hours of immunization is an absolute contraindication to further doses of vaccines containing pertussis. Less serious systemic and local reactions are not common after DTaP and are not contraindications to further doses of pertussis vaccine.

The efficacy of the vaccine in children who have received at least 3 doses is estimated to be 80%; protection is greater against severe disease and begins to wane after about 3 years. Active immunization started after exposure will not protect against disease resulting from that exposure, but it is not contraindicated. The best protection is obtained by adhering to the recommended schedule. Passive immunization is ineffective, and pertussis IG is no longer commercially available. Pertussis vaccine does not protect against infection by *B. parapertussis*.

3) When an outbreak occurs, consider protection of health workers who have been exposed to pertussis cases by using a 14-day course of erythromycin. Although DTaP vaccines, as of late 1999, are not recommended for persons aged 7 or older, new acellular preparations (e.g., dTaP) may be licensed for this purpose.

B. Control of patient, contacts and the immediate environment:

1) Report to local health authority: Case report obligatory in all states (USA) and most countries, Class 2B (see Communicable Disease Reporting). Early reporting permits better outbreak control.

2) Isolation: Respiratory isolation for known cases. Suspected cases should be removed from the presence of young children and infants, especially nonimmunized infants, until the patients have received at least 5 days of a minimum 14-day course of antibiotics. Suspected cases who do not receive antibiotics should be isolated for 3 weeks.

3) Concurrent disinfection: Discharges from nose and throat and articles soiled by them. Terminal cleaning.

4) Quarantine: Inadequately immunized household contacts less than 7 years of age should be excluded from schools, day care centers and public gatherings for 21 days after last exposure or until the cases and contacts have received 5 days of a minimum 14-day course of appropriate antibiotics.

5) Protection of contacts: Passive immunization is not effective, and the initiation of active immunization to protect against infection following recent exposure is also not effective. Close contacts under 7 years of age who have not received 4 DTaP/DTP doses or have not received a DTaP/DTP dose within 3 years should be given a dose as soon after exposure as possible. A 14-day course of erythromycin for household and

other close contacts, regardless of immunization status and age, is recommended.

6) Investigation of contacts and source of infection: A search for early, missed and atypical cases is indicated where a nonimmune infant or young child is or might be at risk.

7) Specific treatment: Erythromycin shortens the period of communicability, but does not reduce symptoms except when given during the incubation period, in the catarrhal stage or early in the paroxysmal stage of the disease.

C. Epidemic measures: A search for unrecognized and unreported cases is indicated to protect preschool children from exposure and to ensure adequate preventive measures for exposed children less than 7 years of age. Accelerated immunization with the first dose at 4-6 weeks of age, and the second and third doses at 4-week intervals, may be indicated; immunizations should be completed for those whose schedule is incomplete.

D. Disaster implications: Pertussis is a potential problem if introduced into crowded refugee camps with many unimmunized children.

E. International measures: Ensure completion of primary immunization of infants and young children before they travel to other countries; review need for a booster dose. WHO Collaborating Centres.

PINTA
(Carate)

ICD-9 103; ICD-10 A67

1. Identification—An acute and chronic nonvenereal treponemal skin infection. A scaling painless papule with satellite lymphadenopathy appears 1-8 weeks after infection, usually on the hands, legs or dorsum of the feet. In 3-12 months a maculopapular, erythematous secondary rash appears and may evolve into tertiary splotches of altered (dyschromic) skin pigmentation of variable size. These treponema containing macules pass through stages of blue to violet to brown pigmentation, finally becoming treponema free depigmented (achromic) scars. Lesions are in different stages of evolution and are most common on the face and extremities. Organ systems are not involved; physical disability and death do not occur.

Spirochetes are demonstrable in dyschromic (but not achromic) lesions by darkfield or direct FA microscopic examination. Serologic tests for syphilis usually become reactive before or during the secondary rash and thereafter behave as in venereal syphilis.

2. Infectious agent—*Treponema carateum,* a spirochete.

3. Occurrence—Found only among isolated rural populations living under crowded unhygienic conditions in the American tropics. Predominantly a disease of older children and adults. Surveys carried out during the mid-1990s by PAHO/WHO in targeted Amazonian populations, in Brazil, Venezuela and Peru found few, mostly old (inactive) cases. WHO has concluded that pinta is a residual problem and that the infection is on its way to elimination and eradication.

4. Reservoir—Humans.

5. Mode of transmission—Presumably person to person transmission by direct and prolonged contact with initial and early dyschromic skin lesions. The location of primary lesions suggests that trauma provides a portal of entry; lesions in children occur in body areas most scratched. Various biting and sucking arthropods, especially black flies, have been suspected but are not proven as biological vectors.

6. Incubation period—Usually 2-3 weeks.

7. Period of communicability—Unknown; potentially communicable while dyschromic skin lesions are active, sometimes for many years. Not highly contagious; several years of intimate contact may be necessary for transmission.

8. Susceptibility and resistance—Undefined; presumably as in other treponematoses.

9. Methods of control—

    A. Preventive meaures: Those applicable to other nonvenereal treponematoses apply to pinta; see Yaws, 9A.

    B. Control of patient, contacts and the immediate environment:

        1) Report to local health authority: In selected endemic areas; in most countries, not a reportable disease, Class 3B (see Communicable Disease Reporting).

        2), 3), 4), 5), 6) and 7) Isolation, Concurrent disinfection, Quarantine, Immunization of contacts, Investigation of contacts and source of infection and Specific treatment: Same as for Yaws, q.v., 9B2 through 9B7.

    C, D. and *E. Epidemic measures, Disaster implications* and *International measures:* See Yaws, C, D and E.

PLAGUE
(Pestis)

ICD-9 020; ICD-10 A20

1. Identification—A specific zoonosis involving rodents and their fleas, which transfer the bacterial infection to various animals and to people. Initial signs and symptoms may be nonspecific with fever, chills, malaise, myalgia, nausea, prostration, sore throat and headache. Commonly a lymphadenitis develops in those lymph nodes that drain the site of the flea bite, where there may be an initial lesion. This is bubonic plague, and it occurs more often in lymph nodes in the inguinal area (90%) and less commonly in those in the axillary and cervical areas. The involved nodes become swollen, inflamed and tender and may suppurate. Fever is usually present. All forms, including instances in which lymphadenopathy is not apparent, may progress to septicemic plague with bloodstream dissemination to diverse parts of the body, that include the meninges. Endotoxic shock and disseminated intravascular coagulation (DIC) may occur without localizing signs of infection. Secondary involvement of the lungs results in pneumonia; mediastinitis or pleural effusion may develop. Secondary pneumonic plague is of special significance, since respiratory droplets may serve as the source of person to person transfer with resultant primary pneumonic or pharyngeal plague; this can lead to localized outbreaks or devastating epidemics. Though naturally acquired plague usually presents as bubonic plague, purposeful aerosol dissemination as a result of biowarfare or a terrorist event would be manifest primarily as pneumonic plague.

Untreated bubonic plague has a case-fatality rate of about 50%-60%. Plague organisms have been recovered from throat cultures of asymptomatic contacts of pneumonic plague patients. Untreated primary septicemic plague and pneumonic plague are invariably fatal. Modern therapy markedly reduces fatality from bubonic plague; pneumonic and septicemic plague also respond if recognized and treated early. However, patients who do not receive adequate therapy for primary pneumonic plague within 18 hours after onset of respiratory symptoms are not likely to survive.

Visualization of characteristic bipolar staining, "safety pin" ovoid, gram-negative organisms in direct microscopic examination of material aspirated from a bubo, sputum or CSF is suggestive, but not conclusive, evidence of plague infection. Examination by FA test or antigen capture ELISA is more specific and is particularly useful in sporadic cases. Diagnosis is confirmed by culture and identification of the causal organism from exudate aspirated from buboes, from blood, CSF or sputum, or by a fourfold or greater rise or fall in antibody titer. Slow growth of the organism at normal incubation temperatures may lead to misidentification by automated systems. The passive hemagglutination test (PHA) using *Yersinia pestis* Fraction-1 antigen is most frequently used for serodiagnosis. Medical personnel should be aware of areas where the disease is endemic and entertain the diagnosis of plague early; unfortunately, plague is often misdiagnosed, especially in travelers who develop illness after returning from an endemic area.

2. Infectious agent—*Yersinia pestis,* the plague bacillus.

3. Occurrence—Plague continues to be a threat because of vast areas of persistent wild rodent infection; contact of wild rodents with domestic rats occurs frequently in some enzootic areas. Wild rodent plague exists in the western half of the USA; large areas of South America; north central, eastern and southern Africa; central and southeast Asia, and extreme southeastern Europe near the Caspian Sea. There are several natural plague foci within the Russian Federation and Kazakhstan. While urban plague has been controlled in most of the world, human plague has occurred in the 1990s in several African countries that include Botswana, Kenya, Madagascar, Malawi, Mozambique, Tanzania, Uganda, Zambia, Zimbabwe, and Democratic Republic of the Congo. Plague is endemic in China, Laos, Mongolia, Myanmar (Burma), India and especially in Vietnam where thousands of cases of bubonic plague, both urban and rural, with scattered outbreaks of pneumonic plague, were reported between 1962 and 1972. In the Americas, foci in northeastern Brazil and the Andean region (Peru, Ecuador and Bolivia) continue to produce sporadic cases and occasional outbreaks including an outbreak of pneumonic plague in Ecuador in 1998.

Human plague in the western USA is sporadic, with only single cases or small common source clusters in an area, usually following exposure to wild rodents or their fleas. Over the 10 year period 1987–1996, there was an annual average of 10 plague cases (range 2 to 15). No human to human transmission has occurred in the USA since 1925, although secondary plague pneumonia has occurred in about 20% of bubonic cases in recent years. Seventeen cases of primary plague pneumonia were acquired from pet cats with plague pneumonia in the interval 1977–1994.

4. Reservoir—Wild rodents (especially ground squirrels) are the natural vertebrate reservoir of plague. Lagomorphs (rabbits and hares), wild carnivores and domestic cats may also be a source of infection to people. Though the organism may remain viable for several weeks in water and moist meals and grains, it is killed with several hours of exposure to sunlight.

5. Mode of transmission—Naturally acquired plague in people occurs as a result of human intrusion into the zoonotic (also termed sylvatic or rural) cycle during or following an epizootic, or by the entry of sylvatic rodents or their infected fleas into man's habitat with infection in commensal rodents and their fleas; this may result in the development of a domestic rat epizootic and epidemic plague. Domestic pets, particularly house cats and dogs, may carry plague infected wild rodent fleas into homes, and cats may occasionally transmit infection by their bites or scratches; cats develop plague abscesses that have been a source of infection to veterinarians.

The most frequent source of exposure that results in human disease worldwide has been the bite of infected fleas (especially *Xenopsylla cheopis,* the oriental rat flea). Other important sources include the handling of tissues of infected animals, especially rodents and rabbits, but also carnivores; rarely airborne droplets from human patients or household cats with plague pharyngitis or pneumonia; or careless manipulation of laboratory cultures. In a bioterrorist setting plague bacilli would probably be transmitted as an aerosol. Person to person transmission by *Pulex irritans* fleas, the "human" flea, is presumed to be important in the Andean region of South America and in other places where plague occurs and this flea is abundant on domestic animals. Certain occupations and lifestyles (including hunting, trapping, cat ownership and rural residence) carry an increased risk of exposure.

6. Incubation period—From 1 to 7 days; may be a few days longer in immunized individuals. For primary plague pneumonia, 1–4 days, usually short.

7. Period of communicability—Fleas may remain infective for months under suitable conditions of temperature and humidity. Bubonic plague is not usually transmitted directly from person to person unless there is contact with pus from suppurating buboes. Pneumonic plague may be highly communicable under appropriate climatic conditions; overcrowding facilitates transmission.

8. Susceptibility and resistance—Susceptibility is general. Immunity after recovery is relative; it may not protect against a large inoculum.

9. Methods of control —

A. *Preventive measures:* The basic objective is to reduce the likelihood of people being bitten by infected fleas, having direct contact with infective tissues and exudates, or of being exposed to patients with pneumonic plague.

1) Educate the public in enzootic areas on the modes of human and domestic animal exposure; the importance of rat proofing buildings, preventing access to food and shelter by peridomestic rodents through appropriate storage and disposal of food, garbage and refuse; and the importance of avoiding flea bites by use of insecticides and repellents. In sylvatic or rural plague areas, the public should be advised to use insect repellents and warned not to camp near rodent burrows and to avoid handling of rodents, but to report dead or sick animals to health authorities or park rangers. Dogs and cats in such areas should be treated periodically with appropriate insecticides.

2) Survey rodent populations periodically to determine the effectiveness of sanitary programs and to evaluate the potential for epizootic plague. Rat suppression by poisoning (see 9B6, below) may be necessary to augment basic environmental sanitation measures; rat control should always be preceded by measures to control fleas. Maintain surveillance of natural foci by bacteriologic testing of sick or dead wild rodents and by serologic studies of wild carnivore and outdoor ranging dog and cat populations in order to define areas of plague activity. Collection and testing of fleas from wild rodents and their nests or burrows may also be appropriate.

3) Control rats on ships and docks and in warehouses by rat proofing or periodic fumigation, combined when necessary with destruction of rats and their fleas in vessels and in cargoes, especially containerized cargoes, before shipment and on arrival from plague endemic locations.

4) Wear gloves when hunting and handling wildlife.

5) Active immunization with a vaccine of killed bacteria confers some protection against bubonic plague (but not primary pneumonic plague) in most recipients for at least several months when administered in a primary series of 3 doses with doses 1 and 2 1-3 months apart followed by dose 3 5-6 months later; booster injections are necessary every 6 months if high risk exposure continues. After the third booster dose, the intervals can be extended to every 1 to 2 years. Immunization of visitors to epidemic localities and of laboratory and field workers handling plague bacilli or infected animals is justifiable but should not be relied upon as the sole preventive measure. Routine immunization is not indicated though for most persons living in enzootic areas such as the western USA. Live attenuated vaccines are used in some countries, but may produce more adverse reactions and there is no evidence that they are more protective.

B. *Control of patient, contacts and the immediate environment:*

1) Report to local health authority: Case report of suspected and confirmed cases universally required by *International Health Regulations*, Class 1 (see Communicable Disease Reporting). Because of the rarity of naturally acquired primary plague pneumonia, even a single case should inititate prompt consideration by both public health and law enforcement authorities of a bioterrorist/biowarfare exposure.

2) Isolation: Rid patients, and especially their clothing and baggage, of fleas using an insecticide effective against local fleas and known to be safe for people; hospitalize if practical. For patients with bubonic plague (if there is no cough and the chest x-ray is negative) drainage and secretion precautions are

indicated for 48 hours after start of effective therapy. For patients with pneumonic plague, strict isolation with precautions against airborne spread is required until 48 hours of appropriate antibiotic therapy have been completed and there has been a favorable clinical response (see 9B7, below).

3) Concurrent disinfection: Of sputum and purulent discharges and articles soiled therewith. Terminal cleaning. Bodies of people and carcasses of animals that died of plague should be handled with strict aseptic precautions.

4) Quarantine: Those who have been in household or face to face contact with patients with pneumonic plague should be provided chemoprophylaxis (see 9B5, below) and placed under surveillance for 7 days; those who refuse chemoprophylaxis should be maintained in strict isolation with careful surveillance for 7 days.

5) Protection of contacts: In epidemic situations where human fleas are known to be involved, contacts of bubonic plague patients should be disinfested with an appropriate insecticide. All close contacts should be evaluated for chemoprophylaxis. Close contacts of confirmed or suspected plague pneumonia cases (including medical personnel) should be provided with chemoprophylaxis using tetracycline (15–30 mg/kg) or chloramphenicol (30 mg/kg) daily in 4 divided doses for 1 week after exposure ceases.

6) Investigation of contacts and source of infection: Search for people with household or face to face exposure to pneumonic plague, and for sick or dead rodents and their fleas. Flea control must precede or coincide with antirodent measures. Dust rodent runs, harborages and burrows in and around known or suspected plague areas with an insecticide labeled for flea control and known to be effective against local fleas. If nonburrowing wild rodents are involved, insecticide bait stations can be used. If urban rats are involved, disinfest by dusting the houses, outhouses and household furnishings; dust the bodies and clothing of all residents in the immediate vicinity. Suppress rat populations by well-planned and energetic campaigns of poisoning and with vigorous concurrent measures to reduce rat harborages and food sources.

7) Specific treatment: Streptomycin is the drug of choice, gentamicin can be used when streptomycin is not readily available; tetracyclines and chloramphenicol are alternative choices. Chloramphenicol is required for treatment of plague meningitis. All are highly effective if used early (within 8–18 hours after onset of pneumonic plague). After a satisfactory response to drug therapy, reappearance of fever may result from a secondary infection or a suppurative bubo that may require incision and drainage.

C. Epidemic measures:

1) Investigate all suspected plague deaths with autopsy and laboratory examinations when indicated. Develop and carry out case finding. Establish the best possible facilities for diagnosis and treatment. Alert existing medical facilities to report cases immediately and to use full diagnostic and therapeutic services.

2) Attempt to mitigate public hysteria by appropriate informational and educational releases through the press and news media.

3) Institute intensive flea control in expanding circles from known foci.

4) Implement rodent destruction within affected areas **only after satisfactory flea control has been accomplished.**

5) Protect all contacts as noted in 9B5, above.

6) Protect field workers against fleas; dust clothing with insecticide powder and use insect repellents daily.

D. Disaster implications:
Plague could become a significant problem in endemic areas when there are social upheavals, crowding and unhygienic conditions. See preceding and following paragraphs for appropriate actions.

E. International measures:

1) Telegraphic notification within 24 hours by governments to WHO and to adjacent countries of the first imported, first transferred or first nonimported case of plague in any area previously free of the disease. Report newly discovered or reactivated foci of plague among rodents.

2) Measures applicable to ships, aircraft and land transport arriving from plague areas are specified in *International Health Regulations.* These regulations are being revised, but the new regulations will not be in effect until the year 2002 or after.

3) All ships should be free of rodents or periodically deratted.

4) Rat proof buildings at seaports and airports; apply appropriate insecticide; eliminate rats with effective rodenticide.

5) For international travelers, international regulations require that prior to their departure on an international voyage from an area where there is an epidemic of pulmonary plague, those suspected of significant exposure shall be placed in isolation for 6 days after last exposure. On arrival of an infested or suspected infested ship, or an infested aircraft, travelers may be disinsected and kept under surveillance for a period of not more than 6 days from the date of arrival. Immunization

against plague cannot be required as a condition of admission to a territory.

6) WHO Collaborating Centres.

F. Bioterrorism measures:

Y. pestis is distributed worldwide; techniques for mass production and aerosol dissemination are available; and the fatality rate of primary pneumonic plague is high and there is a real potential for secondary spread. For these reasons, a biological attack with plague is considered to be of serious public health concern. A few sporadic cases will likely be missed or at least not attributed to a deliberate bioterrorist act. Any suspect case of plague should be reported immediately by telephone to the local health department. The sudden appearance of many patients presenting with fever, cough, a fulminant course and high case-fatality rate should provide a suspect alert for anthrax or plague; if cough is primarily accompanied by hemoptysis, this presentation favors the tentative diagnosis of pneumonic plague. For a suspected or confirmed outbreak of pneumonic plague, follow the treatment and containment measures outlined in 9B above.

PNEUMONIA
I. PNEUMOCOCCAL
PNEUMONIA   ICD-9 481; ICD-10 J13

1. Identification—An acute bacterial infection characterized typically by sudden onset with a shaking chill, fever, pleural pain, dyspnea, tachypnea, a cough productive of "rusty" sputum and leukocytosis. The onset may be less abrupt, especially in the elderly, and chest x-ray may provide the first evidence of pneumonia. In infants and young children, fever, vomiting and convulsions may be the initial manifestations. Consolidation may be bronchopneumonic, especially in children and the aged, rather than segmental or lobar. Pneumococcal pneumonia is an important cause of death in infants and the aged. The case-fatality rate, formerly 20%–40% among hospitalized patients, has fallen to 5%–10% with antimicrobial therapy, but remains 20%–40% among patients with substantial underlying disease or alcoholism. In developing countries the case-fatality rates in children are often over 10% and as high as 60% in infants under 6 months of age.

Early etiologic diagnosis is important for guiding specific therapy. The diagnosis can be suspected from the presence in gram stains of sputum of many gram-positive diplococci together with polymorphonuclear leukocytes; it can be confirmed by isolation of pneumococci from blood or from secretions from the lower respiratory tract of adults obtained by percutaneous transtracheal aspiration.

2. Infectious agent—*Streptococcus pneumoniae* (pneumococcus). Out of 83 known capsulas types, 23 account for approximately 90% of bacteremic infections in the USA.

3. Occurrence—A disease of continuing endemicity, particularly in infancy and old age and in individuals with underlying medical conditions; more frequent in lower socioeconomic groups and in developing countries. It occurs in all climates and seasons, but incidence is highest in winter and spring in temperate zones. Usually sporadic in the USA, it may occur in epidemics in closed populations and during rapid urbanization. Recurring epidemics have been described among South African miners; incidence is high in certain geographic areas (e.g., Papua New Guinea) and in many developing countries among children, in whom it is often the most common cause of death. An increased incidence often accompanies epidemics of influenza. High levels of antibiotic resistance to penicillin, and occasionally to third generation cephalosporins, are becoming increasingly common worldwide.

4. Reservoir—Humans. Pneumococci are commonly found in the upper respiratory tract of healthy people throughout the world.

5. Mode of transmission—By droplet spread, by direct oral contact, or indirectly through articles freshly soiled with respiratory discharges. Person to person transmission of the organisms is common, but illness among casual contacts and attendants is infrequent.

6. Incubation period—Not well determined; may be as short as 1-3 days.

7. Period of communicability—Presumably until discharges of mouth and nose no longer contain virulent pneumococci in significant numbers. Penicillin will render patients with susceptible strains noninfectious within 24-48 hours.

8. Susceptibility and resistance—Susceptibility to symptomatic pneumococcal infection is increased by any process affecting the anatomic or physiologic integrity of the lower respiratory tract, including influenza, pulmonary edema of any cause, aspiration following alcoholic intoxication or other causes, chronic lung disease or exposure to irritants in the air. Elderly persons and persons with the following chronic medical conditions are at increased risk: anatomic or functional asplenia, sickle cell disease, chronic cardiovascular disease, diabetes mellitus, cirrhosis, Hodgkin disease, lymphoma, multiple myeloma, chronic renal failure, nephrotic syndrome, HIV infection and recent organ transplantation. Immunity, specific for the infecting capsular serotype, usually follows an attack and may last for years. Malnutrition and low birthweight are important risk cofactors for pneumonia in infants and young children in developing countries.

9. **Methods of control —**

 A. *Preventive measures:*

1) Avoid crowding in living quarters whenever practical, particularly in institutions, barracks and ships.

2) Administer to high risk persons polyvalent vaccine containing the capsular polysaccharides of the 23 pneumococcal types causing 90% of all pneumococcal infections in the USA; this vaccine is not effective in children less than 2 years old. Those at high risk of fatal infection include individuals 65 years of age and older and those with anatomic or functional asplenia, sickle cell disease, HIV infection and a variety of chronic systemic illnesses, including heart and lung disease, cirrhosis of the liver, renal insufficiency and diabetes mellitus. Because risk of infection and case-fatality rates increase with age, benefits of immunization increase also.

 For most eligible patients, the 23-valent pneumococcal vaccine need be given only once; however, reimmunization is generally safe, and vaccine should be offered to eligible patients whose immunization status cannot be determined. Reimmunization once is recommended for persons more than 2 years of age who are at highest risk for serious pneumococcal infection (e.g., asplenic patients) and those who are likely to have a rapid decline in pneumococcal antibody levels, provided that 5 years or more have elapsed since receipt of the first dose of vaccine. Reimmunization after 3 years should also be considered for children with functional or anatomic asplenia (i.e., sickle cell disease or splenectomy) and those with conditions associated with rapid antibody decline after initial immunization (e.g., nephrotic syndrome, renal failure, or renal transplantation) who would be 10 years of age or older at reimmunization. In addition, persons 65 years and older should be given a second dose of vaccine if they received the vaccine more than 5 years previously and were less than 65 at the time of primary immunization. Most of the pneumococcal antigen types in the 23-valent vaccine are poor immunogens in children under 2 years of age. Because of differences in serotype prevalence, the vaccine may have lower efficacy in developing countries. As of late 1999, pneumococcal protein conjugate vaccines are being evaluated in clinical trials and if effective may be approved for pediatric use.

 B. *Control of patient, contacts and the immediate environment:*

1) Report to local health authority: Obligatory report of epidemics; no individual case report, Class 4 (see Communicable

Disease Reporting). Some states have made penicillin resistant isolates reportable.

2) Isolation: In hospitals, respiratory isolation may be warranted for patients with antibiotic resistant infection who may transmit it to other patients at high risk of pneumococcal disease.

3) Concurrent disinfection: Of discharges from nose and throat. Terminal cleaning.

4) Quarantine: None.

5) Immunization of contacts: None. (See 9C, below.)

6) Investigation of contacts and source of infection: Of no practical value.

7) Specific treatment: Where diagnostic facilities are limited and a delay in treatment could prove fatal, antibiotic treatment of infants and young children should be started on a presumptive diagnosis based on clinical signs, in particular tachypnea and chest indrawing. Infants less than 2 months of age should be transferred to hospital care without delay. Penicillin G, parenterally, is the preferred treatment; use erythromycin for those hypersensitive to penicillin. Because pneumococci that are resistant to penicillin and other antimicrobials are increasingly recognized, the sensitivities of strains isolated from normally sterile sites, including blood or CSF, should be determined. In the USA, where beta-lactam resistance is common, vancomycin should be included in initial regimens for treatment of meningitis possibly due to pneumonococci until susceptibilities can be determined. For pneumonia and other pneumococcal infections, parenteral B-lactam antibiotics are likely to be effective in the majority of cases. Vancomycin is rarely if ever indicated for pneumococcal infections not involving the CNS. For developing countries, WHO recommends either TMP-SMX, ampicillin or amoxicillin for home treatment of nonsevere pneumonia (cough and tachypnea, without chest indrawing) for children less than 5 years.

C. *Epidemic measures:* In outbreaks in institutions or in other closed population groups, immunization with the 23-valent vaccine should be carried out unless it is known that the type causing disease is not included in the vaccine.

D. *Disaster implications:* Crowding of populations in temporary shelters bears a risk of disease, especially for the very young and the elderly.

E. *International measures:* None.

II. MYCOPLASMAL
PNEUMONIA   ICD-9 483; ICD-10 J15.7
(Primary atypical pneumonia)

1. Identification—Predominantly a febrile bacterial lower respiratory infection; less often, a pharyngitis that sometimes progresses to bronchitis or pneumonia. Onset is gradual with headache, malaise, cough (often paroxysmal), sore throat and, less often, chest discomfort that may be pleuritic. Sputum, scant at first, may increase later. Early patchy infiltration of the lungs is often more extensive on x-ray than clinical findings suggest. In severe cases, the pneumonia may progress from one lobe to another and may be bilateral. Leukocytosis occurs after the first week in approximately one third of cases. Duration of illness varies from a few days to a month or more. Secondary bacterial infection and other complications, such as CNS involvement and Stevens-Johnson syndrome, are infrequent, and fatalities are rare.

Differentiation is required from pneumonitis due to many other agents: bacteria, adenoviruses, influenza, respiratory syncytial virus, parainfluenza, measles, Q fever, psittacosis, certain mycoses and tuberculosis.

Diagnosis is based on a rise in antibody titers between acute and convalescent sera. Titers rise after several weeks. The ESR is almost always high. Development of cold hemagglutinins (CA) may occur in one half to two thirds of hospitalized cases; however, this is a nonspecific finding. The level of CA titer may reflect the severity of disease. The infectious agent may be cultured on special media.

2. Infectious agent—*Mycoplasma pneumoniae,* bacteria of the family Mycoplasmataceae.

3. Occurrence—Worldwide; sporadic, endemic and occasionally epidemic, especially in institutions and military populations. Attack rates vary from 5 to more than 50/1,000/year in military populations and 1 to 3/1,000/year in civilians. Epidemics occur more often in late summer and fall; endemic disease is not seasonal, but there can be much variation from year to year and in different geographic areas. There is no selectivity for race or gender. The disease occurs at all ages but is asymptomatic or very mild in children under 5 years; recognized disease is most frequent among school aged children and young adults.

4. Reservoir—Humans.

5. Mode of transmission—Probably by droplet inhalation, direct contact with an infected person (probably including those with subclinical infections) or with articles freshly soiled with discharges of nose and throat from an acutely ill and coughing patient. Secondary cases of pneumonia among contacts, family members and attendants are frequent.

6. Incubation period—From 6 to 32 days.

7. Period of communicability—Unknown; probably less than 20 days. Therapy does not eradicate the organism from the respiratory tract where it may persist for as long as 13 weeks.

8. Susceptibility and resistance—Clinical pneumonia occurs in about 3%-30% of infections with *M. pneumoniae,* depending on age. Disease varies from mild afebrile pharyngitis to febrile illness involving the upper or lower respiratory tract. Duration of immunity is uncertain. Second attacks of pneumonia may occur. Resistance has been correlated with humoral antibodies that remain for up to 1 year.

9. Methods of control—

    A. Preventive measures: Avoid crowded living and sleeping quarters whenever possible, especially in institutions, barracks and ships.

    B. Control of patient, contacts and the immediate environment:

      1) Report to local health authority: Obligatory report of epidemics; no individual case report, Class 4 (see Communicable Disease Reporting).
      2) Isolation: None. Respiratory secretions may be infectious.
      3) Concurrent disinfection: Of discharges from nose and throat. Terminal cleaning.
      4) Quarantine: None.
      5) Immunization of contacts: None.
      6) Investigation of contacts and source of infection: Valuable in detecting treatable clinical disease among family members.
      7) Specific treatment: Erythromycin or other macrolides, or a tetracycline. Erythromycin or other macrolides are preferred for children under 8 years of age to avoid tetracycline staining of immature teeth. Neither antibiotic eliminates organisms from the pharynx; during treatment, erythromycin resistant mycoplasmas may be selected.

    C. Epidemic measures: No reliably effective measures for control are available.

    D. Disaster implications: None.

    E. International measures: WHO Collaborating Centres.

III. PNEUMOCYSTIS
    PNEUMONIA   ICD-9 136.3; ICD-10 B59
(Interstitial plasma-cell pneumonia, PCP)

1. Identification—An acute to subacute, often fatal pulmonary disease, especially in malnourished, chronically ill and premature infants. In older children and adults, it occurs as an opportunistic illness associated with the use of immunosuppressants and diseases of the immune system. It is a major disease problem for people with acquired immunodeficiency syndrome (q.v.). Clinically, there is progressive dyspnea, tachypnea and cyanosis; fever may not be present. Auscultatory signs, other than rales, are usually minimal or absent. Chest x-ray typically shows bilateral interstitial infiltrates. Postmortem examination reveals heavy airless lungs, thickened alveolar septa and foamy material containing clumps of parasites in the alveolar spaces.

Diagnosis is established by demonstration of the causative agent in material from bronchial brushings, open lung biopsy and lung aspirates or in smears of tracheobronchial mucus. Organisms can be identified by methenamine silver, toluidine blue O, Giemsa, Gram-Weigert, cresyl-echt-violet or IFA staining methods. There is no satisfactory culture method or serologic test in routine use at present.

2. Infectious agent—*Pneumocystis carinii*. Generally considered a protozoan parasite; recent studies have shown that the organism's DNA sequence closely resembles that of a fungus.

3. Occurrence—The disease has been recognized on all continents; may be endemic and epidemic in debilitated, malnourished or immunosuppressed infants. It affected approximately 60% of patients with AIDS in the USA, Europe and Australia before the routine use of prophylactic medication. Almost no PCP has been reported from AIDS patients in Africa.

4. Reservoir—Humans. Organisms have been demonstrated in rodents, cattle, dogs and other animals, but with the ubiquitous presence of the organism and its subclinical persistence in man, there appears to be little public health significance of these potential animal sources of human infection.

5. Mode of transmission—Animal to animal transmission via the airborne route has been demonstrated in rats. The mode of transmission in people is not known. In one study, approximately 75% of normal individuals were reported to have humoral antibody to *P. carinii* by the age of 4 years, suggesting that subclinical infection is common in the USA. Pneumonitis in the compromised host may result from either a reactivation of latent infection or a newly acquired infection.

6. Incubation period—Unknown. Analysis of data from institutional outbreaks and animal studies indicates that the onset of disease often occurs 1–2 months after establishment of the immunosuppressed state.

7. Period of communicability—Unknown.

8. Susceptibility and resistance—Susceptibility is enhanced by prematurity, by chronic debilitating illness and by disease or therapy in which immune mechanisms are impaired. Infection with HIV is a predominant risk factor for PCP disease.

9. **Methods of control—**

   A. *Preventive measures:* Prophylaxis with either oral TMP-SMX or pentamidine (aerosolized) has proven to be effective (for as long as the patient is receiving the drug) in preventing endogenous reactivation in immunosuppressed patients, especially those with HIV infection, those treated for lymphatic leukemia and those with organ transplants.

   B. *Control of patient, contacts and the immediate environment:*

   1) Report to local health authority: Official report not ordinarily justifiable, Class 5 (see Communicable Disease Reporting). When cases occur in people with evidence of HIV infection, case report is required in most states, Class 2B (see Communicable Disease Reporting).
   2) Isolation: None.
   3) Concurrent disinfection: Insufficient knowledge.
   4) Quarantine: None.
   5) Immunization of contacts: None.
   6) Investigation of contacts and source of infection: None.
   7) Specific treatment: TMP-SMX is the drug of choice. Alternate drugs are pentamidine (IM or IV) and trimetrexate with leucovorin; several drugs are currently under intensive evaluation.

   C. *Epidemic measures:* Knowledge of source of the organism and mode of transmission is so incomplete that there are no generally accepted measures.

   D. *Disaster implications:* None.

   E. *International measures:* None.

IV. CHLAMYDIAL PNEUMONIAS
IV.A. PNEUMONIA DUE TO
CHLAMYDIA TRACHOMATIS

ICD-9 482.8;
ICD-10 P23.1

(Neonatal eosinophilic pneumonia, Congenital pneumonia due to *Chlamydia*)

1. **Identification**—A subacute chlamydial pulmonary disease occurring in early infancy among infants whose mothers have infection of the uterine cervix. Clinically, the disease is characterized by insidious onset, cough (characteristically staccato), lack of fever, patchy infiltrates on chest

x-ray with hyperinflation, eosinophilia and elevated IgM and IgG. About half of infant cases have a prodrome of rhinitis and conjunctivitis. Duration of illness is commonly 1–3 weeks but may extend as long as 2 months. The spectrum of illness is quite broad, ranging from rhinitis to severe pneumonia. Many infants with pneumonia ultimately develop asthma or obstructive lung disease.

Diagnosis is usually made by direct IF technique. Definition of the infecting immunotype is based on cell culture isolation of the causative agent from the posterior nasopharynx or demonstration of specific serum antibody at a titer of 1:32 or greater by micro-IF. A high titer of specific IgG antibody supports the diagnosis.

2. Infectious agent—*Chlamydia trachomatis* of immunotypes D to K (excluding immunotypes that cause lymphogranuloma venereum).

3. Occurrence—Probably coincides with the worldwide distribution of genital chlamydial infection. The disease has been recognized in the USA and a number of European countries. Epidemics have not been recognized.

4. Reservoir—Humans. Experimental infection with *C. trachomatis* has been induced in nonhuman primates and mice, but animal infections are not known to occur in nature.

5. Mode of transmission—Transmitted from the infected cervix to an infant during birth, with resultant nasopharyngeal infection (and occasionally chlamydial conjunctivitis). Respiratory transmission has not been established.

6. Incubation period—Not known, but pneumonia may occur in infants from 1 to 18 weeks of age (more commonly between 4 and 12 weeks). Nasopharyngeal infection is usually not recognized before 2 weeks of age.

7. Period of communicability—Unknown.

8. Susceptibility and resistance—Unknown. Maternal antibody does not protect the infant from infection.

9. Methods of control—

    A. Preventive measures: Same as for Chlamydial Conjunctivitis (see Conjunctivitis, section IV).

    B. Control of patient, contacts and the immediate environment:

       1) Report to local health authority: Official report not ordinarily justifiable, Class 5 (see Communicable Disease Reporting).
       2) Isolation: Universal precautions.
       3) Concurrent disinfection: Of discharges from nose and throat.
       4) Quarantine: None.

5) Immunization of contacts: None.
6) Investigation of contacts and source of infection: Examine parents for infection and treat if positive.
7) Specific treatment: Oral erythromycin (50 mg/kg/day) is the drug of choice for these infants. Sulfisoxazole is a possible alternative.

C. Epidemic measures: No epidemic occurrence recognized.

D. Disaster implications: None.

E. International measures: None.

IV.B. PNEUMONIA DUE TO
CHLAMYDIA PNEUMONIAE
ICD-9 482.8; ICD-10 J16.0

1. Identification—An acute chlamydial respiratory disease with cough, frequently a sore throat and hoarseness, and fever at the onset. Sputum is scanty; few patients complain of chest pain. Pulmonary rales are usually present. The clinical picture is similar to infection caused by mycoplasma. A variety of radiographic abnormalities have been described including bilateral infiltrates; pleural effusions may occur. Illness is usually mild, but recovery is relatively slow, with cough persisting for 2-6 weeks; in older adults, bronchitis and sinusitis may become chronic. Death is very rare in uncomplicated cases.

Laboratory diagnosis is primarily serologic: the CF test detects antibodies to chlamydia group antigens, and a specific micro-IF test for IgM and IgG (on sera obtained 3 weeks after initial infection) identifies antibodies to the agent. In cases of reinfection, IgG antibody appears early and rises to a high level. Those treated early with tetracycline may have a poor antibody response. The organism can be isolated from throat swab specimens in the yolk sac of embryonated eggs, and can be cultured in special cell lines.

2. Infectious agent—*Chlamydia pneumoniae,* strain TWAR, is the species name for the organism that has distinct morphologic and serologic differences from *C. psittaci* and *C. trachomatis.*

3. Occurrence—Presumably worldwide. Illness has been confirmed in Finland, Denmark, Norway, Sweden, the UK, Hungary, Germany, Spain, Canada, Australia, Japan, the Philippines and the USA. The original isolation was made in Taiwan. Antibodies are rare in children under 5 years of age; prevalence increases among teenagers and young adults to a plateau of about 50% by age 20-30; prevalence remains high into old age. While clinical disease has been seen most frequently in young adults, disease has occurred in all ages; 8 of 18 cases reported from Canada were in persons over 70 years of age, and the oldest (with recovery) was 90. No seasonality has been noted.

4. Reservoir—Presumably people. No avian association has been found; no isolations or antibodies were found in pigeons and other birds captured at the site of an outbreak, nor in dogs or cats.

5. Mode of transmission—Not defined; possibilities include direct contact with secretions, spread via fomites and airborne spread.

6. Incubation period—Unknown; may be at least 10 days.

7. Period of communicability—Not defined but presumed to be prolonged based on military outbreaks that lasted as long as 8 months.

8. Susceptibility and resistance—Susceptibility is presumed to be universal with increased likelihood of clinical disease in the presence of preexisting chronic disease. Serologic evidence of recall type immune response suggests immunity after infection; however, second episodes of pneumonia have been observed in military recruits, with a secondary type of serologic response to the second attack.

9. Methods of control—

    A. Preventive measures:

        1) Avoid crowding in living and sleeping quarters.
        2) Apply personal hygiene measures: cover mouth when coughing and sneezing, dispose of discharges from mouth and nose in a sanitary manner and wash hands frequently.

    B. Control of patient, contacts and the immediate environment:

        1) Report to local health authority: Obligatory report of epidemics; no individual case report, Class 4 (see Communicable Disease Reporting).
        2) Isolation: None. Universal precautions should be practiced.
        3) Concurrent disinfection: Of discharges from nose and throat.
        4) Quarantine: None.
        5) Immunization of contacts: None.
        6) Investigation of contacts and source of infection: Examine all members of the family for infection and treat if positive.
        7) Specific treatment: Oral tetracycline or erythromycin, 2 g/day for 10-14 days. The new macrolides, azithromycin and clarithromycin may be used as well. The new fluoroquinolones may also prove effective.

    C. Epidemic measures: Case finding and appropriate treatment.

D. Disaster implications: None.

E. International measures: None.

OTHER PNEUMONIAS

ICD-9 480, 482;
ICD-10 J12, J13, J15, J16.8, J18

Among the known viruses, the adenoviruses, respiratory syncytial virus, the parainfluenza viruses and probably others as yet unidentified may produce a pneumonitis. Because these infectious agents cause upper respiratory disease more often than pneumonia, they are presented under Respiratory Disease, Acute Viral. Viral pneumonia occurs in measles, influenza and chickenpox. The chlamydial infection by *C. psittaci* is presented as psittacosis (q.v.). Pneumonia is also caused by infection with rickettsiae (see Q Fever) and *Legionella*. It can also be associated with the invasive phase of nematode infections, such as ascariasis, and with mycoses such as aspergillosis, histoplasmosis and coccidioidomycosis.

Various pathogenic bacteria commonly found in the mouth, nose and throat, such as *Haemophilus influenzae, Staphylococcus aureus, Klebsiella pneumoniae, Streptococcus pyogenes* (group A hemolytic streptococci), *Neisseria meningitidis* (notably group Y), *Bacteroides* species, *Moraxella catarrhalis* and anaerobic cocci, may produce pneumonia, especially in association with influenza, as superinfection following broad-spectrum antibiotic therapy, as a complication of chronic pulmonary disease and after aspiration of gastric contents or tracheostomy. *H. influenzae* pneumonia is the second most common cause of pneumonia in developing countries and a major cause of death in children under 5 years of age. With increased use of antimicrobial and immunosuppressive therapy, pneumonias caused by enteric gram-negative bacilli have become more common, especially those caused by *Escherichia coli, Pseudomonas aeruginosa* and *Proteus* species. Management depends on the specific organism involved.

POLIOMYELITIS, ACUTE

ICD-9 045; ICD-10 A80

(Polioviral fever, Infantile paralysis)

1. Identification—A viral infection most often recognized by the acute onset of flaccid paralysis. Poliovirus infection occurs in the GI tract with spread to the regional nodes and in a minority of cases, to the nervous system. Flaccid paralysis occurs in less than 1% of poliovirus infections; greater than 90% of infections are either inapparent or a nonspecific fever. Aseptic meningitis occurs in about 1% of infections. A minor illness is recognized with symptoms that include fever, malaise, headache, nausea and vomiting. If the disease progresses to major illness, severe muscle pain and stiffness of the neck and back with flaccid paralysis may occur. The paralysis of poliomyelitis is characteristically asymmetric with fever present at the onset. The maximum extent of paralysis is reached in a short period, usually within 3-4 days. The site of paralysis depends on the location of nerve cell destruction in the spinal cord or brain stem. The legs are affected more often than the arms. Paralysis of the muscles of respiration and/or swallowing is life threatening. Some improvement in paralysis may be seen during convalescence, but any paralysis still present after 60 days is likely to be permanent. Infrequently, recurrence of muscle weakness following recovery may occur many years after the original infection has resolved ("postpolio syndrome"); this is not believed to be related to persistence of the virus itself.

In highly endemic countries, typical polio cases can be recognized on clinical grounds. In countries where polio is absent or occurs at low levels, poliomyelitis must be distinguished from other paralytic conditions by isolation of virus from stool. Other enteroviruses (notably types 70 and 71), echoviruses and coxsackieviruses can cause an illness simulating paralytic poliomyelitis.

The most frequent cause of acute flaccid paralysis (AFP) that must be distinguished from poliomyelitis is Guillain-Barré syndrome (GBS). The paralysis of GBS is typically symmetrical and may progress for periods as long as 10 days. The fever, headache, nausea, vomiting and pleocytosis characteristic of poliomyelitis are usually absent in GBS; high protein and low cell counts in the CSF and sensory changes in the majority of cases are seen in GBS. Acute motor axonal neuropathy ("China paralytic syndrome") is an important cause of AFP in northern China and is probably present elsewhere; it is seasonally epidemic and closely resembles poliomyelitis. Fever and CSF pleocytosis are usually absent, but paralysis may persist for several months. Other important causes of AFP include transverse myelitis, traumatic neuritis, infectious and toxic neuropathies, tick paralysis, myasthenia gravis, porphyria, botulism, insecticide poisoning, polymyositis, trichinosis and periodic paralysis.

The differential diagnosis of acute nonparalytic poliomyelitis includes other forms of acute nonbacterial meningitis, purulent meningitis, brain abscess, tuberculous meningitis, leptospirosis, lymphocytic choriomeningitis, infectious mononucleosis, the encephalitides, neurosyphilis and toxic encephalopathies.

Definitive laboratory diagnosis is made by isolation of the virus from stool samples, CSF or oropharyngeal secretions in cell culture systems of human or monkey origin (primate cells). Differentiation of "wild" from vaccine virus strains can be made in specialized laboratories. Presumptive diagnosis may be made by fourfold or greater rises in antibody levels; however, type specific neutralizing antibodies may already be present when paralysis develops, so that significant titer rises may not be demonstrable in paired sera. Also, the antibody response following immunization mimics the response following infection with wild type viruses and the widespread use of live polio vaccines makes interpretation of antibody difficult, except for ruling out polio in cases where no antibody has developed in immunocompetent children.

2. Infectious agent—Poliovirus (genus *Enterovirus)* types 1, 2 and 3; all types can cause paralysis. Type 1 is isolated from paralytic cases most often, type 3 less so, and type 2 least commonly. Type 1 most frequently causes epidemics. Most vaccine associated cases are due to type 2 or 3.

3. Occurrence—Prior to the advent of immunization, polio occurred worldwide. As a result of improved immunization programs worldwide and WHO's global initiative to eradicate poliomyelitis, circulation of polioviruses is limited to a decreasing number of countries. The last culture confirmed case of poliomyelitis due to indigenous wild poliovirus in the Western Hemisphere was detected in Peru in August 1991. Poliomyelitis is on the verge of worldwide eradication. The greatest risk of polio now occurs on the Indian subcontinent and, to a lesser extent, in the countries of west and central Africa. War torn countries in this region where the health infrastructure has been destroyed are at particular risk of epidemics. WHO has set the end of the year 2000 as the target for worldwide eradication, but many experts believe that it is likely to take a little longer to accomplish this goal.

Although wild poliovirus transmission has probably ceased in most industrialized countries, importation remains a threat. An outbreak of poliomyelitis occurred in 1992-1993 in the Netherlands among members of a religious group that refuse immunization. The virus was also found among members of a related religious group in Canada, although no cases occurred. Cases of poliomyelitis are also recognized in industrialized countries among tourists who have never been immunized as well as nonimmunized immigrants revisiting their country of origin. With the exception of these rare imported cases, all of the very few cases of poliomyelitis recognized in industrialized countries are caused by vaccine virus strains. In the USA, 5-10 cases of vaccine associated poliomyelitis occurred each year when oral poliovirus vaccine (OPV) was the primary vaccine used. About half of these cases occurred among adult contacts of vaccinees.

In endemic areas, cases of polio occur both sporadically and in epidemics with an increase in cases during the late summer and autumn in temperate countries. In tropical countries, a seasonal peak occurs in the hot and rainy season, but is less pronounced.

Polio remains primarily a disease of infants and young children. In many polio endemic countries, 70%-80% of cases are less than 3 years of age and 80%-90% of cases are less than 5 years of age. Clusters of susceptible persons, including groups that refuse immunization, minority populations, economic migrants and other unregistered children, nomads, refugees and urban poor are at high risk.

4. Reservoir—Humans, most frequently people with inapparent infections, especially children. Long term carriers of wild type viruses have not been found (see below).

5. Mode of transmission—Primarily person to person spread, principally through the fecal-oral route; virus is more easily detectable, and for a longer period, in feces than in throat secretions. However, where sanitation is good, pharyngeal spread may be relatively more important. In rare instances, milk, foodstuffs and other materials contaminated with feces have been incriminated as vehicles. No reliable evidence of spread by insects exists; water and sewage are rarely implicated.

6. Incubation period—Commonly 7-14 days for paralytic cases, with a reported range of 3 to possibly 35 days.

7. Period of communicability—Not precisely defined, but transmission is possible as long as the virus is excreted. Poliovirus is demonstrable in throat secretions as early as 36 hours and in the feces 72 hours after exposure to infection in both clinical and inapparent cases. Virus typically persists in the throat for approximately 1 week and in the feces for 3-6 weeks or longer. Cases are most infectious during the first few days before and after onset of symptoms.

8. Susceptibility and resistance—Susceptibility to infection is universal, but paralysis occurs in only about 1% of infections. Some of these patients recover and residual paralysis is observed in 0.1% to 1%. The rate of paralysis among infected, nonimmune adults is higher than that among nonimmunized infants and young children. Type specific immunity, apparently of lifelong duration, follows both clinically recognizable and inapparent infections. Second attacks are rare and result from infection with a poliovirus of a different type. Infants born of immune mothers have transient passive immunity.

Intramuscular injections, trauma or surgery during the incubation period or prodromal illness may provoke paralysis in the affected extremity. Tonsillectomy increases the risk of bulbar involvement. Excessive muscular activity in the prodromal period may predispose to paralysis.

9. Methods of control—

  A. Preventive measures:

  1) Educate the public on the advantages of immunization in early childhood.
  2) As of late 1999, both a trivalent live, attenuated oral (OPV) and an injectable, inactivated poliovirus vaccine (IPV) are commercially available. Their use varies in different countries.

  OPV simulates natural infection by inducing both circulating antibody and intestinal resistance, and immunizes some susceptible contacts through secondary spread. In developing countries, lower rates of seroconversion and reduced vaccine efficacy for OPV have been reported, but this can be overcome by administration of extra doses in supplemental campaigns. Breast feeding does not cause a significant reduction in the protection provided by OPV. WHO recommends the use of OPV alone for immunization programs in developing countries because of low cost, ease of administration and superior capacity to provide population immunity.

IPV, like OPV, provides excellent individual protection by inducing circulating antibody that blocks spread of the virus to the CNS. Both IPV and OPV induce intestinal immunity. Many industrialized countries switched to IPV alone for routine immunization when it was clear after many years that wild type polioviruses had been eliminated.

Five individuals with underlying primary immune deficiency disorders have been identified who excreted OPV for 4 to 7 or more years. The significance of these cases with regard to the possibility of eventually stopping polio immunization is under review and studies are in place to look for additional instances in developing countries.

3) Recommendations for routine immunization:

From 1962 to 1997, OPV was the vaccine of choice for routine immunization in the USA. In January 1997, the CDC recommended giving IPV at 2 and 4 months of age and OPV at 12–18 months and 4–6 years of age. Effective January 2000, all children in the USA should receive 4 doses of IPV at ages 2 months, 4 months, 6–18 months and 4–6 years. OPV should be used only for the following special circumstances: (1) mass immunization campaigns to control outbreaks of paralytic polio; (2) unimmunized children who will be traveling in less than 4 weeks to areas where polio is endemic; and (3) children of parents who do not accept the recommended number of vaccine injections. These children may receive OPV only for the third or fourth dose or both; in this situation, health care providers should administer OPV only after discussing the risk for vaccine associated paralytic polio (VAPP) with parents or caregivers. It is anticipated that the availability of OPV will be limited in the future in the USA. In developing countries, WHO recommends OPV at 6, 10 and 14 weeks of age. In polio endemic countries, an additional dose of OPV is recommended at birth.

In polio endemic countries, WHO recommends the use of national immunization campaigns that administer 2 doses of OPV, 1 month apart, to all children less than 5 years of age regardless of prior immunization status. These campaigns are ideally conducted during the cool, dry season to achieve maximum effect. When a high level of control has been achieved in a country, targeted immunization campaigns in high risk areas are recommended.

Contraindications to OPV include congenital immunodeficiency

(B-lymphocyte deficiency, thymic dysplasia), current immunosuppressive therapy, disease states associated with immunosuppression (HIV/AIDS, lymphoma, leukemia, generalized malignancy) and the presence of immunodeficient individuals in the household of potential vaccine recipients. (IPV should be used in such people.) However, where polio is still a problem, WHO recommends the use of OPV for infants who may be infected with HIV. Diarrhea is not considered a contraindication to OPV.

When OPV was the recommended vaccine, OPV caused paralytic poliomyelitis in vaccine recipients or their healthy contacts at a rate of approximately one in every 2.5 million doses in the USA. In Romania, multiple injections of antibiotics were associated with an increased risk of vaccine associated poliomyelitis.

Immunization of adults: Routine immunization for adults residing in the continental USA and Canada is not considered necessary, but primary immunization is advised for previously nonimmunized adults traveling to polio endemic countries, for members of communities or population groups in which poliovirus disease is present, for laboratory workers who may handle specimens containing poliovirus and for health care workers who may be exposed to patients excreting wild type polioviruses. IPV is recommended for adult primary immunization; 2 doses are given with a 1-2 month interval and a third dose given 6-12 months later. Those who have previously completed a course of immunization and now will be at increased risk of exposure may be given an additional dose of IPV.

B. Control of patient, contacts and the immediate environment:

1) Report to local health authority: Obligatory case report of paralytic cases as a Disease under Surveillance by WHO, Class 1A. In countries undertaking polio eradication, each case of acute flaccid paralysis (AFP), including Guillain-Barré syndrome, in children less than 15 years of age, should be reported. Results of virus culture of stools, demographic information, immunization history, clinical examination and examination for residual paralysis after 60 days will be reported by supplemental reports. Immunization history and vaccine lot numbers should be recorded. Nonparalytic cases are also reported to the local health authority, Class 2A (see Communicable Disease Reporting).

2) Isolation: Enteric precautions in the hospital for wild virus disease; of little value under home conditions because many household contacts are infected before poliomyelitis has been diagnosed.

3) Concurrent disinfection: Throat discharges, feces and articles soiled therewith. In communities with modern and adequate

sewage disposal systems, feces and urine can be discharged directly into sewers without preliminary disinfection. Terminal cleaning.

4) Quarantine: Of no community value.

5) Protection of contacts: Immunization of familial and other close contacts is recommended but may not contribute to immediate control; often the virus has already infected susceptible close contacts by the time the first case is recognized.

6) Investigation of contacts and source of infection: Occurrence of a single paralytic case in a community should prompt an immediate investigation. Thorough search for additional cases of AFP in the area around the case assures early detection, facilitates control and permits appropriate treatment of unrecognized and unreported cases.

7) Specific treatment: None; attention during the acute illness to the complications of paralysis requires expert knowledge and equipment, especially for patients in need of respiratory assistance. Physical therapy is used to attain maximum function after paralytic poliomyelitis and can prevent many deformities that are late manifestations of the illness.

C. Epidemic measures:

1) In countries undertaking polio eradication, a single case of poliomyelitis is considered a public health emergency. At the time of case investigation, public health authorities will determine the need for supplemental immunization programs in the community.

D. Disaster implications: Overcrowding of nonimmune groups and collapse of the sanitary infrastructure pose an epidemic threat.

E. International measures:

1) Poliomyelitis is a Disease under Surveillance by WHO and is targeted for eradication by the end of the year 2000. National health administrations are expected to inform WHO of outbreaks promptly by telephone or electronic communication, and to supplement these reports as soon as possible with details of the nature and extent of the outbreak. Primary isolation of the virus is often best accomplished in the national laboratory designated to be part of the Global Polio Eradication Laboratory Network. Once identified, molecular epidemiology can often be used to trace the source of the outbreak. Countries are expected to submit monthly reports on polio and AFP cases to their respective WHO offices.

The Pan American Health Organization (PAHO) had set the goal of eradicating polio from the Americas by the end of

1990. An independent international commission has certified that no locally acquired cases of polio have occurred in the Americas since August 1991.

2) International travelers visiting areas of high prevalence should be adequately immunized.

3) WHO Collaborating Centres.

PSITTACOSIS   ICD-9 073; ICD-10 A70
(*Chlamydia psittaci* infection, Ornithosis, Parrot fever, Avian chlamydiosis)

1. Identification—An acute, generalized chlamydial disease with variable clinical presentations; fever, headache, rash, myalgia, chills and upper or lower respiratory tract disease are common. Respiratory symptoms are often disproportionately mild when compared with the extensive pneumonia demonstrable by x-ray. Cough is initially absent or nonproductive; when present, sputum is mucopurulent and scant. Pleuritic chest pain and splenomegaly occur infrequently; the pulse may be slow in relation to temperature. Encephalitis, myocarditis and thrombophlebitis are occasional complications; relapses may occur. Although usually mild or moderate in character, human disease can be severe, especially in untreated elderly persons.

The diagnosis may be suspected in patients with appropriate symptoms who have a history of exposure to birds and elevated or increasing antibodies to chlamydial antigens collected 2–3 weeks apart. Diagnosis is confirmed, under suitably safe laboratory conditions only, by isolation of the infectious agent from sputum, blood or postmortem tissues in mice, eggs or cell culture. Recovery of the agent may be difficult, especially if the patient has received broad-spectrum antibiotics.

2. Infectious agent—*Chlamydia psittaci.*

3. Occurrence—Worldwide. May be associated with obviously sick or apparently healthy pet birds. Outbreaks occasionally occur in individual households, pet shops, aviaries, avian exhibits in zoos and pigeon lofts. Most human cases are sporadic; many infections are probably not diagnosed.

4. Reservoir—Principally in parakeets, parrots and love birds; less often in poultry, pigeons, canaries and sea birds. Birds that appear to be healthy can be carriers and shed the infectious agent, particularly when subjected to the stresses of crowding and shipping.

5. Mode of transmission—By inhaling the agent from desiccated droppings, secretions and dust from feathers of infected birds. Imported psittacine birds are the most frequent source of exposure, followed by turkey, squab and duck farms; processing and rendering plants have also been sources of occupational disease. Geese and pigeons are occasionally responsible for human disease. Laboratory infections have occurred. Rare person to person transmission has been reported to occur during the acute illness with paroxysmal coughing; however, these cases may have been caused by the recently described *C. pneumoniae* rather than *C. psittaci* organisms.

6. Incubation period—From 1 to 4 weeks.

7. Period of communicability—Diseased as well as seemingly healthy birds may shed the agent intermittently, and sometimes continuously, for weeks or months.

8. Susceptibility and resistance—Susceptibility is general; immunity following infection is incomplete and transitory. Older adults may be more severely affected. There is no evidence that persons with antibodies at any given concentration are protected.

9. Methods of control—

A. Preventive measures:

1) Educate the public to the danger of household or occupational exposure to infected pet birds. Medical personnel responsible for occupational health in processing plants should be aware that febrile respiratory illness with headache or myalgia among the employees may be psittacosis.

2) Regulate the importation of, raising of and trafficking in birds of the parrot family. Prevent or eliminate infections of birds by quarantine and appropriate antibiotic treatment.

3) Psittacine birds offered in commerce should be raised under psittacosis free conditions and handled in such manner as to prevent infection. Tetracyclines can be effective in controlling disease in psittacines and other companion birds if properly administered to ensure adequate intake for at least 30 days and preferably for 45 days. Treatment failures can occur.

4) Conduct surveillance of pet shops and aviaries where psittacosis has occurred or where birds epidemiologically linked to cases were obtained, and of farms or processing plants to which human psittacosis was traced epidemiologically. Infected birds should be treated or destroyed and the area where they were housed thoroughly cleaned and disinfected with a phenolic compound.

B. Control of patient, contacts and the immediate environment:

1) Report to local health authority: Obligatory case report in most states (USA) and countries, Class 2A (see Communicable Disease Reporting).

2) Isolation: None. Coughing patients should be instructed to cough into paper tissue.

3) Concurrent disinfection: Of all discharges. **Terminal cleaning.**

4) Quarantine: Of infected farms or premises with infected birds until diseased birds have been destroyed or adequately treated with tetracycline and the buildings disinfected.

5) Immunization of contacts: None.

6) Investigation of contacts and source of infection: Trace origin of suspected birds. Kill suspected birds and immerse bodies in 2% phenolic or equivalent disinfectant. Place in plastic bag, close securely and ship frozen (on dry ice) to nearest laboratory capable of isolating *Chlamydia.* If suspected birds cannot be killed, swab-cultures of their cloacae or droppings should be shipped to the laboratory in appropriate transport media and shipping containers in compliance with postal regulations; after the cultures are taken, the birds should be treated with a tetracycline drug.

7) Specific treatment: Antibiotics of the tetracycline group, given for 10–14 days after temperature returns to normal. Erythromycin is an alternative when tetracycline is contraindicated (pregnancy, children less than 9 years of age).

C. *Epidemic measures:* While cases are usually sporadic or confined to family outbreaks, epidemics related to infected aviaries or bird suppliers may be extensive. Report outbreaks of psittacosis in turkey and duck flocks to state agriculture and health authorities. Large doses of tetracycline can suppress, but not eliminate, infection in poultry flocks and thus may complicate investigations.

D. *Disaster implications:* None.

E. *International measures:* Reciprocal compliance with national regulations to control importation of psittacine birds.

Q FEVER
(Query fever)

ICD-9 083.0; ICD-10 A78

1. Identification—An acute febrile rickettsial disease; onset may be sudden with chills, retrobulbar headache, weakness, malaise and severe sweats. There is considerable variation in severity and duration; infections may be inapparent or present as a nonspecific "fever of unknown origin." A pneumonitis is found on x-ray in some cases, but cough, expectoration, chest pain and physical findings in the lungs are not prominent. Abnormal liver function tests are common. Acute and chronic granulomatous hepatitis, which can be confused with tuberculous hepatitis, has been reported. Chronic Q fever manifests primarily as endocarditis and this form of the disease can occur on abnormal native (e.g., bicuspid aortic) or prosthetic cardiac valves; these infections have an indolent course, extending over years. Other rare clinical syndromes, including neurologic, have been described. The case-fatality rate in untreated acute cases is usually less than 1% but has been reported as high as 2.4%; it is negligible in treated cases, except in individuals who develop endocarditis, in whom protracted antibiotic courses are the rule and valve replacement operations are often required.

Laboratory diagnosis is made by demonstration of a rise in specific antibodies between acute and convalescent stages by IF, microagglutination, CF or ELISA tests; high antibody titers to phase I of the infective organism may indicate chronic infection, such as endocarditis. Recovery of the infectious agent from blood is diagnostic but poses a hazard to laboratory workers. Q fever Coxiellae may be identified in tissues (liver biopsy or heart valve) by immunostains and EM.

2. Infectious agent—*Coxiella burnetii,* an organism with two antigenic phases: phase I is found in nature and phase II after multiple laboratory passages in eggs or cell cultures. The organism has unusual stability, can reach high concentrations in animal tissues, particularly placentae, and is highly resistant to many disinfectants.

3. Occurrence—Reported from all continents; the incidence is greater than that reported because of the mildness of many cases, limited clinical suspicion and nonavailability of testing laboratories. It is endemic in areas where reservoir animals are present, and affects veterinarians, meat workers, sheep (and occasionally dairy) workers and farmers. Epidemics have occurred among workers in stockyards, meat packing and rendering plants, laboratories and in medical and veterinary centers that use sheep (especially pregnant ewes) in research. Thousands of cases occurred in US troops in Europe during World War II. Individual cases may occur where no direct animal contact can be demonstrated. Evidence of previous infection is common among researchers working with *C. burnetii* and cases have occurred among casual visitors to such facilities.

4. Reservoir—Sheep, cattle, goats, cats, dogs, some wild animals (bandicoots and many species of feral rodents), birds and ticks are natural reservoirs. Transovarial and transstadial transmission are common in ticks that participate in wildlife cycles in rodents, larger animals and birds. Ticks were not considered a major source of human infection in the USA. Infected animals, including sheep and cats, are usually asymptomatic, but shed massive numbers of organisms in placental tissues at parturition.

5. Mode of transmission—Commonly by airborne dissemination of Coxiellae in dust from premises contaminated by placental tissues, birth fluids and excreta of infected animals; in establishments processing infected animals or their byproducts and in necropsy rooms. Airborne particles containing organisms may be carried downwind for a considerable distance (one-half mile or more); also by direct contact with infected animals and other contaminated materials, such as wool, straw, fertilizer and laundry. Raw milk from infected cows contains organisms and may be responsible for some cases, but this has not been proven. Direct transmission by blood or marrow transfusion has been reported.

6. Incubation period—Depends on the size of the infecting dose; usually 2-3 weeks.

7. Period of communicability—Direct transmission from person to person occurs rarely, if ever. However, contaminated clothing may be a source of infection.

8. Susceptibility and resistance—Susceptibility is general. Immunity following recovery from clinical illness is probably lifelong, with cell mediated immunity lasting longer than humoral. Antibodies detected by CF persist for 3-5 years: antibodies detected by IF may persist as long as 10-15 years.

9. Methods of control —

   A. Preventive measures:

     1) Educate persons in high risk occupations (sheep and dairy farmers, veterinary researchers, abbatoir workers) on sources of infection and the necessity for adequate disinfection and disposal of animal products of conception; restrict access to cow and sheep sheds, barns and laboratories with potentially infected animals, and stress the value of inactivation procedures such as pasteurization of milk.

     2) Pasteurizing milk from cows, goats and sheep at 62.7°C (145°F) for 30 minutes or at 71.6°C (161°F) for 15 seconds, or boiling, inactivates Q fever Coxiellae.

     3) No commercially available vaccine currently exists in the USA. Immunization with an investigational inactivated vaccine prepared from *C. burnetii* phase I-infected yolk sac is useful in protecting laboratory workers and is strongly recommended for those knowingly working with live *C. burnetii.* It should also be considered for abattoir workers and others in hazardous occupations, including those carrying out medical research with pregnant sheep. To avoid severe local reactions, vaccine administration should be preceded by a skin sensitivity test with a small dose of diluted vaccine; vaccine should not be given to individuals with a positive skin or antibody test or a documented history of Q fever. Vaccine may be obtained under IND by contacting the Commanding Officer, U.S. Army

Medical Research and Materiel Command, ATTN: MCMR-UMP, Fort Detrick, Frederick, MD 21702-5009; telephone 301-619-2051.

4) Research workers using pregnant sheep should be identified and enrolled in a medical surveillance and health education program. This program should include a baseline serum evaluation, followed by periodic evaluations. Persons at risk (i.e., those with valvular heart disease, women of child bearing age, persons who are immunosuppressed) should be advised of the risk of serious illness that may result from Q fever. Animals used in research should also be assessed for Q fever infection by serology. Laboratory clothes must be appropriately bagged and washed to prevent infection of laundry personnel. Sheep-holding facilities should be away from populated areas and measures should be implemented to prevent air flow to other occupied areas; no casual visitors should be permitted.

B. Control of patient, contacts and the immediate environment:

1) Report to local health authority: In the USA, in areas where disease is endemic; in many countries not a reportable disease, Class 3B (see Communicable Disease Reporting).

2) Isolation: None.

3) Concurrent disinfection: Of sputum and blood and articles freshly soiled by these substances, using 0.05% hypochlorite, 5% peroxide or a 1:100 solution of Lysol. Use precautions at postmortem examination of suspected cases in humans or animals.

4) Quarantine: None.

5) Immunization of contacts: Unnecessary.

6) Investigation of contacts and source of infection: Search for history of contact with sheep, cattle or goats on farms or in research facilities, parturient cats, consumption of raw milk, or direct or indirect association with a laboratory that handles *C. burnetii.*

7) Specific treatment: Acute disease: Tetracyclines (particularly doxycycline) administered orally and continued for 15–21 days; reinstitute if relapse occurs. Chronic disease (endocarditis): Doxycycline and oflaxacin for several years, or doxycycline in combination with hydroxychloroquine for several years. Surgical replacement of the infected valve may be necessary in some patients for cure.

C. Epidemic measures: Outbreaks are generally of short duration; control measures are limited essentially to elimination of sources of infection, observation of exposed people and antibiotic therapy for those becoming ill.

D. Disaster implications: None.

E. International measures: Control the importation of goats, sheep and cattle, and their products (e.g., wool). WHO Collaborating Centres.

RABIES
(Hydrophobia, Lyssa)

ICD-9 071; ICD-10 A82

1. Identification—An almost invariably fatal, acute viral encephalomyelitis; onset is often heralded by a sense of apprehension, headache, fever, malaise and indefinite sensory changes often referred to the site of a preceding animal bite. Excitability and aerophobia are frequent symptoms. The disease progresses to paresis or paralysis; spasm of swallowing muscles leads to fear of water (hydrophobia); delirium and convulsions follow. Without medical intervention, the usual duration is 2–6 days, sometimes longer; death is often due to respiratory paralysis.

Diagnosis is made by specific FA staining of brain tissue or by virus isolation in mouse or cell culture systems. Presumptive diagnosis may be made by specific FA staining of frozen skin sections taken from the back of the neck at the hairline. Serologic diagnosis is based on neutralization tests in mice or cell culture.

2. Infectious agent—Rabies virus, a rhabdovirus of the genus *Lyssavirus*. All members of the genus are antigenically related, but use of monoclonal antibodies and nucleotide sequencing of the virus demonstrates differences according to the animal species or the geographic location from which they originate. Rabies related viruses that exist in Africa (Mokola and Duvenhage) have been associated rarely with fatal rabies-like human illness. A new lyssavirus, first identified in 1996 in several species of flying foxes and bats in Australia, has been associated with two human deaths with rabies-like illnesses. This virus has been provisionally named Australian bat lyssavirus. It is closely related to, but not identical to classical rabies virus. Some of the illnesses due to these rabies related viruses may be diagnosed as rabies by the standard FA test.

3. Occurrence—Worldwide, with an estimated 35,000–40,000 deaths a year, almost all in developing countries. From 1980 through 1997, in the USA, 36 human deaths from rabies have been reported; 12 of these were probably acquired outside the USA. Of those who were probably infected within the USA, more than half died of bat associated rabies. Since the 1950s human rabies deaths in the USA have been gradually decreasing as a result of routine rabies immunization of domestic dogs and cats, and the increasing effectiveness of postexposure prophylaxis regimens.

Rabies is a disease primarily of animals. The only areas currently free of rabies in the animal population include Australia, New Zealand, New Guinea, Japan, Hawaii, Taiwan, Oceania, the UK, Ireland, Iceland, mainland Norway, Sweden, Finland, Portugal, Greece and some of the West Indies and Atlantic islands. Urban (or canine) rabies is transmitted by dogs, whereas sylvatic rabies is a disease of wild carnivores and bats, with sporadic spillover to dogs, cats and livestock. In Europe, fox rabies was widespread, but has decreased since 1978 when oral rabies immunization was begun; in western Europe the number of cases has decreased drastically since 1992, except for bat rabies. Since 1986, bat rabies cases have been reported in Denmark, Holland and West Germany. In the USA and Canada, wildlife rabies most commonly involves raccoons, skunks, foxes, coyotes and bats. There has been a progressive epizootic among raccoons in the eastern USA for more than a decade, now reaching New England, and currently among coyotes and dogs in south Texas; spread of the virus to domestic animals most frequently involves cats.

4. Reservoir—Many wild and domestic *Canidae,* including dogs, foxes, coyotes, wolves and jackals; also skunks, raccoons, mongooses and other biting mammals. Infected populations of vampire, frugivorous and insectivorous bats are found in Mexico, Central and South America; infected insectivorous bats are found in the USA, Canada and now in Europe. In developing countries, dogs remain the principal reservoir. Rabbits, opossums, squirrels, chipmunks, rats and mice are rarely infected, and their bites rarely, if ever, call for rabies prophylaxis.

5. Mode of transmission—Virus laden saliva of a rabid animal is introduced by a bite or scratch (or, very rarely, into a fresh break in the skin or through intact mucous membranes). Transmission from person to person is theoretically possible since the saliva of the infected person may contain virus, but this has never been documented. Organ (corneal) transplants taken from persons dying of undiagnosed CNS disease have resulted in rabies in the recipients. Airborne spread has been demonstrated in a cave where myriad of bats were roosting and in laboratory settings, but this occurs very rarely. In Latin America, transmission from infected vampire bats to domestic animals is common. In the USA, rabid insectivorous bats rarely transmit rabies to terrestrial animals, wild or domestic.

6. Incubation period—Usually 3-8 weeks, rarely as short as 9 days or as long as 7 years; depends on the severity of the wound, site of the wound in relation to the richness of the nerve supply and its distance from the brain, amount and strain of virus introduced, protection provided by clothing and other factors. Prolonged incubation periods have occurred in prepubertal individuals.

7. Period of communicability—In dogs and cats, usually for 3-7 days before onset of clinical signs (rarely over 4 days) and throughout the course of the disease. Longer periods of excretion before onset of clinical signs (14 days) have been observed with Ethiopian dog rabies strains. In one study, bats shed virus for 12 days before evidence of illness; in another study, skunks shed virus for at least 8 days before onset of clinical signs. Skunks may shed virus for up to 18 days before death.

8. Susceptibility and resistance—All mammals are susceptible to varying degrees, which may be influenced by the virus strain. Humans are more resistant to infection than several animal species; only approximately 40% of untreated Iranians bitten by proven rabid animals developed the disease.

9. **Methods of control —**

A. *Preventive measures:*

1) Register, license and immunize all dogs in enzootic countries; collect and euthanize ownerless animals and strays. Immunize all cats. Educate pet owners and the public that restrictions for dogs and cats are important (e.g., that pets be leashed in congested areas when not confined on owner's premises; that strange acting or sick animals of any species, domestic or wild, may be dangerous and should not be picked up or handled; that it is necessary to report such animals and animals that have bitten a person or another animal to the police and/or the local health department; that confinement and observation of such animals is a preventive measure against rabies); and that wild animals should not be kept as pets. Where dog control is sociologically impractical, repetitive total dog population immunization has been effective.

2) Maintain active surveillance for rabies in animals. Laboratory capacity should be developed to perform FA testing on all wild animals involved in human or domestic animal exposures and all domestic animals clinically suspected of having rabies. Educate physicians, veterinarians and animal control officials to obtain/euthanize/test animals involved in human and domestic animal exposures.

3) Detain and clinically observe for 10 days any healthy-appearing dog or cat known to have bitten a person (unwanted dogs and cats may be euthanized immediately and examined for rabies by fluorescent microscopy); dogs and cats showing suspicious signs of rabies should be sacrificed and tested for rabies. If the biting animal were infective at the time of the bite, signs of rabies will usually follow within 4–7 days, with a change in behavior and excitability or paralysis, followed by death. All wild mammals that have bitten a person should be sacrificed immediately and the brain examined for

evidence of rabies. In the case of bites by a normal behaving, very valuable pet or zoo animal, it may be appropriate to consider postexposure prophylaxis for the human victim, and, instead of sacrificing the animal, hold it in quarantine for 3–12 weeks.

4) Submit immediately to a laboratory the intact heads, packed in ice (not frozen), of animals that die of suspected rabies, for viral antigen testing by FA staining, or, if this is not available, by microscopic examination for Negri bodies, followed by mouse inoculation.

5) Euthanize immediately nonimmunized dogs or cats bitten by known rabid animals; if detention is elected, hold the animal in an approved secure pound or kennel for at least 6 months under veterinary supervision, and immunize against rabies 30 days before release. If previously immunized, reimmunize and detain (leashing and confinement) for at least 45 days.

6) Oral immunization of wildlife animal reservoirs using attenuated or recombinant vector vaccines has been effective in eliminating fox rabies from parts of Europe and Canada. The technique is being evaluated in the USA, using air drop of bait containing recombinant vaccine.

7) Cooperative programs with wildlife conservation authorities to reduce fox, skunk, raccoon and other terrestrial wildlife hosts of sylvatic rabies may be used in circumscribed enzootic areas near campsites and areas of human habitation. If such focal depopulation is undertaken, it must be maintained to prevent repopulation from the periphery.

8) Individuals at high risk (e.g., veterinarians, wildlife conservation personnel and park rangers in enzootic or epizootic areas, staff of quarantine kennels, laboratory and field personnel working with rabies, and long term travelers to rabies endemic areas) should receive preexposure immunization. Three types of rabies vaccine are currently available in the USA: Human Diploid Cell rabies Vaccine (HDCV), an inactivated vaccine prepared from virus grown in human diploid cell culture; Rabies Vaccine, Adsorbed (RVA), an inactivated vaccine grown in rhesus diploid cells; and Purified Chick Embryo Cell Vaccine (PCEC), an inactivated vaccine grown in primary cultures of chicken fibroblasts. (Other potent cell culture vaccines are available in other countries.) Each vaccine can be given in three 1.0 ml (IM) doses on days 0, 7 and 21 or 28: This regimen has been so satisfactory that routine postimmunization serologic testing is not routinely recommended but may be advisable for groups at high risk of exposure or immunodeficient persons.

If risk of exposure continues, either single booster doses are given, or preferably serum is tested for neutralizing antibody every 2 years, with booster doses given when indicated. HDCV has also been approved for preexposure immunization at an intradermal (ID) dose of 0.1 ml given on days 0, 7 and 21 or 28. If immunization is given in preparation for travel to a rabies endemic area, 30 or more days should elapse after the 3-dose series before departure; otherwise, the IM regimen should be used. Results with ID immunization have generally been good in the USA, but the mean antibody response is somewhat lower and may be of shorter duration than with the 1.0 ml dose given IM. However, the antibody response to ID immunization has been erratic in some groups who were on chloroquine for antimalarial chemoprophylaxis; therefore, ID immunization should not be used in this situation unless facilities are available for testing sera for development of neutralizing antibodies. Although immune response has not been evaluated for antimalarials structurally related to chloroquine (e.g. mefloquine, hydroxychloroquine), similar precautions for individuals receiving these drugs should be followed. RVA and PCEC should not be given intradermally.

9) Prevention of rabies after animal bites ("postexposure prophylaxis") consists of the following:

a) **Treatment of bite wound:** The most effective rabies prevention is immediate and thorough cleaning with soap or detergent and flushing with water all wounds caused by an animal bite or scratch. The wound should not be sutured unless unavoidable for cosmetic or tissue support reasons. Sutures, if required, should be placed after local infiltration of antiserum (see 9b, next below); they should be loose and not interfere with free bleeding and drainage.

b) **Specific immunologic protection:** Immunologic prevention of rabies in humans is provided by administration of human rabies immune globulin (HRIG) as soon as possible after exposure to neutralize the virus at the bite wound site, and then by giving vaccine at a different site to elicit active immunity. Only HRIG is licensed in the USA, purified equine (ERIG) IG is available in other countries. Animal studies suggest that human disease caused by the Australian bat lyssavirus may be prevented by rabies vaccine and rabies immune globulin, and such post exposure prophylaxis is recommended for persons bitten or scratched by any bat in Australia. In contrast, rabies vaccine is not effective for the treatment of African bat lyssaviruses.

Passive immunization: HRIG should be used in a single dose of 20 IU/kg; half should be infiltrated into and around the bite wound if possible, and the rest given IM. If serum of animal origin is used, an intradermal or subcutaneous test dose should precede its administration to detect allergic sensitivity, and the dose should be increased to a total of 40 IU/kg.

Vaccine: Preferably HDCV (or RVA) in five 1.0 ml IM doses in the deltoid region; the first as soon as possible after the bite (at the same time as the single dose of HRIG is given), and the other doses 3, 7, 14 and 28–35 days after the first dose. (The intradermal dose/route at multiple sites is being used in several countries for postexposure prophylaxis, but this has not been approved in the USA.) In individuals with possible immunodeficiency, a serum specimen should be collected at the time the last dose of vaccine is administered and tested for rabies antibodies. If sensitization reactions appear in the course of immunization, consult health department or infectious disease consultants for guidance. If the person has had a previous full course of antirabies immunization with an approved vaccine, or had developed neutralizing antibodies after preexposure immunization (see 9A8, above) or after a postexposure regimen, only 2 doses of vaccine need to be given— one immediately and one 3 days later. With severe exposure (e.g., head bites), a third dose may be given on day 7. HRIG is not used with this regimen.

c) The following is a general guide to prophylaxis in different circumstances: If a bite were unprovoked, the animal not apprehended, and rabies present in that species in the area, administer HRIG and vaccine. Bites of wild carnivorous mammals and bats are considered potential rabies exposures unless negated by laboratory tests. If available, the biting animal may be euthanized immediately (with the owner's and health authorities' concurrence) and its brain examined by FA technique to determine whether antirabies treatment is necessary. The decision whether to administer HRIG and vaccine immediately after exposure to dogs and cats or during the observation period (see 9A3, above) should be based on the behavior of the animal, the presence of rabies in the area, and the circumstances of the bite. (See Guide, below.)

d) Immunization with current rabies vaccines carries a very small risk of postimmunization encephalitis; only 2 cases of transient neuroparalytic illness have been reported in the USA. Local reactions, such as pain, erythema, swelling or itching at the injection site were reported in 25% of those receiving five 1.0 ml doses. Mild systemic reactions of headache, nausea, muscle aches, abdominal pain and dizziness were reported in about 20%. "Serum sickness-like" reactions, including primarily urticaria with generalized itching and wheezing, were reported infrequently.

However, among those receiving booster doses for preexposure prophylaxis, hypersensitivity reactions occur in approximately 6% of recipients 2–21 days after HDCV, presenting as a generalized pruritic rash, urticaria, possible arthralgia, arthritis, angioedema, nausea, vomiting, fever and malaise. These symptoms have responded to antihistamines; a few have required corticosteroids or epinephrine. Persons exposed to rabies who develop these symptoms should complete the required number of injections but in a setting where reactions can be treated. Systemic allergic reactions in those receiving booster doses of RVA have been rare (reported in less than 1%). No significant reactions have been attributed to HRIG (of human origin); however, antiserum from a nonhuman source produces serum sickness in 5%–40% of recipients. Newer purified animal globulins, in particular equine globulin, have only a 1% risk of reactions. These risks must be weighed against the risk of contracting rabies.

e) Management of animal bites—adapted from the Eighth Report of the WHO Expert Committee on Rabies, 1992 and from the USPHS Advisory Committee on Immunization Practices (*MMWR*, Rabies Prevention–United States, 1999;48 No. RR-1:January 1999)—should include:

Checklist for Treatment of Animal Bites

1. Clean and flush the wound immediately (first aid).
2. Thorough wound cleansing under medical supervision.
3. Rabies immune globulin and/or vaccine as indicated.
4. Tetanus prophylaxis and antibacterial treatment when required.
5. No sutures or wound closure advised unless unavoidable.

B. Control of patient, contacts and the immediate environment:

1) Report to local health authority: Obligatory case report required in most states and countries, Class 2A (see Communicable Disease Reporting).
2) Isolation: Contact isolation for respiratory secretions for duration of the illness.
3) Concurrent disinfection: Of saliva and articles soiled therewith. Although transmission from a patient to attending personnel has not been documented, immediate attendants should be warned of the potential hazard of infection from saliva, and should wear rubber gloves, protective gowns, and protection to avoid exposure from a patient coughing saliva in the attendant's face.

4) Quarantine: None.

5) Immunization of contacts: Contacts who have an open wound or mucous membrane exposure to the patient's saliva should receive antirabies specific treatment (see 9A 9b, above).

6) Investigation of contacts and source of infection: Search for rabid animal and for people and other animals bitten.

7) Specific treatment: For clinical rabies, intensive supportive medical care.

C. *Epidemic (epizootic) measures:* Applicable only to animals; a sporadic disease in humans.

1) Establish area control under authority of state laws, public health regulations and local ordinances, in cooperation with appropriate wildlife conservation and animal health authorities.

2) Immunize dogs and cats through officially sponsored, intensified mass programs that provide immunizations at temporary and emergency stations. For protection of other domestic animals, approved vaccines appropriate for each animal species must be used.

3) In urban areas of the USA and other developed countries, strict enforcement of regulations requiring collection, detention and euthanasia of ownerless and stray dogs, and of nonimmunized dogs found off owners' premises; control of the dog population by castration, spaying or drugs have been effective in breaking transmission cycles.

4) Immunization of wildlife by using baits containing vaccine has successfully contained fox rabies in western Europe and Canada and is in clinical trials in the USA; this should prove effective in controlling disease spread in epizootic areas.

D. *Disaster implications:* A potential problem if the disease is freshly introduced or enzootic in an area where there are many stray dogs or wild reservoir animals.

E. *International measures:*

1) Strict compliance by common carriers and travelers with national laws and regulations in most rabies free countries or states that require quarantine for 4-6 months. Immunization of animals, certificates of health and origin, or microchip identification of animals may be required.

2) WHO Collaborating Centres.

RABIES POSTEXPOSURE PROPHYLAXIS GUIDE[1]

The following recommendations are only a guide. In applying them, take into account the animal species involved, the circumstances of the bite or other exposure, immunization status of the animal and presence of rabies in the region. Local or state health officials should be consulted if questions arise about the need for rabies prophylaxis.

Animal type	Evaluation and disposition of animal	Postexposure prophylaxis recommendations
Dogs, cats and ferrets	Healthy and available for 10 days of observation	Persons should not begin prophylaxis unless animal develops clinical signs of rabies.*
	Rabid or suspected rabid	Immediately immunize
	Unknown (e.g., escaped)	Consult public health official
Skunks, raccoons, foxes and most other carnivores; bats	Regard as rabid unless animal proven negative by laboratory tests†	Consider immediate immunization
Livestock, small rodents, lagomorphs (hares and rabbits), large rodents (woodchucks and beavers) and other mamals	Consider individually	Consult public health officials. Bites of squirrels, hamsters, guinea pigs, gerbils, chipmunks, rats, mice, other small rodents, rabbits and hares almost never require antirabies postexposure prophylaxis.

*During the 10-day observation period, begin postexposure prophylaxis at the first sign of rabies in a dog, cat or ferret that has bitten someone. If the animal exhibits clinical signs of rabies, it should be euthanized immediately and tested.
†The animal should be euthanized and tested as soon as possible. Holding for observation is not recommended. Discontinue vaccine if immunofluorescence test results of the animal are negative.
[1]Adapted from recommendations of the Immunization Practices Advisory Committee (ACIP), MMWR Recommendations and Reports, Vol. 48 / No. RR-1; 1999.

RAT BITE FEVER   ICD-9 026; ICD-10 A25

Two bacterial diseases, rare in the USA, are included under the general term of rat bite fever; streptobacillosis is caused by *Streptobacillus moniliformis (Haverhillia multiformis)* and spirillary fever or sodoku by *Spirillum minus (minor)*. Because they have clinical and epidemiologic similarities, only streptobacillosis is presented in detail; variations manifested by *Spirillum minus* infection (which is even rarer in the USA) are noted in a brief summary.

I. STREPTOBACILLOSIS   ICD-9 026.1; ICD-10 A25.1
(Streptobacillary fever, Haverhill fever, Epidemic arthritic erythema, Rat bite fever due to *Streptobacillus moniliformis*)

1. Identification—An abrupt onset of chills and fever, headache and muscle pain, is followed within 1-3 days by a maculopapular rash most marked on the extremities. The rash may also be petechial, purpuric or pustular. One or more large joints then usually become swollen, red and painful. There is usually a history of a rat bite within 10 days that healed normally. Relapses are common. Bacterial endocarditis, pericarditis, parotitis, tenosynovitis and focal abscesses of soft tissues or the brain may occur late in untreated cases, with a case-fatality rate of 7%-10%.

Laboratory confirmation is made by isolation of the organism by inoculating material from the primary lesion, lymph node, blood, joint fluid or pus into the appropriate bacteriologic medium or laboratory animals (guinea pigs or mice that are not naturally infected). Serum antibodies may be detected by agglutination tests.

2. Infectious agent—*Streptobacillus moniliformis.*

3. Occurrence—Worldwide, but uncommon in North and South America and most European countries. Recent cases in the USA have followed bites by laboratory rats and rarely by pet rats.

4. Reservoir—An infected rat, rarely other animals (squirrel, weasel, gerbil).

5. Mode of transmission—Infection is transmitted by urine or secretions of mouth, nose or conjunctival sac of an infected animal, most frequently introduced by biting. Sporadic cases occur without history of a bite. Blood from an experimental laboratory animal has infected humans. Direct contact with rats is not necessary; infection has occurred in people working or living in rat infested buildings. In outbreaks, contaminated milk or water has usually been suspected as the vehicle of infection.

6. Incubation period—From 3 to 10 days, rarely longer.

7. Period of communicability—Not directly transmitted from person to person.

8. **Susceptibility and resistance**—No information.

9. **Methods of control**—

A. *Preventive measures:* Ratproof dwellings and reduce rat populations. Penicillin or doxycycline could be used as prophylaxis following a rat bite.

B. *Control of patient, contacts and the immediate environment:*

1) Report to local health authority: Obligatory report of epidemics; no case report required, Class 4 (see Communicable Disease Reporting).
2) Isolation: No special precautions are recommended.
3) Concurrent disinfection: None.
4) Quarantine: None.
5) Immunization of contacts: None.
6) Investigation of contacts and source of infection: Only to establish whether there are additional unrecognized cases.
7) Specific treatment: Penicillin or tetracyclines for 7–10 days.

C. *Epidemic measures:* A cluster of cases requires search for a common source, possibly contaminated food and water.

D. *Disaster implications:* None.

E. *International measures:* None.

II. SPIRILLOSIS   ICD-9 026.0; ICD-10 A25.0
(Spirillary fever, Sodoku, Rat bite fever due to *Spirillum minus*)

Rat bite fever caused by *Spirillum minus* is the common form of sporadic rat bite fever in Asia, predominantly in Japan. Untreated, the case-fatality rate is approximately 10%. Clinically, *Spirillum minus* disease differs from streptobacillary fever in the rarity of arthritic symptoms and the distinctive rash of reddish or purplish plaques. The incubation period is 1–3 weeks, and the previously healed bite wound reactivates when symptoms appear. Laboratory methods are essential for differentiation; animal inoculation is used for isolation of the *Spirillum*.

RELAPSING FEVER   ICD-9 087; ICD-10 A68

1. **Identification**—A systemic spirochetal disease in which periods of fever lasting 2–9 days alternate with afebrile periods of 2–4 days; the number of relapses varies from 1 to 10 or more. Each febrile period

terminates by crisis. The total duration of the louseborne disease averages 13-16 days; the tickborne disease usually lasts longer. Transitory petechial rashes are common during the initial febrile period. The overall case-fatality rate in untreated cases is between 2% and 10%.

Diagnosis is made by demonstration of the infectious agent in darkfield preparations of fresh blood or stained thick or thin blood films, by intraperitoneal inoculation of laboratory rats or mice with blood taken during the febrile period or by blood culture in special media.

2. Infectious agents—In louseborne disease, *Borrelia recurrentis*, a Gram-negative spirochete. In tickborne disease, many different strains have been distinguished by area of first isolation and/or vector, rather than by inherent biologic differences. Strains isolated during a relapse often show antigenic differences from those obtained during the immediately preceding paroxysm.

3. Occurrence—Characteristically, epidemic where it is spread by lice; endemic where it is spread by ticks. Louseborne relapsing fever occurs in limited areas in Asia, eastern Africa (Ethiopia and the Sudan), the highland areas of central Africa and South America. Tickborne disease is endemic throughout tropical Africa; foci exist in Spain, northern Africa, Saudi Arabia, Iran, India and parts of central Asia, as well as in North and South America. Sporadic human cases and occasional outbreaks of tickborne disease occur in limited areas of several western states (USA) and western Canada.

4. Reservoir—For *B. recurrentis*, humans; for tickborne relapsing fever borreliae, wild rodents and argasid (soft) ticks through transovarian transmission.

5. Mode of transmission—Vectorborne; not directly transmitted from person to person. Louseborne relapsing fever is acquired by crushing an infective louse, *Pediculus humanus*, so that it contaminates the bite wound or an abrasion of the skin. In tickborne disease, people are infected by the bite or coxal fluid of an argasid tick, principally *Ornithodoros hermsi* and *O. turicata* in the USA, *O. rudis* and *O. talaje* in Central and South America, *O. moubata* and *O. hispanica* in Africa and *O. tholozani* in the Near and Middle East. These ticks usually feed at night, rapidly engorge and leave the host; they have a longevity of 2-5 years and remain infective for their lifespan.

6. Incubation period—From 5 to 15 days; usually 8 days.

7. Period of communicability—The louse becomes infective 4-5 days after ingestion of blood from an infective person and remains so for life (20-40 days). Infected ticks can live for several years without feeding; they remain infective during this period and pass the infection transovariantly to their progeny.

8. Susceptibility and resistance—Susceptibility is general. Duration and degree of immunity after clinical attack are unknown; repeated infections may occur.

9. Methods of control—

A. *Preventive measures:*

1) Control lice by measures prescribed for louseborne typhus fever (see Typhus fever, Epidemic louseborne, 9A).
2) Control ticks by measures prescribed for Rocky Mountain spotted fever, 9A. Tick-infested human habitations may present problems, and eradication may be difficult. Rodent-proofing structures to prevent future colonization by rodents and their soft ticks is the mainstay of prevention and control. Spraying with approved acaricides such as diazinon, chlorpyrifos, propoxur or permethrin may be tried.
3) Use personal protective measures, including repellents and permethrin on clothing and bedding for people with exposure in endemic foci.
4) Antibiotic chemoprophylaxis with tetracyclines may be taken after exposure (arthropod bites) when the risk of acquiring the infection is high.

B. *Control of patient, contacts and the immediate environment:*

1) Report to local health authority: Report of louseborne relapsing fever required as a Disease under Surveillance by WHO, Class 1A; tickborne disease, in selected areas, Class 3B (see Communicable Disease Reporting).
2) Isolation: Blood/body fluid precautions. The patients, their clothing, all household contacts and the immediate environment should be deloused or freed of ticks.
3) Concurrent disinfection: None, if proper disinfestation has been carried out.
4) Quarantine: None.
5) Immunization of contacts: None.
6) Investigation of contacts and source of infection: For the individual tickborne case, search for additional associated cases and for sources of infection; for louseborne disease, application of appropriate lousicidal preparation to infested contacts (see Pediculosis, 9B6 and 9B7).
7) Specific treatment: Tetracyclines.

C. *Epidemic measures:* For louseborne relapsing fever, when reporting has been good and cases are localized, apply 1% permethrin dust or spray (an insecticide with residual effect) to contacts and their clothing, and permethrin spray at 0.003–0.3 kg/hectare (2.47 acres) to the immediate environment of all reported cases.

Provide clothes washing and bathing facilities for the affected population; establish active surveillance. Where infection is known to be widespread, apply permethrin systematically to all people in the community. For tickborne relapsing fever, apply permethrin or other acaricide to target areas where vector ticks are thought to be present; for sustained control, a treatment cycle of 1 month is recommended during the transmission season.

D. *Disaster implications:* A serious potential hazard among louse-infested populations. Epidemics are common in wars, famine and other situations where the prevalence of pediculosis is enhanced, as among overcrowded, malnourished populations with poor personal hygiene.

E. *International measures:*

1) Telegraphic notification by governments to WHO and adjacent countries of the occurrence of an outbreak of louseborne relapsing fever in an area previously free of the disease.

2) Louseborne relapsing fever is not a disease subject to the International Health Regulations, but the measures outlined in 9E1, above, should be followed since it is a Disease under Surveillance by WHO.

RESPIRATORY DISEASE, ACUTE VIRAL
(Excluding influenza)
(Acute viral rhinitis, Pharyngitis, Laryngitis)

Numerous acute respiratory illnesses of known and presumed viral etiology are grouped here. Clinically and by CIOMS taxonomy, infections of the upper respiratory tract (above the epiglottis) can be designated as acute viral rhinitis or acute viral pharyngitis (common cold, upper respiratory infections) and infections involving the lower respiratory tract (below the epiglottis) can be designated as croup (laryngotracheitis), acute viral tracheobronchitis, bronchitis, bronchiolitis or acute viral pneumonia. These respiratory syndromes are associated with a large number of viruses, each of which is capable of producing a wide spectrum of acute respiratory illness and which differ in etiology between children and adults.

The illnesses caused by known agents have important common epidemiologic attributes, such as reservoir and mode of transmission. Many of the viruses invade any part of the respiratory tract; others show a predilection for certain anatomic sites. Some predispose to bacterial complications. Morbidity and mortality from acute respiratory diseases are especially significant in children. In adults, the relatively high incidence and resulting disability, with consequent economic loss, make acute respiratory diseases a major health problem worldwide. As a group, acute respiratory diseases are one of the leading causes of death from any infectious disease.

Several other infections of the respiratory tract are recognized as disease entities and are presented as separate chapters because they are sufficiently distinctive in their clinical and epidemiologic manifestations and occur in such regular association with a single infectious agent: influenza, psittacosis, hantavirus pulmonary syndrome, chlamydial pneumonia, vesicular pharyngitis (herpangina) and epidemic myalgia (pleurodynia) are examples. Particularly in pediatric practice, influenza must be considered in cases of acute respiratory tract disease.

Symptoms of upper respiratory tract infection, mainly pharyngotonsillitis, can be produced by bacterial agents, of which group A streptococcus is the most common. Viral infections should be differentiated from bacterial or other infections for which specific antimicrobial measures are available. For instance, although viral pharyngotonsillitis is more common, group A streptococcal infection should be ruled out by rapid streptococcal antigen test and culture, particularly in children over 2 years of age. In addition, in nonstreptococcal outbreaks, it is important to identify the cause in a representative sample of cases by appropriate clinical and laboratory methods to rule out other diseases (e.g., mycoplasmal pneumonia, chlamydial pneumonia, legionellosis and Q fever, for which specific treatments may be effective).

I. ACUTE VIRAL RHINITIS—
THE COMMON COLD   ICD-9 460; ICD-10 J00
(Rhinitis, Coryza [acute])

1. Identification—An acute catarrhal infection of the upper respiratory tract characterized by coryza, sneezing, lacrimation, irritated nasopharynx, chilliness and malaise lasting 2–7 days. Fever is uncommon in children over 3 years old and rare in adults. No fatalities have been reported, but disability is important because it affects work performance and industrial and school absenteeism; illness may be accompanied by laryngitis, tracheitis or bronchitis and may predispose to more serious complications such as sinusitis and otitis media. WBC counts are usually normal, and bacterial flora of the respiratory tract are within normal limits in the absence of complications.

Cell or organ culture studies of nasal secretions may demonstrate a known virus in 20%–35% of cases. Specific clinical, epidemiologic and other manifestations aid differentiation from similar diseases due to toxic, allergic, physical or psychologic stimuli.

2. Infectious agents—Rhinoviruses, of which there are more than 100 recognized serotypes, are the major known etiologic agents of the common cold in adults; they account for 20%–40% of cases, especially in the fall season. Coronaviruses, such as 229E, OC43 and B814, are responsible for about 10%–15% and influenza for 10%–15% of the common colds in adults; they appear to be especially important in the winter and early spring, when the prevalence of rhinoviruses is low. Other known respiratory viruses account for a small proportion of common colds in adults. In infants and children, parainfluenza viruses, respiratory syncytial viruses (RSV), influenza, adenoviruses, certain enteroviruses and coronaviruses cause common cold-like illnesses. The etiology of about half of common colds has not been identified.

3. Occurrence—Worldwide, both endemic and epidemic. In temperate zones, incidence rises in fall, winter and spring; in tropical settings, incidence is highest in the rainy season. Many people, except in small isolated communities, have one to six colds yearly. Incidence is highest in children under 5 years and gradually declines with increasing age.

4. Reservoir—Humans.

5. Mode of transmission—Presumably by direct contact or by inhalation of airborne droplets; more importantly, indirectly by hands and articles freshly soiled by discharges of nose and throat of an infected person. Rhinovirus, RSV and probably other similar viruses are transmitted by contaminated hands carrying virus to the mucous membranes of the eye or nose.

6. Incubation period—Between 12 hours and 5 days, usually 48 hours, varying with the agent.

7. Period of communicability—Nasal washings taken 24 hours before onset and for 5 days after onset have produced symptoms in experimentally infected volunteers.

8. Susceptibility and resistance—Susceptibility is universal. Inapparent and abortive infections occur; frequency of healthy carriers is undetermined but known to be rare with some viral agents, notably rhinoviruses. The frequently repeated attacks are most likely due to the multiplicity of agents, but may be due to a short duration of homologous immunity to different serotypes of the same virus, or to other causes.

9. Methods of control—

   A. Preventive measures:

     1) Educate the public in personal hygiene, such as frequent handwashing, covering the mouth when coughing and sneezing, and sanitary disposal of oral and nasal discharges.

     2) When possible, avoid crowding in living and sleeping quarters, especially in institutions, in barracks and on shipboard. Provide adequate ventilation.

3) Oral live adenovirus vaccines have proven effective against adenovirus 4, 7 and 21 infections in military recruits, but are not indicated in civilian populations because of the low incidence of specific disease.

4) Avoid smoking in households with children, whose risk of pneumonia increases when exposed to passive smoke.

B. Control of patient, contacts and the immediate environment:

1) Report to local health authority: Official report not ordinarily justifiable, Class 5 (see Communicable Disease Reporting).

2), 3), 4), 5), 6) and 7): Isolation, Concurrent disinfection, Quarantine, Immunization of contacts, Investigation of contacts and source of infection and Specific treatment: See section II, 9B2 through 9B7, below.

C., D. and **E. Epidemic measures, Disaster implications** and **International measures:** See section II, 9C, 9D and 9E, below.

II. ACUTE FEBRILE RESPIRATORY DISEASE   ICD-9 461–466; 480; ICD-10 J01–J06; J12
(Excluding Streptococcal pharyngitis, q.v., JO2.0)

1. Identification—Viral diseases of the respiratory tract may be characterized by fever and one or more systemic reactions, such as chills or chilliness, headache, general aching, malaise and anorexia; occasionally in infants by GI disturbances. Localizing signs also occur at various sites in the respiratory tract, either alone or in combination, such as rhinitis, pharyngitis or tonsillitis, laryngitis, laryngotracheitis, bronchitis, bronchiolitis, pneumonitis or pneumonia. There may be associated conjunctivitis. Symptoms and signs usually subside in 2–5 days without complications; infection may, however, be complicated by bacterial sinusitis, otitis media or, more rarely, bacterial pneumonia. WBC counts and respiratory bacterial flora are within normal limits unless modified by complications.

In very young infants, it may be difficult to distinguish between pneumonia, sepsis and meningitis. Specific diagnosis depends on isolation of the etiologic agent from respiratory secretions in appropriate cell or organ cultures, identification of viral antigen in nasopharyngeal cells by FA, ELISA and RIA tests and/or antibody studies of paired sera.

2. Infectious agents—Parainfluenza virus, types 1, 2, 3 and rarely type 4; respiratory syncytial virus (RSV); adenovirus, especially types 1-5, 7, 14 and 21; rhinoviruses; certain coronaviruses; certain types of coxsackievirus groups A and B; and echoviruses are considered etiologic agents of acute febrile respiratory illnesses. Influenza virus (see Influenza) can produce the same clinical picture, especially in children. Some of these agents have a greater tendency to cause more severe illnesses; others have a predilection for certain age groups and populations. RSV, the major viral respiratory tract pathogen of early infancy, produces illness with greatest frequency during the first 2 years of life; it is the major known etiologic agent of bronchiolitis and is a cause of pneumonia, croup, bronchitis, otitis media and febrile upper respiratory illness. The parainfluenza viruses are the major known etiologic agents of croup and also cause bronchitis, pneumonia, bronchiolitis and febrile upper respiratory illness in pediatric populations. RSV and the parainfluenza viruses may cause symptomatic disease in adults, particularly the debilitated elderly. Adenoviruses are associated with several forms of respiratory disease; types 4, 7 and 21 are common causes of acute respiratory disease in nonimmunized military recruits; in young infants, adenoviruses are the most aggressive viral agents that cause significant mortality.

3. Occurrence—Worldwide. Seasonal in temperate zones, with greatest incidence during fall and winter and occasionally spring. In tropical zones, respiratory infections tend to be more frequent in wet and colder weather. In large communities, some viral illnesses are constantly present, usually with little seasonal pattern (e.g., adenovirus type 1); others tend to occur in sharp outbreaks (e.g., RSV).

Annual incidence is high, particularly in infants and children, with 2-6 episodes per child per year, and depends on the number of susceptibles and the virulence of the agent. During autumn, winter and spring, attack rates for preschool children may average 2% per week, as compared to 1% per week for school aged children and 0.5% per week for adults. Under special host and environmental conditions, certain viral infections may disable more than half of a closed community within a few weeks (e.g., outbreaks of adenovirus type 4 or 7 in military recruits). In the USA, two-thirds of all infants will be infected with RSV by 12 months, of whom one-third will develop lower respiratory tract symptoms. Of these symptomatic RSV infected infants, 2.5% will be hospitalized and 1/1,000 infants will die.

4. Reservoir—Humans. Many known viruses produce inapparent infections; adenoviruses may remain latent in tonsils and adenoids. Viruses of the same group cause similar infections in many animal species but are of minor importance as sources of human infections.

5. Mode of transmission—Directly by oral contact or by droplet spread; indirectly by hands, handkerchiefs, eating utensils or other articles freshly soiled by respiratory discharges of an infected person. Viruses discharged in the feces, including enteroviruses and adenoviruses, may be transmitted by the fecal-oral route. Outbreaks of illness due to adenovirus types 3, 4 and 7 have been related to swimming pools.

6. Incubation period—From 1 to 10 days.

7. Period of communicability—Shortly prior to and for the duration of active disease; little is known about subclinical or latent infections. Especially in infants, RSV shedding may very rarely persist for several weeks or longer after clinical symptoms subside.

8. Susceptibility and resistance—Susceptibility is universal. Illness is more frequent and more severe in infants, children and the elderly. Infection induces specific antibodies that are usually short lived. Reinfection with RSV and parainfluenza viruses is common, but the illness is generally milder. Individuals with compromised cardiac, pulmonary or immune systems are at increased risk of severe illness.

9. Methods of control—

A. *Preventive measures:* See section I, 9A, above. Infants at high risk of RSV related complications include infants and children younger than 2 years with chronic lung disease who have required medical therapy for lung disease within 6 months of the RSV season and premature infants 32 to 35 weeks gestation at birth. These high risk infants may benefit from RSV immune globulin intravenous (RSV-IGIV). In addition, palivizumab, an RSV monoclonal antibody preparation that is given IM, has reduced RSV related hospitalization by about half in these infants. Of importance, RSV-IGIV is contraindicated and palivizumab is not recommended for those with cyanotic congenital heart disease because of possible safety concerns.

B. *Control of patient, contacts and the immediate environment:*

1) Report to local health authority: Obligatory report of epidemics; no individual case report, Class 4 (see Communicable Disease Reporting).
2) Isolation: Contact isolation is desirable in children's hospital wards. Outside of hospitals, ill people should avoid direct and indirect exposure of young children, debilitated or aged people or patients with other illnesses.
3) Concurrent disinfection: Of eating and drinking utensils; sanitary disposal of oral and nasal discharges.
4) Quarantine: None.
5) Immunization of contacts: None.
6) Investigation of contacts and source of infection: Not generally indicated.
7) Specific treatment: None. Indiscriminate use of antibiotics is to be discouraged; they should be reserved for patients with group A streptococcal pharyngitis and for patients with identified bacterial complications such as otitis media, pneumonia or sinusitis. There is a lack of consensus regarding appropriate management of the infant with RSV infection, specifically with respect to the use of aerosolized ribavirin.

Despite a number of studies in the USA and Canada, no clear improvement in clinical outcomes attributed to the use of aerosolized ribavirin is consistent across all studies of both ventilated and nonventilated infants with RSV infection. Cough medicines, decongestants and antihistaminics are of questionable effectiveness and may be hazardous, especially in children.

C. Epidemic measures: No effective measures known. Some nosocomial transmission can be prevented by good infection control procedures, including handwashing; procedures such as ultraviolet irradiation, aerosols and dust control have not proven useful. Avoid crowding (see section I, 9A2, above).

D. Disaster implications: None.

E. International measures: WHO Collaborating Centres.

RICKETTSIOSES, TICKBORNE ICD-9 082; ICD-10 A77
(Spotted fever group)

Rickettsioses are a group of clinically similar diseases caused by closely related rickettsiae. They are transmitted by ixodid (hard) ticks, which are widely distributed throughout the world; tick species differ markedly by geographic area. For all of these rickettsial fevers, control measures are similar, and the tetracyclines and chloramphenicol are effective.

Enzyme immunoassays and IFA tests become positive generally in the second week of illness; CF tests using group specific spotted fever antigens become positive somewhat later. The Weil-Felix tests using *Proteus* OX-19 and *Proteus* OX-2 antigens are much less specific and should be confirmed by more specific serologic tests.

I. ROCKY MOUNTAIN SPOTTED
   FEVER   ICD-9 082.0; ICD-10 A77.0
(North American tick typhus, New World spotted fever, Tickborne typhus fever, São Paulo fever)

1. Identification—This prototype disease of the spotted fever group rickettsiae is characterized by sudden onset of moderate to high fever, which ordinarily persists for 2–3 weeks in untreated cases, significant malaise, deep muscle pain, severe headache, chills and conjunctival injection. A maculopapular rash generally appears on the extremities on the third to fifth day; this soon includes the palms and soles and spreads rapidly to much of the body. A petechial exanthem occurs in 40% to 60% of patients, generally on or after the sixth day. The case-fatality rate ranges between 13% and 25% in the absence of specific therapy; with prompt recognition and treatment, death is uncommon, yet 3%–5% of cases reported in the USA during recent years have been fatal. Risk factors associated with more severe disease and death include delayed antibiotic therapy and patient age greater than 40 years. Absence, delayed appearance or failure to recognize the typical rash, especially in dark-skinned individuals contribute to delay in diagnosis and increased fatality.

Early Rocky Mountain spotted fever (RMSF) may be confused with ehrlichiosis, meningococcemia (see Meningitis) and enteroviral infection.

Diagnosis is confirmed by serologic response to specific antigens. During the early stages, rickettsiae may be detected in blood by PCR and in skin biopsies using immunostains or PCR.

2. Infectious agent—*Rickettsia rickettsii.*

3. Occurrence—Throughout the USA, primarily from April through September. Nearly 50% of cases reported in 1993 were from the south Atlantic region and over 20% from the western south-central region; the highest incidence rates were seen in North Carolina and Oklahoma. Few cases are reported from the Rocky Mountain region. In the western USA, adult males are infected most frequently, while in the east, the incidence is higher in children; the difference relates to conditions of exposure to infected ticks. Infection also has been documented in Canada, western and central Mexico, Panamá, Costa Rica, Colombia, Argentina and Brazil.

4. Reservoir—Maintained in nature in ticks by transovarial and transstadial passage. The rickettsiae can be transmitted to dogs, various rodents and other animals; animal infections are usually subclinical, but disease in rodents and dogs has been observed.

5. Mode of transmission—Ordinarily by bite of an infected tick. At least 4–6 hours of attachment and feeding on blood by the tick are required before the rickettsiae become reactivated and infectious for people. Contamination of breaks in the skin or mucous membranes with crushed tissues or feces of the tick may also lead to infection. In eastern and southern USA, the common vector is the American dog tick, *Dermacentor variabilis,* and in northwestern USA, the Rocky Mountain wood tick, *D. andersoni.* The principal vector in Latin America is *A. cajennense.*

6. Incubation period—From 3 to about 14 days.

7. Period of communicability—Not directly transmitted from person to person. The tick remains infective for life, commonly as long as 18 months.

8. Susceptibility and resistance—Susceptibility is general. One attack probably confers lasting immunity.

9. Methods of control —

A. Preventive measures:

1) See also Lyme disease, 9A. Remove attached or crawling ticks after exposures to tick infested habitats.
2) Deticking dogs and using tick repellent collars on them minimizes the tick population near residences.
3) No vaccine is presently licensed in the USA. The trial of a conventional killed organism vaccine failed to prevent infection in 75% of challenged recipients.

B. Control of patient, contacts and the immediate environment:

1) Report to local health authority: Case report obligatory in most states (USA) and most countries, Class 2B (see Communicable Disease Reporting).
2) Isolation: None.
3) Concurrent disinfection: Carefully remove all ticks from patients.
4) Quarantine: None.
5) Immunization of contacts: Unnecessary.
6) Investigation of contacts and source of infection: Not profitable except as a community measure. (See Lyme disease, 9C.)
7) Specific treatment: Tetracyclines (usually doxycyline) in daily oral or intravenous doses for 5–7 days and for at least 48 hours once the patient is afebrile. Chloramphenical may also be used, but is administered only when there is an absolute contraindication for using tetracyclines. Treatment should be initiated on clinical and epidemiologic considerations without waiting for laboratory confirmation of the diagnosis.

C. Epidemic measures: See Lyme disease, 9C.

D. Disaster implications: None.

E. International measures: WHO Collaborating Centres.

II. BOUTONNEUSE FEVER   ICD-9 082.1; ICD-10 A77.1
(Mediterranean tick fever, Mediterranean spotted fever, Marseilles fever, Kenya tick typhus, India tick typhus, Israeli tick typhus)

1. Identification—A mild to severe febrile illness of a few days to 2 weeks; there may be a primary lesion or eschar at the site of a tick bite. This eschar (tâche noire), often evident at the onset of fever, is a small ulcer 2–5 mm in diameter with a black center and red areola; regional lymph nodes are often enlarged. In some areas, such as the Negev in Israel, primary lesions are rarely seen. A generalized maculopapular erythematous rash usually involving palms and soles appears about the fourth to fifth day and persists for 6–7 days; with antibiotic treatment, fever lasts no more than 2 days. The case-fatality rate is very low (less than 3%) even without specific therapy.

Diagnosis is confirmed by using serologic tests or by PCR or immunostains of biopsied tissues. Culturing blood on human fibroblast monolayers permits demonstration of the organisms by DFA testing.

2. Infectious agent—*Rickettsia conorii* and closely related organisms.

3. Occurrence—Widely distributed throughout the African Continent, in India and in those parts of Europe and the Middle East adjacent to the Mediterranean, and Black and Caspian Seas. Expansion of the European endemic zone to the north occurs because tourists often carry their dogs with them; the dogs acquire infected ticks, which establish tick colonies when they return home, and transmission occurs. In more temperate areas, the highest incidence is during warmer months when ticks are numerous; in tropical areas, throughout the year.

4. Reservoir—As in RMSF (see section I, 4, above).

5. Mode of transmission—In the Mediterranean area, by bite of infected *Rhipicephalus sanguineus,* the brown dog tick.

6. Incubation period—Usually 5–7 days.

7., 8. and **9. Period of communicability, Susceptibility and resistance** and **Methods of control**—As in RMSF (see section I, 7, 8 and 9, above).

III AFRICAN TICK BITE FEVER ICD-9 082.8; ICD-10 A77.8

1. Identification—Clinically similar to Boutonneuse fever (see section II, above), however diffuse rash is frequently subtle or absent in African tick bite fever. Multiple eschars, lymphangitis, lymphadenopathy, and edema localized to the eschar site are seen more commonly with African tick bite fever than with Boutonnuese fever. Outbreaks of disease may occur when groups of travelers (such as persons on safari in Africa) are bitten by ticks. Cases are often imported to United States and Europe.

2. Infectious agent—*Rickettsia africae.*

3. Occurrence—Sub-Saharan Africa, including Botswana, Zimbabwe, Swaziland, and South Africa.

4. Reservoir—As in RMSF (see section 1, 4, above).

5. Mode of transmission—As in RMSF (see section 1, 5 above). *Amblyomma hebreum* appears to be the major vector.

6. Incubation period—1 to 15 days (median, 4 days after tick bite).

7., 8, and 9. Period of communicability, Susceptibility and resistance and Methods of control.—As in RMSF (see section 1, 7, 8 and 9, above).

IV. QUEENSLAND TICK
TYPHUS   ICD-9 082.3; ICD-10 A77.3

1. Identification—Clinically similar to Boutonneuse fever (see section II, above).

2. Infectious agent—*Rickettsia australis.*

3. Occurrence—Queensland, New South Wales, Tasmania and coastal areas of eastern Victoria, Australia.

4. Reservoir—As in RMSF (see section I, 4, above).

5. Mode of transmission—As in RMSF (see section I, 5, above). *Ixodes holocyclus*, that infests small marsupials and wild rodents, is probably the major vector.

6. Incubation period—About 7–10 days.

7., 8. and 9. Period of communicability, Susceptibility and resistance and **Methods of control** —As in RMSF (see section I, 7, 8 and 9, above).

V. NORTH ASIAN TICK
FEVER   ICD-9 082.2; ICD-10 A77.2
(Siberian tick typhus)

1. Identification—Clinically similar to Boutonneuse fever (see section II, above).

2. Infectious agent—*Rickettsia sibirica.*

3. Occurrence—Asiatic areas of the former Soviet Union, north China and the Mongolian People's Republic.

4. Reservoir—As in RMSF (see section I, 4, above).

5. Mode of transmission—By the bite of ticks in the genera *Dermacentor* and *Haemaphysalis*, which infest certain wild rodents.

6. Incubation period—2 to 7 days.

7., 8. and 9. **Period of communicability, Susceptibility and resistance** and **Methods of control**—As in RMSF (see section I, 7, 8 and 9, above).

VI. RICKETTSIALPOX   ICD-9 083.2; ICD-10 A79.1
(Vesicular rickettsiosis)

An acute febrile illness transmitted by mites. An initial skin lesion at the site of a mite bite, often associated with lymphadenopathy, is followed by fever; a disseminated vesicular skin rash appears, which generally does not involve the palms and soles and lasts only a few days. It may be confused with chickenpox. Death is uncommon and the infection is responsive to tetracyclines. Diagnosis is made by serology or by PCR or immunostains of biopsied tissues. The disease, caused by *Rickettsia akari*, a member of the spotted fever group of rickettsiae, is transmitted to humans from mice *(Mus musculus)* by a mite *(Liponyssoides sanguineus)*. It occurs primarily in urban areas of the eastern USA; most cases have been described from New York City and in the former Soviet Union. The incidence has been markedly reduced by changes in management of garbage in tenement housing, so that few cases have been diagnosed in recent years. In the former Soviet Union, commensal rats are reported to be the reservoir. Isolations of *R. akari* have been made in Africa and Korea. Prevention is by rodent elimination and mite control.

RUBELLA   ICD-9 056; ICD-10 B06
(German measles)
CONGENITAL RUBELLA   ICD-9 771.0; ICD-10 P35.0
(Congenital rubella syndrome)

1. **Identification**—Rubella is a mild febrile viral disease with a diffuse punctate and maculopapular rash somewhat resembling that of measles or scarlet fever. Children usually present few or no constitutional symptoms, but adults may experience a 1-5 day prodrome of low grade fever, headache, malaise, mild coryza and conjunctivitis. Postauricular, occipital and posterior cervical lymphadenopathy is the most characteristic clinical feature and precedes the rash by 5-10 days. Up to half the infections occur without recognized rash. Leukopenia is common and thrombocytopenia can occur, but hemorrhagic manifestations are rare. Arthralgia and, less commonly, arthritis complicate a substantial proportion of infections, particularly among adult females. Encephalitis and thrombocytopenia are rare complications in children; encephalitis occurs more frequently in adults.

Rubella is important because of its ability to produce anomalies in the developing fetus. Congenital rubella syndrome (CRS) occurs in up to 90% of infants born to women who are infected with rubella during the first trimester of pregnancy; the risk of a single congenital defect falls to approximately 10%-20% by the 16th week, and defects are rare when the maternal infection occurs after the 20th week of gestation.

Fetuses infected early are at greatest risk of intrauterine death, spontaneous abortion and congenital malformations of major organ systems. These include single or combined defects such as deafness, cataracts, microphthalmia, congenital glaucoma, microcephaly, meningoencephalitis, mental retardation, patent ductus arteriosus, atrial or ventricular septal defects, purpura, hepatosplenomegaly, jaundice and radiolucent bone disease. Moderate and severe cases of CRS are usually recognizable at birth; mild cases with only slight cardiac involvement or partial deafness may not be detected for months or even years after birth. Insulin dependent diabetes mellitus is recognized as a frequent late manifestation of CRS. Congenital malformations and even fetal death may occur following inapparent maternal rubella.

Differentiation of rubella from measles (q.v.), scarlet fever (see Streptococcal diseases) and other similar exanthems (e.g., see Erythema infectiosum and Exanthem subitum) is often necessary. Macular and maculopapular rashes also occur in 1%-5% of patients with infectious mononucleosis (especially if given ampicillin), in infections with certain enteroviruses and after certain drugs.

Clinical diagnosis of rubella is often inaccurate. Laboratory confirmation is the only reliable evidence of acute infection. Rubella infection can be confirmed by a significant rise in specific antibody titer between acute and convalescent phase serum specimens by ELISA, HAI, passive HA or LA testing, or by the presence of rubella specific IgM indicating a recent infection.

Sera should be collected as early as possible (within 7-10 days) after onset of illness, and again at least 7-14 days (preferably 2-3 weeks) later. Virus may be isolated from the pharynx 1 week before and up to 2 weeks after onset of rash. Blood, urine or stool specimens may yield virus. However, virus isolation is a lengthy procedure requiring 10-14 days. The diagnosis of CRS in the newborn is confirmed by the presence of specific IgM antibodies in a single specimen, by the persistence of a rubella specific antibody titer beyond the time expected from passive transfer of maternal IgG antibody, or by isolation of the virus that may be shed from the throat and urine for as long as a year. Virus may also be detected in cataracts for up to the first 3 years of life.

2. Infectious agent—Rubella virus (family Togaviridae; genus *Rubivirus*).

3. Occurrence—Worldwide; universally endemic except in remote and isolated communities, especially on certain island groups that have epidemics every 10-15 years. It is prevalent in winter and spring. Extensive epidemics occurred in the USA in 1935, 1943 and 1964, and in Australia in 1940. Before vaccine was licensed in 1969, peaks of rubella incidence occurred in the USA every 6-9 years. Throughout the 1990s the incidence of rubella in the USA declined steadily. However, the percent of cases among the foreign born increased steadily during the same period. During the 1990s, rubella outbreaks occurred in the USA in workplace settings, institutions, communities, and other environments where adolescents and young adults congregate, and have been primarily sustained by persons who have not been included in vaccine programs.

4. Reservoir—Humans.

5. Mode of transmission—Contact with nasopharyngeal secretions of infected people. Infection is by droplet spread or direct contact with patients. In closed environments such as among military recruits, all exposed susceptibles may be infected. Infants with CRS shed large quantities of virus in their pharyngeal secretions and in urine, and serve as a source of infection to their contacts.

6. Incubation period—From 14-17 days with a range of 14-21 days.

7. Period of communicability—For about 1 week before and at least 4 days after onset of rash; highly communicable. Infants with CRS may shed virus for months after birth.

8. Susceptibility and resistance—Susceptibility is general after loss of transplacentally acquired maternal antibodies. Active immunity is acquired by natural infection or by immunization; it is usually permanent after natural infection and thought to be long term, probably lifelong, after immunization, but this may depend on contact with endemic cases. In the USA, about 10% of the general population remain susceptible. Infants born to immune mothers are ordinarily protected for 6-9 months, depending on the amount of maternal antibodies acquired transplacentally.

9. Methods of control—Rubella control is needed primarily to prevent defects in the offspring of women who acquire the disease during pregnancy.

A. Preventive measures:

1) Educate the general public on modes of transmission and the need for rubella immunization. Education by health care providers should encourage rubella immunization for all susceptible persons. Efforts should be intensified to immunize susceptible adolescents and young adults; assessment of the immunity status of those born outside of the USA should be given particular attention.
2) A single dose of live, attenuated rubella virus vaccine (Rubella Virus Vaccine, Live) elicits a significant antibody response in

approximately 98%–99% of susceptibles. The vaccine is in dried form and after reconstitution must be kept at 2°–8°C (35.6°–46.4°F) or colder and protected from light to retain potency. Vaccine virus may be recovered from the nasopharynx of some recipients during the second to the fourth week postimmunization, more commonly for only several days, but is not communicable. In the USA, immunization of all children is recommended at 12–15 months of age as part of a combined vaccine containing measles and mumps vaccine (MMR), with a second dose of MMR at school entry or at adolescence. The continuing occurrence of rubella among those born outside the USA indicates that emphasis should be placed on immunizing this population. Vaccine is recommended for all susceptible nonpregnant females without contraindications. Susceptible young adults who have contact with young children or congregate at colleges and other types of institutions should be immunized. All medical personnel should be immune to rubella, in particular those who are in contact with patients in prenatal clinics. Proof of immunity is indicated by presence of rubella specific antibodies or written documentation of receiving rubella vaccine on or after the first birthday.

Vaccine should not be given to anyone with an immunodeficiency or on immunosuppressive therapy; however, MMR is recommended for persons with asymptomatic HIV infection. MMR should be considered for persons with symptomatic HIV infections. Because of theoretical concerns, women known to be pregnant or who are planning to get pregnant in the next 3 months, should not be immunized. However, results from a registry at CDC indicated that of 321 women who received rubella vaccine during pregnancy, all gave birth to full-term, healthy infants.

Reasonable precautions in a rubella immunization program include asking postpubertal females if they are pregnant, excluding those who say they are, and explaining the theoretical risks to the others and emphasizing the need to prevent pregnancy for the next 3 months. The immune status of an individual can be determined reliably only by serologic testing, but this is not necessary before immunization since vaccine can be given safely to an immune person. In some countries, routine immunization is given to girls between 11 and 13 years of age with or without prior antibody testing. In many countries, including the USA, Australia and the Nordic countries, a second dose of MMR vaccine is recommend for teenagers of both genders. For greater general detail, see Measles, 9A1.

3) In case of natural infection early in pregnancy, abortion should be considered because of high risk of damage to the fetus. In

studies carried out among pregnant women inadvertently immunized, congenital defects in live born infants have not been found; therefore, immunization of a woman subsequently discovered to be pregnant need not be considered an indication for abortion, but the potential risks should be explained. The final decision rests with the individual woman and her physician.

4) IG given after exposure early in pregnancy may not prevent infection or viremia, but it may modify or suppress symptoms. It is sometimes given in huge doses (20 ml) to a susceptible pregnant woman exposed to the disease who would not consider abortion under any circumstances, but its value has not been established.

B. *Control of patient, contacts and the immediate environment:*

1) Report to local health authority: All cases of rubella and of CRS should be reported. In the USA, report is obligatory, Class 3B (see Communicable Disease Reporting). Early reporting of suspected cases will permit early establishment of control measures.

2) Isolation: In hospitals and institutions, patients suspected of having rubella should be managed under contact isolation precautions and placed in a private room; attempts should be made to prevent exposure of nonimmune pregnant women. Exclude children from school and adults from work for 7 days after onset of rash. Infants with CRS may shed virus for prolonged periods of time. All persons having contact with infants with CRS should be immune to rubella, and these infants should be placed in contact isolation. Isolation precautions should be regulated during any admission before the first birthday, unless pharyngeal and urine cultures are negative for virus after 3 months of age.

3) Concurrent disinfection: None.

4) Quarantine: None.

5) Immunization of contacts: Immunization, while not contraindicated (except during pregnancy), will not necessarily prevent infection or illness. Passive immunization with IG is not indicated (except possibly as in 9A4, above).

6) Investigation of contacts and source of infection: Identify pregnant female contacts, especially those in the first trimester. Such contacts should be tested serologically for susceptibility or early infection (IgM antibody) and advised accordingly.

7) Specific treatment: None.

C. *Epidemic measures:*

1) Prompt reporting of all confirmed and suspected cases and

immunization of all susceptible contacts are needed for outbreak control.

2) The medical community and general public should be informed about rubella epidemics in order to identify and protect susceptible pregnant women.

D. Disaster implications: None.

E. International measures: None.

SALMONELLOSIS   ICD-9 003; ICD-10 A02.0

1. Identification—A bacterial disease commonly manifested by an acute enterocolitis, with sudden onset of headache, abdominal pain, diarrhea, nausea and sometimes vomiting. Dehydration, especially among infants or in the elderly, may be severe. Fever is almost always present. Anorexia and diarrhea often persist for several days. Infection may begin as acute enterocolitis and develop into septicemia or focal infection. Occasionally, the infectious agent may localize in any tissue of the body, produce abscesses and cause septic arthritis, cholecystitis, endocarditis, meningitis, pericarditis, pneumonia, pyoderma or pyelonephritis. Deaths are uncommon, except in the very young, the very old, the debilitated and the immunosuppressed. However, morbidity and associated costs of salmonellosis may be high.

In cases of septicemia, *Salmonella* may be isolated on enteric media from feces and blood during the acute stages of illness. In cases of enterocolitis, fecal excretion usually persists for several days or weeks beyond the acute phase of illness; administration of antibiotics may not decrease the time that organisms are excreted. For detection of asymptomatic infections, 3–10 g of fecal material is preferred to rectal swabs and should be inoculated first into an appropriate enrichment medium; specimens should be collected over several days since excretion of the organisms may be intermittent. Serologic tests are not useful in diagnosis.

2. Infectious agents—A new nomenclature for *Salmonella* has been proposed based on DNA relatedness. According to the proposed nomenclature, only two species would be recognized—*Salmonella bongori* and *Salmonella enterica* (both genus and species italicized). All human pathogens would be regarded as serovars within subspecies I of *S. enterica*. The proposed nomenclature would change *S. typhi* to *S. enterica* serovar Typhi, abbreviated *S.* Typhi (note that Typhi is not italicized and a capital letter is used). Some official agencies have adopted the new nomenclature although it had not been officially approved as of mid-1999. This new nomenclature is used in this chapter.

Numerous serotypes of *Salmonella* are pathogenic for both animals and people (strains of human origin that cause typhoid and paratyphoid fevers are presented in a separate chapter). There is much variation in the relative prevalence of the different serotypes from country to country; in most countries that maintain *Salmonella* surveillance, *Salmonella enterica* serovar Typhimurium (*S. Tyhpimurium*) and *Salmonella enterica* serovar Enteritidis (*S. Enteritidis*) are the two most commonly reported. Of more than 2,000 known serotypes, only about 200 are detected in the USA in any given year. In most areas, a small number of serotypes account for the majority of confirmed cases.

3. Occurrence—Worldwide; more extensively reported in North America and Europe due to better reporting systems in these regions. Salmonellosis is classified as a foodborne disease because contaminated food, mainly of animal origin, is the predominant mode of transmission. Only a small proportion of cases are recognized clinically, and in industrialized countries as few as 1% of clinical cases are estimated to be reported. The incidence rate of infection is highest in infants and young children. Epidemiologically, *Salmonella* gastroenteritis may occur in small outbreaks in the general population. About 60%–80% of all cases occur sporadically; however, large outbreaks in hospitals, institutions for children, restaurants and nursing homes are not uncommon and usually arise from food contaminated at its source, or less often, during handling by an ill person or a carrier, but person to person spread can occur. It is estimated that about 5 million cases of salmonellosis occur annually in the USA. An epidemic in the USA that involved 25,000 cases resulted from a nonchlorinated municipal water supply; the largest single epidemic due to improperly pasteurized milk affected 285,000 persons.

4. Reservoir—A wide range of domestic and wild animals, including poultry, swine, cattle, rodents and pets such as iguanas, tortoises, turtles, terrapins, chicks, dogs and cats; also humans, i.e., patients, convalescent carriers and, especially, mild and unrecognized cases. Chronic carriers are rare in humans but prevalent in animals and birds.

5. Mode of transmission—By ingestion of the organisms in food derived from infected animals or contaminated by feces of an infected animal or person. This includes raw and undercooked (inadequate time for a given temperature) eggs and egg products, raw milk and raw milk products, contaminated water, meat and meat products, poultry and poultry products. In addition, pet turtles, iguanas and chicks, and unsterilized pharmaceuticals of animal origin are potential sources of these bacteria. Recently, several outbreaks of salmonellosis have been traced to consumption of raw fruits and vegetables that were contaminated during slicing. Infection is transmitted to farm animals by feeds and fertilizers prepared from contaminated meat scraps, tankage, fish meal and bones; the infection spreads by bacterial multiplication during rearing and slaughter. Fecal-oral transmission from person to person is important, especially when diarrhea is present; infants and stool incontinent adults pose a greater risk of transmission than do asymptomatic carriers. With several serotypes, only a few organisms ingested in vehicles that buffer gastric acid can cause infection, but usually $>10^{2-3}$ organisms are required.

Epidemics are usually traced to foods such as processed meat products, inadequately cooked poultry and poultry products; uncooked or lightly cooked foods containing eggs and egg products, raw milk and dairy products, including dried milk; and foods contaminated with feces by an infected food handler. Epidemics may also be traced to foods such as meat and poultry products that have been processed or prepared with contaminated utensils or on work surfaces or tables contaminated in previous use. S. Enteritidis infection of chickens and eggs has caused outbreaks and single cases, especially in the northeastern USA and Europe, and is responsible for the majority of cases of this serotype in the USA. The organisms can multiply in a variety of foods, especially milk, to attain a very high infective dose; temperature abuse of food during its preparation and cross contamination during food handling are the most important risk factors. Hospital epidemics tend to be protracted, with organisms persisting in the environment; these epidemics often start with contaminated food and continue through person to person transmission via the hands of personnel or contaminated instruments. Maternity units with infected (at times asymptomatic) infants are sources of further spread. Fecal contamination of nonchlorinated public water supplies has caused some extensive outbreaks. In recent years, geographically widespread outbreaks due to ingestion of tomatoes or melons from single suppliers have been recognized.

6. Incubation period—From 6 to 72 hours, usually about 12–36 hours.

7. Period of communicability—Throughout the course of infection; extremely variable, usually several days to several weeks. A temporary carrier state occasionally continues for months, especially in infants. Depending on the serotypes, approximately 1% of infected adults and 5% of children aged <5 years may excrete the organism for >1 year.

8. Susceptibility and resistance—Susceptibility is general and is usually increased by achlorhydria, antacid therapy, GI surgery, prior or current broad-spectrum antibiotic therapy, neoplastic disease, immunosuppressive therapy and other debilitating conditions including malnutrition. Severity of the disease is related to the serotype, the number of organisms ingested and host factors. HIV infected persons are at risk for recurrent nontyphoidal *Salmonella* septicemia. Septicemia in people with sickle cell disease increases the risk of focal systemic infection, e.g., osteomyelitis.

9. Methods of control—

A. Preventive measures:

1) Educate food handlers and preparers about the importance of

a) hand-washing before, during and after food preparation; b) refrigerating prepared foods in small containers; c) thoroughly cooking all foodstuffs derived from animal sources, particularly poultry, pork, egg products and meat dishes; d) avoiding recontamination within the kitchen after cooking is completed; and e) maintaining a sanitary kitchen and protecting prepared foods against rodent and insect contamination.

2) Educate the public to avoid consuming raw or incompletely cooked eggs, as in eggs cooked "over easy" or "sunny side up," in eggnogs or homemade ice cream, and using dirty or cracked eggs.

3) Pasteurized or irradiated egg products should be used to prepare dishes in which eggs would otherwise be pooled before cooking or when the dish containing eggs is not subsequently cooked.

4) Exclude individuals with diarrhea from food handling and from care of hospitalized patients, the elderly and children.

5) Indoctrinate known carriers on the need for very careful handwashing after defecating (and before handling food) and discourage them from handling food for others as long as they shed organisms.

6) Recognize the risk of *Salmonella* infections in pets. Chicks, ducklings and turtles are particularly dangerous pets for small children.

7) Establish the facilities and encourage the use of food irradiation for meats and eggs.

8) Inspect for sanitation and adequately supervise abattoirs, food processing plants, feed blending mills, egg grading stations and butcher shops.

9) Establish *Salmonella* control programs (feed control, cleaning and disinfection, vector control and other sanitary and hygienic measures).

10) Adequately cook or heat treat (including pasteurization or irradiation) animal derived foods prepared for animal consumption (meat meal, bone meal, fish meal, pet food) to eliminate pathogens; follow by measures to avoid recontamination.

B. *Control of patient, contacts and the immediate environment:*

1) Report to local health authority: Obligatory case report, Class 2B (see Communicable Disease Reporting).

2) Isolation: For hospitalized patients, enteric precautions in handling feces and contaminated clothing and bed linen. Exclude symptomatic individuals from food handling and from direct care of infants, elderly, immunocompromised and institutionalized patients. Exclusion of asymptomatic infected individuals is indicated for those

with questionable hygienic habits and may be required by local or state regulations. When exclusion is mandated, release to return to work handling food or in patient care generally requires 2 consecutive negative stool cultures for *Salmonella* collected not less than 24 hours apart; if antibiotics have been given, the initial culture should be taken at least 48 hours after the last dose. Proper handwashing should be stressed.

3) Concurrent disinfection: Of feces and articles soiled therewith. In communities with a modern and adequate sewage disposal system, feces can be discharged directly into sewers without preliminary disinfection. Terminal cleaning.

4) Quarantine: None.

5) Immunization of contacts: No immunization available.

6) Investigation of contacts and source of infection: Culture stools of any household contacts who are involved in food handling, direct patient care, or care of young children or elderly people in institutional settings.

7) Specific treatment: For uncomplicated enterocolitis, none generally indicated except rehydration and electrolyte replacement with oral rehydration solution (see Cholera, 9B7). Antibiotics may not eliminate the carrier state and may lead to resistant strains or more severe infections. However, infants under 2 months of age, the elderly, the debilitated, those with sickle cell disease, persons infected with HIV, or patients with continued or high fever or manifestations of extraintestinal infection, should be given antibiotic therapy. Antimicrobial resistance of nontyphoidal salmonellae is variable; in adults, ciprofloxacin is highly effective but its use is not approved for children; ampicillin or amoxicillin may also be used. TMP-SMX and chloramphenicol are alternatives when antimicrobial resistant strains are involved. Patients infected with HIV may require life-long therapy to prevent *Salmonella* septicemia.

C. **Epidemic measures:** See Foodborne diseases, Staphylococcal food intoxication, 9C1 and 9C2. Search for a history of food handling errors, such as use of unsafe raw ingredients, inadequate cooking, time-temperature abuses and cross contamination. In the USA, in *S.* Enteritidis outbreaks in which dishes containing eggs are implicated, initiate trace back to the egg source; report to the U.S. Department of Agriculture is advised.

D. **Disaster implications:** A danger in a situation with mass feeding and poor sanitation.

E. **International measures:** WHO Collaborating Centres.

SCABIES   ICD-9 133.0; ICD-10 B86
(Sarcoptic itch, Acariasis)

1. Identification—A parasitic infestation of the skin caused by a mite, whose penetration is visible as papules, vesicles or tiny linear burrows containing the mites and their eggs. Lesions are prominent around finger webs, anterior surfaces of wrists and elbows, anterior axillary folds, belt line, thighs and external genitalia in men; nipples, abdomen and the lower portion of the buttocks are frequently affected in women. In infants, the head, neck, palms and soles may be involved; these areas are usually spared in older individuals. Itching is intense, especially at night, but complications are limited to lesions secondarily infected by scratching. In immuno-deficient individuals and in senile patients, infestation often appears as a generalized dermatitis more widely distributed than the burrows, with extensive scaling, and sometimes vesiculation and crusting ("Norwegian scabies"); the usual severe itching may be reduced or absent. When scabies is complicated by β-hemolytic streptococcal infection, risk of acute glomerulonephritis is present.

Diagnosis may be established by recovering the mite from its burrow and identifying it microscopically. Care should be taken to choose lesions for scraping or biopsy that have not been excoriated by repeated scratching. Prior application of mineral oil facilitates collecting the scrapings and examining them under a cover slip. Applying ink to the skin and then washing it off will disclose the burrows.

2. Etiologic agent—*Sarcoptes scabiei,* a mite.

3. Occurrence—Widespread. Past epidemics were attributed to poverty, poor sanitation and crowding due to war, movement of refugees and economic crises. The recent wave of infestation in the USA and Europe has evolved in the absence of major social disturbances and has affected people of all socioeconomic levels without regard to age, gender, race or standards of personal hygiene. It is endemic in many developing countries.

4. Reservoir—Humans; *Sarcoptes* species and other mites of animals can live on humans but do not reproduce on them.

5. Mode of transmission—Transfer of parasites is by direct contact with infested skin and can be acquired during sexual contact. Transfer from undergarments and bedclothes occurs only if these have been contaminated by infested people immediately beforehand. Mites can burrow beneath the skin surface in 2.5 minutes. Persons with the Norwegian scabies syndrome are highly contagious because of the large number of mites that are present in the exfoliating scales.

6. Incubation period—Two to six weeks before onset of itching in people without previous exposure. People who have been previously infested develop symptoms 1–4 days after reexposure.

7. Period of communicability—Until mites and eggs are destroyed by treatment, ordinarily after 1 or occasionally 2 courses of treatment, a week apart.

8. Susceptibility and resistance—Some resistance is suggested since immunologically compromised people are susceptible to hyperinfestation; fewer mites succeed in establishing themselves on people previously infested than on those with no prior exposure.

9. Methods of control —

    A. Preventive measures: Educate the public and medical community on mode of transmission, early diagnosis and treatment of infested patients and contacts.

    B. Control of patient, contacts and the immediate environment:

      1) Report to local health authority: Official report not ordinarily justifiable, Class 5 (see Communicable Disease Reporting).
      2) Isolation: Exclude infested individuals from school or work until the day after treatment. For hospitalized patients, contact isolation for 24 hours after start of effective treatment.
      3) Concurrent disinfestation: Laundering underwear, clothing and bedsheets worn or used by the patient in the 48 hours prior to treatment using hot cycles of both washer and dryer will kill mites and eggs, but may not be needed for most infestations. Laundering bedding and clothing is important for patients with Norwegian scabies because the potential for fomite transmission is high.
      4) Quarantine: None.
      5) Immunization of contacts: None.
      6) Investigation of contacts and source of infestation: Search for unreported and unrecognized cases among companions and household members; single infestations in a family are uncommon. Treat prophylactically those who have had skin to skin contact with infested people (including family members and sexual contacts).
      7) Specific treatment: The treatment of choice for children is 5% permethrin. Alternatively, apply 1% gamma benzene hexachloride (lindane and Kwell® are contraindicated in premature neonates and used with caution in infants less than 1 year of age and in pregnant women); crotamiton (Eurax®); tetraethylthiuram monosulfide (Tetmosol®, not available in the USA) in 5% solution twice daily; or an emulsion of benzyl benzoate to the whole body except the head and neck. (Treatment details vary with the drug.) On the next day, a cleansing bath is taken and a change made to fresh clothing and bedclothes. Itching may persist for 1–2 weeks; during this period it should not be

regarded as a sign of drug failure or reinfestation. Overtreatment is common and should be avoided because of toxicity of some of these agents, especially gamma benzene hexachloride. In about 5% of cases, a second course of treatment may be necessary after an interval of 7–10 days if eggs survived the first treatment. Close supervision of treatment, including bathing, is necessary.

C. *Epidemic measures:*

1) Provide treatment and educate infested individuals and others at risk. Cooperation of civilian or military authorities, often both, is needed.
2) Treatment is undertaken on a coordinated mass basis.
3) Case-finding efforts are extended to screen whole families, military units or institutions, with segregation of infested individuals if possible.
4) Soap and facilities for mass bathing and laundering are essential. Tetmosol soap, where available, helps to prevent infestation.

D. *Disaster implications:* A potential nuisance in situations of overcrowding.

E. *International measures:* None.

SCHISTOSOMIASIS　　　　ICD-9 120; ICD-10 B65
(Bilharziasis, Snail fever)

1. Identification—A blood fluke (trematode) infection with adult male and female worms living within mesenteric or vesical veins of the host over a life span of many years. Eggs produce minute granulomata and scars in organs where they lodge or are deposited. Symptoms are related to the number and location of the eggs in the human host: *Schistosoma mansoni* and *S. japonicum* give rise primarily to hepatic and intestinal signs and symptoms, including diarrhea, abdominal pain and hepatosplenomegaly; *S. haematobium* to urinary manifestations, including dysuria, urinary frequency and hematuria at the end of urination.

The most important pathologic effects are the complications that arise from chronic infection: liver fibrosis, portal hypertension and its sequelae and possibly colorectal malignancy in the intestinal forms; obstructive uropathy, superimposed bacterial infection, infertility and possibly bladder cancer in the urinary form of schistosomiasis. Eggs of all three *Schistosoma* species can be deposited at ectopic sites, including the brain, spinal cord, skin, pelvis and vulvovaginal areas.

The larvae of certain schistosomes of birds and mammals may penetrate the human skin and cause a dermatitis, sometimes known as "swimmer's itch"; these schistosomes do not mature in humans. Such infections may be prevalent among bathers in lakes in many parts of the world, including the Great Lakes region of North America and certain California coastal beaches. However, the clinical entity of "seabather's eruption," a pruritic dermatitis that appears principally where the bathing suit had been worn (that occurs particularly among swimmers on south Florida, Caribbean and Long Island, New York, beaches) has been shown to be caused by the larval stage of some jellyfish species.

Definitive diagnosis of schistosomiasis depends on demonstration of eggs in the stool microscopically by direct smear or on a Kato thick smear, in urine by nuclearpore filtration or in biopsy specimens. Nuclearpore filtration of urine is especially useful for *S. haematobium* infections. Useful immunologic tests include immunoblot analysis, the circumoval precipitin test, IFA and ELISA with egg or adult worm antigen, and RIA with purified egg or adult antigens; positive results on serologic tests indicate prior infection and are not proof of current infection.

2. Infectious agents—*Schistosoma mansoni, S. haematobium* and *S. japonicum* are the major species causing human disease. *S. mekongi, S. malayensis, S. mattheei* and *S. intercalatum* are of importance only in limited areas.

3. Occurrence—*S. mansoni* is found in Africa (including Madagascar); the Arabian Peninsula; Brazil, Suriname and Venezuela in South America; and in some Caribbean islands. *S. haematobium* is found in Africa (including Madagascar and Mauritius) and the Middle East. *S. japonicum* is found in China, Taiwan, the Philippines and Sulawesi (Celebes), in Indonesia; no new cases have been found in Japan since 1978 after an intensive control program. *S. mekongi* is found in the Mekong River area of Laos, Cambodia and Thailand. *S. intercalatum* occurs in parts of west Africa, including Cameroon, Central African Republic, Chad, Gabon, São Tomé and Zaire. *S. mattheei* is found in southern Africa. *S. malayensis* is known only from peninsular Malaysia. None of these species is indigenous to North America.

4. Reservoir—Humans are the principal reservoir of *S. haematobium, S. intercalatum* and *S. mansoni.* People, dogs, cats, pigs, cattle, water buffalo, horses and wild rodents are potential hosts of *S. japonicum;* their relative epidemiologic importance varies in different regions. *S. malayensis* appears to be a rodent parasite that occasionally infects humans. Epidemiologic persistence of the parasite depends on the presence of an appropriate snail as intermediate host, i.e., species of the genera *Biomphalaria* for *S. mansoni; Bulinus* for *S. haematobium, S. intercalatum* and *S.*

mattheei; Oncomelania for *S. japonicum; Neotricula* for *S. mekongi;* and *Robertsiella* for *S. malayensis.*

5. Mode of transmission—Infection is acquired from water containing free swimming larval forms (cercariae) that have developed in snails. The eggs of *S. haematobium* leave the mammalian body mainly in the urine, those of the other species in the feces. The eggs hatch in water and the liberated larvae (miracidia) penetrate into suitable freshwater snail hosts. After several weeks, the cercariae emerge from the snail and penetrate human skin, usually while the person is working, swimming or wading in water; they enter the bloodstream, are carried to blood vessels of the lungs, migrate to the liver, develop to maturity and then migrate to veins of the abdominal cavity.

Adult forms of *S. mansoni, S. japonicum, S. mekongi, S. mattheei* and *S. intercalatum* usually remain in mesenteric veins; those of *S. haematobium* usually migrate through anastomoses into the vesical plexus of the urinary bladder. Eggs are deposited in venules and escape into the lumen of the bowel or urinary bladder or lodge in other organs, including the liver and the lungs.

6. Incubation period—Acute systemic manifestations (Katayama fever) may occur in primary infections 2–6 weeks after exposure, immediately preceding and during initial egg deposition. Acute systemic manifestations are uncommon but can occur with *S. haematobium* infections.

7. Period of communicability—Not communicable from person to person, but people with chronic schistosomiasis may spread the infection by discharging eggs in urine and/or feces into bodies of water for as long as they excrete eggs; it is common for human infections with *S. mansoni* and *S. haematobium* to last in excess of 10 years. Infected snails will release cercariae for as long as they live, a period that may last from several weeks to about 3 months.

8. Susceptibility and resistance—Susceptibility is universal; any resistance developing as a result of infection is variable and poorly defined.

9. Methods of control—

    A. Preventive measures:

        1) Educate the public in endemic areas regarding mode of transmission and methods of protection.

        2) Dispose of feces and urine so that viable eggs will not reach bodies of fresh water containing intermediate snail hosts. Control of animals infected with *S. japonicum* is desirable but usually not practical.

        3) Improve irrigation and agriculture practices; reduce snail habitats by removing vegetation or by draining and filling.

4) Treat snail breeding sites with molluscicides. (Cost may limit use of these agents.)

5) Prevent exposure to contaminated water (e.g., use rubber boots). To minimize cercarial penetration after brief or accidental water exposure, towel dry, vigorously and completely, skin surfaces that are wet with suspected water. Apply 70% alcohol immediately to the skin to kill surface cercariae.

6) Provide water for drinking, bathing and washing clothes from sources free of cercariae or treated to kill them. Effective measures for inactivating cercariae include water treatment with iodine or chlorine, or the use of paper filters. Allowing water to stand 48-72 hours before use is also effective.

7) Treat patients in endemic areas with praziquantel to prevent disease progression and to reduce transmission by reducing egg passage.

8) Travelers visiting endemic areas should be advised of the risks and informed about preventive measures.

B. Control of patient, contacts and the immediate environment:

1) Report to local health authority: In selected endemic areas; in many countries, not a reportable disease, Class 3C (see Communicable Disease Reporting).

2) Isolation: None.

3) Concurrent disinfection: Sanitary disposal of feces and urine.

4) Quarantine: None.

5) Immunization of contacts: None.

6) Investigation of contacts and source of infection: Examine contacts for infection from a common source. The search for a source is a community effort (see 9C, below).

7) Specific treatment: Praziquantel (Biltricide®) is the drug of choice against all species. Alternative drugs are oxamniquine for *S. mansoni* and metrifonate for *S. haematobium*.

C. Epidemic measures:
Examine for schistosomiasis and treat all who are infected, but especially those with moderate to heavy intensities of egg passage; pay particular attention to children. Provide clean water, warn people against contact with water potentially containing cercariae and prohibit contamination of water. Treat areas that have high snail densities with molluscicides.

D. Disaster implications: None.

E. International measures: WHO Collaborating Centres.

APHA

SHIGELLOSIS
(Bacillary dysentery)

ICD-9 004; ICD-10 A03

1. Identification—An acute bacterial disease involving the large and distal small intestine and characterized by diarrhea accompanied by fever, nausea and sometimes toxemia, vomiting, cramps and tenesmus. In typical cases, the stools contain blood and mucus (dysentery) resulting from mucosal ulcerations and confluent colonic crypt microabscesses caused by the invasive organisms; however, many cases present with a watery diarrhea. Convulsions may be an important complication in young children. Bacteremia is uncommon. Mild and asymptomatic infections occur. Illness is usually self-limited, lasting an average of 4–7 days. The severity of illness and the case-fatality rate are functions of the host (age and preexisting nutritional state) and the serotype. *Shigella dysenteriae* 1 (Shiga bacillus) is often associated with serious disease and severe complications that include toxic megacolon and the hemolytic-uremic syndrome; case-fatality rates have been as high as 20% among hospitalized cases even in recent years. In contrast, many infections with *S. sonnei* result in a short clinical course and an almost negligible case-fatality rate except in compromised hosts. Certain strains of *S. flexneri* can cause a reactive arthropathy (Reiter syndrome), especially in persons who are genetically predisposed by having HLA-B27 antigen.

Bacteriologic diagnosis is made by isolation of *Shigella* from feces or rectal swabs. Prompt laboratory processing of specimens and use of appropriate media (a differential, low selectivity—MacConkey agar—together with one of high selectivity—XLD or S/S agar) increase the likelihood of *Shigella* isolation. Particular effort is needed to isolate *S. dysenteriae* type 1, as this organism is inhibited by some selective media, including S/S agar. Infection is usually associated with the presence of copious numbers of fecal leukocytes detected by microscopic examination of stool mucus stained with methylene blue or gram stain.

2. Infectious agents—The genus *Shigella* is comprised of four species or serogroups: Group A, *S. dysenteriae;* Group B, *S. flexneri;* Group C, *S. boydii;* and Group D, *S. sonnei.* Groups A, B and C, and D are further divided into 12, 14, and 18 serotypes and subtypes, respectively, designated by arabic numbers and lower case letters (e.g., *S. flexneri* 2a). In contrast, *S. sonnei* consists of only a single serotype. A specific virulence plasmid is necessary for the epithelial cell invasiveness manifested by *Shigellae.* The infectious dose for humans is low (10–100 bacteria caused disease in volunteers).

3. Occurrence—Worldwide; it is estimated that shigellosis causes about 600,000 deaths per year in the world. Two thirds of the cases, and most of the deaths, are in children under 10 years of age. Illness in infants under 6 months is unusual. Secondary attack rates in households can be as high as 40%. Outbreaks commonly occur in homosexual men; under conditions of crowding; and where personal hygiene is poor, such as in jails, institutions for children, day care centers, mental hospitals and crowded refugee camps. Shigellosis is endemic in both tropical and temperate climates; reported cases represent only a small proportion of cases, even in developed areas.

More than one serotype is commonly present in a community; mixed infections with other intestinal pathogens also occur. In general, *S. flexneri*, *S. boydii* and *S. dysenteriae* account for most isolates from developing countries. In contrast, *S. sonnei* is most common and *S. dysenteriae* is least common in developed countries. Multiantibiotic resistant *Shigella* (including *S. dysenteriae* 1) have appeared in all areas of the world, and are related to widespread use of antimicrobial agents.

4. Reservoir—The only significant reservoir is humans. However, prolonged outbreaks have occurred in primate colonies.

5. Mode of transmission—Mainly by direct or indirect fecal oral transmission from a symptomatic patient or a short term asymptomatic carrier. Infection may occur after the ingestion of very few (10–100) organisms. Individuals primarily responsible for transmission are those who fail to clean hands and under fingernails thoroughly after defecation. They may then spread infection to others directly by physical contact or indirectly by contaminating food. Water and milk transmission may occur as the result of direct fecal contamination; flies can transfer organisms from latrines to uncovered food items.

6. Incubation period—Usually 1–3 days, but may range from 12–96 hours; up to 1 week for *S. dysenteriae* 1.

7. Period of communicability—During acute infection and until the infectious agent is no longer present in feces, usually within 4 weeks after illness. Asymptomatic carriers may transmit infection; rarely, the carrier state may persist for months or longer. Appropriate antimicrobial treatment usually reduces duration of carriage to a few days.

8. Susceptibility and resistance—Susceptibility is general, with infection following ingestion of a small number of organisms; in endemic areas the disease is more severe in young children than in adults, among whom many infections may be asymptomatic. The elderly, the debilitated and the malnourished of all ages are particularly susceptible to severe disease and death. Breast feeding is protective for infants and young children. Studies with experimental serotype specific live oral vaccines and parenteral polysaccharide conjugate vaccines have shown protection of short duration (1 year) against infection with the homologous serotype.

9. Methods of control—Because of the diverse problems that may be involved in shigellosis, health authorities must be prepared to evaluate the local situation and take appropriate steps to prevent the spread of infection. It is not possible to provide a specific set of guidelines applicable to all situations. General measures to improve hygiene are important but often are difficult to implement because of their cost. An organized effort to promote careful handwashing with soap and water is the single most important control measure to decrease transmission rates in most settings.

The potentially high case-fatality rate in infections with *S. dysenteriae* 1 coupled with antibiotic resistance, calls for measures comparable to those for typhoid fever which include the need to identify source(s) of all infections. In contrast, an isolated infection with *S. sonnei* in a private home would not merit such an approach. Common source foodborne or waterborne outbreaks require prompt investigation and intervention without regard to the infecting species. Institutional outbreaks may require special measures, including separate housing for cases and new admissions, a vigorous program of supervised handwashing, and repeated cultures of patients and attendants. The most difficult outbreaks to control are: those that involve groups of young children (not yet toilet trained); the mentally deficient; and those outbreaks where there is an inadequate supply of water. Closure of affected day care centers may lead to placement of infected children in other centers (with subsequent transmission in those centers) and is not by itself an effective control measure. There is a clear need for an effective and long-lasting protective vaccine.

   A. ***Preventive measures:*** Same as those listed under typhoid fever, 9A1-9A10, except that no commercial vaccine is available.

   B. ***Control of patient, contacts and the immediate environment:***

     1) Report to local health authority: Case report is obligatory in most states and countries, Class 2B (see Communicable Disease Reporting). Recognition and report of outbreaks in child care centers and institutions are especially important.

     2) Isolation: During acute illness, enteric precautions. Because of the extremely small infective dose, patients with known *Shigella* infections should not be employed to handle food or to provide child or patient care until 2 successive fecal samples or rectal swabs (collected 24 or more hours apart, but not sooner than 48 hours following discontinuance of antimicrobials) are found to be free of *Shigella*. Patients must be advised of the importance and effectiveness of handwashing with soap and water after defecation as a means of curtailing transmission of *Shigella* to contacts.

     3) Concurrent disinfection: Of feces and contaminated articles. In communities with a modern and adequate sewage disposal system, feces can be discharged directly into sewers without preliminary disinfection. Terminal cleaning.

     4) Quarantine: None.

     5) Management of contacts: Whenever feasible, ill contacts of shigellosis patients should be excluded from food handling and the care of children or patients until diarrhea ceases and 2

successive negative stool cultures are obtained at least 24 hours apart and at least 48 hours after discontinuance of antibiotics. Thorough handwashing after defecation and before handling food or caring for children or patients must be stressed if such contacts are unavoidable.

6) Investigation of contacts and source of infection: The search for unrecognized mild cases and convalescent carriers among contacts may be unproductive in sporadic cases and seldom contributes to the control of an outbreak. Cultures of contacts should generally be confined to food handlers, attendants and children in hospitals, and other situations where the spread of infection is particularly likely.

7) Specific treatment: Fluid and electrolyte replacement is important when diarrhea is watery or there are signs of dehydration (see Cholera, 9B7). Antibacterials (oral TMP-SMX, ciprofloxacin or ofloxacin in adults; oral TMP-SMX, ampicillin or nalidixic acid or parenteral ceftriaxone in children) shorten the duration and severity of illness and the duration of pathogen excretion; they should be used in individual cases if warranted by the severity of the illness or to protect contacts (i.e., in day care centers or institutions) when epidemiologically indicated. During the past five decades *Shigella* have earned notoriety for the propensity with which they have acquired resistance to newly introduced antimicrobials that were initially highly effective. Multidrug resistance is common, so the choice of specific agents will depend on the antibiogram of the isolated strain or on local antimicrobial susceptibility patterns. In many areas, the high prevalence of *Shigella* resistance to TMP-SMX, ampicillin and tetracycline has resulted in a reliance on fluoroquinolones such as ciprofloxacin as first line therapy. The use of antimotility agents such as loperamide is contraindicated in children and is generally discouraged in adults as these drugs may prolong the illness. Nevertheless, if they are administered in an attempt to alleviate the severe cramps that often accompany shigellosis, antimotility agents should be limited to only 1 or at most 2 doses and should never be given without concomitant antimicrobial therapy.

C. Epidemic measures:

1) Report at once to the local health authority any group of cases of acute diarrheal disorder, even in the absence of specific identification of the causal agent.

2) Investigate food, water and milk supplies, and use general sanitation measures.

3) Prophylactic administration of antibiotics is not recommended.

4) Publicize the importance of handwashing after defecation;

provide soap and individual paper towels if otherwise not available.

D. Disaster implications: A potential problem where personal hygiene and environmental sanitation are deficient (see Typhoid fever).

E. International measures: WHO Collaborating Centres.

SMALLPOX   ICD-9 050; ICD-10 B03

The last naturally acquired case of smallpox in the world occurred in October 1977 in Somalia; global eradication was certified two years later by the WHO and sanctioned by the World Health Assembly (WHA) in May 1980. Except for a laboratory associated smallpox death at the University of Birmingham, England, in 1978, no cases have been identified since. All known variola virus stocks are held under security at the CDC, Atlanta, Georgia, or the State Research Centre of Virology and Biotechnology, Koltsovo, Novosibirsk Region, Russian Federation. In response to concerns that variola stocks may be needed for counterterrorism research in the event that clandestine stocks held by other countries fall into terrorist hands, the WHA in May 1999 authorized that the virus be held at laboratories in USA and Russia until no later than 2002. WHO reaffirmed that destruction of all the remaining virus stocks is still the organization's ultimate goal and will appoint a group of experts to consider what research needs to be carried out before the virus can be destroyed. WHO will also set up an inspection schedule for the two laboratories where the official stocks are kept to make sure that they are secure and that research can be carried out safely.

Because of the potential use of clandestine supplies of variola virus for biowarfare or bioterrorism, it is important that health care workers become familiar with the clinical and epidemiologic features of smallpox and how it was distinguished from chickenpox. Even though strains of virus used for biowarfare might have been engineered so that clinical differences may result, past experience with naturally occurring variola remains the best guide to recognition and management of an epidemic pox virus disease.

1. Identification—Smallpox was a systemic viral disease that generally presented with a characteristic skin eruption. Onset was sudden, with fever, malaise, headache, prostration, severe backache and occasional abdominal pain and vomiting; a clinical picture that resembled influenza. After 2 to 4 days, the fever began to fall and a deep-seated rash developed in which individual lesions containing infectious virus progressed through sucessive stages of macules, papules, vesicles, pustules and crusted scabs which fell off after three to four weeks. The lesions were first evident on the face and extremities and subsequently on the trunk—the so-called centrifugal rash distribution—and were at the same stage of development in a given area.

Two epidemiologic types of smallpox were recognized during the 20th century: variola minor (alastrim), which had a case fatality rate of less than 1% and variola major (ordinary) with a fatality rate among unvaccinated populations of 20–40% or more. Fatalities normally occurred between the 5th and 7th day, occasionally as late as the 2nd week. Less than 3% of variola major cases experienced fulminating disease with a severe pro-drome, prostration, and bleeding into the skin and mucous membranes; such hemorrhagic cases were rapidly fatal. The usual rash did not appear and the disease might have been confused with severe leukemia, meningo-coccemia or idiopathic thrombocytopenic purpura. In previously vaccinated persons, the rash was significantly modified to the extent that only a few highly atypical lesions might be seen. Generally the prodromal illness was not modified but the stages of the lesions were accelerated with crusting by the 10th day.

Most frequently smallpox was confused with chickenpox in which the skin lesions commonly occur in successive crops with several stages of maturity at the same time. The chickenpox rash is more abundant on covered than on exposed parts of the body; the rash is centripetal rather than centrifugal. Smallpox was indicated by a clear-cut prodromal illness; by the appearance of all lesions more or less simultaneously when the fever broke; by the similarity of appearance of all lesions in a given area rather than successive crops; and by more deep-seated lesions, which often involved sebaceous glands and scarring of the pitted lesions. By contrast, the chickenpox lesions are superficial. Smallpox lesions were virtually never seen at the apex of the axilla.

Outbreaks of variola minor (alastrim) appeared in the late 19th century. Although the rash was like that in ordinary smallpox, patients generally experienced less severe systemic reactions, and hemorrhagic cases were virtually unknown. Although the last cases of smallpox in Somalia in the late 1970s were classified as variola minor, DNA studies indicated that the virus was more like that of variola major than true alastrim virus, which suggested that this was an attenuated variola major. Laboratory confirma-tion was by isolation of the virus on chorioallantoic membranes or tissue culture from the scrapings of lesions, from vesicular or pustular fluid, from crusts, and sometimes from blood during the febrile preeruptive stage. A rapid provisional diagnosis was often possible by electron microscopy or the immunodiffusion technique. Now these methods would be superseded by m ore rapid and accurate PCR methods.

2. Infectious agent—Variola virus, a species of *Orthopoxvirus*. Map-ping of endonuclease cleavage sites of several strains of variola has been done, and the complete DNA sequences of two major strains are published.

3. Occurrence—Formerly a worldwide disease; no known humans cases since 1978.

4. Reservoir—Officially, only in designated freezers.

5. Mode of transmission—The secondary attack rate among unvaccinated populations was about 50% depending on the outbreak. If used in biowarfare, the agent would most likely be disseminated in an aerosol cloud.

6. Incubation period—From 7–19 days; commonly 10–14 days to onset of illness and 2–4 days more to onset of rash.

7. Period of communicability—From the time of development of the earliest lesions to disappearance of all scabs; about 3 weeks. The patient is most contagious during the preeruptive period by aerosol droplets from oropharyngeal lesions.

8. Susceptibility and resistance—Susceptibility among the unvaccinated is universal.

9. Methods of control—Control of smallpox is based on immunization with vaccinia virus. Should a nonvaricella, smallpox-like case be suspected, **IMMEDIATE TELEPHONIC COMMUNICATION WITH LOCAL AND STATE HEALTH AUTHORITIES IS OBLIGATORY: CDC SHOULD BE CONTACTED ALSO.** In the USA, smallpox vaccine (vaccinia virus) and human vaccinia immune globulin to treat vaccinal side effects are available through CDC Drug Service (404) 639-3670; the CDC bioterrorism response coordination hotline is (404) 639-0385.

VACCINIA   ICD-9 051.0; ICD-10 B08.0

Vaccinia virus, which was the immunizing agent used to eradicate smallpox, has been genetically engineered into candidate recombinant vaccines (some are in clinical trials), with low potential for spread to nonimmune contacts. The Immunization Practices Advisory Committee (ACIP) recommends vaccination with U.S.A. licensed smallpox vaccine of all laboratory workers at high risk of contracting infection, such as those who directly handle cultures or animals contaminated or infected with vaccinia or other orthopoxviruses that infect humans. It may be considered for other health care personnel who are at much lower risk of infection, such as doctors and nurses, whose contact with these viruses is limited to contaminated dressings. Vaccination is contraindicated in persons with deficient immune systems (e.g., AIDS and certain transplant and cancer patients); persons with eczema; certain other dermatitis disorders; and pregnant women. In the USA the vaccine immune globulin can be obtained for laboratory workers by contacting the CDC Drug Service, 1600 Clifton Road (Mailstop D09), Atlanta, GA 30333; telephone (404) 639-3670. If vaccine is approved for dispensing, the instructions (outlining vaccination methods, contraindications, reactions and complications) that accompany the vaccine should be followed rigorously. Vaccination may be repeated unless a major reaction (one that is indurated and erythematous 7 days after vaccination) has developed. Booster vaccinations are recommended within 10 years if the person remains in a category for which vaccine is rfecommended. The WHO maintains a supply of the vaccine seedlot (vaccinia virus strain Lister Elstree) for emergency use at the WHO Collaborating Center for Smallpox Vaccine at the National Institute of Public Health and Environmental Protection in Bilthoven, The Netherlands.

MONKEYPOX
ICD-9 051.9; ICD-10 B04

Human monkeypox is a sporadic zoonosic infection that has been reported from remote rural villages in central and west African rainforest countries. Clinically the disease closely resembles ordinary or modified smallpox, but lymphadenopathy is a more prominent feature in many cases and occurs in the early stage of the disease. Pleomorphism and "cropping," similar to that seen in chickenpox, are observed in 20% of patients. The natural history of the virus is unclear, but humans, primates and squirrels appear to be involved in the enzootic cycle. The disease affects all age groups, but children under 16 years of age constitute the greatest proportion of cases. The case-fatality rate among children not vaccinated against smallpox ranges in various studies from 1–3% to 10–14%. Between 1970 and 1994, over 400 cases were reported from west and central Africa; the Democratic Republic of Congo (DRC, formerly Zaire) accounted for about 95% of reported cases during a WHO prospective 5-year surveillance from 1981–1986. Over 70 suspect human cases with 6 deaths reported in 1996 led to three WHO sponsored retrospective studies in central DRC that covered about 0.5 million people and 800 suspect cases. About 20 monkeypox virus isolates were made from active cases and sera collected and analyzed from suspect cases showed both monkeypox and concurrent chickenpox. Because of the poor public health infrastructure and other factors complicating accurate case reporting, the exact number of cases and proportion of primary and secondary cases is unclear.

In the 1980s about 75% of reported cases were attributable to contact with affected animals; recent studies suggest that about 75% of cases are from human contact, but in both periods cascades of cases were very rare. The longest chain of person to person transmission consisted of only seven reported serial cases, but serial transmission usually did not extend beyond secondary. The limited epidemiologic data suggests a secondary attack rate of about 8%. Most cases have occurred either singly or in small clusters in small remote villages close to, or in the tropical rainforest, where the population usually has multiple contacts with a variety of wild animals. Ecologic studies in the 1980s indicated that squirrels (*Funisciurus* and *Heliosciurus*), abundant among the oil palms surrounding the villages, appear to be a significant reservoir host contributing to the occurrence of human monkeypox virus in the DRC. Maintenance of an animal reservoir and animal contact is required to sustain the disease among humans. Thus, human infection may be controllable by education to limit contact with infected cases and potentially infected animals.

Monkeypox virus is a species of the genus *Orthopoxvirus,* with biological properties and a genome map distinct from variola virus. There is no evidence that monkeypox will become a public health threat outside of enzootic areas. Cross-protective vaccination against smallpox was stopped in the DRC by 1982; reestablishment of vaccination is not recommended by WHO. A WHO Technical Advisory Committee on monkeypox has recently recommended continued studies, in particular, intensified prospective surveillance and ecological studies.

SPOROTRICHOSIS   ICD-9 117.1; ICD-10 B42

1. Identification—A fungal disease, usually of the skin, often of an extremity, which begins as a nodule. As the nodule grows, lymphatics draining the area become firm and cord-like and form a series of nodules, which in turn may soften and ulcerate. Osteoarticular, pulmonary and disseminated multifocal infections are rare. Fatalities are uncommon.

Laboratory confirmation is made by culture of a biopsy, pus or exudate. Organisms are rarely visualized by direct smear. Biopsied tissue should be examined with fungal stains.

2. Infectious agent—*Sporothrix schenckii,* a dimorphic fungus.

3. Occurrence—Reported from all parts of the world, an occupational disease of farmers, gardeners and horticulturists. The disease is characteristically sporadic and relatively uncommon. An epidemic among gold miners in South Africa involved some 3,000 people; fungus was growing on mine timbers. In 1988, in 14 states (USA), 84 cases occurred in people who handled conifer seedlings packed with sphagnum moss.

4. Reservoir—Soil, decaying vegetation, wood, moss and hay.

5. Mode of transmission—Introduction of fungus through the skin by pricks of thorns or barbs, the handling of sphagnum moss or by slivers from wood or lumber. Outbreaks have occurred among children playing in and adults working with baled hay. Pulmonary sporotrichosis is assumed to arise by inhalation of conidia.

6. Incubation period—The lymphatic form may develop 1 week to 3 months after injury.

7. Period of communicability—Transmission from person to person has been documented in only one case.

8. Susceptibility and resistance—Unknown.

9. Methods of control—

    *A. **Preventive measures:*** Treat lumber with fungicides in industries where disease occurs. Wear gloves and long sleeves when working with sphagnum moss.

B. *Control of patient, contacts and the immediate environment:*

1) Report to local health authority: Official report not ordinarily justifiable, Class 5 (see Communicable Disease Reporting).
2) Isolation: None.
3) Concurrent disinfection: Of discharges and dressings. Terminal cleaning.
4) Quarantine: None.
5) Immunization of contacts: None.
6) Investigation of contacts and source of infection: Seek undiagnosed and untreated cases.
7) Specific treatment: Orally administered iodides or itraconazole are effective in lymphocutaneous infection; in extracutaneous forms, amphotericin B (Fungizone®) is considered the drug of choice, but itraconazole is also useful.

C. *Epidemic measures:* Determine source to limit future exposures. In the South African epidemic, mine timbers were sprayed with a mixture of zinc sulfate and triolith. This and other sanitary measures controlled the epidemic.

D. *Disaster implications:* None.

E. *International measures:* None.

STAFFYLOCOCCAL DISEASES

Staphylococci produce a variety of syndromes with clinical manifestations ranging from a single pustule to sepsis and death. A lesion (or lesions) containing pus is the primary clinical finding, abscess formation the typical pathologic manifestation. Virulence of bacterial strains varies greatly. The most important pathogen of humans is *Staphylococcus aureus*. Most strains ferment mannitol and are coagulase positive. However, coagulase negative strains are increasingly more important, especially in bloodstream infections in patients with intravascular catheters, in urinary tract infections of women and in hospital acquired infections.

Staphylococcal disease has distinctly different clinical and epidemiologic patterns in the general community, in newborns, in menstruating women and among hospitalized patients. Therefore, each will be presented separately. Staphylococcal food poisoning, an intoxication and not an infection, is discussed separately (see Foodborne Intoxications, section I, Staphylococcal).

I. STAPHYLOCOCCAL DISEASE IN THE COMMUNITY

BOILS, CARBUNCLES, FURUNCLES, ABSCESSES	ICD-9 680, 041.1; ICD-10 L02; B95.6–B95.8
IMPETIGO	ICD-9 684, 041.1; ICD-10 L01
CELLULITIS	ICD-9 682.9; ICD-10 L03
STAPHYLOCOCCAL SEPSIS	ICD-9 038.1; ICD-10 A41.0–A41.2
STAPHYLOCOCCAL PNEUMONIA	ICD-9 482.4; ICD-10 J15.2
ARTHRITIS	ICD-9 711.0, 041.1; ICD-10 M00.0
OSTEOMYELITIS	ICD-9 730, 041.1; ICD-10 M86
ENDOCARDITIS	ICD-9 421.0, 041.1; ICD-10 I33.0

1. Identification—The common bacterial skin lesions are impetigo, folliculitis, furuncles, carbuncles, abscesses and infected lacerations. The basic lesion of impetigo is described in section II, 1, below; in addition, a distinctive "scalded skin" syndrome is associated with certain strains of *Staphylococcus aureus,* most often those of phage group II, which elaborate an epidermolytic toxin. The other skin lesions are localized and discrete. Constitutional symptoms are unusual; if lesions extend or are widespread, fever, malaise, headache and anorexia may develop. Usually, lesions are uncomplicated, but seeding of the bloodstream may lead to pneumonia, lung abscess, osteomyelitis, sepsis, endocarditis, pyarthrosis, meningitis or brain abscess. In addition to primary lesions of the skin, staphylococcal conjunctivitis occurs in newborns and the elderly. Staphylococcal pneumonia is a well-recognized complication of influenza. Staphylococcal endocarditis and other complications of staphylococcal bacteremia may result from parenteral use of illicit drugs or be acquired nosocomially from intravenous catheters and other devices. Embolic skin lesions are frequent complications of endocarditis and/or bacteremia.

Coagulase negative staphylococci may cause sepsis, meningitis, endocarditis or urinary tract infections and are increasingly involved in the etiology of disease, usually in connection with prosthetic devices or indwelling catheters.

Diagnosis is confirmed by isolation of the organism.

2. Infectious agent—Various coagulase positive strains of *Staphylococcus aureus.* When indicated, most strains of staphylococci may be characterized by molecular methods such as pulsed-field gel electrophoresis, phage type, antibiotic resistance profile or serologic agglutination; epidemics are caused by relatively few specific strains. The majority of clinical isolates of *S. aureus,* both community and hospital acquired, are resistant to penicillin G, and multiresistant (including methicillin resistant) strains have become widespread. Some evidence suggests that slime-producing strains of coagulase negative staphylococci may be more pathogenic, but the data are inconclusive. *S. saprophyticus* is a common cause of urinary tract infection in young women.

3. Occurrence—Worldwide. Highest incidence is in areas where personal hygiene (especially the use of soap and water) is suboptimal and people are crowded; common among children, especially in warm weather. The disease occurs sporadically and as small epidemics in families and summer camps, with various members developing recurrent illness due to the same staphylococcal strain.

4. Reservoir—Humans and rarely animals.

5. Mode of transmission—The major site of colonization is the anterior nares; 20%-30% of the general population are nasal carriers of coagulase positive staphylococci. Autoinfection is responsible for at least one third of infections. Persons with a draining lesion or any purulent discharge are the most common sources of epidemic spread. Transmission is through contact with a person who either has a purulent lesion or is an asymptomatic (usually nasal) carrier of a pathogenic strain. Some carriers are more effective disseminators of infection than others. The role of contaminated objects has been overstressed; the hands are the most important instrument for transmitting infection. Airborne spread is rare but has been demonstrated in infants with associated viral respiratory disease.

6. Incubation period—Variable and indefinite; commonly 4-10 days.

7. Period of communicability—As long as purulent lesions continue to drain or the carrier state persists. Autoinfection may continue for the period of nasal colonization or duration of active lesions.

8. Susceptibility and resistance—Immune mechanisms are not well understood. Susceptibility is greatest among the newborn and the chronically ill. Elderly and debilitated people, drug abusers, and those with diabetes mellitus, cystic fibrosis, chronic renal failure, agammaglobulinemia, any disorder of neutrophil function (such as agranulocytosis, chronic granulomatous disease), neoplastic disease and burns are particularly susceptible. Use of steroids and antimetabolites also increases susceptibility.

9. Methods of control—

  A. Preventive measures:

    1) Educate the public in personal hygiene, especially handwashing and the importance of avoiding sharing toilet articles.
    2) Treat initial cases in children and families promptly.

  B. Control of patient, contacts and the immediate environment:

    1) Report to local health authority: Obligatory report of outbreaks in schools, summer camps and other population

groups; also any recognized concentration of cases in the community. No individual case report, Class 4 (see Communicable Disease Reporting).

2) Isolation: Not practical in most communities; infected people should avoid contact with infants and debilitated people.

3) Concurrent disinfection: Place dressings from open lesions and discharges in disposable bags and dispose in a practical and safe manner.

4) Quarantine: None.

5) Immunization of contacts: None.

6) Investigation of contacts and source of infection: Search for draining lesions; occasionally, determination of nasal carrier status of the pathogenic strain among family members is useful.

7) Specific treatment: In localized skin infections, systemic antimicrobials are not indicated unless infection spreads significantly or complications ensue; local skin cleaning followed by application of an appropriate topical antimicrobial (such as mupirocin, 4 times a day) is adequate. Avoid wet compresses, which may spread infection; hot dry compresses may help localized infections. Abscesses should be incised to permit drainage of pus. For severe staphylococcal infections, use a penicillinase-resistant penicillin; when hypersensitivity to penicillin is present, use a cephalosporin active against staphylococci (unless there is a history of immediate hypersensitivity to penicillin) or clindamycin. In severe systemic infections, the selection of antibiotics should be governed by results of susceptibility tests on isolates. Vancomycin is the treatment of choice for severe infections caused by coagulase negative staphylococci and methicillin resistant *S. aureus;* prompt parenteral treatment is important.

Strains of *Staphylococcus aureus* with decreased susceptibility to vancomycin and other glycopeptide antibiotics, so-called GISA strains, have been reported from Japan and the USA during the late 1990s. These strains were recovered from patients treated with vancomycin for extended periods of time (months). These isolates may have been the first evidence of the emergence of strains of *S. aureus* that eventually became resistant to this antibiotic.

C. Epidemic measures:

1) Search for and treat those with clinical illness, especially with draining lesions. Institute strict personal hygiene with emphasis on handwashing. Culture for nasal carriers of the epidemic strain and treat locally with mupirocin and, if this fails, with orally administered antimicrobials.

2) Investigate any unusual or abrupt increase in prevalence of staphylococcal infections in the community for a possible common source, such as an unrecognized hospital epidemic.

D. Disaster implications: None.

E. International measures: WHO Collaborating Centres.

II. STAPHYLOCOCCAL DISEASE IN HOSPITAL NURSERIES

IMPETIGO NEONATORUM	ICD-9 684, 041.1; ICD-10 L00
STAPHYLOCOCCAL SCALDED SKIN SYNDROME (SSSS, Ritter's disease)	ICD-9 695.81
ABSCESS OF THE BREAST	ICD-9 771.5, 041.1; ICD-10 P39.0

1. Identification—Impetigo or pustulosis of the newborn and other purulent skin manifestations are the most frequent nursery acquired staphylococcal diseases. Characteristic skin lesions develop secondary to colonization of the nose, umbilicus, circumcision site, rectum or conjunctivae. (Colonization of these sites with strains of staphylococci is a normal occurrence and does not imply disease.)

Lesions are most commonly found in diaper and intertriginous areas but may be distributed anywhere on the body. They are initially vesicular, rapidly turning seropurulent, surrounded by an erythematous base; bullae may form (bullous impetigo). Rupture of pustules favors their spread. Complications are unusual, although lymphadenitis, furunculosis, breast abscess, pneumonia, sepsis, arthritis, osteomyelitis and other serious diseases have been reported.

Though uncommon, staphylococcal scalded skin syndrome (SSSS, Ritter's disease, pemphigus neonatorum) may occur, with clinical manifestations ranging from diffuse scarlatiniform erythema to generalized bullous desquamation of the skin. This condition, like bullous impetigo, is caused by strains of *S. aureus,* usually of phage type II, which produce an epidermolytic toxin.

2. Infectious agent—Same as for staphylococcal disease in the community (see section I, 2, above).

3. Occurrence—Worldwide. Problems occur mainly in hospitals, are promoted by laxity in aseptic techniques and are exaggerated by development of antibiotic resistant strains of the infectious agent (i.e., hospital strains).

4. Reservoir—Same as for staphylococcal disease in the community (see section I, 4, above).

5. Mode of transmission—Primary mode is spread by hands of hospital personnel; rarely airborne.

6. Incubation period—Commonly 4-10 days, but disease may not occur until several months after colonization.

7. Period of communicability—Same as for staphylococcal disease in the community (see section I, 7, above).

8. Susceptibility and resistance—Susceptibility in the newborn appears to be general. Infants remain at risk of disease for duration of colonization with pathogenic strains.

9. Methods of control—

A. Preventive measures:

1) Use aseptic techniques when necessary and adequate hand-washing before contact with each infant in nurseries.
2) Do not permit hospital personnel with minor lesions (pustules, boils, abscesses, paronychia, conjunctivitis, severe acne, otitis externa or infected lacerations) to work in the nursery.
3) Surveillance and supervision through an active hospital infection control committee are indicated, and include a regular system for investigating, reporting and reviewing all hospital acquired infections. Illness developing after discharge from hospital should also be investigated and recorded, preferably by active surveillance of all discharged newborns at about 1 month of age.
4) Some advocate routine application of antibacterial substances, such as gentian violet, acriflavine, chlorhexidine or bacitracin ointment, to the umbilical cord stump while the baby is in the hospital.

B. Control of patient, contacts and the immediate environment:

1) Report to local health authority: Obligatory report of epidemics; no individual case report, Class 4 (see Communicable Disease Reporting).
2) Isolation: Without delay, place all known or suspected cases in the nursery on contact isolation precautions.
3) Concurrent disinfection: Same as for staphylococcal disease in the community (see section I, 9B3, above).
4) Quarantine: None.
5) Immunization of contacts: None.
6) Investigation of contacts and source of infection: See epidemic measures in 9C, below.

7) Specific treatment: For localized impetigo: cleanse skin and apply topical mupirocin ointment 4 times a day; widespread lesions may be treated orally with an antistaphylococcal antimicrobial such as cephalexin or cloxacillin. Parenteral therapy is indicated for serious infections (see section I, 9B7, above).

C. Epidemic measures:

1) The occurrence of 2 or more concurrent cases of staphylococcal disease related to a nursery or a maternity ward is presumptive evidence of an outbreak and warrants investigation. Culture all lesions to determine antibiotic resistance pattern and type of epidemic strain. Clinically important isolates should be kept by the laboratory for 6 months before discarding to support possible epidemiologic investigation using antibiotic sensitivity patterns or pulsed-field gel electrophoresis.

2) In a nursery outbreak, institute isolation precautions for cases and contacts until all have been discharged. Use a rotational system ("cohorting") in which one unit (A) is filled and subsequent babies are admitted to a second nursery (B) while the initial unit (A) discharges infants and is cleaned before new admissions. If facilities are present for baby rooming with mother, this may reduce risk. Colonized or infected infants should be grouped in another cohort. Assignments of nursing and other ward personnel should be restricted to specific cohorts.

   Before admitting new patients, wash cribs, beds, isolettes and other furniture with an EPA approved disinfectant. Autoclave instruments that enter sterile body sites, wipe mattresses and thoroughly launder bedding and diapers (or use disposable diapers).

3) Examine all patient care personnel, including physicians, nurses, aides and attendants, for draining lesions anywhere on the body. Perform an epidemiologic investigation, and if one or more personnel are associated with the disease, culture nasal specimens from them and all others in contact with infants. With continuing disease, it may become necessary to exclude and treat all carriers of the epidemic strain until cultures are negative. Treatment of asymptomatic carriers is directed at suppression of the nasal carrier state, usually accomplished by local application of appropriate antibiotic ointments to the nasal vestibule, sometimes with concurrent rifampin systemically.

4) Investigate adequacy of nursing procedures and particularly availability of handwashing facilities. Emphasize strict hand-

washing; if facilities are inaccessible or inadequate, consider use of a hand antiseptic agent (e.g., alcohol) at the bedside. Personnel assigned to infected or colonized infants should not work with noncolonized newborns.

5) Although prohibited for routine use in the USA, preparations containing 3% hexachlorophene may be used during an outbreak. Full-term infants may be bathed (in the diaper area only) as soon after birth as possible and daily until they are discharged. After bathing is completed, the hexachlorophene should be washed off thoroughly because CNS damage may result from systemic absorption.

D. Disaster implications: None.

E. International measures: WHO Collaborating Centres.

III. STAPHYLOCOCCAL DISEASE ON HOSPITAL MEDICAL AND SURGICAL WARDS ICD-9 998.5; ICD-10 T81.4

1. Identification—Lesions vary from simple furuncles or stitch abscesses to extensively infected bedsores or surgical wounds, septic phlebitis, chronic osteomyelitis, fulminating pneumonia, meningitis, endocarditis or sepsis. Postoperative staphylococcal disease is a constant threat to the convalescence of the hospitalized surgical patient. The increasing complexity of surgical operations, with greater organ exposure and more prolonged anesthesia, promotes entry of staphylococci. Increased use of prosthetic devices and indwelling catheters accounts for an increased incidence of nosocomial staphylococcal infections. Frequent and sometimes injudicious use of antimicrobial therapy has increased the prevalence of antibiotic resistant staphylococci. Verification depends on isolation of *Staphylococcus aureus,* associated with a clinical illness compatible with the bacteriologic findings.

2. Infectious agent—*Staphylococcus aureus;* see section I, 2, above. Ninety-five percent of strains are resistant to penicillin, and increasing proportions are resistant to semisynthetic penicillin (e.g., methicillin) and the aminoglycosides (e.g., gentamicin).

3. Occurrence—Worldwide. Staphylococcal infection is a major form of acquired sepsis in the general wards of hospitals. At times, attack rates assume epidemic proportions. Spread to the community may occur when patients infected in the hospital are discharged.

4., 5., 6. and **7. Reservoir, Mode of transmission, Incubation period** and **Period of communicability:** Same as for staphylococcal disease in the community (see section I, 4, 5, 6 and 7, above).

8. Susceptibility and resistance—Same as section I. The widespread use of continuous intravenous therapy with indwelling catheters and parenteral injections has opened new portals of entry for infectious agents.

9. Methods of control—

A. Preventive measures:

1) Educate hospital medical staff to use common, narrow-spectrum antimicrobials for simple staphylococcal infections and reserve certain antibiotics (e.g., cephalosporins for penicillin resistant and vancomycin for β-lactam resistant staphylococcal infections).

2) A hospital infection control committee should enforce strict aseptic technique and provide programs for monitoring nosocomial infections.

3) Replace all indwelling peripheral venous catheters at least every 72 hours; change sites of IV needle infusions every 48 hours.

B. Control of patient, contacts and the immediate environment:

1) Report to local health authority: Obligatory report of epidemics; no individual case report, Class 4 (see Communicable Disease Reporting).

2) Isolation: Whenever a moderate or heavy abundance of staphylococci is known or suspected to be present in draining pus or the sputum of a patient with pneumonia, the patient should be placed in a private room; this is not required when wound drainage is scanty, provided that an occlusive dressing is used and care is taken in changing dressings to prevent contamination of the environment. Health care workers should practice appropriate handwashing, gloving and gowning techniques.

3) Concurrent disinfection: As in staphylococcal disease in the community (see section I, 9B3, above).

4) Quarantine: None.

5) Immunization of contacts: None.

6) Investigation of contacts and source of infection: Not practical for sporadic cases (see 9C, below).

7) Specific treatment: Appropriate antimicrobials as determined by antibiotic sensitivity tests. Life threatening infections should be treated with vancomycin pending test results.

C. Epidemic measures:

1) The occurrence of 2 or more cases with epidemiologic association is sufficient to suspect epidemic spread and to initiate investigation.

2) Same as section II, 9C3, above.

3) Review and enforce rigid aseptic techniques.

D. Disaster implications: None.

E. International measures: WHO Collaborating Centres.

IV. TOXIC SHOCK
SYNDROME ICD-9 785.5; ICD-10 A48.3

Toxic shock syndrome (TSS) is a severe illness characterized by sudden onset of high fever, vomiting, profuse watery diarrhea and myalgia, followed by hypotension and, in severe cases, shock. An erythematous "sunburn-like" rash is present during the acute phase; about 1–2 weeks after onset, there is desquamation of the skin, especially of palms and soles. Fever is usually higher than 38.8°C (102°F), systolic blood pressure is less than 90 mm mercury and three or more of the following organ systems are involved: **GI**; **muscular** (severe myalgia and/or creatine phosphokinase level greater than twice the normal upper limit); **mucous membranes** (hyperemia of vaginal, pharyngeal and/or conjunctival); **renal** (blood urea nitrogen or creatinine more than twice normal and/or sterile pyuria); **hepatic** (AST or ALT greater than twice normal); **hematologic** (platelets less than 100,000/cu mm; SI units less than 100×10^9/L); and the **CNS** (disorientation or alterations in consciousness without focal neurologic signs).

Blood, throat and CSF cultures are negative for pathogens, although the recovery of *S. aureus* from any of these sites does not invalidate a case. Serologic tests for Rocky Mountain spotted fever, leptospirosis and measles are negative.

Most cases of TSS have been associated with strains of *S. aureus* producing toxic shock syndrome toxin 1. These strains are rarely present in vaginal cultures from healthy women but are regularly recovered from women with menstrually associated TSS or in those with TSS following gynecologic surgery.

Although almost all early cases of TSS occurred in women during menstruation, and most with vaginal tampon use, only 55% of cases now reported are associated with menses. Other risk factors include use of contraceptive diaphragms and vaginal contraceptive sponges, and infection following childbirth or abortion. A recent study demonstrated a significantly increased risk of TSS in users of contraceptive diaphragms and vaginal contraceptive sponges. Instructions for sponge use, which advise they should not be left in place for more than 30 hours, should be heeded. Cases have occurred in men and women in whom *S. aureus* was isolated from focal lesions of the skin, bone, the respiratory tract and surgical sites. In one-third of cases no source of infection could be found.

Menstrual TSS can be almost entirely prevented by avoiding use of highly absorbent vaginal tampons; risk may be reduced by using tampons intermittently during each menstrual cycle (that is, not used all day and all night during the period) and by using less absorbent tampons. Women who develop a high fever and vomiting or diarrhea during menstruation should discontinue tampon use immediately and consult a physician. It is not known when those who have had an episode of menstrual TSS can safely resume tampon use.

A syndrome virtually identical to that occurring with *S. aureus* infection occurs with infection caused by group A beta-hemolytic streptococci.

Treatment of TSS is largely supportive. Efforts should be made to eradicate any potential focus of *S. aureus* infection through drainage of wounds, removal of vaginal or other foreign bodies (e.g., wound packing) and use of β-lactam resistant antistaphylococcal antimicrobial therapy.

STREPTOCOCCAL DISEASES CAUSED BY GROUP A (BETA HEMOLYTIC) STREPTOCOCCI ICD-9 034, 035, 670; ICD-10 A49.1, J02.0, A38, L01.0, A46, 085
(Streptococcal sore throat, Streptococcal infection, Scarlet fever, Impetigo, Erysipelas, Puerperal fever, Rheumatic fever)

1. Identification—Group A streptococci cause a variety of diseases. The most frequently encountered conditions are streptococcal sore throat (ICD-10 J02.0) and streptococcal skin infections (impetigo or pyoderma). Other diseases include scarlet fever (ICD-10 A38), puerperal fever (ICD-10 085), septicemia, erysipelas, cellulitis, mastoiditis, otitis media, pneumonia, peritonsillitis, wound infections and rarely, necrotizing fasciitis, rheumatic fever and a toxic shock-like syndrome. In outbreaks, one form of clinical disease often predominates.

Patients with **streptococcal sore throat** typically exhibit the sudden onset of fever, sore throat, exudative tonsillitis or pharyngitis and tender, enlarged anterior cervical lymph nodes. The pharynx, the tonsillar pillars and soft palate may be injected and edematous; petechiae may be present against a background of diffuse redness. Symptoms may be minimal or absent. Coincident or subsequent otitis media or peritonsillar abscess may occur; after 1–5 weeks acute glomerulonephritis (mean = 10 days) or acute rheumatic fever (mean = 19 days) may appear. In contrast to the other manifestations of rheumatic fever, Sydenham chorea may occur several months following the streptococcal infection; rheumatic heart disease occurs days to weeks after acute streptococcal infection.

Streptococcal skin infection (pyoderma, impetigo) is usually superficial and may proceed through vesicular, pustular and encrusted stages. Scarlatiniform rash is unusual and rheumatic fever is not a sequel; however, glomerulonephritis may occur later, usually 3 weeks after the skin infection.

Scarlet fever is a form of streptococcal disease characterized by a skin rash; it occurs when the infecting strain of streptococcus produces a pyrogenic exotoxin (erythrogenic toxin) and the patient is sensitized but not immune to the toxin. Clinical characteristics may include all symptoms associated with a streptococcal sore throat (or those associated with a wound, skin or puerperal infection) as well as enanthem, strawberry tongue and exanthem. The rash is usually a fine erythema, commonly punctate, blanching on pressure, often felt (like sandpaper) better than seen and appearing most often on the neck, chest, in folds of the axilla, elbow, groin, and on inner surfaces of the thighs.

Typically, the scarlet fever rash does not involve the face, but there is flushing of the cheeks and circumoral pallor. High fever, nausea and vomiting often accompany severe infections. During convalescence, desquamation of the skin occurs at the tips of fingers and toes, less often over wide areas of trunk and limbs, including palms and soles; it is more pronounced where the exanthem was severe. The case-fatality rate in some parts of the world has occasionally been as high as 3%. Scarlet fever may be followed by the same sequelae as streptococcal sore throat.

Erysipelas is an acute cellulitis characterized by fever, constitutional symptoms, leukocytosis and a red, tender, edematous, spreading lesion of the skin, often with a definite raised border. The central point of origin tends to clear as the periphery extends. Face and legs are common sites. Recurrences are frequent. The disease is more common in women and may be especially severe, with bacteremia, in patients suffering from debilitating disease. Case-fatality rates vary greatly depending on the part of the body affected and whether there is an associated disease. Erysipelas due to group A streptococci is to be distinguished from erysipeloid, caused by *Erysipelothrix rhusiopathiae,* a localized cutaneous infection seen primarily as an occupational disease of people handling freshwater fish or shellfish, infected swine or turkeys or their tissues, or rarely sheep, cattle, chickens or pheasants.

Perianal cellulitis due to group A streptococci has been recognized more frequently in recent years.

Streptococcal puerperal fever is an acute disease, usually febrile, accompanied by local and general symptoms and signs of bacterial invasion of the genital tract and sometimes the bloodstream in the postpartum or postabortion patient. Case-fatality rate is low when streptococcal puerperal fever is adequately treated. Puerperal infections may be caused by organisms other than hemolytic streptococci; while clinically similar, they differ bacteriologically and epidemiologically. (See Staphylococcal disease.)

Toxic shock syndrome (TSS) in people with invasive group A streptococcal infection has been increasingly recognized in the USA since 1987. Predominant clinical features include hypotension and any of the following: renal impairment; thrombocytopenia; disseminated intravascular coagulation (DIC); SGOT or bilirubin elevation; adult respiratory distress syndrome; a generalized erythematous macular rash or soft-tissue necrosis (necrotizing fasciitis), the last labeled the "flesh-eating bacteria" by the news media. TSS may occur with either systemic or focal (i.e., throat, skin, lung sites) group A streptococcal infections.

Streptococci of other groups can produce human disease. Beta-hemolytic organisms of group B are frequently found in the human vagina and may cause neonatal sepsis and suppurative meningitis (see group B Streptococcal Disease of the Newborn, below), as well as urinary tract infections, postpartum endometritis and other systemic disease in adults, especially those with diabetes mellitus. Group D organisms (including enterococci), hemolytic or nonhemolytic, are involved in subacute bacterial endocarditis and urinary tract infections. Groups C and G have produced outbreaks of streptococcal tonsillitis, usually foodborne; their role in sporadic cases is less well-defined. Glomerulonephritis has followed group C infections, but has been reported very rarely following group G infection; neither group causes rheumatic fever. Groups C and G infections are more common in adolescents and young adults. Alpha-hemolytic streptococci are also a common cause of subacute bacterial endocarditis.

Provisional laboratory findings that support group A streptococcal disease are based on the isolation of the organisms from the affected tissues on blood agar or other appropriate media, or the identification of group A streptococcal antigen in pharyngeal secretions (the rapid strep test). In cultures, streptococci are identified by the morphology of colonies and production of clear β-hemolysis on blood agar made with sheep's blood; tentative identification is shown by inhibition by special antibiotic discs containing 0.02–0.04 units of bacitracin. Definitive identification depends on specific serogrouping procedures. Antigen detection tests are also available for rapid identification. A rise in serum antibody titer (antistreptolysin O, antihyaluronidase, anti-DNA-ase B) may be demonstrated between acute and convalescent stages of illness; high titers may persist for several months.

In the USA, the current recommended practice is to first do a rapid strep test (which has high specificity but low sensitivity) and, if positive, assume the patient has a group A streptococcal infection. If the result is negative or equivocal, a throat culture should be done to guide management.

2. Infectious agent—*Streptococcus pyogenes,* group A streptococci of approximately 80 serologically distinct types that may vary greatly by geographic and time distributions. Group A streptococci producing skin infections are usually of different serologic types from those associated with throat infections. In scarlet fever, three immunologically different types of erythrogenic toxin (pyrogenic exotoxins A, B and C) have been demonstrated. In TSS, 80% of isolates produce pyrogenic exotoxin A. While β-hemolysis is characteristic of group A streptococci, strains of groups B, C and G are most often also β-hemolytic. M type mucoid strains are involved in recent outbreaks of rheumatic fever and in invasive necrotizing fasciitis.

3. Occurrence—Streptococcal sore throat and scarlet fever are common in temperate zones, well recognized in semitropical areas and less frequently recognized in tropical climates. Inapparent infections are at least as common in tropical as in temperate zones. In the USA, streptococcal diseases may be endemic, epidemic or sporadic in character. Streptococcal pharyngitis is unusual under 2-3 years of age, peaks in age group 6-12 and declines after that. Cases occur year round but peak in late winter and early spring. Group A streptococcal infections due to a few specific types of M protein (M-types), especially types 1, 3, 4, 12 and 25, have frequently been associated with the development of acute glomerulonephritis.

Acute rheumatic fever may occur as a nonsuppurative complication following infection with group A serotypes that have the capacity to produce clinical infection of the upper respiratory tract. This complication had virtually disappeared from industrialized countries until several outbreaks appeared in the USA in 1985; increased numbers from many areas of the country are still being reported in the 1990s. Many of the reported cases have followed infections by specific group A serotypes, such as M-types 1, 3 and 18, which seem to be rheumatogenic.

Rheumatic fever remains a great problem in the developing world. The highest incidence is during late winter and spring and corresponds to that of pharyngitis. The group aged 3-15 years is most often affected; military and school populations are also frequently affected. Together with reappearance of rheumatic fever, more severe streptococcal infections have also been reported; these include generalized infections and toxic shock syndrome. In the USA, an estimated 10,000-15,000 cases of severe group A strep occur each year, 5%-19% of which (between 500 and 1,500 cases) develop necrotizing fasciitis.

The highest incidence of **streptococcal impetigo** occurs in young children in late summer and fall in hot climates. Nephritis following skin infections is associated with a limited number of streptococcal M-types (e.g., types 2, 49, 55, 57, 58, 59, 60 and other higher types), which generally differ from those associated with nephritis following infections of the upper respiratory tract.

Geographic and seasonal distribution of **erysipelas** are similar to those for scarlet fever and streptococcal sore throat; erysipelas is most common in infants and those over 20 years of age. Occurrence is sporadic, even during epidemics of streptococcal infection.

Reliable morbidity data do not exist for **puerperal fever.** In developed countries, morbidity and mortality have declined precipitously since the advent of antibiotics. It is now chiefly a sporadic disease, although epidemics may occur in institutions where aseptic technique is faulty.

4. Reservoir—Humans.

5. Mode of transmission—Large respiratory droplets or direct contact with patients or carriers, rarely by indirect contact through objects. Nasal carriers are particularly likely to transmit disease. Casual contact rarely leads to infection. In populations where impetigo is prevalent, group A streptococci may be recovered from the normal skin for 1-2 weeks before skin lesions develop; the same strain may appear in the throat (without clinical evidence of throat infection) usually late in the course of the skin infection.

Anal, vaginal, skin and pharyngeal carriers have been responsible for nosocomial outbreaks of serious streptococcal infection, particularly following surgical procedures. Many of these outbreaks have been traced to operating room personnel who were carriers of the streptococcal strain involved. Identification of the carrier often involves intensive epidemiologic and microbiologic investigation; eradication of the carrier state is often difficult and may require multiple courses of various antibiotics. Dried streptococci reaching the air via contaminated items (floor dust, lint from bedclothing, handkerchiefs) are viable but apparently noninfectious for mucous membranes and intact skin.

Explosive outbreaks of streptococcal sore throat may follow ingestion of contaminated food. Milk and milk products have been associated most frequently with foodborne outbreaks; egg salad and deviled hard-boiled eggs have recently been implicated with increasing frequency. Group A streptococci may be transmitted to cattle from human carriers, then spread through raw milk from these cattle; group B organisms that cause human and bovine disease differ biochemically. Contamination of milk or egg products by humans appears to be the important source of foodborne episodes. Milkborne group C outbreaks have been traced to infected cows.

6. **Incubation period**—Short, usually 1-3 days, rarely longer.

7. **Period of communicability**—In untreated, uncomplicated cases, 10-21 days; in untreated conditions with purulent discharges, weeks or months. With adequate penicillin therapy, transmissibility generally is terminated within 24 hours. Patients with untreated streptococcal pharyngitis may carry the organism in the pharynx for weeks or months, usually in decreasing numbers; the contagiousness of these carriers decreases sharply in 2-3 weeks after onset of infection.

8. **Susceptibility and resistance**—Susceptibility to streptococcal sore throat and scarlet fever is general, although many people develop either antitoxin or type specific antibacterial immunity, or both, through inapparent infection. Antibacterial immunity develops only against the specific M-type of group A streptococcus that induced infection and may last for years. Antibiotic therapy may interfere with the development of type specific immunity. No gender or racial differences in susceptibility have been defined; reports of racial differences probably relate to differing environmental factors.

Repeated attacks of sore throat or other streptococcal disease due to different types of streptococci are relatively frequent. Immunity against erythrogenic toxin, and hence to rash, develops within a week after onset of scarlet fever and is usually permanent; second attacks of scarlet fever are rare, but may occur because of the three immunologic forms of toxin. Passive immunity to group A streptococcal disease occurs in newborns with transplacental maternal type specific antibodies.

Patients who have had one attack of rheumatic fever have a significant risk of recurrence of rheumatic fever with further cardiac damage following group A streptococcal infections. Individuals who have had erysipelas appear to be predisposed to subsequent attacks. Recurrence of glomerulonephritis is unusual.

9. **Methods of control—**

   A. *Preventive measures:*

   1) Educate the public and health workers about modes of transmission; about the relationship of streptococcal infection to acute rheumatic fever, Sydenham chorea, rheumatic heart disease and glomerulonephritis; and about the necessity for prompt diagnosis and completion of the full course of antibiotic therapy prescribed for streptococcal infections.

   2) Provide easily accessible laboratory facilities for recognition of group A hemolytic streptococci.

   3) Pasteurize milk and exclude infected people from handling milk likely to become contaminated.

   4) Prepare other foods, such as deviled eggs, just prior to serving or adequately refrigerate in small quantities at 5°C (41°F) or less.

   5) Exclude people with skin lesions from food handling.

   6) Secondary prevention of complications: To prevent streptococcal reinfection and possible recurrence of rheumatic fever, erysipelas or chorea, monthly injections of long acting benzathine penicillin G (or daily penicillin orally, if the patient is compliant) should be given for at least 5 years. Those who do not tolerate penicillin may be given sulfisoxazole orally.

   B. *Control of patient, contacts and the immediate environment:*

   1) Report to local health authority: Obligatory report of epidemics, Class 4. Acute rheumatic fever and/or streptococcal TSS reportable in some localities, Class 3B (see Communicable Disease Reporting).

   2) Isolation: Drainage and secretion precautions; may be terminated after 24 hours' treatment with penicillin or other effective antibiotics; therapy should be continued for 10 days to avoid development of rheumatic heart disease.

   3) Concurrent disinfection: Of purulent discharges and all articles soiled therewith. Terminal cleaning.

   4) Quarantine: None.

   5) Immunization of contacts: None.

   6) Investigation of contacts and source of infection: Culture

symptomatic contacts. Search for and treat carriers in well-documented epidemics of streptococcal infection and in high risk situations (e.g., evidence of streptococcal infection in families with multiple cases of rheumatic fever or streptococcal TSS, occurrence of cases of rheumatic fever or acute nephritis in a population group such as a school, outbreaks of postoperative wound infections).

7) Specific treatment: Penicillin; several forms are acceptable for treatment: benzathine penicillin G, IM (treatment of choice), or penicillin G (PO) or penicillin V (PO). Penicillin resistant strains of streptococci have not occurred. Therapy should provide adequate penicillin levels for 10 days. Such treatment initiated within the first 24–48 hours may ameliorate the acute illness; however, the bacteria may persist in the pharynx in up to 30% of patients. Therapy will reduce the frequency of suppurative complications and prevent the development of most cases of acute rheumatic fever.

Therapy may also reduce the risk of acute glomerulonephritis and prevent further spread of the organism in the community. Erythromycin is the preferred treatment for penicillin sensitive patients, but strains resistant to this antibiotic have been reported. Clindamycin or a cephalosporin can be used when penicillin and erythromycin are contraindicated. Sulfonamides are not effective in eliminating the streptococcus from the throat or in preventing nonsuppurative complications. Many strains are resistant to the tetracyclines.

C. *Epidemic measures:*

1) Determine the source and manner of spread (i.e., person to person, by milk or food). Outbreaks can often be traced to an individual with an acute or persistent streptococcal infection or carrier state (nose, throat, skin, vagina or perianal area) through identification of the serologic type of the streptococcus.

2) Investigate promptly any unusual grouping of cases to identify possible common sources, such as contaminated milk or foods.

3) For outbreaks in special groups in which individuals have especially close contact, such as military populations and newborn nurseries, it may be necessary to administer penicillin to the entire group to terminate spread.

D. *Disaster implications:* Patients with thermal burns or wounds are highly susceptible to streptococcal infections of the affected area.

E. *International measures:* WHO Collaborating Centres.

GROUP B STREPTOCOCCAL SEPSIS OF THE NEWBORN   ICD-9 038.0; ICD-10 P36.0

Human subtypes of group B streptococci *(S. agalactiae)* produce important diseases in newborn infants. Two distinct forms of illness occur: early onset disease (from 1–7 days) is characterized by sepsis, respiratory distress, apnea, shock, pneumonia and meningitis; it has a case-fatality rate of about 50%, is acquired in utero or during delivery, and occurs more frequently in low birthweight infants. Late onset disease (from 7 days to several months) is characterized by sepsis and meningitis; it has a case-fatality rate of about 25%, is acquired by person to person contact, and occurs in full-term infants. Survivors of meningitis may have speech, hearing or visual problems, psychomotor retardation or seizure disorders.

While the manner of acquisition is unclear, approximately 10%–30% of pregnant women harbor group B streptococci in the genital tract. Approximately 1% of their offspring develop symptomatic infection; risk of serious disease is greatest among premature infants. The group B streptococci found in bovine mastitis are not a cause of this disease.

Attempts to use oral antibiotics to eradicate genital tract group B streptococci in women during pregnancy have been only partially successful. There are high relapse rates when antibiotics have been discontinued, possibly due to reinfection from rectal carriage of the organism or by possible reacquisition from culture positive sexual partners.

The administration of intravenous penicillin or ampicillin at the onset and throughout labor to women who are colonized with group B streptococci and who are at high risk of delivering an infected infant (premature labor at less than 37 weeks, premature rupture of membranes at less than 37 weeks, intrapartum fever, prolonged rupture of membranes of more than 18 hours, or a sibling affected by symptomatic group B infection) interrupts transmission of group B streptococci to newborn infants and decreases infection and mortality. While group B streptococci are sensitive to penicillin G and ampicillin, penicillin tolerant strains have been described, which suggests that severe infections should be treated with a penicillin plus an aminoglycoside, preferably gentamicin. A vaccine for pregnant women to stimulate antibody production against invasive disease in newborns is under development.

DENTAL CARIES OF EARLY CHILDHOOD, STREPTOCOCCAL   ICD-9 521.0; ICD-10 K02
(Nursing bottle caries, Baby bottle tooth decay)

While the cause of dental caries in young children is multifactorial, the subject is included in this section on streptococcal diseases because of the involvement of a streptococcal species.

A characteristic pattern of dental caries occurs in early childhood in which the maxillary primary incisors are routinely affected with carious lesions, but the mandibular primary incisors are rarely involved; involvement of other primary teeth is variable. Because of the association of this distinctive pattern of early childhood caries with a specific feeding habit, the process was called nursing bottle caries or baby bottle tooth decay, but it also occurs in children using feeding cups.

Streptococcus mutans organisms are present in these carious lesions. These organisms have been shown to produce caries in young experimental animals in the presence of dietary sugar. These gram-positive facultative anaerobes are members of the viridans group of streptococci; hemolysis of blood agar is usually alpha or gamma. The organisms require a nonshedding oral surface for colonization; they are common residents of dental plaque.

Early childhood caries occurs globally, with highest prevalence in developing countries. Disadvantaged children, regardless of ethnicity or culture, and those with low birthweights, are most frequently involved; enamel hypoplasia, which may be the consequence of compromised nutritional status during formative stages of primary dentition, is often associated. The major reservoir from which an infant acquires mutans streptococci is its mother; strains isolated from mothers and their babies exhibit similar or identical bacteriocin profiles and identical plasmid or chromosomal DNA patterns.

Transmission from mother to child occurs by transfer of infected saliva by kissing the baby on the mouth or, more likely, by moistening the nipple or pacifier or tasting food on the baby's spoon before serving it. Colonization by the maternal organisms is largely dependent on the size of the inoculum; mothers with extensive dental caries usually have high levels of mutans streptococci in their saliva.

To prevent dental caries of early childhood, promote good oral hygiene in mothers and encourage early weaning from the bottle. Counsel parents and caretakers about the dangers of dental caries from feeding children milk and other beverages containing sugar and of transferring saliva to a baby's mouth when mothers and other caretakers have untreated carious teeth.

STRONGYLOIDIASIS   ICD-9 127.2; ICD-10 B78

1. Identification—An often asymptomatic helminthic infection of the duodenum and upper jejunum. Clinical manifestations include transient dermatitis when larvae of the parasite penetrate the skin on initial infection; cough, rales and sometimes a demonstrable pneumonitis when larvae pass through the lungs; or abdominal symptoms caused by the adult female worm in the mucosa of the intestine. Symptoms of chronic infection may be mild or severe, depending on the intensity of the infection.

Classic symptoms are abdominal pain (usually epigastric and often suggesting peptic ulcer), diarrhea and urticaria; they may also include nausea, weight loss, vomiting, weakness and constipation. Intensely pruritic dermatitis (larva currens) radiating from the anus may occur; stationary wheals lasting 1-2 days may occur as well as a migrating serpiginous rash moving several centimeters per hour across the trunk. Rarely, intestinal autoinfection with increasing worm burden may lead to disseminated strongyloidiasis with wasting, pulmonary involvement and death, particularly but not exclusively in the immunocompromised host. In these cases, secondary gram-negative sepsis is common. Eosinophilia is usually moderate (10%-25%) in the chronic stage and in those with intercurrent infections, especially in persons infected with human T-cell lymphotrophic virus (HTLV-1) and those receiving chemotherapy for malignancies, but may be normal or low with dissemination.

Diagnosis is made by identifying larvae in concentrated stool specimens (motile in freshly passed feces), in the agar plate method, in duodenal aspirates or, occasionally, in sputum. Repeat examinations may be necessary to rule out the diagnosis. Held at room temperature for 24 hours or more, feces may show developing stages of the parasite, including rhabditiform larvae (noninfectious) and filariform (infective) larvae (which must be distinguished from larvae of hookworm species) and free living adults. Serologic tests, such as EIA, based on larval stage antigens are positive in 80%-85% of infected patients.

2. Infectious agents—*Strongyloides stercoralis* and *S. fülleborni*, nematodes.

3. Occurrence—Throughout tropical and temperate areas; more common in warm, wet regions. Prevalence in endemic areas is not accurately known. May be prevalent in residents of institutions where personal hygiene is poor. *S. fülleborni* has been reported only in Africa and Papua New Guinea.

4. Reservoir—Humans are the principal reservoir of *S. stercoralis*, with only occasional transmission of dog and cat strains to humans. Nonhuman primates are the reservoir of *S. fülleborni* in Africa. Person to person transmission may also occur.

5. Mode of transmission—Infective (filariform) larvae, which develop in feces or moist soil contaminated with feces, penetrate the skin, enter the venous circulation and are carried to the lungs. They penetrate capillary walls, enter the alveoli, ascend the trachea to the epiglottis and descend into the digestive tract to reach the upper part of the small intestine, where development of the adult female is completed.

The adult worm, a parthenogenetic female, lives embedded in the mucosal epithelium of the intestine, especially the duodenum, where eggs are deposited. They hatch and liberate rhabditiform (noninfective) larvae that migrate into the lumen of the intestine, exit the host in the feces and develop into either infective filariform larvae (which may infect the same or a new host) or free living male and female adults after reaching the soil. The free living, fertilized females produce eggs that soon hatch and liberate rhabditiform larvae, which may become filariform larvae within 24-36 hours. In some individuals, rhabditiform larvae may develop to the infective stage before leaving the body and penetrate through the intestinal mucosa or perianal skin; the resulting autoinfection can cause persistent infection for many years.

6. Incubation period—From penetration of the skin by filariform larvae until rhabditiform larvae appear in the feces is 2-4 weeks; the period until symptoms appear is indefinite and variable.

7. Period of communicability—As long as living worms remain in the intestine; up to 35 years in cases of autoinfection.

8. Susceptibility and resistance—Susceptibility is universal. Acquired immunity has been demonstrated in laboratory animals but not in humans. Patients with AIDS, with malignant disease or on immunosuppressive medication are at risk of dissemination.

9. Methods of control—

   A. Preventive measures:

   1) Dispose of human feces in a sanitary manner.
   2) Pay rigid attention to hygienic habits, including use of footwear in endemic areas.
   3) Rule out strongyloidiasis before initiating immunosuppressive therapy.
   4) Examine and treat infected dogs, cats and monkeys that are in contact with people.

   B. Control of patient, contacts and the immediate environment:

   1) Report to local health authority: Official report not ordinarily justifiable, Class 5 (see Communicable Disease Reporting).
   2) Isolation: None.
   3) Concurrent disinfection: Sanitary disposal of feces.
   4) Quarantine: None.
   5) Immunization of contacts: None.
   6) Investigation of contacts and source of infection: Members of the same household or institution should be examined for evidence of infection.
   7) Specific treatment: Because of the potential for autoinfection and dissemination, all infections, regardless of worm burden,

should be treated, preferably with ivermectin (Mectizan®), thiabendazole (Mintezol®), or albendazole (Zentel®). Repeated courses of treatment may be required.

C. Epidemic measures: Not applicable; a sporadic disease.

D. Disaster implications: None.

E. International measures: None.

SYPHILIS
I. SYPHILIS   ICD-9 090–096; ICD-10 A50–A52
(Lues)

1. Identification—An acute and chronic treponemal disease characterized clinically by a primary lesion, a secondary eruption involving skin and mucous membranes, long periods of latency, and late lesions of skin, bone, viscera, the CNS and cardiovascular system. The primary lesion (chancre) usually appears about three weeks after exposure as an indurated, painless ulcer with a serous exudate at the site of initial invasion. Invasion of the bloodstream precedes the initial lesion, and a firm, nonfluctuant, painless satellite lymph node (bubo) commonly follows.

Infection may occur without a clinically evident chancre; i.e., it may be in the rectum or on the cervix. After 4–6 weeks, even with specific treatment, the chancre begins to involute and, in approximately one third of untreated cases, a generalized secondary eruption appears, often accompanied by mild constitutional symptoms. This symmetrical maculopapular rash involving the palms and soles, with associated lymphadenopathy, is classic. Secondary manifestations resolve spontaneously within weeks to 12 months; again, about one third of untreated cases of secondary syphilis will become clinically latent for weeks to years. In the early years of latency, there may be recurrence of infectious lesions of the skin and mucous membranes.

CNS disease, manifested as acute syphilitic meningitis, may occur at any time in secondary or early latent syphilis, later as meningovascular syphilis, and finally as paresis or tabes dorsalis. Latency sometimes continues through life. In other instances, and unpredictably, 5–20 years after initial infection, disabling lesions occur in the aorta (cardiovascular syphilis) or gummas may occur in the skin, viscera, bone and/or mucosal surfaces. Death or serious disability rarely occurs during early stages; late manifestations shorten life, impair health and limit occupational efficiency. Concurrent HIV infection may increase the risk of CNS syphilis; neurosyphilis must be considered in the differential diagnosis of an HIV infected individual with CNS symptoms.

Fetal infection occurs with high frequency in untreated early infections of pregnant women and with lower frequency later in latency. It frequently causes abortion or stillbirth and may cause infant death due to preterm delivery of low birthweight infants or from generalized systemic disease. Congenital infection may result in late manifestations that include involvement of the CNS and occasionally cause such stigmata as Hutchinson teeth, saddlenose, saber shins, interstitial keratitis and deafness. Congenital syphilis can be asymptomatic, especially in the first weeks of life.

The laboratory diagnosis of syphilis is usually made by serologic tests of blood and CSF when indicated. Reactive tests with nontreponemal antigens (e.g., RPR [rapid plasma reagin] or VDRL [Venereal Disease Research Laboratory]) need to be confirmed by tests that employ treponemal antigens (i.e., FTA-Abs [fluorescent treponemal antibody absorbed], MHA-TP [microhemagglutination assay for antibody to *Treponema pallidum*] or TPHA [*T. pallidum* hemagglutinating antibody]), when available, to aid in excluding biological false-positive reactions. For screening newborn infants, serum is preferred over cord blood, which produces more false-positive reactions. Primary and secondary syphilis can be confirmed by darkfield or phase-contrast examination or by FA antibody staining of exudates from lesions or aspirates from lymph nodes if no antibiotic has been administered. Serologic tests are usually nonreactive during the early primary stage while the chancre is still present; a darkfield examination of all genital ulcerative lesions can be useful, particularly in suspected early seronegative primary syphilis.

2. Infectious agent—*Treponema pallidum,* subspecies *pallidum,* a spirochete.

3. Occurrence—Widespread; in the USA sexually active young people between 20 and 29 years of age are primarily involved. Racial differences in incidence reflect social rather than biological factors. Syphilis is usually more prevalent in urban than rural areas, and in some cultures, in males more than in females. The high prevalence among homosexual men seen in the late 1970s and early 1980s has declined since 1983.

In many areas of the USA, especially urban areas and the rural South, reported rates of syphilis and congenital syphilis increased beginning in 1986 and continued into 1990, then subsequently declined. This increase occurred primarily among those in lower socioeconomic classes and especially among teenagers; risk factors include illicit drug use, prostitution, AIDS and earlier age at first sexual intercourse. 1991 was the first year since 1985 in which the number of reported syphilis cases declined; the reasons for this decline are unclear. Early venereal and congenital syphilis have increased significantly throughout much of the world since 1957.

4. Reservoir—Humans.

5. Mode of transmission—By direct contact with infectious exudates from obvious or concealed, moist, early lesions of skin and mucous membranes of infected people during sexual contact; exposure nearly always occurs during sexual intercourse. Transmission by kissing or fondling children with early congenital disease occurs rarely. Transplacental infection of the fetus occurs during the pregnancy of an infected woman.

Transmission can occur through blood transfusion if the donor is in the early stages of disease. Infection by contact with contaminated articles may be theoretically possible but is extraordinarily rare. Health professionals have developed primary lesions on the hands following clinical examination of infectious lesions.

6. Incubation period—From 10 days to 3 months, usually 3 weeks.

7. Period of communicability—Communicability exists when moist mucocutaneous lesions of primary and secondary syphilis are present. However, the distinction between the infectious primary and secondary stages and the noninfectious early latent stage of syphilis is somewhat arbitrary with regard to communicability, since primary and secondary stage lesions may not be apparent to the infected individual. The lesions of secondary syphilis may recur with decreasing frequency up to four years after infection. However, transmission of infection is rare after the first year. Consequently, in the United States infectious early syphilis is usually defined as ending after the first year of infection.

Transmission of syphilis from mother to fetus is most probable during early maternal syphilis but can occur throughout the latent period. Infected infants may have moist mucocutaneous lesions that are more widespread than in adult syphilis and are a potential source of infection.

8. Susceptibility and resistance—Susceptibility is universal, though only approximately 30% of exposures result in infection. Infection leads to gradual development of immunity against *T. pallidum* and, to some extent, against heterologous treponemes; immunity often fails to develop because of early treatment in the primary and secondary stages. Concurrent HIV infection may reduce the normal host response to *T. pallidum*.

9. Methods of control—

    A. Preventive measures: In general, the following preventive measures are applicable to all STDs: syphilis, HIV infection, chancroid, lymphogranuloma venereum, granuloma inguinale, gonorrhea, herpes simplex virus infection, genital human papillomavirus infections (genital warts), trichomoniasis, bacterial vaginosis, sexually transmitted hepatitis B, chlamydial infections and genital mycoplasma.

        Emphasis on early detection and effective treatment of patients with transmissible syphilis and their contacts should not preclude search for people with latent syphilis to prevent relapse and disability due to late manifestations.

1) Educate the community in general health promotion measures; provide health and sex instruction that teaches the value of delaying sexual activity until onset of sexual maturity as well as the importance of establishing mutually monogamous relationships and reducing numbers of sexual partners. Syphilis serology should be included in the workup of all cases of STD and as a routine part of prenatal examination. Congenital syphilis is prevented by serologic examination in early pregnancy and again in late pregnancy and at delivery in high prevalence populations; treat those who are reactive.

2) Protect the community by preventing and controlling STDs in sex workers and their clients by discouraging multiple sexual partners and anonymous or casual sexual activity. Teach methods of personal prophylaxis applicable before, during and after exposure, especially the correct and consistent use of condoms.

3) Provide health care facilities for early diagnosis and treatment of STDs; encourage their use through education of the public about symptoms of STDs and modes of spread; make these services culturally appropriate and readily accessible and acceptable, regardless of economic status. Establish intensive case-finding programs that include interviewing patients and partner notification; for syphilis, repeated serologic screening within special populations with known high incidence of STDs. Follow cases serologically to exclude other STD infections such as HIV.

B. Control of patient, contacts and the immediate environment:

1) Report to local health authority: Case report of early infectious syphilis and congenital syphilis is required in all states and variously in other countries, Class 2A (see Communicable Disease Reporting); laboratories are required to report reactive serology and positive darkfield examinations in most states. Confidentiality of the individual must be safeguarded.

2) Isolation: For hospitalized patients, universal precautions for blood and body secretions should be applied. Patients should refrain from sexual intercourse until treatment is completed and lesions disappear; to avoid reinfection, they should refrain from sexual activity with previous partners until they have been examined and treated.

3) Concurrent disinfection: None in adequately treated cases; care to avoid contact with discharges from open lesions and articles soiled therewith.

4) Quarantine: None.

5) Immunization of contacts: None available.

6) Investigation of contacts and source of infection: A fundamen-

tal feature of programs for syphilis control is the interviewing of patients to identify sexual contacts from whom infection was acquired in addition to those whom the patient may have infected. Trained interviewers obtain best results. The stage of disease determines the criteria for partner notification: a) for primary syphilis, all sexual contacts during the 3 months preceding onset of symptoms; b) for secondary syphilis, contacts during the preceding 6 months; c) for early latent syphilis, those of the preceding year, if time of primary and secondary lesions cannot be established; d) for late and late latent syphilis, marital partners and children of infected mothers; and e) for congenital syphilis, all members of the immediate family. All identified sexual contacts of confirmed cases of early syphilis exposed within 90 days of examination should receive treatment. Patients and their partners should be encouraged to obtain HIV counseling and testing.

Infants born to all seroreactive mothers should be treated with penicillin, if adequate treatment of the mother prior to the last month of pregnancy cannot be established.

7) Specific treatment: Long acting penicillin G (benzathine penicillin), 2.4 million units given in a single IM dose on the day that primary, secondary or early latent syphilis, is diagnosed; this assures effective therapy even if the patient fails to return.

Alternative therapy for nonpregnant penicillin allergic patients: either doxycycline PO, 100 mg twice daily for 14 days, or tetracycline PO, 500 mg 4 times/day for 14 days.

Serologic testing is important to ensure adequate therapy; tests are repeated at 3 and 6 months after treatment and later as needed. In HIV infected patients, testing should be repeated at 1, 2 and 3 months, and at 3-month intervals thereafter. Any fourfold titer rise indicates the need for retreatment.

Failure of nontreponemal tests to decline fourfold by 3 months after therapy for primary or secondary syphilis identifies those at risk of treatment failure. Increased dosages and longer periods of therapy are indicated for the late stages of syphilis (i.e., benzathine penicillin G, 7.2 million units total, administered as 3 doses of 2.4 million units IM at 1-week intervals). Consideration should be given to analysis of the CSF, especially if increased risk of neurosyphilis exists: those who have failed therapy, those who are infected with HIV, and those with neurologic findings.

For neurosyphilis, aqueous crystalline penicillin G, 18–24 million units a day administered as 3–4 million units IV every 4 hours for 10–14 days. An alternative therapy is procaine penicillin, 2–4 million units IM daily, plus probenecid PO, 500 mg orally, 4 times/day, both for 10–14 days. Success in therapy should be checked by following serologic titers and appropriate CSF examinations every 6 months until cell count is normal.

Penicillin sensitive pregnant women should have their allergy confirmed with skin tests to the major and minor penicillin determinants, if the test antigens are available. Erythromycin can be used for penicillin sensitive pregnant women but this has high failure rates. Patients with confirmed penicillin allergy can be desensitized and then given the dose of penicillin indicated by the stage of their syphilis.

For early congenital syphilis, aqueous crystalline penicillin G, 50,000 units/kg/dose, given IV or IM every 12 hours during the first 7 days of life, and every 8 hours thereafter for 10–14 days. For late congenital syphilis, if the CSF is normal and there is no neurologic involvement, children can be treated as for latent syphilis. If the CSF is abnormal, treatment for neurosyphilis is required: 200,000 units/kg/d of aqueous crystalline penicillin G every 6 hours for 10–14 days.

C. Epidemic measures: Intensification of measures outlined under 9A and 9B, above.

D. Disaster implications: None.

E. International measures:

1) Examine groups of adolescents and young adults who move from areas of high prevalence of treponemal infections.
2) Adhere to agreements among nations (e.g., Brussels Agreement) as to records, provision of diagnostic and treatment facilities and contact interviews at seaports for foreign merchant seamen.
3) Provide for rapid international exchange of information on contacts.
4) WHO Collaborating Centres.

II. NONVENEREAL ENDEMIC SYPHILIS ICD-9 104.0; ICD-10 A65
(Bejel, Njovera)

1. Identification—An acute disease of limited geographic distribution, characterized clinically by an eruption of skin and mucous membranes, usually without an evident primary sore. Mucous patches of the mouth are often the first lesions, soon followed by moist papules in skin folds and by drier lesions of the trunk and extremities. Other early skin lesions are macular or papular, often hypertrophic, and frequently circinate; lesions resemble those of venereal syphilis. Plantar and palmar hyperkeratoses occur frequently, often with painful fissuring; patchy depigmentation and hyperpigmentation of the skin and alopecia are common. Inflammatory or destructive lesions of skin, long bones and nasopharynx are late manifestations. Unlike venereal syphilis, the nervous and cardiovascular systems are rarely involved. The case-fatality rate is low.

Organisms are demonstrable in lesions by darkfield examination during early disease. Serologic tests for syphilis are reactive in the early stages and remain so for many years then gradually tend toward reversal; response to treatment as in venereal syphilis.

2. Infectious agent—*Treponema pallidum*, subspecies *endemicum*, a spirochete indistinguishable from that of syphilis.

3. Occurrence—A common disease of childhood in localized areas where poor socioeconomic conditions and primitive sanitary and dwelling arrangements prevail. Present in eastern Mediterranean and Asian countries; numerous foci exist in Africa, particularly in arid regions.

4. Reservoir—Humans.

5. Mode of transmission—Direct or indirect contact with infectious early lesions of skin and mucous membranes; the latter is favored by common use of eating and drinking utensils and generally unsatisfactory hygienic conditions. Congenital transmission does not occur.

6. Incubation period—From 2 weeks to 3 months.

7. Period of communicability—Until moist eruptions of skin and mucous patches disappear; sometimes several weeks or months.

8. Susceptibility and resistance—Similar to venereal syphilis.

9. Methods of control —

    A. Preventive measures: Those of the nonvenereal treponematoses. See Yaws, 9A.

    B. Control of patient, contacts and the immediate environment:

      1) Report to local health authority: In selected endemic areas; in most countries not a reportable disease, Class 3B (see Communicable Disease Reporting).

      2), 3), 4), 5), 6) and 7) Isolation, Concurrent disinfection, Quarantine, Immunization of contacts, Investigation of contacts and source of infection, and Specific treatment: See Yaws, 9B, applicable to all nonvenereal treponematoses.

    C. Epidemic measures: Intensification of preventive and control activities.

    D. Disaster implications: None.

    E. International measures: See Yaws, 9E. WHO Collaborating Centres.

TAENIASIS   ICD-9 123; ICD-10 B68
TAENIA SOLIUM TAENIASIS
   INTESTINAL FORM   ICD-9 123.0; ICD-10 B68.0
(Pork tapeworm)
TAENIA SAGINATA
   TAENIASIS   ICD-9 123.2; ICD-10 B68.1
(Beef tapeworm)
CYSTICERCOSIS   ICD-9 123.I; ICD-10 B69
(Cysticerciasis, *Taenia solium* cysticercosis)

1. **Identification**—Taeniasis is an intestinal infection with the adult stage of large tapeworms; cysticercosis is a tissue infection with the larval stage of one species, *Taenia solium*. Clinical manifestations of infection with the adult worm, if present, are variable and may include nervousness, insomnia, anorexia, weight loss, abdominal pain and digestive disturbances. Except for the annoyance of having segments of worms emerging from the anus, many infections are asymptomatic. Taeniasis is usually a nonfatal infection, but the larval stage of *T. solium* may cause fatal cysticercosis.

Larval infection of humans with the pork tapeworm, cysticercosis, may produce serious somatic disease, usually involving the CNS. When eggs or proglottids of the pork tapeworm are swallowed by people, the eggs hatch in the small intestine and the larvae migrate to the subcutaneous tissues, striated muscles, and other tissues and vital organs of the body, where they form cysticerci. Consequences may be grave when larvae localize in the eye, CNS or heart. In the presence of somatic cysticercosis, epileptiform seizures, headache, signs of intracranial hypertension or psychiatric disturbances strongly suggest cerebral involvement. Neurocysticercosis may cause serious disability but with a relatively low case-fatality rate.

Infection with an adult tapeworm is diagnosed by identification of proglottids (segments), eggs or antigens of the worm in the feces or on anal swabs. Eggs of *T. solium* and *T. saginata* cannot be differentiated from each other morphologically. Specific diagnosis is based on the morphology of the scolex (head) and/or gravid proglottids.

Specific serologic tests should support the clinical diagnosis of cysticercosis. Subcutaneous cysticerci may be visible or palpable; microscopic examination of an excised cysticercus confirms the diagnosis. Cysticercosis in intracerebral and other tissues may be recognized by CAT scan or MRI, or by x-ray when the cysticerci are calcified.

2. **Infectious agents**—*Taenia solium,* the pork tapeworm, causes both intestinal infection with the adult worm and somatic infection with the larvae (cysticerci). *T. saginata,* the beef tapeworm, causes only intestinal infection with the adult worm in humans.

3. Occurrence—Worldwide; particularly frequent wherever beef or pork is eaten raw or insufficiently cooked and where sanitary conditions permit pigs and cattle to have access to human feces. Prevalence is highest in parts of Latin America, Africa, southeast Asia and eastern Europe, and infection is common in immigrants from these areas. Transmission of *T. solium* is rare in the USA and Canada, and exceedingly rare in the UK and Scandinavia. Transmission associated with fecal-oral contact with immigrants with imported *T. solium* infections has been reported with increasing frequency in the USA. Immigrants from endemic areas are unlikely to spread infection in countries with good sanitation.

4. Reservoir—Humans are the definitive host of both species of *Taenia;* cattle are the intermediate hosts for *T. saginata,* and pigs for *T. solium.*

5. Mode of transmission—Eggs of *T. saginata* passed in the stool of an infected person are infectious only to cattle, in the flesh of which the parasites develop into cysticercus bovis, the larval stage of *T. saginata.* In humans, infection follows ingestion of raw or undercooked beef containing cysticerci; in the intestine, the adult worm develops attached to the jejunal mucosa.

Intestinal infection in humans (taeniasis due to *T. solium)* follows ingestion of raw or undercooked infected pork ("measly pork"), with subsequent development of the adult worm in the intestine. However, human cysticercosis may occur by direct transfer of *T. solium* eggs from the feces of people harboring an adult worm to their own (autoinfection) or another's mouth or indirectly by ingestion of food or water contaminated with eggs. When the eggs of *T. solium* are ingested by either humans or pigs, the embryos escape from the shells, penetrate the intestinal wall into lymphatics or blood vessels and are carried to the various tissues, where they develop to produce cysticercosis.

6. Incubation period—Symptoms of cysticercosis may appear from weeks to 10 years or more after infection. Eggs appear in the stool 8-12 weeks after infection with the adult *T. solium* tapeworm, 10-14 weeks with *T. saginata.*

7. Period of communicability—*T. saginata* is not directly transmitted from person to person, but *T. solium* may be. Eggs of both species are disseminated into the environment as long as the worm remains in the intestine, sometimes more than 30 years; eggs may remain viable in the environment for months.

8. Susceptibility and resistance—Susceptibility is general. No apparent resistance follows infection, but more than one tapeworm in a person has rarely been reported.

9. **Methods of control—**

A. *Preventive measures:*

1) Educate the public to prevent fecal contamination of soil, water, and human and animal food; to avoid use of sewage effluents for pasture irrigation; and to cook beef and pork thoroughly.
2) Identification and immediate treatment or institution of enteric precautions for people harboring adult *T. solium* is essential to prevent human cysticercosis. *T. solium* eggs are infective immediately on leaving the host and are capable of producing a severe human illness. Appropriate measures to protect patients from themselves and their contacts are necessary.
3) Freezing pork or beef at a temperature below –5°C (23°F) for more than 4 days kills the cysticerci effectively. Irradiation is very effective at 1 kGy.
4) Inspection of the carcasses of cattle and swine will detect only a proportion of infected carcasses; these should be condemned, irradiated or processed into cooked products.
5) Deny swine access to latrines and human feces.

B. *Control of patient, contacts and the immediate environment:*

1) Report to local health authority: Selectively reportable, Class 3C (see Communicable Disease Reporting).
2) Isolation: None recommended. Stools of patients with untreated taeniasis due to *T. solium* may be infective (see 9A2, above).
3) Concurrent disinfection: Dispose of feces in a sanitary manner; emphasize rigid sanitation, with handwashing after defecating and before eating, especially for *T. solium.*
4) Quarantine: None.
5) Immunization of contacts: None.
6) Investigation of contacts and source of infection: Evaluate symptomatic contacts.
7) Specific treatment: Praziquantel (Biltricide®) is effective in the treatment of *T. saginata* and *T. solium* intestinal infections. Niclosamide (Niclocide®, Yomesan®) is now a secondary choice and is no longer widely available. For cysticercosis, surgical intervention may relieve some symptoms. Patients with active CNS cysticercosis should be treated with praziquantel or albendazole under hospitalization; a short course of corticosteroids is usually given to control cerebral edema from dying cysticerci.

C. *Epidemic measures:* None.

D. Disaster implications: None.

E. International measures: None.

ASIAN TAENIASIS

Human infections have been reported from the Philippines, Korea, Taiwan, Indonesia and Thailand with a *T. saginata*-like tapeworm acquired by eating uncooked liver and other viscera of pigs; in experimental studies this organism produced cysticerci only in the livers of pigs, cattle, goats and monkeys. This organism has been established to be genetically distinct and is variously named as a separate species or subspecies.

TETANUS   ICD-9 037; ICD-10 A35
(Lockjaw)
(Obstetrical tetanus: ICD-10 A34)

1. Identification—An acute disease induced by an exotoxin of the tetanus bacillus, which grows anaerobically at the site of an injury. The disease is characterized by painful muscular contractions, primarily of the masseter and neck muscles, secondarily of trunk muscles. A common first sign suggestive of tetanus in older children and adults is abdominal rigidity, though rigidity is sometimes confined to the region of injury. Generalized spasms occur, frequently induced by sensory stimuli; typical features of the tetanic spasm are the position of opisthotonus and the facial expression known as "risus sardonicus." History of an injury or apparent portal of entry may be lacking. The case-fatality rate ranges from 10% to 90%, it is highest in infants and the elderly, and varies inversely with the length of the incubation period and the availability of experienced intensive care unit personnel and resources.

Attempts at laboratory confirmation are of little help. The organism is rarely recovered from the site of infection, and usually there is no detectable antibody response.

2. Infectious agent—*Clostridium tetani,* the tetanus bacillus.

3. Occurrence—Worldwide. Sporadic and relatively uncommon in the USA and most industrial countries. During the period 1995-1997, there were 124 cases reported from 33 states in the USA; 60% occurred in persons aged 20-59 years; 35% were 60 years of age or older; and 5% were less than 20 years old. The case-fatality rate increased with age from 2.3% in those aged 20-39 years to 18% for persons over 60 years of age. Tetanus in injecting drug users with no known acute injury accounted for 11% of the

124 cases compared with 3.6% during 1991–1994. An average of 50 cases per year continue to be reported to CDC. The disease is more common in agricultural regions and in underdeveloped areas where contact with animal excreta is more likely and immunization is inadequate; an important cause of death in many countries of Asia, Africa and South America, especially in rural and tropical areas where tetanus neonatorum is common (see below). Parenteral use of drugs by addicts, particularly intramuscular or subcutaneous use, can result in individual cases and occasional circumscribed outbreaks.

4. Reservoir—Intestines of horses and other animals, including humans, in which the organism is a harmless normal inhabitant. Soil or fomites contaminated with animal and human feces. Tetanus spores are ubiquitous in the environment and can contaminate wounds of all types.

5. Mode of transmission—Tetanus spores are introduced into the body, usually through a puncture wound contaminated with soil, street dust or animal or human feces; through lacerations, burns and trivial or unnoticed wounds; or by injected contaminated street drugs. Tetanus occasionally follows surgical procedures, which include circumcision. The presence of necrotic tissue and/or foreign bodies favors growth of the anaerobic pathogen. Cases have followed injuries considered too trivial for medical consultation.

6. Incubation period—Usually 3–21 days, although it may range from 1 day to several months, depending on the character, extent and location of the wound; average 10 days. Most cases occur within 14 days. In general, shorter incubation periods are associated with more heavily contaminated wounds, more severe disease and a worse prognosis.

7. Period of communicability—Not directly transmitted from person to person.

8. Susceptibility and resistance—Susceptibility is general. Active immunity is induced by tetanus toxoid and persists for at least 10 years after full immunization; transient passive immunity follows injection of tetanus immune globulin (TIG) or tetanus antitoxin (equine origin). Infants of actively immunized mothers acquire passive immunity that protects them from neonatal tetanus. Recovery from tetanus may not result in immunity; second attacks can occur. Primary immunization is indicated after recovery.

9. Methods of control—

   A. *Preventive measures:*

   1) Educate the public on the necessity for complete immunization with tetanus toxoid, the hazards of puncture wounds and closed injuries that are particularly liable to be complicated by

tetanus, and the potential need after injury for active and/or passive prophylaxis.

2) Universal active immunization with adsorbed tetanus toxoid, which gives durable protection for at least 10 years; after the initial basic series has been completed, single booster doses elicit high levels of immunity. The toxoid is generally administered together with diphtheria toxoid and pertussis vaccine as a triple (DTP or DTaP) antigen (or double [DT] antigen for children under 7 years with contraindications to pertussis vaccine), or Td for older people. For children 7 years or older, preparations that include *Haemophilus influenzae* type b conjugate vaccines (DTP–Hib) are available in the USA, as are preparations that include acellular pertussis vaccine (DTaP). In some countries, DTP, DT and T are available combined with inactivated polio vaccine. In countries with incomplete immunization programs for children, all pregnant women should receive 2 doses of tetanus toxoid. Nonadsorbed ("plain") preparations are less immunogenic for primary immunization or booster shots. Minor local reactions following tetanus toxoid injections are relatively frequent; severe local and systemic reactions are infrequent but do occur, particularly after excessive numbers of prior doses have been given.

a) The schedule recommended for tetanus immunization is the same as for diphtheria (see Diphtheria, 9A).

b) While tetanus toxoid is recommended for universal use regardless of age, it is especially important for workers in contact with soil, sewage and domestic animals; members of the military forces; policemen and others with greater than usual risk of traumatic injury; and older adults who are currently at highest risk for tetanus and tetanus related mortality. Vaccine induced maternal immunity is important in preventing neonatal tetanus.

c) Active protection should be maintained by administering booster doses of Td every 10 years.

d) For children and adults who are severely immunocompromised or infected with HIV, tetanus toxoid is indicated in the same schedule and dose as for immunocompetent persons even though the immune response may be suboptimal.

3) Prophylaxis in wound management: Tetanus prophylaxis in patients with wounds is based on careful assessment of whether the wound is clean or contaminated, the immunization status of the patient, proper use of tetanus toxoid and/or TIG (see table, below), wound cleaning and, where required, surgical debridement and the proper use of antibiotics.

a) Those who have been completely immunized who sustain minor and uncontaminated wounds require a booster dose of toxoid only if more than 10 years have elapsed since the last dose was given. For major and/or contaminated wounds, a single booster injection of a tetanus toxoid (preferably Td) should be administered promptly on the day of injury if the patient has not received tetanus toxoid within the preceding 5 years.

b) Persons who have not completed a full primary series of tetanus toxoid require a dose of toxoid as soon as possible following the wound and may require passive immunization with human TIG if it is a major wound and/or it is contaminated with soil containing animal excreta. DTP/ DTaP, DT or Td, as determined by the age of the patient and previous immunization history, should be used at the time of the wound, and ultimately, to complete the primary series.

Passive immunization with at least 250 IU of TIG IM (or 1,500 to 5,000 IU of antitoxin of animal origin if TIG is not available) is indicated for patients with other than clean, minor wounds and a history of no, unknown or fewer than three previous tetanus toxoid doses. When tetanus toxoid and TIG or antitoxin are given concurrently, separate syringes and separate sites must be used.

When antitoxin of animal origin is given, it is essential to avoid anaphylaxis by first injecting 0.02 ml of a 1:100 dilution in physiologic saline intradermally, with a syringe containing adrenaline on hand. Pretest with a 1:1,000 dilution if there has been prior animal serum exposure, together with a similar injection of physiologic saline as a negative control. If after 15-20 minutes there is a wheal with surrounding erythema at least 3 mm larger than the negative control, it is necessary to desensitize the individual. Penicillin given for 7 days may kill *C. tetani* in the wound, but this does not obviate the need for prompt treatment of the wound together with appropriate immunization.

B. Control of patient, contacts and the immediate environment:

1) Report to local health authority: Case report required in all states (USA) and in most countries, Class 2B (see Communicable Disease Reporting).
2) Isolation: None.
3) Concurrent disinfection: None.
4) Quarantine: None.
5) Immunization of contacts: None.
6) Investigation of contacts and source of infection: Case investigation to determine circumstances of injury.
7) Specific treatment: TIG IM in doses of 3,000-6,000 IU. If TIG is not available, tetanus antitoxin (equine origin) in a single large

dose should be given IV following appropriate testing for hypersensitivity; IV metronidazole in large doses should be given for 7–14 days. The wound should be debrided widely and excised if possible. Wide debridement of the umbilical stump in neonates is not indicated. Maintain an adequate airway and employ sedation as indicated; muscle relaxant drugs together with tracheostomy or nasotracheal intubation and mechanically assisted respiration may be lifesaving. Active immunization should be initiated concurrently with therapy.

C. *Epidemic measures:* In the rare outbreak, search for contaminated street drugs.

D. *Disaster implications:* Social upheaval (military conflicts, riots) and natural disasters (floods, hurricanes, earthquakes) that cause many traumatic injuries in nonimmunized populations will result in an increased need for TIG or tetanus antitoxin and toxoid for injured patients.

E. *International measures:* Up-to-date immunization against tetanus is advised for international travelers.

TETANUS NEONATORUM   ICD-9 771.3; ICD-10 A33

Tetanus neonatorum is a serious health problem in many developing countries where maternity care services are limited and immunization against tetanus is inadequate. In the past 5 years the incidence of tetanus neonatorum declined considerably in many developing countries due to immunization of women of childbearing age with tetanus toxoid. However, in spite of this decline, WHO estimates that more than 500,000 deaths due to tetanus neonatorum still occur annually in the developing world. Most newborn infants with tetanus have been born to nonimmunized mothers delivered by a traditional birth attendant outside a hospital.

The disease usually occurs through introduction via the umbilical cord of tetanus spores during delivery through the use of an unclean instrument to cut the cord, or after delivery by ''dressing'' the umbilical stump with substances heavily contaminated with tetanus spores, frequently as part of natal rituals.

In neonates, inability to nurse is the most common presenting sign. Tetanus neonatorum is typified by a newborn infant who sucks and cries well for the first few days after birth and subsequently develops progressive difficulty and then inability to feed because of trismus, generalized stiffness with spasms or convulsions and opisthotonus. The average incubation period is about 6 days, with a range from 3 to 28 days. Overall, neonatal tetanus case-fatality rates are very high; exceeding 80% among cases with short incubation periods.

Prevention of tetanus neonatorum can be achieved by a combination of two approaches: by improving maternity care with emphasis on increasing the tetanus toxoid immunization coverage of women of childbearing age (especially pregnant women), and by increasing the proportion of deliveries attended by trained attendants.

Important control measures include licensing of midwives; providing professional supervision and education as to methods, equipment and techniques of asepsis in childbirth; and educating mothers, relatives and attendants in the practice of strict asepsis of the umbilical stump of newborn infants. The latter is especially important in many lesser-developed areas where strips of bamboo are used to sever the umbilical cord and where ashes, cow dung poultices or other contaminated substances are traditionally applied to the umbilicus. In those areas, any woman of childbearing age visiting a health facility should be screened and offered immunization, no matter what the reason for the visit.

Nonimmunized women should receive at least 2 doses of tetanus toxoid according to the following schedule: the first at initial contact or as early as possible during pregnancy, the second 4 weeks after the first and preferably at least 2 weeks before delivery. A third dose could be given 6–12 months after the second, or during her next pregnancy. An additional 2 doses should be given at annual intervals when the mother is in contact with the health service or during her subsequent pregnancies. A total of 5 doses should protect the previously unimmunized woman through her entire childbearing period. Women whose infants have a risk of neonatal tetanus, but who themselves have received 3 or 4 doses of DTP/DTaP as children, need only receive two doses of tetanus toxoid during their first pregnancy.

Summary Guide to Tetanus Prophylaxis in Routine Wound Management[1]

History of tetanus immunization (doses)	Clean, minor wounds		All other wounds	
	Td[2]	TIG	Td[2]	TIG
Uncertain or <3	Yes	No	Yes	Yes
3 or more	No[3]	No	No[4]	No

[1]Important details in the text.
[2]For children less than 7 years old, DTaP or DTP (DT, if pertussis vaccine is contraindicated) is preferred to tetanus toxoid alone. For persons 7 years old or older, Td is preferred to tetanus toxoid alone.
[3]Yes, if more than 10 years since last dose.
[4]Yes, if more than 5 years since last dose. (More frequent boosters are not needed and can accentuate side effects.)

TOXOCARIASIS

ICD-9 128.0; ICD-10 B83.0

(Visceral larva migrans, Larva migrans visceralis, Ocular larva migrans, *Toxocara [canis] [cati]* infection)

1. Identification—A chronic infection and usually mild disease, predominantly of young children but increasingly recognized in adults, caused by migration of larval forms of *Toxocara* species in the organs and tissues. It is characterized by eosinophilia of variable duration, hepatomegaly, hyperglobulinemia, pulmonary symptoms and fever. With an acute and heavy infection, the WBC count may reach 100,000/cu mm or more (SI units more than 100×10^9/L), with 50%-90% eosinophils. Symptoms may persist for a year or longer. Pneumonitis, chronic abdominal pain, a generalized rash and focal neurologic disturbances may occur. Endophthalmitis (caused by larvae entering the eye) may occur, usually in older children, and can result in loss of vision in the affected eye. Retinal lesions must be differentiated from retinoblastoma and other retinal masses. The disease is rarely fatal.

ELISA testing with larval-stage antigens is 75%-90% sensitive in VLM and in ocular infections. Western blotting procedures can be used to increase specificity of the ELISA screening test.

2. Infectious agents—*Toxocara canis* and *T. cati,* predominantly the former.

3. Occurrence—Worldwide. Severe disease occurs sporadically and affects mainly children aged 14-40 months, but it also occurs in older age groups. Siblings often have eosinophilia or other evidence of light or residual infection. Serologic studies in asymptomatic children have shown a wide range in different populations, with an average of 3% in the USA, but with some subpopulations reaching 23%. Internationally, seroprevalence ranges from lows of 0-4% in Madrid and Germany; to 31% in Irish children; 66% in rural Spain; and up to 83% in some Caribbean subpopulations. Adults are less frequently acutely infected.

4. Reservoir—For dogs and cats, *T. canis* and *T. cati,* respectively. Puppies are infected by transplacental and transmammary migration of larvae and pass eggs in their stools by the time they are 3 weeks old. Infection in the female dog may end or become dormant with sexual maturity; with pregnancy, however, *T. canis* larvae become active and infect the fetuses and the newborn pups through the milk. Gender and age differences are less marked for cats; older animals are somewhat less susceptible than young.

5. Mode of transmission—For most infections in children, by direct or indirect transmission of infective *Toxocara* eggs from contaminated soil to the mouth, directly by contact with infected soil or indirectly by eating unwashed raw vegetables. Some infections may occur from ingestion of larvae in raw liver from infected chickens, cattle and sheep.

Eggs are shed in the feces of infected dogs and cats; up to 30% of soil samples from certain parks in the USA and the UK contained eggs. In certain parks in Japan, up to 75% of sandboxes contained eggs. The eggs require 1–3 weeks' incubation to become infective, but remain viable and infective in soil for many months; they are adversely affected by desiccation.

After ingestion, embryonated eggs hatch in the intestine; larvae penetrate the wall and migrate to the liver and other tissues by the lymphatic and circulatory systems. From the liver, larvae spread to other tissues, particularly to the lungs and abdominal organs (visceral larva migrans) or the eyes (ocular larva migrans), and cause damage by migration and induce granulomatous lesions. The parasites cannot replicate in the human or other end-stage (paratenic) hosts; however, viable larvae may remain in tissues for years, usually in the absence of symptomatic disease. When the tissues of paratenic hosts are eaten, the larvae may be infective for the new host.

6. Incubation period—In children, weeks or months, depending on intensity of infection, reinfection and sensitivity of the patient. Ocular manifestations may occur as late as 4–10 years after initial infection. In infections acquired by ingestion of raw liver, very short (hours or days) incubation periods have been reported.

7. Period of communicability—Not directly transmitted from person to person.

8. Susceptibility and resistance—The lower incidence in older children and adults relates mainly to less exposure. Reinfection can occur.

9. Methods of control—

A. Preventive measures:

1) Educate the public, especially pet owners, concerning sources and origin of the infection, particularly the danger of pica, of exposure to areas contaminated with the feces of untreated puppies and of ingestion of raw or undercooked liver of animals exposed to dogs or cats. Parents of toddlers should be made aware of the risk associated with pets in the household and how to minimize them.

2) Prevent contamination of soil by dog and cat feces in areas immediately adjacent to houses and children's play areas, especially in urban areas and multiple housing projects. Encourage cat and dog owners to practice responsible pet ownership, which includes prompt removal of their pets' feces from areas of public access. Control stray dogs and cats.

3) Require removal of canine and feline feces passed in play areas. Children's sandboxes offer an attractive site for defecating cats; cover when not in use.

4) Deworm dogs and cats beginning at 3 weeks of age, repeated 3 times at 2-week intervals, and every 6 months thereafter. Also treat lactating bitches. Dispose of feces passed as a result of treatment, as well as other stools, in a sanitary manner.

5) Always wash hands after handling soil and before eating.

6) Teach children not to put dirty objects into their mouths.

B. Control of patient, contacts and the immediate environment:

1) Report to local health authority: Official report not ordinarily justifiable, Class 5 (see Communicable Disease Reporting).

2) Isolation: None.

3) Concurrent disinfection: None.

4) Quarantine: None.

5) Immunization of contacts: None.

6) Investigation of contacts and source of infection: Search for site of infection of index case; identify others exposed. Intensify preventive measures (see 9A, above). Treatment of asymptomatic, ELISA positive individuals is not indicated; one may consider treatment for those with hypereosinophilia.

7) Specific treatment: Mebendazole or albendazole is the antihelminthic of choice because of relative safety. Diethylcarbamazine and thiabendazole have been used; effectiveness of antihelminthics is questionable at best.

C. Epidemic measures: Not applicable.

D. Disaster implications: None.

E. International measures: None.

GNATHOSTOMIASIS ICD-9 128.1; ICD-10 B83.1

Another visceral larva migrans, common in Thailand and elsewhere in southeast Asia, is caused by *Gnathostoma spinigerum,* a nematode parasite of dogs and cats. Following ingestion of undercooked fish and poultry containing third stage larvae, the parasites migrate through the tissue of people or animals, forming transient inflammatory lesions or abscesses in various parts of the body. Larvae may invade the brain, producing focal cerebral lesions associated with eosinophilic pleocytosis. The effectiveness of antihelminthic drugs, including albendazole and mebendazole, is questionable, and these drugs are considered investigational.

CUTANEOUS LARVA MIGRANS
ICD-9 126; ICD-10 B76.9
DUE TO *ANCYLOSTOMA BRAZILIENSE*
ICD-9 126.2; ICD-10 B76.0
DUE TO *ANCYLOSTOMA CANINUM*
ICD-9 126.8; ICD-10 B76.0
(Creeping eruption)

Infective larvae of dog and cat hookworms, *Ancylostoma braziliense* and *A. caninum,* cause a dermatitis in people called "creeping eruption." This is a disease of utility workers, gardeners, children, sea bathers and others who come in contact with damp sandy soil contaminated with dog and cat feces; in the USA, most prevalent in the southeast. The larvae enter the skin and migrate intracutaneously for long periods; eventually they may penetrate to deeper tissues. Each larva causes a serpiginous track, advancing several millimeters to a few centimeters a day, with intense itching more marked at night. The cutaneous disease is self-limited, with spontaneous cure after several weeks or months. Individual larvae can be killed by freezing the area with ethyl chloride spray. Thiabendazole is effective as a topical ointment, and albendazole or ivermectin is effective systemically. Occasionally, *A. caninum* larvae migrate to the small intestine where they may cause eosinophilic enteritis; these zoonotic infections respond to treatment with pyrantel pamoate, mebendazole or albendazole.

TOXOPLASMOSIS
ICD-9 130; ICD-10 B58
CONGENITAL TOXOPLASMOSIS
ICD-9 771.2; ICD-10 P37.1

1. Identification—A systemic coccidian protozoan disease; infections are frequently asymptomatic or present as an acute disease with only lymphadenopathy, or one resembling infectious mononucleosis, with fever, lymphadenopathy and lymphocytosis persisting for days or weeks. With development of an immune response, the parasitemia decreases, but *Toxoplasma* cysts remaining in the tissues contain viable organisms. These tissue cysts may reactivate if the immune system becomes compromised. Among immunodeficient individuals, primary or reactivated infection may cause cerebritis, chorioretinitis, pneumonia, generalized skeletal muscle involvement, myocarditis, a maculopapular rash and/or death. Cerebral toxoplasmosis is a frequent component of AIDS.

A primary infection during early pregnancy may lead to fetal infection with death of the fetus or chorioretinitis, brain damage with intracerebral calcification, hydrocephaly, microcephaly, fever, jaundice, rash, hepatosplenomegaly, xanthochromic CSF and convulsions evident at birth or shortly thereafter. Later in pregnancy, maternal infection results in mild or subclinical fetal disease with delayed manifestations, such as recurrent or chronic chorioretinitis. In immunosuppressed pregnant women who are *Toxoplasma* seropositive, there may be reactivation of the latent infection that may rarely result in congenital toxoplasmosis. Dormant organisms from a latent infection can reactivate and cause cerebral toxoplasmosis, particularly among immunodeficient individuals, such as AIDS patients.

Diagnosis is based on clinical signs and supportive serologic results, demonstration of the agent in body tissues or fluids by biopsy or necropsy, or isolation in animals or cell culture. Rising antibody levels are corroborative of active infection; the presence of specific IgM and/or rising IgG titers in sequential sera of infants is conclusive evidence of congenital infection. High IgG antibody levels may persist for years with no relation to active disease.

2. Infectious agent—*Toxoplasma gondii,* an intracellular coccidian protozoan of cats, belonging to the family Sarcocystidae, grouped in the class Sporozoa.

3. Occurrence—Worldwide in mammals and birds. Infection in humans is common.

4. Reservoir—The definitive hosts of *T. gondii* are cats and other felines, which acquire infection mainly from eating infected mammals (especially rodents) or birds and rarely from feces of infected cats. Only felines harbor the parasite in the intestinal tract, where the sexual stage of its life cycle takes place, which results in excretion of oocysts in feces for 10–20 days or, rarely, longer.

The intermediate hosts of *T. gondii* include sheep, goats, rodents, swine, cattle, chickens and birds; all may carry an infective stage (cystozoite or bradyzoite) of *T. gondii* encysted in tissue, especially muscle and brain. Tissue cysts remain viable for long periods, perhaps for the life of the animal.

5. Mode of transmission—Transplacental infection in humans occurs when a pregnant woman has rapidly dividing tachyzoites circulating in the bloodstream, usually in the primary infection. Children may become infected by ingesting infective oocysts from dirt in sandboxes, playgrounds and yards in which cats have defecated. Infections may be acquired by eating raw or undercooked infected meat (pork or mutton, more rarely beef) containing tissue cysts, or by ingestion of infective oocysts in food or water contaminated with feline feces. Inhalation of sporulated oocysts was associated with one outbreak. Milk of infected goats and cattle may contain tachyzoites; one outbreak was associated epidemiologically with consumption of raw goat's milk. Infection may rarely be acquired by blood transfusion or organ transplantation from an infected donor.

6. Incubation period—From 10 to 23 days in one common source outbreak from ingestion of undercooked meat; 5–20 days in an outbreak associated with cats.

7. Period of communicability—Not directly transmitted from person to person except in utero. Oocysts shed by cats sporulate and become infective 1–5 days later and may remain infective in water or moist soil for over a year. Cysts in the flesh of an infected animal remain infective as long as the meat is edible and uncooked.

8. Susceptibility and resistance—Susceptibility to infection is general, but immunity is readily acquired and most infections are asymptomatic. Duration and degree of immunity are unknown but assumed to be long lasting or permanent; antibodies persist for years, probably for life. Patients undergoing cytotoxic or immunosuppressive therapy or patients with AIDS are at high risk of developing illness from reactivated infection.

9. Methods of control—

A. Preventive measures:

1) Educate pregnant women about these preventive measures:
   a) Use irradiated meats or cook them to 150°F (66°C) before eating. Freezing meat reduces infectivity but does not eliminate it.
   b) Unless they are known to have antibodies to *T. gondii*, pregnant women should avoid cleaning litter pans and contact with cats of unknown feeding history. Wear gloves during gardening and wash hands thoroughly after work and before eating.
2) Feed cats dry, canned or boiled food and discourage hunting (i.e., keep them as indoor pets only).
3) Dispose of cat feces and litter daily (before sporocysts become infective). Feces can be flushed down the toilet, burned or deeply buried. Disinfect litter pans daily by scalding; wear gloves or wash hands thoroughly after handling potentially infective material. Dried litter should be disposed of without shaking, to avoid dispersal of oocysts in the air.
4) Wash hands thoroughly before eating and after handling raw meat or having contact with soil possibly contaminated with cat feces.
5) Control stray cats and prevent them from gaining access to sandboxes and sand piles used by children for play. Sandboxes should be covered when not in use.
6) Patients with AIDS who have severe symptomatic toxoplasmosis should receive prophylactic treatment throughout life with pyrimethamine, sulfadiazine and folinic acid.

B. Control of patient, contacts and the immediate environment:

1) Report to local health authority: Not ordinarily required, but reportable in some states (USA) and countries to facilitate

further understanding of the epidemiology of the disease, Class 3C (see Communicable Disease Reporting).

2) Isolation: None.

3) Concurrent disinfection: None.

4) Quarantine: None.

5) Immunization of contacts: None.

6) Investigation of contacts and source of infection: In congenital cases, determine antibody titers in mother; in acquired cases, determine antibody titers in members of the household and common exposure to cat feces, soil, raw meat or infected animals.

7) Specific treatment: Treatment is not routinely indicated for a healthy immunocompetent host, except in an initial infection during pregnancy or the presence of active chorioretinitis, myocarditis or other organ involvement. Pyrimethamine (Daraprim®) combined with sulfadiazine and folinic acid (to avoid bone marrow depression) for 4 weeks is the preferred treatment for those with severe symptomatic disease. Clindamycin, in addition to these agents, has been used to treat ocular toxoplasmosis. In ocular disease, systemic corticosteroids are indicated when irreversible loss of vision can occur from lesional involvement of the macula, papillomacular bundle or optic nerve.

Treatment of pregnant women is problematic. Spiramycin is commonly used to prevent placental infection; pyrimethamine and sulfadiazine should be considered if ultrasound or other studies indicate that fetal infection has occurred. Because of concerns about possible teratogenicity, however, pyrimethamine should not be given during the first 16 weeks of pregnancy; sulfadiazine may be administered alone in this circumstance. Infants whose mothers had primary infections or were HIV positive during pregnancy should be treated with pyrimethamine-sulfadiazine–folinic acid during their first year of life or until congenital infection is ruled out to prevent chorioretinitis and other sequelae. There are no clear guidelines for the management of infants born to HIV infected mothers who are *Toxoplasma* seropositive.

C. Epidemic measures: None.

D. Disaster implications: None.

E. International measures: None.

TRACHOMA   ICD-9 076; ICD-10 A71

1. Identification—A chlamydial conjunctivitis of insidious or abrupt onset; the infection may persist for a few years if untreated, but the characteristic lifetime duration of active disease in hyperendemic areas is the result of frequent reinfection. The disease is characterized by the presence of lymphoid follicles and diffuse conjunctival inflammation (papillary hypertrophy), particularly on the tarsal conjunctiva lining the upper eyelid. The inflammation produces superficial vascularization of the cornea (pannus) and scarring of the conjunctiva. This scarring increases with the severity and duration of the inflammatory disease.

The marked conjunctival scarring causes in-turned eyelashes and lid deformities (trichiasis and entropion) that in turn cause chronic abrasion of the cornea and scarring with visual impairment and blindness later in adult life. Secondary bacterial infections are common in populations with endemic trachoma and contribute to the communicability and severity of the disease.

Early trachoma in some developing countries is an endemic childhood disease in families or communities. However, the early stages of trachoma may be indistinguishable from conjunctivitis caused by other bacteria (including genital stains of *Chlamydia trachomatis*) The differential diagnosis includes molluscum contagiosum nodules of the eyelids, toxic reactions to chronically administered eye drops and chronic staphylococcal lid-margin infection. An allergic reaction to contact lens wear (giant papillary conjunctivitis) may produce a trachoma-like syndrome with tarsal nodules (giant papillae), conjunctival scarring and corneal pannus.

Laboratory diagnosis is made by detection of intracellular chlamydial elementary bodies in epithelial cells of conjunctival scrapings by Giemsa-stained smears, or by IF after methanol fixation of the smear; by detection of chlamydial antigen by EIA or DNA by probe; or by isolation of the agent in special cell culture.

2. Infectious agent—*Chlamydia trachomatis* of serovars A, B, Ba and C. Some strains are indistinguishable from those of chlamydial conjunctivitis (q.v.), and serovars B, Ba and C have been isolated from genital chlamydial infections.

3. Occurrence—Worldwide, occurring as an endemic disease most often in poorer rural communities in developing countries. In endemic areas, trachoma presents in childhood, then subsides in adolescence, leaving varying degrees of potentially disabling scarring. Blinding trachoma is still widespread in the Middle East, northern and sub-Saharan Africa, parts of the Indian subcontinent, southeast Asia and China. Pockets of blinding trachoma occur in Latin America, Australia (among Aboriginals) and the Pacific islands.

The disease is rare in the USA; it occurs among population groups with poor hygiene, poverty and crowded living conditions, particularly in dry dusty regions such as some Native American reservations in the southwest. The late complications of trachoma (in-turned lids and corneal scarring) occur in older people who had infectious trachoma in childhood; these people are rarely infectious.

4. **Reservoir**—Humans.

5. **Mode of transmission**—Through direct contact with infectious ocular or nasopharyngeal discharges on fingers or indirect contact with contaminated fomites such as towels, clothes and nasopharyngeal discharges from infected people and materials soiled therewith. Flies, especially *Musca sorbens* in Africa and the Middle East and *Hippelates* species in the southern USA, contribute to the spread of the disease. In children with active trachoma, *Chlamydia* can be recovered from the nasopharynx and rectum, but the trachoma serovars do not appear to have a genital reservoir in endemic communities.

6. **Incubation period**—From 5 to 12 days (based on volunteer studies).

7. **Period of communicability**—As long as active lesions are present in the conjunctivae and adnexal mucous membranes; this may last a few years. Concentration of the agent in the tissues is greatly reduced with cicatrization, but increases again with reactivation and recurrence of infective discharges. Infectivity is terminated within 2–3 days of the start of antibiotic treatment, long before the clinical disease improves.

8. **Susceptibility and resistance**—Susceptibility is general; there is no evidence that infection confers immunity or that experimental vaccines are useful in preventing infection or in reducing the severity of established cases. In endemic areas, children have active disease more frequently than adults. The severity of disease often is related to living conditions, particularly poor hygiene; exposure to dry winds, dust and fine sand may also contribute.

9. **Methods of control**—

A. *Preventive measures:*

1) Educate the public on the need for personal hygiene, especially the risk in common use of toilet articles.
2) Improve basic sanitation, including availability and use of soap and water; encourage washing the face; avoid common-use towels.
3) Provide adequate case finding and treatment facilities, with emphasis on preschool children.
4) Conduct epidemiologic investigations to determine important factors in the occurrence of the disease in each specific situation.

B. *Control of patient, contacts and the immediate environment:*

1) Report to local health authority: Case report required in some states (USA) and countries of low endemicity, Class 2B (see Communicable Disease Reporting).
2) Isolation: Not practical in most areas where the disease occurs. For hospitalized patients, drainage and secretion precautions.
3) Concurrent disinfection: Of eye and nasal discharges and contaminated articles.
4) Quarantine: None.
5) Immunization of contacts: None.
6) Investigation of contacts and source of infection: Members of family, playmates and schoolmates.
7) Specific treatment: In areas where the disease is severe and highly prevalent, mass treatment of the whole population, especially children, with topical tetracycline or erythromycin ointments can be used with varying schedules, such as twice daily for 5 consecutive days, or once monthly for 6 months. Oral sulfonamides, tetracyclines, erythromycin and azithromycin are also effective in the active stages of the disease.

C. *Epidemic measures:* In regions of hyperendemic prevalence, mass treatment campaigns have been successful in reducing severity and frequency when associated with education of the people in personal hygiene and improvement of the sanitary environment, particularly a good water supply.

D. *Disaster implications:* None.

E. *International measures:* WHO Collaborating Centres.

TRENCH FEVER   ICD-9 083.1; ICD-10 A79.0
(Quintana fever)

1. Identification—A typically nonfatal, febrile bacterial disease varying in manifestations and severity. It is characterized by headache, malaise, pain and tenderness, especially on the shins. Onset is either sudden or slow, with a fever that may be relapsing, typhoid-like or limited to a single febrile episode lasting for several days. Splenomegaly is common, and a transient macular rash may occur. Symptoms may continue to recur many years after the primary infection, which may be subclinical with organisms circulating in the blood for months, with or without repeated recurrence of symptoms. Bacteremia, osteomyelitis, and bacillary angiomatosis can occur among immunocompromised patients, especially those with HIV infection. Endocarditis has been associated with trench fever infections especially among homeless alcoholics.

Laboratory diagnosis is made by culture of patients blood on blood or chocolate agar under 5% CO_2. Microcolonies are visible after 8-21 days incubation at 37°C (98.6°F). Infection evokes genus specific antibodies detectable by serologic tests. An IFA test is available through the CDC.

2. Infectious agent—*Bartonella quintana (formerly Rochalimaea quintana).*

3. Occurrence—Epidemics occurred in Europe during World Wars I and II among troops and prisoners of war living in crowded, unhygienic conditions. Sporadic cases in endemic foci probably are not recognized. The organism probably can be found wherever the human body louse exists. Endemic foci of infection have been detected in Poland, the former Soviet Union, Mexico, Bolivia, Burundi, Ethiopia and North Africa. Two forms of infection have been documented during the 1990s in the USA: one, an opportunistic febrile infection in AIDS patients (sometimes presenting as bacillary angiomatosis, see Cat Scratch Disease); and, the second, louseborne febrile disease in homeless or alcoholic individuals, so-called "urban trench fever" which may be associated with endocarditis.

4. Reservoir—Humans. The intermediate host and vector is the body louse, *Pediculus humanus corporis.* The organism multiplies extracellularly in the gut lumen for the duration of the insect's life, which is approximately 5 weeks after hatching. No transovarial transmission occurs.

5. Mode of transmission—Not directly transmitted from person to person. People are infected by inoculation of the organism in louse feces through a break in the skin, either from the bite of the louse or other means. Infected lice begin to excrete infectious feces 5-12 days after ingesting infective blood; this continues for the remainder of their life span. Nymphal stages may also become infected. The disease spreads when lice leave abnormally hot (febrile) or cold (dead) bodies in search of a normothermic host.

6. Incubation period—Generally 7-30 days.

7. Period of communicability—Organisms may circulate in the blood (by which lice are infected) for weeks, months or years and may recur with or without symptoms. A history of trench fever is a permanent contraindication to blood donation.

8. Susceptibility and resistance—Susceptibility is general. After infection, the degree of protective immunity to either infection or disease is unknown.

9. Methods of control—

A. Preventive measures: Delousing procedures will destroy the vector and prevent transmission to humans. Dust clothing and body with an effective insecticide.

B. ***Control of patient, contacts and the immediate environment:***

1) Report to local health authority: Cases should be reported so that an evaluation of louse infestation in the population may be made and appropriate measures taken, since lice also transmit epidemic typhus and relapsing fever, Class 3B (see Communicable Disease Reporting).

2) Isolation: None after delousing.

3) Concurrent disinfection: Louse infested clothing should be treated to kill the lice.

4) Quarantine: None.

5) Immunization of contacts: None.

6) Investigation of contacts and source of infection: Search the bodies and clothing of people at risk for the presence of lice; delouse if indicated.

7) Specific treatment: Tetracyclines particularly doxycycline should be given or 2–4 weeks. Patients should first be carefully evaluated for endocarditis, as this will change the duration and follow-up of antibiotic treatment. Relapse may occur, despite antibiotic therapy, in both immunocompromised and immunocompetent patients.

C. ***Epidemic measures:*** Systematic application of residual insecticide to the clothing of all people in the affected population (see 9A, above).

D. ***Disaster implications:*** Risk is increased when louse infested people are forced to live in crowded, unhygienic shelters (see 9B1, above).

E. ***International measures:*** WHO Collaborating Centres.

TRICHINELLOSIS ICD-9 124; ICD-10 B75
(Trichiniasis, Trichinosis)

1. Identification—A disease caused by an intestinal roundworm whose larvae (trichinae) migrate to and become encapsulated in the muscles. Clinical illness in humans is highly variable and can range from inapparent infection to a fulminating, fatal disease, depending on the number of larvae ingested. Sudden appearance of muscle soreness and pain together with edema of the upper eyelids and fever are early characteristic signs. These are sometimes followed by subconjunctival, subungual and retinal hemorrhages, pain and photophobia. Thirst, profuse sweating, chills, weakness, prostration and rapidly increasing eosinophilia may follow shortly after the ocular signs.

Gastrointestinal symptoms, such as diarrhea, due to the intraintestinal activity of the adult worms, may precede the ocular manifestations. Remittent fever is usual, sometimes as high as 40°C (104°F); the fever terminates after 1-6 weeks, depending on intensity of infection. Cardiac and neurologic complications may appear in the 3rd to 6th week; in the most severe cases, death due to myocardial failure may occur in either the 1st to 2nd week or between the 4th and 8th weeks.

Serologic tests and marked eosinophilia may aid in diagnosis. Biopsy of skeletal muscle, taken more than 10 days after infection (most often positive after the 4th or 5th week of infection), frequently provides conclusive evidence of infection by demonstrating the uncalcified parasite cyst.

2. Infectious agent—*Trichinella spiralis,* an intestinal nematode. Separate taxonomic designations have been accepted for isolates found in the Arctic *(T. nativa),* Palaearctic *(T. britovi),* in Africa *(T. nelsoni)* and in several regions of the world *(T. pseudospiralis).*

3. Occurrence—Worldwide, but variable in incidence, depending in part on practices of eating and preparing pork or wild animal meat and the extent to which the disease is recognized and reported. Cases usually are sporadic and outbreaks localized, often resulting from eating sausage and other meat products using pork or shared meat from Arctic mammals. Several outbreaks in France and Italy due to infected horse meat have been reported.

4. Reservoir—Swine, dogs, cats, horses, rats and many wild animals, including fox, wolf, bear, polar bear, wild boar and marine mammals in the Arctic, and hyena, jackal, lion and leopard in the tropics.

5. Mode of transmission—By eating raw or insufficiently cooked flesh of animals containing viable encysted larvae, chiefly pork and pork products, and beef products, such as hamburger adulterated either intentionally or inadvertently with raw pork. In the epithelium of the small intestine, larvae develop into adults. Gravid female worms then produce larvae, which penetrate the lymphatics or venules and are disseminated via the bloodstream throughout the body. The larvae become encapsulated in skeletal muscle.

6. Incubation period—Systemic symptoms usually appear about 8-15 days after ingestion of infected meat; varies between 5 and 45 days depending on the number of parasites involved. GI symptoms may appear within a few days.

7. Period of communicability—Not transmitted directly from person to person. Animal hosts remain infective for months, and meat from such animals stays infective for appreciable periods unless cooked, frozen or irradiated to kill the larvae (see 9A, below).

8. Susceptibility and resistance—Susceptibility is universal. Infection results in partial immunity.

9. Methods of control—

A. Preventive measures:

1) Educate the public on the need to cook all fresh pork and pork products and meat from wild animals at a temperature and for a time sufficient to allow all parts to reach at least 71°C (160°F), or until meat changes from pink to grey, which allows a sufficient margin of safety. This should be done unless it has been established that these meat products have been processed either by heating, curing, freezing or irradiation adequate to kill trichinae.

2) Grind pork in a separate grinder or clean the grinder thoroughly before and after processing other meats.

3) Adopt regulations to encourage commercial irradiation processing of pork products. Testing carcasses for infection with a digestion technique is useful. Immunodiagnosis of pigs with an approved ELISA test is also useful.

4) Adopt and enforce regulations that allow only certified trichinae free pork to be used in raw pork products that have a cooked appearance or in products that traditionally are not heated sufficiently to kill trichinae during final preparation.

5) Adopt laws and regulations to require and enforce the cooking of garbage and offal before feeding to swine.

6) Educate hunters to cook thoroughly the meat of walrus, seal, wild boar, bear and other wild animals.

7) Freezing temperatures maintained throughout the mass of the infected meat are effective in inactivating trichinae i.e., holding pieces of pork up to 15 cm thick at a temperature of –15°C (5°F) for 30 days or –25°C (–13°F) or lower for 10 days will effectively destroy all common types of trichinae cysts. Hold thicker pieces at the lower temperature for at least 20 days. These temperatures will not inactivate the cold-resistant Arctic strains *(T. nativa)* found in walrus and bear meat and rarely in swine.

8) Exposure of pork cuts or carcasses to low-level gamma irradiation effectively sterilizes and, at higher doses, kills trichinae encysted larvae.

B. Control of patient, contacts and the immediate environment:

1) Report to local health authority: Case report required in most

states (USA) and countries, Class 2B (see Communicable Disease Reporting).
2) Isolation: None.
3) Concurrent disinfection: None.
4) Quarantine: None.
5) Immunization of contacts: None.
6) Investigation of contacts and source of infection: Check other family members and persons who have eaten meat suspected as the source of infection. Confiscate any remaining suspected food.
7) Specific treatment: Albendazole (Zentel®) or mebendazole (Vermox®) are effective in the intestinal stage and in the muscular stage. Corticosteroids are indicated only in severe cases to alleviate symptoms of the inflammatory reaction when the CNS or heart is involved; however, they delay elimination of the adult worms from the intestine. In rare situations in which known infected meat has been consumed, prompt administration of antihelminthic treatment may prevent development of symptoms.

C. Epidemic measures: Institute epidemiologic study to determine the common food involved. Confiscate remainder of suspected food and correct faulty practices. Eliminate infected swine herds.

D. Disaster implications: None.

E. International measures: WHO Collaborating Centres.

TRICHOMONIASIS   ICD-9 131; ICD-10 A59

1. Identification—A common and persistent protozoal disease of the genitourinary tract, characterized in women by vaginitis, with small petechial or sometimes punctate red ''strawberry'' spots and a profuse, thin, foamy, greenish-yellow discharge with foul odor. The disease may cause a urethritis or cystitis but is frequently asymptomatic; it may also cause obstetric complications and may facilitate HIV infection. In men, the infectious agent invades and persists in the prostate, urethra or seminal vesicles, and often causes only mild symptoms, but may cause as much as 5%–10% of the cases of nongonococcal urethritis in some areas.

Trichomoniasis often coexists with gonorrhea, in up to 40% of cases in some studies; a full assessment for STD pathogens (''STD check'') should be carried out when trichomoniasis is diagnosed.

Diagnosis is made through identification of the motile parasite, either by microscopic examination of discharges or by culture, which is more sensitive. The organisms can be seen on a Pap smear.

2. Infectious agent—*Trichomonas vaginalis,* a flagellate protozoan.

3. Occurrence—Widespread; a frequent disease of all continents and all races, primarily of adults, with the highest incidence among females 16-35 years. Overall, about 20% of females may become infected during their reproductive years.

4. Reservoir—Humans.

5. Mode of transmission—By contact with vaginal and urethral discharges of infected people during sexual intercourse.

6. Incubation period—From 4 to 20 days, average 7 days; many are symptom free carriers for years.

7. Period of communicability—For the duration of the persistent infection, which may last for years.

8. Susceptibility and resistance—Susceptibility to infection is general, but clinical disease is seen mainly in females.

9. Methods of control—

    A. Preventive measures: Educate the public to seek medical advice whenever there is an abnormal discharge from the genitalia and to refrain from sexual intercourse until investigation and treatment of self and partner(s) are completed. Promotion of "safer sex" behavior, including condom use, for all nonmutually monogamous sexual contacts is indicated.

    B. Control of patient, contacts and the immediate environment:

        1) Report to local health authority: Official report not ordinarily justifiable, Class 5 (see Communicable Disease Reporting).

        2) Isolation: None; avoid sexual relations during period of infection and treatment.

        3) Concurrent disinfection: None; the organism cannot withstand drying.

        4) Quarantine: None.

        5) Immunization of contacts: None.

        6) Investigation of contacts and source of infection: Sexual partners should be evaluated for other STDs and should be treated concurrently.

        7) Specific treatment: Metronidazole (Flagyl®), tinidazole (Fasigyn®) or ornidazole (Tiberal®) by mouth is effective in both male and female patients; they are contraindicated during the

first trimester of pregnancy. Clotrimazole, which will produce symptomatic relief and may cure up to 50% of patients, may be used. Concurrently treat sexual partner(s) to prevent reinfection. Cases of metronidazole resistance have been reported and may be treated with topical intravaginal paromomycin.

C. Epidemic measures: None.

D. Disaster implications: None.

E. International measures: None.

TRICHURIASIS   ICD-9 127.3; ICD-10 B79
(Trichocephaliasis, Whipworm disease)

1. Identification—A nematode infection of the large intestine, usually asymptomatic. Heavy infections may cause bloody, mucoid stools and diarrhea. Rectal prolapse, clubbing of the fingers, hypoproteinemia, anemia and growth retardation may occur in heavily infected children.

Diagnosis is made by demonstration of eggs in feces or by sigmoidoscopic observation of worms attached to the wall of the lower colon in heavy infections. Eggs must be differentiated from those of *Capillaria* species.

2. Infectious agent—*Trichuris trichiura (Trichocephalus trichiurus),* a nematode; the human whipworm.

3. Occurrence—Worldwide, especially in warm, moist regions.

4. Reservoir—Humans. Animal whipworms do not infect humans.

5. Mode of transmission—Indirect, particularly through pica or ingestion of contaminated vegetables; not immediately transmissible from person to person. Eggs passed in feces require a minimum of 10–14 days in warm moist soil to become infective. Ingestion of infective eggs from contaminated soil is followed by hatching of the larvae, their attachment to the mucosa of the cecum and proximal colon, and development into mature worms. Eggs appear in the feces 70–90 days after ingestion of the embryonated eggs; symptoms may appear much earlier.

6. Incubation period—Indefinite.

7. Period of communicability—Several years in untreated carriers.

8. Susceptibility and resistance—Susceptibility is universal.

9. **Methods of control—**

A. *Preventive measures:*

1) Educate all members of the family, particularly children, in the use of toilet facilities.
2) Provide adequate facilities for feces disposal.
3) Encourage satisfactory hygienic habits, especially handwashing before food handling; avoid ingestion of soil by thorough washing of vegetables and other foods contaminated with soil.

B. *Control of patient, contacts and the immediate environment:*

1) Report to local health authority: Official report not ordinarily justifiable, Class 5 (see Communicable Disease Reporting). Advise school health authorities of unusual frequency in school populations.
2) Isolation: None.
3) Concurrent disinfection: None; sanitary disposal of feces.
4) Quarantine: None.
5) Immunization of contacts: None.
6) Investigation of contacts and source of infection: Examine feces of all symptomatic members of the family group, especially children and playmates.
7) Specific treatment: Mebendazole (Vermox®) is the drug of choice. Albendazole (Zentel®) and oxantel (not available in the USA) are alternative drugs. As a general rule, pregnant women should not be treated in the first trimester unless there are specific medical indications.

C. *Epidemic measures:* Not applicable.

D. *Disaster implications:* None.

E. *International measures:* None.

TRYPANOSOMIASIS   ICD-9 086; ICD-10 B56–B57
I. AFRICAN
TRYPANOSOMIASIS   ICD-9 086.3–086.5; ICD-10 B56
(Sleeping sickness)

1. **Identification**—A systemic protozoal disease. In the early stages, a painful chancre, which originated as a papule and then evolved into a nodule, may be found at the primary tsetse fly bite site; there may also be

fever, intense headache, insomnia, painless enlarged lymph nodes, anemia, local edema and rash. In the late stage, there is body wasting, somnolence and signs referable to the CNS. The gambiense disease (ICD-9 086.3; ICD-10 B56.0) may run a protracted course of several years; the rhodesiense disease (ICD-9 086.4; ICD-10 B56.1) is lethal within weeks or a few months without treatment. Both forms are always fatal without treatment.

Diagnosis is made by finding trypanosomes in blood, lymph or CSF. Parasite-concentration techniques, such as capillary tube centrifugation, quantitative buffy coat (QBC) or minianion exchange centrifugation, are almost always required in the gambiense and less often in the rhodesiense disease. Inoculation of laboratory rats or mice is sometimes useful in rhodesiense disease. Lymph node aspirates may help in detecting the parasite. Specific antibodies may be demonstrated by ELISA, IFA and agglutination tests; high levels of immunoglobulins, especially IgM, are common in African trypanosomiasis. Circulating antigens can be detected with various immunologic techniques such as the TrypTech CIATT card indirect agglutination test.

2. Infectious agents—*Trypanosoma brucei gambiense* and *T. b. rhodesiense,* hemoflagellates. Criteria for species differentiation are not absolute; isolates from cases of virulent, rapidly progressive disease are considered to be *T. b. rhodesiense,* especially if contracted in east Africa; west and central African cases are usually more chronic and considered to be due to *T. b. gambiense.*

3. Occurrence—The disease is confined to tropical Africa between 15°N and 20°S latitude, corresponding to the distribution of the tsetse fly. In endemic regions, infection has been found in 0.1%–2% of the population; during epidemic outbreaks, prevalence can reach up to 70%. Outbreaks can occur when, for any reason, human fly contact is intensified, or when virulent strains of trypanosomes are introduced into a tsetse infested area by movement of infected flies or reservoir hosts. Where flies of the *Glossina palpalis* group are the principal vectors, as in west and central Africa, infection occurs mainly along streams where forest galleries border the rivers and brooks.

In east Africa and around Lake Victoria, where the main vectors are of the *G. morsitans* group, disease occurs over the broader dry savannas. *G. fuscipes,* which belongs to the palpalis group, has been responsible for outbreaks of rhodesiense sleeping sickness in Kenya and Zaire and has been the vector involved in peridomestic transmission in Uganda since 1976.

4. Reservoir—In *T. b. gambiense,* humans are the major reservoir; however, the role of domestic and wild animals is not clear. Wild animals, especially bushbucks and antelopes, and domestic cattle are the chief animal reservoirs of *T. b. rhodesiense.*

5. Mode of transmission—By the bite of infective *Glossina,* the tsetse fly. Six species are the principal vectors in nature: *G. palpalis, G. tachinoides, G. morsitans, G. pallidipes, G. swynnertoni* and *G. fuscipes.* The tsetse fly is infected by ingesting blood of a human or animal that carries trypanosomes. The parasite multiplies in the fly for 12–30 days, depending on temperature and other factors, until infective forms develop in the salivary glands. Once infected, a tsetse fly remains infective for life (average 3 months but as long as 10 months); infection is not passed from generation to generation in flies. Congenital transmission can occur in humans. Direct mechanical transmission is possible by blood on the proboscis of *Glossina* and other biting insects, such as horseflies, or in laboratory accidents.

6. **Incubation period**—In the more virulent *T. b. rhodesiense* infections, usually 3 days to a few weeks; in the more chronic *T. b. gambiense* infections, there is a longer incubation period that may last several months or even years.

7. **Period of communicability**—Communicable to the tsetse fly as long as the parasite is present in the blood of the infected person or animal. Parasitemia occurs in waves of varying intensity in untreated cases and occurs in all stages of the disease. In one study of rhodesiense disease, parasitemia was detected in only 60% of infected cases.

8. **Susceptibility and resistance**—Susceptibility is general. Occasional inapparent infections have been documented with both *T. b. gambiense* and *T. b. rhodesiense.* Spontaneous recovery in cases with the gambiense form without CNS involvement has been claimed, but this has not been confirmed.

9. **Methods of control**—

   A. *Preventive measures:* Selection of appropriate methods of prevention must be based on knowledge of the local ecology of the vectors and infectious agents. Thus, in a given geographic area, priority must be given to one or more of the following:

   1) Educate the public on personal protective measures against tsetse fly bites.
   2) Reduce the parasite population by surveying the human population for infection; treat those infected.
   3) Destroy vector tsetse fly habitats if necessary, but indiscriminate destruction of vegetation is not recommended. Clearing bushes and tall grasses around villages is useful when peridomestic transmission occurs. If cleared areas can be reclaimed for agricultural use, a permanent solution to the vector problem may result.
   4) Reduce the fly population by appropriate use of traps and screens impregnated with deltamethrine and by local use of residual insecticides (synthetic pyrethroids, 5% DDT and 3%

dieldrin are effective); in emergency situations, use aerosol insecticides sprayed by helicopter and fixed wing aircraft.

5) Prohibit blood donation from those who have visited or lived in endemic areas in Africa.

B. Control of patient, contacts and the immediate environment:

1) Report to local health authority: In selected endemic areas, establish records of prevalence and encourage control measures; not a reportable disease in most countries, Class 3B (see Communicable Disease Reporting).

2) Isolation: Not practicable. Prevent tsetse flies from feeding on patients with trypanosomes in their blood. In some countries, legal restrictions are placed on the movement of untreated patients.

3) Concurrent disinfection: None.

4) Quarantine: None.

5) Immunization of contacts: None.

6) Investigation of contacts and source of infection: If the case is a member of a tour group, others in the group should be alerted and investigated.

7) Specific treatment: If the CSF shows no changes in cellular or protein content, suramin is the drug of choice for *T. b. rhodesiense* infections and pentamidine for *T. b. gambiense* infections. However, these drugs do not cross the blood-brain barrier. *T. b. rhodesiense* may be resistant to pentamidine. Melarsoprol (Mel-B®) has been used effectively for treatment of patients with abnormal CSF with either parasite, but severe adverse side effects may occur in 5%–10% of patients. Suramin and melarsoprol are available from CDC Drug Service, Atlanta, on an investigational basis. While studies have shown that eflornithine (difluoromethylornithine (DFMO), Ornidyl®) may be preferable for the treatment of gambiense CNS disease, this drug is, as of late 1999, no longer available from CDC and its future availability from WHO is uncertain. All treated patients should be checked at 3, 6, 12 and 24 months after treatment for possible relapsed infections.

C. Epidemic measures:
Well-organized and implemented mass surveys, urgent treatment for identified infections and tsetse fly control. If epidemics recur in an area despite initial control measures, the measures recommended in 9A, above, should be more vigorously pursued.

D. Disaster implications:
None.

E. International measures:
Promote cooperative efforts of governments in endemic areas. Disseminate information and increase the availability of simple diagnostic tests for screening and simple

means of vector control. Develop systems for effective distribution of reagents and drugs. Stimulate training at national and international levels. WHO Collaborating Centres.

II. AMERICAN
   TRYPANOSOMIASIS   ICD-9 086.2; ICD-10 B57
(Chagas' disease)

1. Identification—The acute disease generally occurs in children, while irreversible chronic manifestations generally appear later in life. Many infected people have no clinical manifestations. The acute disease is characterized by variable fever, malaise, lymphadenopathy and hepatosplenomegaly. An inflammatory response at the site of infection (chagoma) may last up to 8 weeks. Unilateral bipalpebral edema (Romaña sign) occurs in a small percentage of acute cases. Life threatening or fatal manifestations include myocarditis and meningoencephalitis.

Chronic irreversible sequelae include myocardial damage with cardiac dilatation, arrhythmias and major conduction abnormalities, and intestinal tract involvement with megaesophagus and megacolon. Megaviscera occurs mainly in central Brazil. Cardiac involvement is not as common north of Ecuador as in southern areas. In patients with AIDS, severe multifocal or diffuse meningoencephalitis with necrosis and hemorrhage, and acute myocarditis occur as relapses of chronic infection. This has also been reported in cases of chronic Chagas' disease with non-AIDS immunosuppression.

Infection with *Trypanosoma rangeli* occurs in focal areas of endemic Chagas' disease, that extend from Central America to Colombia and Venezuela; a prolonged parasitemia occurs, sometimes coexisting with *T. cruzi* flagellates (with which *T. rangeli* shares reservoir hosts), but no clinical manifestations attributable to this infection have been noted.

Diagnosis of Chagas' disease in the acute phase is established by demonstration of the organism in blood (rarely, in a lymph node or skeletal muscle) by direct examination or after hemoconcentration, culture or xenodiagnosis (feeding noninfected triatomid bugs on the patient and finding the parasite in the bugs' feces several weeks later).

Parasitemia is most intense during febrile episodes early in the course of infection. In the chronic phase, xenodiagnosis and blood culture on diphasic media may be positive, but other methods rarely reveal parasites. Parasites are differentiated from those of *T. rangeli* by their shorter length (20mm v. 36mm) and larger kinetoplast. Serologic tests are valuable for individual diagnosis as well as for screening purposes.

2. Infectious agent—*Trypanosoma cruzi (Schizotrypanum cruzi),* a protozoan that occurs in humans as a hemoflagellate and as an intracellular parasite without an external flagellum.

3. Occurrence—The disease is confined to the Western Hemisphere, with wide geographic distribution in rural Mexico and Central and South America; highly endemic in some areas. Five acute vectorborne human infections acquired within the USA have been reported (4 in Texas, 1 in California); 3 additional infections were acquired by blood transfusion. Reactivated infection in AIDS patients may cause meningoencephalitis.

Serologic studies suggest the possible occurrence of other asymptomatic cases. *T. cruzi* has been found in small mammals in Alabama, Arizona, Arkansas, California, Florida, Georgia, Louisiana, Maryland, New Mexico, Texas and Utah. Recent studies found serologic evidence of infection in 4.9% of migrants from Central America living in the Washington, D.C., area.

4. Reservoir—Humans, and over 150 species of domestic and wild animals, including dogs, cats, rats, mice and other domestic animals; plus marsupials, edentates, rodents, chiropters, carnivores and primates.

5. Mode of transmission—Infected vectors, i.e., blood-sucking species of *Reduviidae* (cone-nosed bugs or kissing bugs), especially various species from the genera *Triatoma, Rhodnius* and *Panstrongylus,* have the trypanosomes in their feces. Defecation occurs during feeding; infection of humans and other mammals occurs when the freshly excreted bug feces contaminate conjunctivae, mucous membranes, abrasions or skin wounds (including the bite wound). The bugs become infected when they feed on a parasitemic animal; the parasites multiply in the bug's gut.

Transmission may also occur by blood transfusion, with an increasing rate of infected donors in cities due to migrants from rural areas. Organisms may also cross the placenta to cause congenital infection; transmission through breast feeding seems highly unlikely, so there is currently no reason to restrict breast feeding by chagasic mothers. Accidental laboratory infections occur occasionally; transplantation of organs from chagasic donors presents a growing risk of *T. cruzi* transmission.

6. Incubation period—About 5-14 days after bite of the insect vector; 30-40 days if infected through blood transfusion.

7. Period of communicability—Organisms are present regularly in the blood during the acute period and may persist in very small numbers throughout life in symptomatic and asymptomatic people. The vector becomes infective 10-30 days after biting an infected host, and the gut infection in the bug persists for life (as long as 2 years).

8. Susceptibility and resistance—All ages are susceptible, but the disease is usually more severe in younger people. Immunosuppressed people, especially those with AIDS, are at risk of serious infections and complications.

9. Methods of control—

 A. Preventive measures:

  1) Educate the public on the mode of spread and methods of prevention.

2) Systematically attack vectors infesting poorly constructed houses and those with thatched roofs by use of effective insecticides with residual action, by spraying or by use of insecticidal paints or fumigant canisters.

3) Construct or repair living areas to eliminate lodging places for the insect vector and shelter for domestic and wild reservoir animals.

4) Use bed nets in houses infested by the vector.

5) Screen blood and organ donors living in or coming from endemic areas by appropriate serologic tests to prevent infection by transfusion or transplants, as required by law in several South American countries. Addition of gentian violet (25 ml of 0.5% solution/500 ml of blood 24 hours before use) may prevent transmission.

B. Control of patient, contacts and the immediate environment:

1) Report to local health authority: In selected endemic areas; not a reportable disease in most countries, Class 3B (see Communicable Disease Reporting).

2) Isolation: Not generally practical. Blood and body fluid precautions for hospitalized patients.

3) Concurrent disinfection: None.

4) Quarantine: None.

5) Immunization of contacts: None.

6) Investigation of contacts and source of infection: Search thatched roofs, bedding and rooms for the vector. All members of the family of a case should be examined. Perform serologic tests and blood examinations on all blood and organ donors implicated as possible sources of transfusion or transplant acquired infection.

7) Specific treatment: Nifurtimox, a nitrofurfurylidene derivative, is most useful in treatment of acute cases and is available from the CDC Drug Service, Atlanta, on an investigational basis and from major hospitals in endemic areas. Benznidazole, a 2-nitroimidazole derivative, has also proven to be effective in acute cases.

C. Epidemic measures: In areas of high incidence, field survey to determine distribution and density of vectors and animal hosts.

D. Disaster implications: None.

E. International measures: None.

TUBERCULOSIS   ICD-9 010–018; ICD-10 A15–A19
(TB, TB disease)

1. Identification—A mycobacterial disease that is important as a major cause of disability and death in many parts of the world. The initial infection usually goes unnoticed; tuberculin skin test sensitivity appears within 2–10 weeks. Early lung lesions commonly heal, and leave no residual changes except occasional pulmonary or tracheobronchial lymph node calcifications. Approximately 90%–95% of those initially infected enter this latent phase from which there is lifelong risk of reactivation. Appropriate completion of preventive chemotherapy can reduce the lifetime risk of clinical tuberculosis (TB disease) by 95% and is effective in persons with HIV infection. In approximately 5% of apparently normal hosts and as many as 50% of persons with advanced HIV infection, the initial infection may progress directly to pulmonary tuberculosis or, by lymphohematogenous dissemination of bacilli, to pulmonary, miliary, meningeal or other extrapulmonary involvement. Serious outcome of the initial infection is more frequent in infants, adolescents, young adults and the immunosuppressed.

Extrapulmonary TB occurs less commonly than pulmonary TB. Children and persons with immunodeficiencies such as from HIV infection have a higher proportion of extrapulmonary TB, but pulmonary disease remains the most common type of TB disease worldwide, even in these more susceptible groups. TB disease may affect any organ or tissue such as the lymph nodes, pleura, pericardium, kidneys, bones and joints, larynx, middle ear, skin, intestines, peritoneum and eyes.

Progressive pulmonary TB arises from exogenous reinfection or endogenous reactivation of a latent focus remaining from the initial infection. If untreated, about half the patients will die within 5 years, a majority of these within 18 months. Clinical status is based mainly on the presence or absence of tubercle bacilli in the sputum and chest radiographs. Abnormal radiographic densities indicative of pulmonary infiltration, cavitation and fibrosis can occur before clinical manifestations. Fatigue, fever, night sweats and weight loss may occur early, while localizing symptoms of cough, chest pain, hemoptysis and hoarseness become prominent in advanced stages.

Immunocompetent people who are or have been infected with *Mycobacterium tuberculosis*, *M. africanum* or *M. bovis* will usually react to an intermediate strength tuberculin skin test, i.e., bioequivalent to 5 IUs of the International Standard of Purified Protein Derivative-Standard (PPD-S). A positive reaction is defined as either 5, 10, or 15 mm in duration based on the risk of exposure or disease. Ten to 20% of persons with active TB disease may not have any reaction to PPD. Therefore, a negative skin test does not rule out active TB disease. Induration of more than 5 mm is considered positive for household and/or close contacts of infectious TB disease cases, persons with an abnormal chest radiograph suggesting old healed TB disease, and persons with HIV infection. A diameter of 10 mm is considered positive for persons with medical risk factors (including diabetes mellitus, alcoholism and drug abuse), persons from high prevalence areas for tuberculosis, from areas of low socioeconomic status, residents and staff of long term care facilities (including jails and prisons), and children younger than 4 years of age.

A PPD of 15 mm or greater in diameter is considered positive for adults and children (4 years of age or older) who have no risk factors and who live in areas with few cases tuberculosis.

Cutaneous skin tests for anergy are no longer recommended, even for high risk patients such as those with HIV infection. Routine skin testing of all children is no longer recommended in the USA. Children who should be tested immediately include those who are suspected of having active TB disease, those exposed to an active case, those who are immigrating from an endemic country, or those who have recently traveled to an endemic country and had close contact to local persons from those countries. Incarcerated individuals and persons with HIV infection or children residing in a household with an HIV infected person should be tested annually. Children should be tested every 2-3 years if they are exposed to persons at high risk of disease. Testing at 4-6 and 11-12 years of age is indicated if their parents immigrated from a high risk area or if the children reside in high risk communities.

In some persons with TB infection, delayed type hypersensitivity to tuberculin may wane with time. When these individuals are skin tested many years after their initial infection, they may have a negative reaction. However, the skin test may stimulate (i.e., boost) their ability to react to tuberculin and cause a positive reaction to subsequent tests. This "boosted" reaction may be mistaken as new infection. Boosting has also been reported in persons who have received BCG vaccine. A 2 step testing procedure is used to distinguish boosted reactions and reactions due to new infection. If the reaction to the first test is classified as negative, a second test should be performed 1-3 weeks later. A positive reaction to the second test probably represents a boosted reaction. On the basis of the second test result, the person should be classified as previously infected and managed accordingly. This would not be considered a skin test conversion. If the second test result is also negative, the person should be classified as uninfected. Two step testing should be used for the initial skin testing of adults who will be retested periodically, such as health care workers.

A presumptive diagnosis of active TB disease is made by demonstration of acid-fast bacilli in stained smears from sputum or other body fluids; a positive sputum smear justifies initiation of antituberculosis therapy. The diagnosis is confirmed, where resources permit, by isolation of organisms of the *Mycobacterium tuberculosis* complex on culture; this also permits determination of the drug susceptibility of the infecting organism. In the absence of bacteriologic confirmation, active disease can be presumed if there is strong clinical evidence of an ongoing disease process by histologic or radiologic studies in a patient with a positive tuberculin skin test.

2. Infectious agents—*Mycobacterium tuberculosis* complex. This complex includes *M. tuberculosis* and *M. africanum* primarily from humans, and *M. bovis* primarily from cattle. Other mycobacteria occasionally produce disease clinically indistinguishable from tuberculosis; the etiologic agents can be identified only by culture of the organisms. Genetic sequence analyses using PCR offers the potential for nonculture identification.

3. Occurrence—Worldwide; industrialized countries had shown downward trends of mortality and morbidity for many years, but in the late 1980s reported cases reached a plateau and then increased in areas and population groups with a high prevalence of HIV infection or with large numbers of persons from areas with a high prevalence of tuberculosis. Mortality and morbidity rates increase with age, and in older people rates are higher in males than in females. TB morbidity rates are much higher among the poor, and usually higher in cities than in rural areas.

In the USA, the incidence of TB disease has declined since 1994, when the reported incidence of TB disease was 9.4/100,000 population (over 24,000 verified cases). In low incidence areas, including many areas in the USA, most TB disease in adults results from reactivation of latent foci that remain from an initial TB infection. In some large urban areas about 1/3 of TB disease cases resulted from recent infection. Although TB disease ranks low among communicable diseases in infectiousness per unit time of exposure, the long exposure of some contacts, notably household associates, may lead to a 30% risk of becoming infected. For infected children, the lifetime risk of developing disease may approach 10%. For people coinfected with HIV, the annual risk has been estimated at 2%–7% and the cumulative risk at about 60–80%. Epidemics have been reported among people congregated in enclosed spaces, such as nursing homes, shelters for the homeless, hospitals, schools, prisons and office buildings. From 1989 to the early 1990s, extensive propagated outbreaks of multidrug resistant TB, usually defined as resistant to at least isoniazid and rifampin, have been recognized in settings where many HIV infected persons are congregated (hospitals, correctional facilities, drug treatment clinics and HIV residences). These outbreaks have been associated with high mortality rates and with transmission of *M. tuberculosis* to health care workers. Strict enforcement of infection control guidelines have been effective in combating and preventing these outbreaks.

The prevalence of TB infection detected by tuberculin testing increases with age. The incidence of infection in developed countries has declined rapidly in recent decades; in the USA, the annual risk of new infection is estimated to average about 10/100,000 people or less, although there probably are areas in the USA with a relatively high annual risk of new infection. In areas where human infection with mycobacteria other than tubercle bacilli is prevalent, cross reactions complicate interpretation of the tuberculin reaction.

Infection with *M. bovis*, the bovine tubercle bacillus, in humans is rare in the USA, but is still a problem in some areas, such as the border with Mexico, where the disease in cattle has not been controlled and milk and milk products are consumed raw.

4. Reservoir—Primarily humans, rarely primates; in some areas, diseased cattle, badgers, swine, and other mammals are infected.

5. Mode of transmission—Exposure to tubercle bacilli in airborne droplet nuclei produced by people with pulmonary or laryngeal tuberculosis during expiratory efforts, such as coughing, singing or sneezing. Health care workers are exposed during medical procedures such as bronchoscopy, autopsy and intubation. Laryngeal tuberculosis is highly contagious. Prolonged close exposure to an infectious case may lead to infection of contacts. Direct invasion through mucous membranes or breaks in the skin may occur but is extremely rare. Bovine tuberculosis results from exposure to tuberculous cattle, usually by ingestion of unpasteurized milk or dairy products, and sometimes by airborne spread to farmers and animal handlers. Except for rare situations where there is a draining sinus, extrapulmonary tuberculosis (other than laryngeal) is generally not communicable.

6. Incubation period—From infection to demonstrable primary lesion or significant tuberculin reaction, about 2-10 weeks. While the subsequent risk of progressive pulmonary or extrapulmonary TB is greatest within the first year or two after infection, latent infection may persist for a lifetime. HIV infection appears to increase the risk greatly and shorten the interval for the development of TB disease.

7. Period of communicability—Theoretically, as long as viable tubercle bacilli are being discharged in the sputum. Some untreated or inadequately treated patients may be sputum positive intermittently for years. The degree of communicability depends on the number of bacilli discharged, the virulence of the bacilli, adequacy of ventilation, exposure of the bacilli to sun or UV light, and opportunities for their aerosolization by coughing, sneezing, talking or singing, or during high risk medical procedures such as autopsies, intubations or bronchoscopies. Effective antimicrobial chemotherapy usually eliminates communicability within a few weeks, at least in the household setting. Children with primary tuberculosis are generally not infectious.

8. Susceptibility and resistance—The risk of infection with the tubercle bacillus is directly related to the degree of exposure and does not appear to be related to genetic or other host factors. The most hazardous period for development of clinical disease is the first 6-12 months after infection. The risk of developing disease is highest in children under 3 years old, lowest in later childhood, and high again among adolescents, young adults, the very old and the immunosuppressed. Reactivation of long latent infections accounts for a large proportion of TB disease cases in older people. For infected persons, susceptibility to TB disease is markedly increased by HIV infection and other forms of immunosuppression, those underweight or undernourished, those with a debilitating disease such as chronic renal failure, cancer, silicosis, diabetes or postgastrectomy, or those who are substance abusers.

For adults with latent TB infection who are also infected with HIV, the lifetime risk of developing TB disease rises from an estimated 10% to 60-80%. This interaction has resulted in a parallel pandemic of TB disease: in some urban sub-Saharan African populations where 10-15% of the adult population have HIV and TB infections, annual TB disease rates have increased from 5-10 fold during the latter half of the 1990s.

9. Methods of control—

A. *Preventive measures:*

1) Promptly identify, diagnose and treat potentially infectious patients with TB disease. Establish case finding and treatment facilities for infectious cases to reduce transmission.

2) Make available medical, laboratory and x-ray facilities for prompt examination of patients, contacts and suspects; facilities for early treatment of cases and people at high risk of infection; and beds for those needing hospitalization.

    In high incidence areas, examination of sputum by direct microscopy (by culture when possible) of those presenting at health facilities because of chest symptoms may give a high yield of infectious tuberculosis. In many situations, direct microscopy may be the most cost effective method of case finding and is the first priority in developing countries. Because of recent outbreaks of multidrug resistant tuberculosis, all initial isolates in the USA should be submitted for drug susceptibility testing. In countries with limited resources or laboratory capacity, drug susceptibility testing may be limited to treatment failures and former defaulters.

3) Educate the public in mode of spread and methods of control and the importance of early diagnosis.

4) Reduce or eliminate those social conditions that increase the risk of infection, such as overcrowding.

5) TB prevention and control programs should be established in all institutional settings in which health care is provided and/or immunocompromised patients such as HIV infected persons may be congregated (e.g., hospitals, drug treatment programs, correctional facilities and homeless shelters).

6) Use preventive treatment with isoniazid, which has been shown to be effective in preventing the progression of latent TB infection to TB disease in a high proportion of individuals. Studies in adults with HIV infection have demonstrated the effectiveness of alternative regimens including shorter courses

of rifampin and pyrazinamide. Preventive therapy is routinely indicated for infected persons under 35 years of age. It is important to rule out active TB disease before starting preventive therapy, especially in immunocompromised persons such as HIV infected individuals.

Because of the increased risk of isoniazid associated hepatitis with increasing age, isoniazid is not routinely advised for persons with TB infection over 35 years of age unless one or more of the following is present: recent infection (determined by recent tuberculin skin test conversion); close or household association with a current case; an abnormal chest radiograph consistent with old healed TB disease, diabetes, silicosis, prolonged therapy with corticosteroids or other immunosuppressive drugs; or immunosuppressive disease such as HIV infection.

Persons started on preventive treatment should be informed of possible adverse effects, such as hepatitis, drug fever or severe rash, and advised to discontinue treatment and seek medical advice if any suggestive symptoms develop. Most health care providers obtain baseline liver function tests on all patients; it is especially important in those 35 years of age or older and those who abuse alcohol. Directly observed, supervised preventive therapy (DOPT) should be used when possible (e.g., in correctional facilities, some drug treatment programs, schools). No more than one month's supply of medication should be given at any time. Patients should be queried at least monthly about adverse effects. Biochemical monitoring for hepatitis need not be done routinely, but is mandatory if symptoms or signs of hepatitis occur.

Isoniazid preventive therapy is contraindicated where there is a history of a previous severe adverse reaction to the drug or when there is acute liver disease of any etiology. During pregnancy, it may be wise to postpone preventive treatment until after delivery except in high risk individuals, and then it should be administered with caution. Isoniazid should be given with added caution to people who use alcohol regularly and those with chronic liver disease. Persons with hepatitis C infection may be at increased risk of isoniazid toxicity.

A policy of preventive treatment is unrealistic and unsuitable for mass application in most community health programs unless there is a well-organized program to supervise and encourage adherence to therapy and the treatment program for patients with active TB disease can achieve a high rate of cure. Persons with HIV infection and a positive PPD who do not have active TB disease should receive preventive therapy.

7) Provide public health nursing and outreach services for direct supervision of patient therapy, and arrange for the examination and preventive treatment of contacts.

8) Persons infected with HIV should be skin tested by the Mantoux method, using intermediate strength PPD at the time their HIV infection is identified and started on prophylactic treatment if they are PPD positive (5 mm or more of induration) and active TB disease has been ruled out. Conversely, all people with evidence of TB disease or TB infection should be considered for counseling and tested for HIV infection if appropriate counseling is available.

9) In the USA and other industrialized areas where BCG immunization is not routinely carried out, groups at high risk of TB infection and/or HIV infection may be selectively tuberculin tested as a case finding measure, e.g., health care workers, foreign born persons from areas where tuberculosis is highly prevalent and groups at high risk for HIV infection such as prison inmates and injecting drug users. In population groups where disease still occurs, systematic tuberculin test surveys may be used to monitor trends in the incidence of infection. X-ray examination is especially indicated whenever persistent chest symptoms are noted and bacteriologic tests are negative. Prior BCG immunization may complicate the interpretation of a positive skin test in a child or a recently immunized adult. However, skin test reactions from BCG wane over time and strongly positive reactions or significant increases in reactivity in such individuals should be considered indicative of TB infection.

10) BCG immunization of uninfected (tuberculin negative) people can induce tuberculin reactivity in more than 90% of vaccinees. The protection conferred has varied markedly in different field trials, and is perhaps related to some special characteristics of the population, the quality of the vaccine, or the strain of BCG employed. Some controlled trials have provided evidence that protection may persist for as long as 20 years in high incidence situations, while others have shown no protection at all.

Case-control and contact studies have consistently demonstrated protection against TB meningitis and disseminated disease in children less than 5 years old. Because the risk of infection is very low in the USA, BCG is not routinely used. BCG should be considered only for children with a negative PPD skin test who cannot be placed on preventive therapy but have continuous exposure to people with untreated or ineffectively treated active disease, or who have continuous exposure to patients infected by organisms resistant to isoniazid and rifampin and the child cannot be removed from the exposure. BCG is contraindicated for people with immunodeficiency diseases including HIV infection. WHO has permitted the administration of BCG to asymptomatic HIV infected children and those at high risk of acquiring HIV infection.

11) Eliminate bovine tuberculosis among dairy cattle by tuberculin testing and slaughter of reactors; pasteurize or boil milk.

12) Take measures to prevent silicosis among those working in industrial plants and mines.

B. Control of patient, contacts and the immediate environment:

1) Report to local health authority when diagnosis is suspected: Obligatory case report in all states (USA) and most countries, Class 2A (see Communicable Disease Reporting). Case report should indicate if it is bacteriologically positive or based on positive tuberculin reaction and clinical and/or x-ray findings. Health departments should maintain a current register of cases requiring treatment and be actively involved with planning and monitoring the course of therapy.

2) Isolation: For pulmonary tuberculosis, control of infectivity is best achieved by prompt specific drug therapy, which usually produces sputum conversion within 4–8 weeks. Hospital treatment is necessary only for patients with severe illness and for those whose medical or social circumstances make treatment at home impossible. Adult patients with sputum positive pulmonary tuberculosis need to be placed in a private room with negative pressure ventilation. Patients should be taught to cover both mouth and nose when coughing or sneezing. Persons entering the room should wear personal respiratory protective devices capable of filtering submicron particles. Isolation is unnecessary for patients whose sputum is bacteriologically negative, who do not cough and who are known to be on adequate chemotherapy (based on known or probable drug susceptibility and a clear clinical response to therapy). Children with active TB disease and no cough and negative sputum smears are not contagious and do not require isolation. Adolescents should be managed as adults. The need to adhere to the prescribed chemotherapeutic regimen must be reemphasized repeatedly to all patients. Directly observed therapy should be used when logistically and financially feasible and in particular for persons with suspected drug resistance, a previous history of poor compliance to therapy, or who live in conditions in which relapse would result in exposure of many other persons.

3) Concurrent disinfection: Handwashing and good housekeeping practices should be maintained according to routine

policy. There are no special precautions necessary for handling fomites (dishes, laundry, bedding, clothes and personal effects). Decontamination of air may be achieved by ventilation; this may be supplemented by ultraviolet light.

4) Quarantine: None.

5) Management of contacts: In the USA, preventive treatment for 3 months is recommended (see 9A6, above) for skin test negative close contacts; the skin test should then be repeated to determine the need for additional preventive therapy. BCG immunization of tuberculin negative household contacts may be warranted under special circumstances (see above).

6) Investigation of contacts and source of infection: PPD testing of all members of the household and other close contacts is recommended in the USA. If negative, a repeat skin test should be performed 2–3 months after exposure has ended. Chest radiographs should be obtained on positive reactors when they are identified. Preventive treatment is indicated (see 9A6, above) for contacts who are positive reactors and for some initially negative reactors at high risk of developing active disease, especially young (5 years old or younger) and HIV infected close contacts, at least until the repeat skin test is shown to remain negative. Unfortunately, in many developing countries, investigation of household contacts is limited to sputum microscopy of those contacts who have symptoms suggestive of TB disease.

7) Specific treatment: Directly observed therapy has been shown to be highly effective and is recommended for treatment of TB disease in the USA. Patients with TB disease should be given prompt treatment with an appropriate combination of antimicrobial drugs, with regular monitoring of sputum smears. For drug susceptible disease, a 6 month regimen consisting of isoniazid (INH), rifampin (RIF), and pyrazinamide (PZA) is recommended for the first 2 months followed by INH and PZA for 4 months. A 4 drug initial therapy (including ethambutol (EMB) or streptomycin (SM)) is recommended if the infection was acquired in areas where an increased prevalence of INH resistance has been reported. After drug susceptibility results are available, a specific drug regimen can be selected.

If sputum fails to become negative after 2–3 months of regular therapy or reverts to positive after a series of negatives, or if clinical response is poor, examination for drug taking compliance and for bacterial drug resistance is indicated. Treatment failure is usually the result of irregularity in taking drugs and may not necessitate a change in regimen; a change in supervision may well be required if a favorable clinical response is not observed. At least two drugs to which the organisms are susceptible should be included in the regimen; a single new drug should never be added to a failing regimen. If INH or RIF cannot be included in the regimen, the minimum duration of therapy is 18 months after cultures have become negative.

For newly diagnosed smear positive patients in developing countries, WHO recommends that treatment should include 2 months of daily doses of INH, RIF, PZA and EMB followed by 4 months of twice weekly INH and RIF. All treatment should be supervised or directly observed; if treatment cannot be directly observed in the second phase, 6 months of INH and EMB may be substituted. Even though these short, intensive regimens are more expensive than those employing fewer drugs for 12–18 months, they are much more effective and allow for better compliance.

Children are treated with the same regimens as adults with some modifications. In children, susceptibility of the causitive organism can often be inferred from testing isolates of the adult source case. Children with hilar adenopathy only can be treated with only INH and RIF for 6 months. Therapy for children with meningitis, miliary disease, or bone/joint disease should last for at least 9–12 months; some experts recommend a total of only 9 months of therapy. EMB is not used until the child is old enough for color vision to be checked (usually 5 years of age or older). Children with life threatening disease should receive the initial 4 drug regimen. Streptomycin is contraindicated during pregnancy.

All drugs occasionally cause adverse reactions. Thoracic surgery is occasionally indicated, usually in multidrug resistant cases.

C. Epidemic measures: Alertness to recognize and treat aggregations of new infections resulting from contact with an unrecognized infectious case, and intensive search for and treatment of the source of infection.

D. Disaster implications: None.

E. International measures: Chest radiograph screening, PPD testing, and smear and culture testing of symptomatic PPD positive persons from high prevalence countries is suggested on immigration. WHO Collaborating Centres.

DISEASES DUE TO OTHER
MYCOBACTERIA   ICD-9 031; ICD-10 A31
(Mycobacterioses, Nontuberculous mycobacterial disease)

Mycobacteria other than *Mycobacterium tuberculosis, M. africanum, M. bovis* and *M. leprae* are ubiquitous in nature and may produce disease in humans. These acid-fast bacilli in the past have been variously termed atypical, unclassified mycobacteria or mycobacteria other than tuberculosis (MOTT). Of the numerous identified species only about 15 are recognized as being pathogenic to people.

Clinical syndromes associated with the pathogenic species of mycobacteria can be classified broadly as follows:

1) disseminated disease (in the presence of severe immunodeficiency as in AIDS)—*M. avium* complex, *M. kansasii, M. haemophilum, M. chelonae;*

2) pulmonary disease resembling tuberculosis—*M. kansasii, M. avium* complex, *M. abscessus, M. xenopi, M. simiae;*

3) lymphadenitis (primarily cervical)—*M. avium* complex, *M. scrofulaceum, M. kansasii;*

4) skin ulcers—*M. ulcerans* (Buruli ulcer), *M. marinum;*

5) post-traumatic wound infections—*M. fortuitum, M. chelonae, M. abscessus, M. marinum, M. avium* complex;

6) nosocomial disease: surgical wound infections (sternal following cardiac surgery, mammaplasty wounds), catheter related infections (bacteremia, peritonitis and post injection abscesses)—*M. fortuitum, M. chelonae, M. abscessus;* and

7) Crohn disease—*M. paratuberculosis* has been suggested as the causative agent in some cases of regional enteritis.

The epidemiology of the diseases attributable to these organisms has not been well delineated, but the organisms have been found in soil, milk and water; other factors, such as host tissue damage and immunodeficiency, may predispose to infection. With the exception of organisms causing skin lesions, there is no evidence of person to person transmission. A single isolation of these bacilli from sputum, or gastric washing can occur in the absence of signs or symptoms of clinical disease. A single positive culture from a wound or tissue is generally considered diagnostic.

In general, the diagnosis of disease requiring treatment is based on repeated isolations of many colonies from symptomatic patients with progressive illness. Where human infections with nontuberculous mycobacteria are prevalent, cross reactions may interfere with the interpretation of the skin test for *M. tuberculosis* infection. Chemotherapy is relatively effective in treating *M. kansasii* and *M. marinum* disease, but traditional antituberculosis drugs (especially PZA) may not be effective for the other mycobacterioses. For selection of an efficient drug combination, drug susceptibility tests should be performed on the isolated organisms. Surgery should be given more serious consideration than in TB disease, especially when the disease is limited, as in localized pulmonary disease, cervical lymphadenitis or a subcutaneous abscess.

Disseminated *Mycobacterium avium* complex (MAC) infection is a major problem in HIV infected persons and was considered poorly amenable to treatment until recently. For disseminated MAC infections, drug regimens containing rifabutin and clarithromycin have shown some therapeutic potential. Rifabutin has been approved for MAC prophylaxis in HIV infected patients whose CD4 counts are below 100.

TULAREMIA   ICD-9 021; ICD-10 A21
(Rabbit fever, Deer-fly fever, Ohara disease, Francis disease)

1. Identification—A zoonotic bacterial disease with a variety of clinical manifestations related to the route of introduction and the virulence of the disease agent. Most often it presents as an indolent ulcer at the site of introduction of the organism, together with swelling of the regional lymph nodes (ulceroglandular type). There may be no apparent primary ulcer, but only one or more enlarged and painful lymph nodes that may suppurate (glandular type). Ingestion of organisms in contaminated food or water may produce a painful pharyngitis (with or without ulceration), abdominal pain, diarrhea and vomiting (oropharyngeal type). Inhalation of infectious material may be followed by pneumonic involvement or a primary septicemic syndrome with a 30%–60% case-fatality rate if untreated (typhoidal type); bloodborne organisms may localize in the lung and pleural spaces (pleuropulmonary type). The conjunctival sac is a rare route of introduction that results in a clinical disease of painful purulent conjunctivitis with regional lymphadenitis (oculoglandular type). Pneumonia may complicate all clinical types and requires prompt identification and specific treatment to prevent a fatal outcome.

Two biovars with differing pathogenicity cause human disease. Jellison type A organisms are more virulent, with an untreated case-fatality rate of 5%–15% primarily due to typhoidal or pulmonary disease. With appropriate antibiotic treatment, the case-fatality rate is negligible. Jellison type B organisms are less virulent and, even without treatment, produce few fatalities. Clinically, because of buboes and/or severe pneumonia, tularemia may be confused with plague, as well as many other infectious diseases, including staphylococcal and streptococcal infections, cat-scratch fever and sporotrichosis.

Diagnosis is most commonly made clinically and confirmed by a rise in specific serum antibodies that usually appear in the second week of the disease. Cross-reactions occur with *Brucella* species. Examination of ulcer exudate, lymph node aspirates and other clinical specimens by FA test may provide rapid diagnosis. Diagnostic biopsy of acutely infected lymph nodes should be done only under the cover of specific antibiotic treatment since it will often induce bacteremia. The causative bacteria can be cultured on special media such as cysteine-glucose blood agar or by inoculation of laboratory animals with material from lesions, blood or sputum. The biovars are differentiated by their chemical reactions; type A organisms ferment glycerol and convert citrulline to ornithine. Extreme care must be exercised to avoid laboratory transmission of highly infectious aerosolized organisms; hence, culture identification is performed only in reference laboratories and most cases are diagnosed serologically.

2. Infectious agent—*Francisella tularensis* (formerly *Pasteurella tularensis*), a small, gram-negative nonmotile coccobacillus. All isolates are serologically homogeneous but are differentiated epidemiologically and biochemically into Jellison type A *(F. tularensis* biovar *tularensis)*, which has an LD_{50} in rabbits of fewer than 10 bacteria, or type B strains *(F. tularensis* biovar *palaearctica)*, which have an LD_{50} of greater than 10^7 in rabbits.

3. Occurrence—Tularemia occurs throughout North America and in many parts of continental Europe, the former Soviet Union, China and Japan. In the USA, it occurs in all months of the year; incidence may be higher in adults in early winter during rabbit hunting season and in children during the summer when ticks and deer flies are abundant. *F. tularensis* biovar *tularensis* organisms, restricted to North America, are common in rabbits (cottontail, jack and snowshoe), and are frequently transmitted by tick bite. *F. tularensis* biovar *palaearctica* strains are commonly found in mammals other than rabbits in North America; strains in Eurasia are found in voles, muskrats and water rats; and in rabbits in Japan.

4. Reservoir—Numerous wild animals, especially rabbits, hares, voles, muskrats, beavers and some domestic animals; also various hard ticks. In addition, a rodent-mosquito cycle has been described for *F. tularensis* biovar *palaearctica* in Scandinavia, the Baltic states and Russia.

5. Mode of transmission—Through the bite of arthropods, including the wood tick *Dermacentor andersoni*, the dog tick *D. variabilis*, the lone star tick *Amblyomma americanum*, less commonly the deer fly *Chrysops discalis* and, in Sweden, the mosquito *Aedes cinereus;* by inoculation of skin, conjunctival sac or oropharyngeal mucosa with contaminated water, blood or tissue while handling carcasses of infected animals (e.g., skinning, dressing or performing necropsies); by handling or ingesting insufficiently cooked meat of infected animal hosts; by drinking contaminated water; by inhalation of dust from contaminated soil, grain or hay; rarely, from bites of coyote, squirrel, skunk, hog, cat and dog whose mouth presumably was contaminated from eating an infected animal; and from contaminated pelts and paws of animals. Laboratory infections occur and frequently present as a primary pneumonia or typhoidal tularemia.

6. Incubation period—Related to virulence of infecting strain and to size of inoculum; the range is 1–14 days, usually 3–5 days.

7. Period of communicability—Not directly transmitted from person to person. Unless treated, the infectious agent may be found in the blood during the first 2 weeks of disease and in lesions for a month, sometimes longer. Flies can be infective for 14 days and ticks throughout their lifetime (about 2 years). Rabbit meat frozen at −15°C (5°F) has remained infective longer than 3 years.

8. Susceptibility and resistance—All ages are susceptible, and long-term immunity follows recovery; however, reinfection has been reported in laboratorians.

9. Methods of control—

A. Preventive measures:

1) Educate the public to avoid bites of ticks, flies and mosquitoes and to avoid drinking, bathing, swimming or working in untreated water where infection prevails among wild animals.
2) Use impervious gloves when skinning or handling animals, especially rabbits. Cook the meat of wild rabbits and rodents thoroughly.
3) Prohibit interstate or interarea shipment of infected animals or their carcasses.
4) Live attenuated vaccines applied intradermally by scarification are used extensively in the former Soviet Union, and to a limited extent for occupational risk groups in the USA. Such an investigational live attenuated vaccine for laboratory personnel working with the organism is no longer available in the USA.
5) Wear face masks, gowns and impervious gloves and negative pressure microbiological cabinets when working with cultures of *F. tularensis*.

B. Control of patient, contacts and the immediate environment:

1) Report to local health authority: In selected endemic areas (USA); in many countries, not a reportable disease, Class 3B (see Communicable Disease Reporting).
2) Isolation: Drainage and secretion precautions for open lesions.
3) Concurrent disinfection: Of discharges from ulcers, lymph nodes or conjunctival sacs.
4) Quarantine: None.
5) Immunization of contacts: Not indicated.
6) Investigation of contacts and source of infection: Important in each case, with search for the origin of infection.
7) Specific treatment: Streptomycin or gentamicin given for 7–14 days is the drug of choice; the tetracyclines and chloramphenicol are bacteriostatic and effective when continued for no less than 14 days; relapses are reported to occur more often than with streptomycin. Moreover, fully virulent streptomycin-resistant organisms have been described. Aspiration, incision and drainage, or biopsy of an inflamed lymph node can spread

the infection and must be covered with prompt and specific antibiotics.

C. Epidemic measures: Search for sources of infection related to arthropods, animal hosts, water, soil and crops. Control measures as indicated in 9A, above.

D. Disaster implications: None.

E. International measures: None.

F. Bioterrorism measures: Tularemia is considered to be a potential biowarfare/bioterrorist agent, particularly if used as an aerosol threat. As is true of plague, cases acquired by inhalation would present as primary pneumonia. Such cases require prompt identification and specific treatment to prevent a fatal outcome. All diagnosed cases of pneumonia due to *F. tularensis,* especially any cluster of cases should be reported **immediately** to the local FBI and health department for appropriate investigations.

TYPHOID FEVER   ICD-9 002.0; ICD-10 A01.0
(Enteric fever, Typhus abdominalis)
PARATYPHOID
FEVER   ICD-9 002.1–002.9; ICD-10 A01.1–A01.4

1. Identification—Systemic bacterial diseases characterized by insidious onset of sustained fever, severe headache, malaise, anorexia, a relative bradycardia, splenomegaly, rose spots on the trunk in 25% of white patients, nonproductive cough in the early stage of the illness and constipation more commonly than diarrhea in adults. Many mild and atypical infections occur.

In typhoid fever, ulceration of Peyer patches in the ileum can produce intestinal hemorrhage or perforation (about 1% of cases), especially late in untreated cases. Severe forms have been described with cerebral dysfunction. Nonsweating fever, mental dullness, slight deafness and parotitis may occur. The case-fatality rate of 10%–20% observed in the preantibiotic era can be reduced to less than 1% with prompt antibiotic therapy. Depending on the antimicrobial agent used, (15%–20%) of patients may experience relapses (which are generally much milder than the initial clinical illness). Mild and inapparent illnesses occur, especially in endemic areas.

A new nomenclature for *Salmonella* has been proposed based on DNA relatedness. According to the proposed nomenclature, only two species would be recognized—*Salmonella bongori* and *Salmonella enterica* (both genus and species italicized). All human pathogens would be regarded as serovars within subspecies I of *S. enterica*. The proposed nomenclature would change *S. typhi* to *S. enterica* serovar Typhi, abbreviated *S.* Typhi (note that Typhi is not italicized and a capital letter is used.) Some official agencies have adopted the new nomenclature although it had not been officially approved as of mid-1999. This new nomenclature is used in this chapter.

Paratyphoid fever presents a similar clinical picture, but tends to be milder, and the case-fatality rate is much lower. The ratio of disease caused by *Salmonella enterica* serovar Typhi (*S.* Typhi) to that caused by *S. enterica,* serovar Paratyphi A and B (*S* Paratyphi A, *S* Paratyphi B) is about 10:1. Relapses may occur in approximately 3%–4% of cases. When the salmonella infections are not systemic, they are manifested only by a gastroenteritis (see Salmonellosis).

The etiologic organisms can be isolated from the blood early in the disease and from urine and feces after the first week; bone marrow culture provides the best bacteriologic confirmation (90%–95% recovery) even in patients who have already received antimicrobials. Because of its limited sensitivity and specificity, serologic tests (widal test) are generally of little diagnostic value.

2. Infectious agents—For typhoid fever, *S.* Typhi, the typhoid bacillus. Phage typing and pulsed field gel electrophoresis of *S.* Typhi are valuable laboratory tests for characterizing isolates in epidemiologic studies.

For paratyphoid fever, three serovars of *S. enterica* are recognized: *S.* Paratyphi A, *S.* Paratyphi B, and *S.* Parathyphi C. A number of phage types can be distinguished.

3. Occurrence—Worldwide; the annual incidence of typhoid fever is estimated at about 17 million cases with approximately 600,000 deaths. The number of sporadic cases of typhoid fever has remained relatively constant in the USA, with fewer than 500 cases annually for several years (compared with 2,484 reported in 1950), and, with development of sanitary facilities, has been virtually eliminated from many areas; most USA cases now are imported from endemic areas. Strains resistant to chloramphenicol and other recommended antimicrobials have become prevalent in several areas of the world. The majority of isolates from south and southeast Asia, the Middle East and northeast Africa in the 1990s have been strains carrying an R factor plasmid that encodes resistance to multiple antimicrobial agents that were previously the mainstays of oral therapy including chloramphenicol, amoxicillin and trimethoprim/sulfamethoxazole.

Paratyphoid fever occurs sporadically or in limited outbreaks, probably more frequently than reports suggest. In the USA and Canada, paratyphoid fever is infrequently identified. Of the three bioserotypes, paratyphoid B is most common, A less frequent and C extremely rare.

4. Reservoir—Humans for both typhoid and paratyphoid; rarely, domestic animals for paratyphoid. Family contacts may be transient or permanent carriers. In most parts of the world, short-term fecal carriers are more common than urinary carriers. The carrier state may follow acute illness or mild or even subclinical infections. The chronic carrier state is most common among persons infected during middle age, especially women; carriers frequently have biliary tract abnormalities including gallstones. The chronic urinary carrier state occurs in those with schistosome infections. In one outbreak of paratyphoid fever in England, dairy cows excreted Paratyphi B organisms in milk and feces.

5. Mode of transmission—By food and water contaminated by feces and urine of patients and carriers. Important vehicles in some countries include shellfish taken from sewage contaminated beds (particularly oysters), raw fruits, vegetables fertilized by night soil and eaten raw, contaminated milk and milk products (usually contaminated by hands of carriers) and missed cases. Flies may infect foods in which the organism then multiplies to achieve an infective dose, which is much lower for typhoid than for paratyphoid bacteria.

6. Incubation period—The incubation period depends on the size of the infecting dose; from 3 days to 1 month with a usual range of 8–14 days. For paratyphoid gastroenteritis, 1–10 days.

7. Period of communicability—As long as the bacilli appear in excreta, usually from the first week throughout convalescence; variable thereafter (commonly 1–2 weeks for paratyphoid). About 10% of untreated typhoid fever patients will discharge bacilli for 3 months after onset of symptoms, and 2%–5% become permanent carriers; considerably fewer persons infected with paratyphoid organisms may become permanent gallbladder carriers.

8. Susceptibility and resistance—Susceptibility is general and is increased in individuals with gastric achlorhydria or those who are HIV positive. Relative specific immunity follows recovery from clinical disease, inapparent infection and active immunization. In endemic areas, typhoid fever is most common in preschool and children 5–19 years of age.

9. Methods of control—

 A. Preventive measures:

  1) Educate the public regarding the importance of handwashing. Provide suitable handwashing facilities; this is particularly important for food handlers and attendants involved in the care of patients and children.

  2) Dispose of human feces in a sanitary manner and maintain fly proof latrines. Stress use of sufficient toilet paper to minimize finger contamination. Under field conditions, dispose of

feces by burial at a site distant and downstream from the source of drinking water.

3) Protect, purify and chlorinate public water supplies, provide safe private supplies, and avoid possible back flow connections between water and sewer systems. For individual and small group protection, and while traveling or in the field, treat water chemically or by boiling.

4) Control flies by screening, spraying with insecticides and use of insecticidal baits and traps. Control fly breeding by frequent collection and disposal of garbage, and fly control measures in latrine construction and maintenance.

5) Use scrupulous cleanliness in food preparation and handling; refrigerate as appropriate. Particular attention should be directed to the proper storage of salads and other foods served cold. These provisions apply equally to home and public eating places. If uncertain about sanitary practices, select foods that are cooked and served hot, and fruits peeled by the consumer.

6) Pasteurize or boil all milk and dairy products. Supervise the sanitary aspects of commercial milk production, storage and delivery.

7) Enforce suitable quality-control procedures in industries that prepare food and drink for human consumption. Use chlorinated water for cooling during canned food processing.

8) Limit the collection and marketing of shellfish to supplies from approved sources. Boil or steam (for at least 10 minutes) before serving.

9) Instruct patients, convalescents and carriers in personal hygiene. Emphasize handwashing as a routine practice after defecation and before preparing and serving food.

10) Encourage breast feeding throughout infancy; boil all milk and water used for infant feeding.

11) Exclude typhoid carriers from handling food and from providing patient care. Identify and supervise typhoid carriers; culture of sewage may help in locating carriers. Chronic carriers should not be released from supervision and restriction of occupation until local or state regulations are met, often not until 3 consecutive negative cultures are obtained from authenticated fecal (and urine in schistosomiasis endemic areas) specimens taken at least 1 month apart and at least 48 hours after antimicrobial therapy has stopped. Fresh stool specimens are preferred to rectal swabs; at least 1 of the 3 consecutive negative stool specimens should be obtained by purging.

In recent studies, the new oral quinolones have produced excellent results in the treatment of the carrier, even when biliary disease exists; follow-up cultures are necessary to confirm cure.

12) Typhoid fever: Immunization is not routinely recommended in the USA. Current practice is to immunize those subject to unusual exposure to enteric infections from occupation (e.g., clinical microbiology technicians) or travel to endemic areas, those living in areas of high endemicity, and household members of known carriers. An oral, live vaccine using *S.* Typhi strain Ty21a (requiring 3 or 4 doses, 2 days apart) and a parenteral vaccine containing the polysaccharide Vi antigen (single dose) are available. Since these vaccines are as protective as the whole cell bacteria vaccine and are much less reactogenic, they are the vaccines of choice. However, Ty21a should not be used in patients receiving antibiotics or the antimalarial mefloquine. Because it commonly elicits marked systemic adverse reactions, use of the old inactivated whole cell vaccines is strongly discouraged. Booster doses are desirable for those at continuing risk of infection with an interval between booster doses ranging from 2 to 5 years, depending on the type of vaccine.

Paratyphoid fever: In field trials, oral typhoid vaccine (Ty21a) conferred partial protection against paratyphoid B but not as well as it protected against typhoid.

B. Control of patient, contacts and the immediate environment:

1) Report to local health authority: Obligatory case report in most states and countries, Class 2A (see Communicable Disease Reporting).

2) Isolation: Enteric precautions while ill; hospital care is desirable during acute illness. Release from supervision by local health authority should be based on not fewer than 3 consecutive negative cultures of feces (and urine in patients with schistosomiasis) taken at least 24 hours apart and at least 48 hours after any antimicrobials, and not earlier than 1 month after onset; if any one of these is positive, repeat cultures at intervals of 1 month during the 12 months following onset until at least 3 consecutive negative cultures are obtained.

3) Concurrent disinfection: Of feces and urine and articles soiled therewith. In communities with modern and adequate sewage disposal systems, feces and urine can be disposed of directly into sewers without preliminary disinfection. Terminal cleaning.

4) Quarantine: None.

5) Immunization of contacts: Routine administration of typhoid vaccine is of limited value for family, household and nursing contacts who have been or may be exposed to active cases; it

should be considered for those who may be exposed to carriers. There is no effective immunization for paratyphoid A fever.

6) Investigation of contacts and source of infection: The actual or probable source of infection of every case should be determined by search for unreported cases, carriers or contaminated food, water, milk or shellfish. All members of travel groups in which a case has been identified should be followed.

The presence of elevated antibody titers to purified Vi polysaccharide is highly suggestive of the typhoidal carrier state. Identification of the same phage type in the organisms isolated from patients and a carrier suggests a possible chain of transmission.

Household and close contacts should not be employed in sensitive occupations (e.g., food handlers) until at least 2 negative feces and urine cultures, taken at least 24 hours apart, are obtained.

7) Specific treatment: Increasing prevalence of resistant strains currently dictates therapy. In general, in adults, oral ciprofloxacin should be considered the drug of choice, particularly in patients from Asia. There have been recent reports of Asian strains showing diminished *in vivo* sensitivity. If local strains are known to be sensitive, oral chloramphenicol, amoxicillin or TMP-SMX (particularly in children) have comparable high efficacy for acute infections. Ceftriaxone is a parenteral once daily antibiotic that is useful in obtunded patients or those with complications in whom oral antibiotics cannot be used. Short-term, high dose corticosteroid treatment, combined with specific antibiotics and supportive care, clearly reduce mortality in critically ill patients. (See 9A11, above, for treatment of the carrier state.) Patients with concurrent schistosomiasis must also be treated with praziquantel to eliminate possible carriage of *S.* Typhi bacilli by the schistosomes.

C. Epidemic measures:

1) Search intensively for the case or carrier who is the source of infection and for the vehicle (water or food) by which infection was transmitted.

2) Selectively eliminate suspected contaminated food.

3) Pasteurize or boil milk, or exclude milk supplies and other foods suspected on epidemiologic evidence, until safety is ensured.

4) Chlorinate suspected water supplies adequately under compe-

tent supervision or avoid use. All drinking water must be chlorinated, treated with iodine or boiled before use.

5) Routine use of vaccine is not recommended.

D. *Disaster implications:* With disruption of usual water supply and sewage disposal, and of controls on food and water, transmission of typhoid fever may occur if there are active cases or carriers in a displaced population. Efforts to restore safe drinking water supplies and excreta disposal facilities are recommended. Selective immunization of stabilized groups such as school children, prisoners, and utility, municipal or hospital personnel can be helpful.

E. *International measures:*

1) For typhoid fever: Immunization is advised for international travelers to endemic areas, especially if travel will likely involve exposure to unsafe food and water, or close contact in rural areas to indigenous populations. Immunization is not a legal requirement for entry into any country.

2) For both typhoid and paratyphoid fevers, WHO Collaborating Centres.

TYPHUS FEVER   ICD-10 A75
I. EPIDEMIC LOUSEBORNE
TYPHUS FEVER   ICD-9 080; ICD-10 A75.0
(Louseborne typhus, Typhus exanthematicus, Classic typhus fever)

1. Identification—A rickettsial disease with variable onset; often sudden and marked by headache, chills, prostration, fever and general pains. A macular eruption appears on the fifth to sixth day, initially on the upper trunk, followed by spread to the entire body, but usually not to the face, palms or soles. Toxemia is usually pronounced, and the disease terminates by rapid defervescence after about 2 weeks of fever. The case-fatality rate increases with age and varies from 10% to 40% in the absence of specific therapy. Mild infections may occur without eruption, especially in children and people partially protected by prior immunization. The disease may recrudesce years after the primary attack (Brill-Zinsser disease, ICD-9 081.1; ICD-10 A75.1); this form of disease is milder, has fewer complications, and has a lower case-fatality rate.

The IF test is most commonly used for laboratory confirmation, but it does not discriminate between louseborne and murine typhus (ICD-9 081.0; ICD-10 A75.2) unless the sera are differentially absorbed with the respective rickettsial antigen prior to testing. Other diagnostic methods are

EIA, PCR, immunohistochemical staining of tissues, CF with group specific or washed type specific rickettsial antigens, and the toxin-neutralization test. Antibody tests usually become positive in the second week. In acute disease, the initial antibody is IgM and in Brill-Zinsser disease, IgG.

2. Infectious agent—*Rickettsia prowazekii.*

3. Occurrence—In colder areas where people may live under unhygienic conditions and are louse infested; enormous and explosive epidemics may occur druing war and famine. Endemic foci exist in mountainous regions of Mexico, Central and South America, in central and east Africa and numerous countries of Asia. In the USA, the last outbreak of louseborne typhus occurred in 1921. This rickettsia exists as a zoonosis of flying squirrels *(Glaucomys volans)* and there is serologic evidence that humans have been infected from this source, possibly by the squirrel flea. Most of these have been in the east coast states, cases have also been reported from Indiana, California, Illinois, Ohio, Tennessee and West Virginia.

4. Reservoir—Humans are the reservoir and are responsible for maintaining the infection during interepidemic periods. Although not a major source of human disease, sporadic cases may be associated with flying squirrels.

5. Mode of transmission—The body louse, *Pediculus humanus corporis,* is infected by feeding on the blood of a patient with acute typhus fever. Patients with Brill-Zinsser disease can infect lice and may serve as foci for new outbreaks in louse infested communities. Infected lice excrete rickettsiae in their feces and usually defecate at the time of feeding. People are infected by rubbing feces or crushed lice into the bite or into superficial abrasions. Inhalation of infective louse feces in dust may account for some infections. Transmission from the flying squirrel is presumed to be by the bite of the squirrel flea, but this has not been documented.

6. Incubation period—From 1 to 2 weeks, commonly 12 days.

7. Period of communicability—The disease is not directly transmitted from person to person. Patients are infective for lice during the febrile illness and possibly for 2-3 days after the temperature returns to normal. Infected lice pass rickettsiae in their feces within 2-6 days after the blood meal; it is infective earlier if crushed. The louse invariably dies within 2 weeks after infection; rickettsiae may remain viable in the dead louse for weeks.

8. Susceptibility and resistance—Susceptibility is general. One attack usually confers long-lasting immunity.

9. Methods of control—

A. Preventive measures:

1) Apply an effective residual insecticide powder at appropriate intervals by hand or power blower to clothes and persons of

populations living under conditions favoring louse infestation. The lousicide used should be effective on local lice.

2) Improve living conditions with provisions for bathing and washing clothes.

3) Treat prophylactically those who are subject to risk, by application of residual insecticide to clothing by dusting or impregnation.

B. Control of patient, contacts and the immediate environment:

1) Report to local health authority: Report of louseborne typhus fever required as a Disease under Surveillance by WHO, Class 1A (see Communicable Disease Reporting).

2) Isolation: Not required after proper delousing of patient, clothing, living quarters and household contacts.

3) Concurrent disinfection: Appropriate insecticide powder applied to clothing and bedding of patient and contacts; launder clothing and bedclothes. Lice tend to leave abnormally hot or cold bodies in search of a normothermic clothed body (see 9A1, above). If death from louseborne typhus occurs before delousing, delouse the body and clothing by thorough application of an insecticide.

4) Quarantine: Louse infested susceptibles exposed to typhus fever ordinarily should be quarantined for 15 days after application of an insecticide with residual effect.

5) Management of contacts: All immediate contacts should be kept under surveillance for 2 weeks.

6) Investigation of contacts and source of infection: Every effort should be made to trace the infection to the immediate source.

7) Specific treatment: A single dose of doxycycline 200 mg will usually cure patients in epidemic settings. Tetracyclines or chloramphenicol orally in a loading dose of 2–3 g, followed by daily doses of 1–2 g/day in 4 divided doses until the patient becomes afebrile (usually 2 days) plus 1 day. When faced with a seriously ill patient with possible typhus, suitable therapy should be started without waiting for laboratory confirmation.

C. Epidemic measures:
The measure for rapid control of typhus is application of an insecticide with residual effect to all contacts. Where infestation is known to be widespread, systematic application of residual insecticide to all people in the community is indicated. Treatment of cases in an epidemic may also decrease the spread of disease.

D. Disaster implications:
Typhus can be expected to be a significant problem in louse infested populations in endemic areas if social upheavals and crowding occur.

E. International measures:

1) Telegraphic notification by governments to WHO and to adjacent countries of the occurrence of a case or an outbreak of louseborne typhus fever in an area previously free of the disease.

2) International travelers: No country currently requires immunization against typhus for entry.

3) Louseborne typhus is a Disease under Surveillance by WHO. WHO Collaborating Centres.

II. ENDEMIC FLEABORNE TYPHUS FEVER

ICD-9 081.0;
ICD-10 A75.2

(Murine typhus, Shop typhus)

1. Identification—A rickettsial disease whose course resembles that of louseborne typhus, but is milder. The case-fatality rate for all ages is less than 1% but increases with age. Absence of louse infestation, geographic and seasonal distribution and sporadic occurrence of the disease help to differentiate it from louseborne typhus. For laboratory diagnosis, see section I, 1, above.

2. Infectious agents—*Rickettsia typhi (Rickettsia mooseri); Rickettsia felis.*

3. Occurrence—Worldwide. Found in areas where people and rats occupy the same buildings. In the USA, fewer than 80 cases are reported annually. Seasonal peak occurs in late summer and autumn; cases tend to be scattered, but with a high proportion reported from Texas and southern California. Multiple cases may occur in the same household.

4. Reservoir—Rats, mice and possibly other small mammals. Infection is maintained in nature by a rat flea rat cycle where rats are the reservoir (commonly *Rattus rattus* and *R. norvegicus)* but infection is inapparent. A closely related organism, *Rickettsia felis,* has been found in a cat to cat flea to opossum cycle in southern California and probably occurs elsewhere.

5. Mode of transmission—Infective rat fleas (usually *Xenopsylla cheopis)* defecate rickettsiae while sucking blood, this contaminates the bite site and other fresh skin wounds. An occasional case may follow inhalation of dried infective flea feces. Infection with *Rickettsia felis* occurs in opossums, cats, dogs and other wild and domestic animals; this is self-limited, but these animals may transport infective cat fleas, *Ctenocephalides felis* to humans.

6. Incubation period—From 1 to 2 weeks, commonly 12 days.

7. Period of communicability—Not directly transmitted from person to person. Once infected, fleas remain so for life (up to 1 year).

8. Susceptibility and resistance—Susceptibility is general. One attack confers immunity.

9. Methods of control—

A. Preventive measures:

1) Apply insecticide powders with residual action to rat runs, burrows and harborages.
2) To avoid increased exposure of humans, wait until flea populations have first been reduced by insecticides before instituting rodent control measures (see Plague, 9A2–9A3, 9B6).

B. Control of patient, contacts and the immediate environment:

1) Report to local health authority: Case report obligatory in most states (USA) and countries, Class 2B (see Communicable Disease Reporting).
2) Isolation: None.
3) Concurrent disinfection: None.
4) Quarantine: None.
5) Immunization of contacts: None.
6) Investigation of contacts and source of infection: Search for rodents or opossums around premises or home of patient.
7) Specific treatment: As for Rocky Mountain Spotted Fever (q.v.).

C. Epidemic measures:
In endemic areas with numerous cases, use of a residual insecticide effective against rat or cat fleas will reduce the flea index and the incidence of infection in humans.

D. Disaster implications:
Cases can be expected when people, rats and fleas are forced to coexist, but murine typhus has not been a major contributor to disease rates in such situations.

E. International measures:
WHO Collaborating Centres.

III. SCRUB TYPHUS ICD-9 081.2; ICD-10 A75.3
(Tsutsugamushi disease, Miteborne typhus fever)

1. Identification—A rickettsial disease often characterized by a primary "punched out" skin ulcer (eschar) corresponding to the site of attachment of an infected mite. An acute febrile onset follows within several days, along with headache, profuse sweating, conjunctival injection and lymphadenopathy. Late in the first week of fever, a dull red, maculopapular eruption appears on the trunk, extends to the extremities and disappears in a few days. Cough and x-ray evidence of pneumonitis are common. Without antibiotic therapy, fever lasts for about 14 days. The case-fatality rate in untreated cases varies from 1% to 60%, according to area, strain of rickettsia and previous exposure to disease; it is consistently higher among older people.

Definitive diagnosis is made by isolation of the infectious agent by inoculating the patient's blood into mice. Serologic diagnosis is complicated by antigenic differences of various strains of the causal rickettsia; the IF test is the preferred technique, but EIAs are also available. Many cases develop a positive Weil-Felix reaction with the *Proteus* OXK strain.

2. Infectious agent—*Orientia tsutsugamushi* with multiple serologically distinct strains.

3. Occurrence—Central, eastern and southeast Asia; from southeastern Siberia and northern Japan to northern Australia and Vanuatu, as far west as Pakistan, to as high as 10,000 feet above sea level in the Himalayan Mountains, and particularly prevalent in northern Thailand. Acquired by humans in one of innumerable small, sharply delimited "typhus islands," some covering an area of only a few square feet, where rickettsiae, vectors and suitable rodents exist simultaneously. Occupation greatly influences the gender distribution; restricted mainly to adult workers who frequent scrub overgrown terrain or other mite infested areas, such as forest clearings, reforested areas, new settlements or even newly irrigated desert regions. Epidemics occur when susceptibles are brought into endemic areas, especially in military operations in which 20%–50% of troops have been infected within weeks or months.

4. Reservoir—Infected larval stages of trombiculid mites; *Leptotrombidium akamushi*, *L. deliensis* and related species (varying with area) are the most common vectors for humans. Infection is maintained by transovarian passage in mites.

5. Mode of transmission—By the bite of infected larval mites; nymphs and adults do not feed on vertebrate hosts.

6. Incubation period—Usually 10–12 days; varies from 6 to 21 days.

7. Period of communicability—Not directly transmitted from person to person.

8. Susceptibility and resistance—Susceptibility is general. An attack confers prolonged immunity against the homologous strain of *O. tsutsugamushi* but only transient immunity against heterologous strains. Heterologous infection within a few months results in mild disease, but after a year produces typical illness. Second and even third attacks of naturally acquired scrub typhus (usually benign or inapparent) occur among people who spend their lives in endemic areas or who have not been completely treated (see below). No experimental vaccine has been effective.

9. Methods of control—

A. *Preventive measures:*

1) Prevent contact with infected mites by personal prophylaxis against the mite vector, achieved by impregnating clothes and blankets with miticidal chemicals (permethrin and benzyl benzoate) and application of mite repellents (diethyltoluamide, Deet®) to exposed skin surfaces.

2) Eliminate mites from the specific sites by application of chlorinated hydrocarbons, such as lindane, dieldrin or chlordane, to ground and vegetation in environs of camps, mine buildings and other populated zones in endemic areas.

3) In a small group of volunteers in Malaysia, the administration of 7 weekly doses of doxycycline (200 mg/week in a single dose) was an effective prophylactic regimen.

B. *Control of patient, contacts and the immediate environment:*

1) Report to local health authority: In selected endemic areas (clearly differentiated from murine and louseborne typhus). In many countries, not a reportable disease, Class 3A (see Communicable Disease Reporting).

2) Isolation: None.

3) Concurrent disinfection: None.

4) Quarantine: None.

5) Immunization of contacts: None.

6) Investigation of contacts and source of infection: None (see 9C, below).

7) Specific treatment: One of the tetracyclines orally in a loading dose, followed by divided doses daily until patient is afebrile (average 30 hours). Chloramphenicol is equally effective and should be given if tetracyclines are contraindicated (see section I, 9B7, above). If treatment is started within the first 3 days of illness, recrudescence is likely unless a second course of antibiotic is given after an interval of 6 days. In Malaysia single doses of doxycycline (5 mg/kg) were effective when given on the seventh day, and in the Pescadores Islands (Taiwan area) when given on the fifth day; earlier administration was associated with some relapses. Azithromycin has also been used successfully in pregnant patients.

C. *Epidemic measures:* Rigorously employ procedures described in this section, 9A1–9A2 above, in the affected area; daily observation of all people at risk for fever and appearance of primary lesions; institute treatment on first indication of illness.

D. Disaster implications: Only if refugee centers are sited in or near a "typhus island."

E. International measures: WHO Collaborating Centres.

WARTS, VIRAL ICD-9 078.1; ICD-10 B07
(Verruca vulgaris, Common wart, Condyloma acuminatum, Papilloma venereum)

1. Identification—A viral disease manifested by a variety of skin and mucous membrane lesions. These include: **the common wart,** a circumscribed, hyperkeratotic, rough-textured, painless papule, varying in size from a pinhead to large masses; **filiform warts,** elongated, pointed, delicate lesions that may reach 1 cm in length; **laryngeal papillomas** on vocal cords and the epiglottis in children and adults; **flat warts,** smooth, slightly elevated, usually multiple lesions varying in size from 1 mm to 1 cm; **venereal warts** (condyloma acuminatum), cauliflower like, fleshy growths, most often seen in moist areas in and around the genitalia, around the anus and within the anal canal, which must be differentiated from condyloma lata of secondary syphilis; **flat papillomas** of the cervix; and **plantar warts,** flat, hyperkeratotic lesions of the plantar surface of the feet, which are frequently painful.

Both laryngeal papillomas and genital warts have occasionally become malignant. The warts in epidermodysplasia verruciformis occur usually on the torso and upper extremities, usually appearing in the first decade of life; they often undergo malignant transformation to squamous cell carcinomas in young adulthood.

The diagnosis is usually based on the typical lesion. If there is doubt, it should be excised and examined histologically.

2. Infectious agent—Human papillomavirus (HPV) of the papovavirus group of DNA viruses (the human wart viruses). At least 70 HPV types have been associated with specific manifestations and more than 20 types of HPV can infect the genital tract. Most genital HPV infections are asymptomatic, subclinical, or unrecognized. Visible genital warts are usually caused by HPV types 6 or 11: they can also cause warts on the uterine crevix and in the vagina, urethra, and anus, and are sometimes symptomatic. Other HPV types in the anogenital region, types 16, 18, 31, 33, and 35, have been strongly associated with cervical dysplasia; they have been associated also with vulvar, penile, and anal squamous intraepithelial neoplasia (i.e., squamous cell carcinoma in situ, bowenoid papulosis, Erythroplasia of Queyrat, or Bowen's disease of the genitalia). Type 7 is associated with warts in meat handlers and veterinarians. Types 5 and 8 are associated with epidermodysplasia verruciformis.

3. Occurrence—Worldwide.

4. Reservoir—Humans.

5. Mode of transmission—Usually by direct contact. Warts may be autoinoculated, such as by razors in shaving; contaminated floors are frequently incriminated as the source of infection. Condyloma acuminatum is usually sexually transmitted; laryngeal papillomata are probably transmitted during passage of the infant through the birth canal. The viral types in the genital and respiratory tracts are the same.

6. Incubation period—About 2-3 months; range is 1-20 months.

7. Period of communicability—Unknown, but probably at least as long as visible lesions persist.

8. Susceptibility and resistance—Common and flat warts are most frequently seen in young children, genital warts in sexually active young adults, and plantar warts in school aged children and teenagers. The incidence of warts is increased in immunosuppressed patients.

9. Methods of control—

A. *Preventive measures:* Avoid direct contact with lesions on another person. Recent studies indicate that the male condom does not prevent infection.

B. *Control of patient, contacts and the immediate environment:*

1) Report to local health authority: None, Class 5 (see Communicable Disease Reporting).
2) Isolation: None.
3) Concurrent disinfection: None.
4) Quarantine: None.
5) Immunization of contacts: None.
6) Investigation of contacts and source of infection: Sexual contacts of patients with venereal warts should be examined and treated if indicated.
7) Specific treatment: Treatment of the affected individual will decrease the amount of wart virus available for transmission. Warts usually regress spontaneously within months to years. If treatment is indicated, use freezing with liquid nitrogen for lesions on most of the body surface; salicylic acid plasters and curettage for plantar warts; and 10%-25% podophyllin in tincture of benzoin, trichloroacetic acid or liquid nitrogen for readily accessible genital warts—except in pregnant females.

For widespread genital lesions, 5-fluorouracil has been helpful. Intralesional recombinant interferon alpha-2b (Intron A®, Schering) has been shown to be effective in treatment of condyloma acuminatum and is approved for this use. Surgical removal or laser therapy is required for laryngeal papillomata. Cesarean section may be considered if genital papillomatosis is very extensive.

8) Microscopic examination of cells (Papanicolau smears) is an effective method for detecting cellular abnormalities associated with malignancy in women. Surgical intervention for cervical cancer is curative if the intervention is done early in the disease.

C. Epidemic measures: Usually a sporadic disease.

D. Disaster implications: None.

E. International measures: None.

YAWS　　　　　　　　　　　　　ICD-9 102; ICD-10 A66
(Frambesia tropica)

1. Identification—A chronic, relapsing, nonvenereal treponematosis, characterized by highly contagious, primary and secondary cutaneous lesions, and noncontagious, tertiary/late, destructive lesions. Typical initial lesion (mother yaw) is a papilloma on the face or extremities (usually the leg) that persists for several weeks or months, and which is painless unless secondarily infected. It proliferates slowly and may form a frambesial (raspberry) lesion, or undergo ulceration (ulceropapilloma). Secondary disseminated or satellite papillomata appear before or shortly after the initial lesion heals; these lesions occur in successive crops and are often accompanied by periostitis of the long bones (saber shin) and fingers (polydactylitis), and mild constitutional symptoms. Papillomata and hyperkeratoses on palms and soles may appear in both early and late stages; these lesions are very painful and usually disabling. Lesions heal spontaneously, but relapses may occur at other sites during early and late phases.

The late stage, characterized by destructive lesions of skin and bone, occurs in about 10%–20% of untreated patients, usually 5 or more years after infection. Unlike syphilis, the brain, eyes, heart, aorta and abdominal organs are not involved. Congenital transmission does not occur and the infection is rarely, if ever, fatal, but can be very disfiguring and disabling.

Diagnosis is confirmed by darkfield or direct FA microscopic examination of exudates from primary or secondary lesions. Nontreponemal serologic tests for syphilis (e.g., VDRL [Venereal Disease Research Laboratory], RPR [rapid plasma reagin]) become reactive during the initial stage, remain reactive during the early infection and tend to become nonreactive after many years of latency, even without specific therapy; in some, they remain reactive at low titer for life. Treponemal serologic tests (e.g., FTA-ABS [fluorescent treponemal antibody absorbed], MHA-TP [microhemagglutination assay for antibody to *T. pallidum*]) usually remain reactive for life.

2. Infectious agent—*Treponema pallidum,* subspecies *pertenue,* a spirochete.

3. Occurrence—Predominantly a disease of children living in rural, warm, humid, tropical areas; more frequent in males. Worldwide prevalence was dramatically decreased by mass penicillin treatment campaigns in the 1950s and 1960s, but early yaws has resurged in parts of equatorial and west Africa, with scattered foci of infection persisting in Latin America, the Caribbean islands, India, southeast Asia and the South Pacific islands.

4. Reservoir—Humans and possibly higher primates.

5. Mode of transmission—Principally by direct contact with exudates of early skin lesions of infected people. Indirect transmission by contamination from scratching, skin piercing articles and flies on open wounds is probable but of undetermined importance. Climate influences the morphology, distribution and infectiousness of the early lesions.

6. Incubation period—From 2 weeks to 3 months.

7. Period of communicability—Variable; may extend intermittently over several years while moist lesions are present. The infectious agent is not usually found in late destructive lesions.

8. Susceptibility and resistance—No evidence of natural or racial resistance. Infection results in immunity to reinfection and may offer protection against infection by other pathogenic treponemes.

9. Methods of control—

    A. Preventive measures: The following are applicable to yaws and other nonvenereal treponematoses. Although the infectious agents cannot be differentiated with present techniques, the observed differences in clinical syndromes are unlikely to result only from epidemiological or environmental factors.

        1) General health promotion measures; health education of the public about treponematosis; teach them the value of better sanitation, including liberal use of soap and water and the

importance of improving social and economic conditions over a period of years to reduce incidence.

2) Organize intensive control activities on a community level suitable to the local problem; examine entire populations, and treat patients with active or latent disease. Treatment of asymptomatic contacts is justified, and there may be need to treat the entire population when the prevalence of active disease is more than 10%. Periodic clinical resurveys and continuous surveillance are essential for success.

3) Survey serologically for latent cases, particularly in children, to prevent relapses and development of infective lesions that maintain the disease in the community.

4) Provide facilities for early diagnosis and treatment as part of a plan in which the mass control campaign (9A2, above) is eventually consolidated into permanent local health services.

5) Treat disfiguring and incapacitating late manifestations.

B. Control of patient, contacts and the immediate environment:

1) Report to local health authority: In selected endemic areas; in many countries not a reportable disease, Class 3B (see Communicable Disease Reporting). Differentiation of venereal and nonvenereal treponematoses, with proper reporting of each, has particular importance in evaluation of mass campaigns and the subsequent consolidation period thereafter.

2) Isolation: None; avoid intimate contact and contamination of the environment until lesions are healed.

3) Concurrent disinfection: Care in disposal of discharges and articles contaminated therewith.

4) Quarantine: None.

5) Immunization of contacts: None.

6) Investigation of contacts and source of infection: All familial contacts should be treated; those with no active disease should be regarded as latent cases. In areas of low prevalence, treat all active cases, all children and close contacts of infectious cases.

7) Specific treatment: Penicillin. For patients 10 years or older with active disease and contacts, a single injection of benzathine penicillin G (Bicillin), 1.2 million units IM; 0.6 million units for patients under 10 years.

C. Epidemic measures: Active mass treatment programs in areas of high prevalence. Essential features of these programs are: 1) examination of a high percentage of the population through field surveys; 2) treatment of active cases extended to the family and community contacts based on the demonstrated prevalence of active yaws; and 3) surveys made at yearly intervals for 1–3 years,

as part of the established rural public health activities of the country.

D. Disaster implications: None observed, but potentially a risk in refugee or displaced populations in endemic areas without hygienic facilities.

E. International measures: To protect countries against risk of reinfection where active mass treatment programs are in progress, adjacent countries in the endemic area should institute suitable measures against yaws. Movement of infected people across frontiers may need supervision (see Syphilis, section I, 9E). WHO Collaborating Centres.

YELLOW FEVER   ICD-9 060; ICD-10 A95

1. Identification—An acute infectious viral disease of short duration and varying severity. The mildest cases may be clinically indeterminate; typical attacks are characterized by sudden onset, fever, chills, headache, backache, generalized muscle pain, prostration, nausea and vomiting. The pulse may be slow and weak out of proportion to the elevated temperature (the Faget sign). Jaundice is moderate early in the disease and is intensified later. Albuminuria, sometimes pronounced, and anuria may occur. Leukopenia appears early and is most pronounced about the fifth day. Most infections resolve at this stage. After a brief remission of hours to a day, some cases progress into the ominous stage of intoxication manifested by hemorrhagic symptoms including epistaxis, gingival bleeding, hematemesis (coffee-ground or black), melena, and liver and renal failure; 20%–50% of jaundiced cases are fatal. The overall case-fatality rate among indigenous populations in endemic regions is 5% but may reach 20%–40% in individual outbreaks.

Laboratory diagnosis is made by isolation of virus from blood by inoculation of suckling mice, mosquitoes or cell cultures (especially those of mosquito cells); by demonstration of viral antigen in the blood by ELISA or liver tissue by use of labeled specific antibodies; and by demonstration of viral genome in blood and liver tissue by PCR or hybridization probes. Serologic diagnosis is made by demonstrating specific IgM in early sera or a rise in titer of specific antibodies in paired acute and convalescent sera. Serologic cross-reactions occur with other flaviviruses. Recent infections can often be distinguished from vaccine immunity by complement fixation testing. The diagnosis is supported by demonstration of typical lesions in the liver.

2. Infectious agent—The virus of yellow fever, of the genus *Flavivirus* and family Flaviviridae.

3. Occurrence—Yellow fever exists in nature in two transmission cycles, a sylvatic or jungle cycle that involves mosquitoes and nonhuman primates, and an urban cycle involving *Aedes aegypti* mosquitoes and humans. Sylvatic transmission is restricted to tropical regions of Africa and Latin America, where a few hundred cases occur annually, most frequently among young adult males who are occupationally exposed in forested or transitional areas of Bolivia, Brazil, Colombia, Ecuador and Peru (with 70%-90% of cases reported from Bolivia and Peru). Historically, urban yellow fever occurred in many cities of the Americas. With the exception of a few cases in Trinidad in 1954, no outbreak of urban yellow fever had been transmitted by *Ae. aegypti* in the Americas since 1942. However, reinfestation in many cities with *Ae. aegypti* places them at risk of renewed urban yellow fever transmission. In Africa, the endemic zone includes the area between 15°N and 10°S latitude, extending from the Sahara desert south through northern Angola, Zaire and Tanzania. For the past several decades yellow fever due to *Ae. aegypti* mosquitoes was reported only from Nigeria with nearly 20,000 cases and more than 4,000 deaths between 1986 and 1991. There is no evidence that yellow fever has ever been present in Asia or on the easternmost coast of Africa, although sylvatic yellow fever was reported in 1992-1993 in western Kenya.

4. Reservoir—In urban areas, humans and *Aedes aegypti* mosquitoes; in forest areas, vertebrates other than humans, mainly monkeys and possibly marsupials, and forest mosquitoes. Transovarian transmission in mosquitoes may contribute to maintenance of infection. Humans have no essential role in transmission of jungle yellow fever or in maintaining the virus, but are the primary amplifying host in the urban cycle.

5. Mode of transmission—In urban and certain rural areas, by the bite of infective *Ae. aegypti* mosquitoes. In forests of South America, by the bite of several species of forest mosquitoes of the genus *Haemagogus*. In east Africa, *Ae. africanus* is the vector in the monkey population, while semidomestic *Ae. bromeliae* and *Ae. simpsoni,* and probably other *Aedes* species, transmit the virus from monkeys to humans. In large epidemics in Ethiopia, good epidemiologic evidence incriminated *Ae. simpsoni* as a person to person vector. In west Africa, *Ae. furcifer-taylori, Ae. luteocephalus* and other species are responsible for spread between monkeys and humans. *Ae. albopictus* has been introduced into Brazil and the USA from Asia and has the potential for bridging the sylvatic and urban cycles of yellow fever in the Western Hemisphere. However, no instance of involvement of this species in yellow fever transmission has been documented.

6. Incubation period—Three to six days.

7. Period of communicability—Blood of patients is infective for mosquitoes shortly before onset of fever and for the first 3-5 days of illness. The disease is highly communicable where many susceptible people and abundant vector mosquitoes coexist; not communicable by contact or common vehicles. The extrinsic incubation period in *Ae. aegypti* is commonly 9-12 days at the usual tropical temperatures. Once infected, mosquitoes remain so for life.

8. Susceptibility and resistance—Recovery from yellow fever is followed by lasting immunity; second attacks are unknown. Mild inapparent infections are common in endemic areas. Transient passive immunity in infants born to immune mothers may persist for up to 6 months. In natural infections, antibodies appear in the blood within the first week.

9. Methods of control—

A. Preventive measures:

1) Institute a program for active immunization of all people 9 months of age or older necessarily exposed to infection because of residence, occupation or travel. A single subcutaneous injection of a vaccine containing viable attenuated yellow fever 17D strain virus, cultivated in chick embryo, is effective in almost 99% of recipients. Antibodies appear 7-10 days after immunization and may persist for at least 30-35 years, probably much longer, though immunization or reimmunization within 10 years is required by the *International Health Regulations* for travel from endemic areas.

Since 1989, WHO has recommended that at-risk countries in Africa that fall in the endemic-epidemic belt should incorporate yellow fever vaccine into their routine childhood immunization programs. As of March 1998, there were 17 African countries with such a policy but, only two that have achieved 50% coverage. The vaccine can be given any time after 6 months of age and can be administered with other antigens such as measles vaccine.

The vaccine is contraindicated in the first 4 months of life and should be considered for those aged 4-9 months only if the risk of exposure is judged to exceed the risk of vaccine-associated encephalitis, the principal complication in this age group. The vaccine is also not recommended in circumstances where live virus vaccines are contraindicated, nor in the first trimester of pregnancy, unless the risk of disease is believed to be higher than the theoretical risk to the pregnancy. There is, however, no evidence of fetal damage from the vaccine, but lower rates of maternal seroconversion have been observed, an indication for reimmunization after termination of the pregnancy. The vaccine is recommended for asymptomatic HIV seropositive individuals; there is insufficient evidence to permit a definitive statement on whether the vaccine would pose a risk for symptomatic individuals.

2) For urban yellow fever eradicate or control of *Ae. aegypti* mosquitoes; immunization when indicated.

3) Sylvan or jungle yellow fever, transmitted by *Haemagogus* and forest species of *Aedes,* is best controlled by immunization, which is recommended for all people in rural communities whose occupation brings them into forests in yellow fever areas, and for people who intend to visit those areas. Protective clothing, bed nets and repellents are advised for those not immunized.

B. Control of patient, contacts and the immediate environment:

1) Report to local health authority: Case report universally required by *International Health Regulations* (1969), Third Annotated Edition 1983, Updated and Reprinted 1992, WHO, Geneva; Class 1 (see Communicable Disease Reporting).

2) Isolation: Blood and body fluid precautions. Prevent access of mosquitoes to patient for at least 5 days after onset by screening the sickroom, by spraying quarters with residual insecticide, and by using a bed net.

3) Concurrent disinfection: None; the home of patients and all houses in the vicinity should be sprayed promptly with an effective insecticide.

4) Quarantine: None.

5) Immunization of contacts: Family and other contacts and neighbors not previously immunized should be immunized promptly.

6) Investigation of contacts and source of infection: Inquire about all places, including forested areas, visited by the patient 3–6 days before onset, to locate focus of yellow fever; observe all people visiting that focus. Search premises, and places of the patient's work or visits over the preceding several days for mosquitoes capable of transmitting infection; eradicate them with effective insecticide. Investigate mild febrile illnesses and unexplained deaths suggesting yellow fever.

7) Specific treatment: None.

C. Epidemic measures:

1) Urban or *Ae. aegypti* transmitted yellow fever:
   a) Mass immunization, beginning with people most exposed and those living in *Ae. aegypti* infected areas.
   b) Spraying the inside of all houses in the community with insecticides has shown promise for controlling urban epidemics.

    c) Eliminate or apply larvicide to all actual and potential breeding places of *Ae. aegypti.*

2) Jungle or sylvan yellow fever:

    a) Immediately immunize all people living in or near forested areas or entering such areas.

    b) Ensure that nonimmunized individuals avoid those tracts of forest where infection has been localized, and that those just immunized avoid the areas for the first week after immunization.

3) In regions where yellow fever may occur, a diagnostic viscerotomy service should be organized to collect small specimens of liver post mortem from fatal febrile illnesses of 10 days duration or less; facilities for viral isolation or serologic confirmation are necessary to establish the diagnosis since histopathologic changes in the liver are not pathognomonic of yellow fever.

4) In Central and South America, confirmed deaths of howler and spider monkeys in the forest are presumptive evidence of the presence of yellow fever. Confirmation by the histopathologic examination of livers of moribund or recently dead monkeys or by virus isolation is highly desirable.

5) Immunity surveys by neutralization tests of wild primates captured in forested areas are useful in defining enzootic areas. Serologic surveys of human populations are almost useless where yellow fever vaccine has been widely used.

D. Disaster implications: None.

E. International measures:

1) Telegraphic notification by governments to WHO and to adjacent countries of the first imported, first transferred, or first nonimported case of yellow fever in an area previously free of the disease; and of newly discovered or reactivated foci of yellow fever infection among vertebrates other than man.

2) Measures applicable to ships, aircraft and land transport arriving from yellow fever areas are specified in the *International Health Regulations* (1969), Third Annotated Edition 1983, Updated and Reprinted 1992, WHO, Geneva. These regulations are being revised, but the new regulations are not expected to be available until sometimes in the year 2002 or after.

3) Animal quarantine: Quarantine of monkeys and other wild primates arriving from yellow fever areas may be required until 7 days have elapsed after leaving such areas.

4) International travel: A valid international certificate of immunization against yellow fever is required by many countries for entry of travelers coming from or going to recognized yellow

fever zones of Africa and South America; otherwise, quarantine measures are applicable for up to 6 days. Immunization is recommended by WHO for all travelers to areas other than major cities in countries where the disease occurs in humans or is assumed to be present in nonhuman primates. The International Certificate of Vaccination against Yellow Fever is valid from 10 days after date of immunization for 10 years; if reimmunized within that period, valid from date of reimmunization for 10 years.

YERSINIOSIS   ICD-9 027.8
INTESTINAL YERSINIOSIS   ICD-10 A04.6
EXTRAINTESTINAL YERSINIOSIS   ICD-10 A28.2

1. Identification—An acute bacterial enteric disease typically manifested by acute febrile diarrhea (especially in young children), enterocolitis, acute mesenteric lymphadenitis mimicking appendicitis (especially in older children and adults), complicated in some cases by erythema nodosum (in about 10% of adults, particularly women), postinfectious arthritis and systemic infection; caused by either of two agents, Yersinia enterocolitica or Y. pseudotuberculosis. Bloody diarrhea is reported by up to 1/4 of patients with *Yersinia enteritis.* Whereas infection with either Y. enterocolitica or Y. pseudotuberculosis can result in clinical illness, most reported cases are caused by Y. enterocolitica. Y. pseudotuberculosis has been linked primarily with mesenteric adenitis, although a syndrome of enteritis in children (Izumi fever) has been reported in Japan.

Diagnosis is usually made by stool culture. Cefsulodin irgasan novobiocin (CIN) medium is highly selective and should be used if there is reason to suspect infection with *Yersinia;* it permits identification in 24 hours at 32°C (89.6°F) without cold enrichment. With precautions to prevent overgrowth of fecal flora, the organisms can be recovered on usual enteric media. Cold enrichment in buffered saline at 4°C (39°F) for 2-3 weeks can be used to select for these organisms; however, the sensitivity of the technique may result in identification of very small numbers of organisms that are of uncertain clinical significance. *Yersinia* can be isolated from blood with standard commercial blood culture media. Serologic diagnosis is possible by an agglutination test or by ELISA, but its availability is generally limited to research settings.

2. Infectious agents—Gram-negative bacilli. *Y. pseudotuberculosis* comprises 6 serotypes with 4 subtypes; >90% of infections in humans and animals are O-group I strains. *Y. enterocolitica* comprises over 50 serotypes and 5 biotypes, many of which are nonpathogenic. Strains pathogenic for humans are generally pyrazinamidase negative; this includes strains in serotypes O3, O8, O9, and O5,27, and biotypes 1, 2, 3 and 4. Serotypes causing disease may vary in different geographic areas; types O3, O9 and O5,27 account for most of the cases in Europe. Type O8 strains had been responsible for most outbreaks in the USA; however, type O3 has emerged in the 1990s as the most common serotype in the USA.

3. Occurrence—Worldwide. *Y. pseudotuberculosis* is primarily a zoonotic disease of wild and domesticated birds and mammals, with humans an incidental host. *Y. enterocolitica* has been recovered from a wide variety of animals that show no signs of disease. The most important source of infection may be pork, as the pharynx of pigs may be heavily colonized by *Y. enterocolitica*. Since the 1960s, *Yersinieae* have been recognized as etiologic agents of gastroenteritis (as high as 1%–3% of acute enteritis in some areas) and mesenteric lymphadenitis. Approximately 2/3 of *Y. enterocolitica* cases occur among infants and children; 3/4 of *Y. pseudotuberculosis* cases are aged 5 to 20 years. Human cases have been reported in association with disease in household pets, particularly sick puppies and kittens.

The highest isolation rates have been reported during the cold season in temperate climates, including northern Europe (in particular, Scandinavia), North America and temperate regions of South America. Vehicles implicated in outbreaks attributed to *Y. enterocolitica* have included soybean cake (tofu) and pork chitterlings (pig large intestines). In the USA some outbreaks with milk (including pasteurized milk) as the vehicle have occurred. However, where pasteurized milk was implicated, it was believed to be due to postpasteurization contamination rather than resistance of the agent to the pasteurization process. Studies in Europe suggest that many cases are related to ingestion of raw or undercooked pork. Since 20% of infections in older children and adolescents can mimic acute appendicitis, outbreaks can sometimes be recognized by local increases in appendectomies.

4. Reservoir—Animals are the principal reservoir for *Yersinia*. The pig is the principal reservoir for pathogenic *Y. enterocolitica;* asymptomatic pharyngeal carriage is common in swine, especially in the winter. *Y. pseudotuberculosis* is widespread among many species of avian and mammalian hosts, and particularly among rodents and other small mammals.

5. Mode of transmission—Fecal-oral transmission takes place by eating and drinking contaminated food and water or by contact with infected people or animals. *Y. enterocolitica* has been isolated from a variety of foods; however, pathogenic strains are most commonly isolated from raw pork or pork products. In the USA, chitterlings are a common source of infection; in Europe, cases have been significantly associated with feeding of raw pork to infants. In contrast to many other foodborne pathogens, *Y. enterocolitica* is able to multiply under refrigeration and microaerophilic conditions. Thus, there is an increased risk of infection by *Y. enterocolitica* if uncured meat stored in evacuated plastic bags is undercooked. *Y. enterocolitica* has been recovered from natural bodies of water in the absence of *Escherichia coli* organisms. Nosocomial transmission has been reported, as has transmission by transfusion of stored blood from donors who were asymptomatic or had mild GI illness.

6. Incubation period—Probably 3-7 days, generally under 10 days.

7. Period of communicability—Secondary transmission appears to be rare. There is fecal shedding at least as long as symptoms exist, usually for 2-3 weeks. Untreated cases may excrete the organism for 2-3 months. Prolonged asymptomatic carriage has been reported in both children and adults.

8. Susceptibility and resistance—Gastroenterocolitis (diarrhea) is more severe in children, whereas postinfectious arthritis is more severe in adolescents and older adults. *Y. pseudotuberculosis* exhibits a predilection for male adolescents, while *Y. enterocolitica* attacks both genders equally. Reactive arthritis and the Reiter syndrome have a predilection for people with the HLA-B27 genetic type. Septicemia occurs most often among people with iron overload (e.g., hemochromatosis) or those with underlying immunosuppressive illness or therapy.

9. Methods of control—

A. *Preventive measures:*

1) Prepare meat and other foods in a sanitary manner, avoid eating raw pork and pasteurize milk; irradiation of meat is effective.
2) Wash hands prior to food handling and eating, after handling raw pork and after animal contact.
3) Protect water supplies from animal and human feces; purify appropriately.
4) Control rodents and birds (for *Y. pseudotuberculosis*).
5) Dispose of human, dog and cat feces in a sanitary manner.
6) During the slaughtering of pigs, the head and neck should be removed from the body to avoid contaminating meat from the heavily colonized pharynx.

B. *Control of patient, contacts and the immediate environment:*

1) Report to local health authority: Case reporting obligatory in many states (USA) and countries, Class 2B (see Communicable Disease Reporting).
2) Isolation: Enteric precautions for patients in hospitals. Remove those with diarrhea from food handling, patient care and occupations involving care of young children.

3) Concurrent disinfection: Of feces. In communities with modern and adequate sewage disposal systems, feces can be discharged directly into sewers without preliminary disinfection.

4) Quarantine: None.

5) Immunization of contacts: None.

6) Investigation of contacts and source of infection: A search for unrecognized cases and convalescent carriers among contacts is indicated only when a common-source exposure is suspected.

7) Specific treatment: Organisms are sensitive to many antibiotics, but are generally resistant to penicillin and its semisynthetic derivatives. Therapy may be helpful for GI symptoms; definitely indicated for septicemia and other invasive disease. Agents of choice against *Y. enterocolitica* are the aminoglycosides (for septicemia only) and TMP-SMX. Newer quinolones such as ciprofloxacin may also be effective. Both *Y. enterocolitica* and *Y. pseudotuberculosis* are usually sensitive to the tetracyclines.

C. Epidemic measures:

1) Any group of cases of acute gastroenteritis or cases suggestive of appendicitis should be reported at once to the local health authority, even in the absence of specific identification of the etiology.

2) Investigate general sanitation and search for common-source vehicle; pay attention to consumption of (or possible cross contamination with) raw or undercooked pork; also look for evidence of close contacts with animals, especially pet dogs, cats and other domestic animals.

D. Disaster implications: None.

E. International measures: None.

ZYGOMYCOSIS
(Phycomycosis)

ICD-9 117.7; ICD-10 B46

Zygomycosis is the designation for all infections caused by fungi of the class Zygomycetes. These include mucormycosis and entomophthoramycosis due to either *Conidiobolus* or *Basidiobolus* species.

MUCORMYCOSIS   ICD-10 B46.0–B46.5

1. Identification—A group of mycoses usually caused by fungi of the family Mucoraceae, order Mucorales, class Zygomycetes. These fungi have an affinity for blood vessels, and cause thrombosis and infarction. The craniofacial form of the disease usually presents as nasal or paranasal sinus infection, most often during episodes of poorly controlled diabetes mellitus. Necrosis of the turbinates, perforation of the hard palate, necrosis of the cheek or orbital cellulitis, proptosis and ophthalmoplegia may occur. Infection may penetrate to the internal carotid artery or by direct extension to the brain, and cause infarction. Patients receiving immunosuppression or deferoxamine are susceptible to either craniofacial or pulmonary mucormycosis. In the pulmonary form of disease, the fungus causes thrombosis of pulmonary blood vessels and infarcts of the lung. In the GI form, mucosal ulcers or thrombosis and gangrene of stomach or bowel wall may occur.

Diagnosis is confirmed by microscopic demonstration of distinctive broad nonseptate hyphae in biopsies and by culture of biopsy tissue. Wet preparations and smears may be examined. Cultures alone are not diagnostic because fungi of the order Mucorales are frequently found in the environment.

2. Infectious agents—Some species of *Rhizopus,* especially *R. arrhizus (R. oryzae),* have caused most of the culture positive craniofacial cases of mucormycosis. Probably *Mucor, Rhizomucor, Rhizopus* and *Cunninghamella* spp. are the chief causes of mucormycosis in other sites. *Apophysomyces elegans, Saksenaea vasiformis* and *Absidia* spp. have been reported from a few human cases of mucormycosis.

3. Occurrence—Worldwide. Incidence may be increasing because of longer survival of patients with diabetes mellitus and certain blood dyscrasias, especially acute leukemia and aplastic anemia, as well as the use of deferoxamine for aluminum or iron overload in patients receiving chronic hemodialysis for renal failure.

4. Reservoir—Members of the order Mucorales are common saprophytes in the environment.

5. Mode of transmission—By inhalation or ingestion of spores of the fungal agents by susceptible individuals. Direct inoculation by IV drug abuse and at sites of IV catheters and cutaneous burns is seen occasionally.

6. Incubation period—Unknown. Fungus spreads rapidly in susceptible tissues.

7. Period of communicability—Not directly transmitted from person to person or between animals and people.

8. Susceptibility and resistance—The rarity of infection in healthy individuals despite the abundance of the Mucorales in the environment indicates natural resistance. Corticosteroid use, metabolic acidosis, deferoxamine and immunosuppressive therapy predispose to infection. Malnutrition predisposes to the GI form.

9. Methods of control—

A. *Preventive measures:* Optimal clinical control of diabetes mellitus to avoid acidosis.

B. *Control of patient, contacts and the immediate environment:*

1) Report to local health authority: Official report not ordinarily justifiable, Class 5 (see Communicable Disease Reporting).
2) Isolation: None.
3) Concurrent disinfection: Ordinary cleanliness. Terminal cleaning.
4) Quarantine: None.
5) Immunization of contacts: None.
6) Investigation of contacts and source of infection: Ordinarily not profitable.
7) Specific treatment: In the cranial form, clinical control of diabetes; amphotericin B (Fungizone®) and resection of necrotic tissue have been helpful.

C. *Epidemic measures:* Not applicable; a sporadic disease.

D. *Disaster implications:* None.

E. *International measures:* None.

ENTOMOPHTHORAMYCOSIS DUE TO *BASIDIOBOLUS* spp.   ICD-9 117.7; ICD-10 B46.8
ENTOMOPHTHORAMYCOSIS DUE TO *CONIDIOBOLUS* spp.   ICD-9 117.7; ICD-10 B46.8

These two infections have been recognized principally in tropical and subtropical Asia and Africa, are not characterized by thromboses or infarction, do not usually occur in association with serious preexisting disease, do not usually cause disseminated disease and seldom cause death.

Entomophthoramycosis caused by *Basidiobolus ranarum (haptosporus)* is a granulomatous inflammation of subcutaneous tissue. The fungus is ubiquitous; it occurs in decaying vegetation, soil and the GI tract of amphibians and reptiles. The disease presents as a firm subcutaneous mass, fixed to the skin, principally in children and adolescents, more commonly in males. The infection may heal spontaneously. Recommended therapy is oral potassium iodide.

Entomophthoramycosis due to *Conidiobolus coronatus* (rhinoentomoph-thoramycosis) usually originates in the paranasal skin or nasal mucosa and presents as nasal obstruction or swelling of the nose or adjacent structures. The lesion may spread to involve contiguous areas, such as lip, cheek, palate or pharynx. The disease is uncommon and occurs principally in adult males. Recommended therapy is oral potassium iodide or IV amphotericin B (Fungizone®). The infectious agent, *Conidiobolus corona-tus,* occurs in soil and decaying vegetation. For both forms of entomoph-thoramycosis, incubation periods and modes of transmission are unknown. Person to person transmission does not occur.

Abbreviations Used in
Control of Communicable Diseases Manual

AAP	= American Academy of Pediatrics
ACIP	= Immunization Practices Advisory Committee (CDC)
ALT	= alanine aminotransferase (was SGPT)
AST	= aspartate aminotransferase (was SGOT)
BCG	= Bacille Calmette-Guérin; vaccine
BSL	= Biosafety level (i.e., BSL-1, -2, -3, -4)
CA	= cold hemagglutinins
ca	= circa
CAT scan	= computerized axial tomography
CDC	= Centers for Disease Control and Prevention
CF	= complement fixation
CIE	= counterimmunoelectrophoresis
CIOMS	= Council for International Organizations of Medical Sciences
CIS	= Commonwealth of Independent States
cm	= centimeter
CNS	= central nervous system
CSF	= cerebrospinal fluid
cu mm	= cubic millimeter (mm^3)
dL	= deciliter
DNA	= deoxyribonucleic acid
DTP	= Diphtheria and Tetanus Toxoids and Pertussis Vaccine Adsorbed USP
EIA	= enzyme immunoassay
ELISA	= enzyme-linked immunosorbent assay
EM	= electron microscopy
EPI	= Expanded Programme of Immunizations, WHO
ESR	= erythrocyte sedimentation rate
FA	= direct fluorescent or immunofluorescent antibody test
FAO	= Food and Agriculture Organization of the United Nations
g	= gram
GI	= gastrointestinal
HA	= hemagglutination
HAI/HI	= hemagglutination inhibition
HIV	= human immunodeficiency virus
IEM	= immune electron microscopy
IF	= immunofluorescent testing
IFA	= indirect immunofluorescent antibody test
IG	= immune globulin (serum)
IgA	= immunoglobulin class

IgG	=	immunoglobulin class
IgM	=	immunoglobulin class
IHA	=	indirect hemagglutination
IM	=	intramuscular
IU	=	international unit
IV	=	intravenous
kb	=	kilobase
kg	=	kilogram
kGy	=	kiloGray
km	=	kilometer
L	=	liter
LA	=	latex agglutination
lbs	=	pounds
m	=	meter
µg	=	microgram
µL	=	microliter
µm	=	micrometer
m.u.	=	million units
mEq	=	milliequivalents
mg	=	milligram
mIU	=	milli-IU (international units)
ml	=	milliliter
mm	=	millimeter
nm	=	nanometer
PAHO	=	Pan American Health Organization
PCR	=	polymerase chain reaction
PO	=	oral (per os)
ppm	=	parts per million
RBC	=	red blood cell
RIA	=	radioimmunoassay
RNA	=	ribonucleic acid
SC	=	subcutaneous
SI	=	Système International d'Unités (International System of Units)
sp. or spp.	=	species
ssp.	=	subspecies
STDs	=	sexually transmitted disease(s)
TMP-SMX	=	co-trimoxazole (trimethoprim-sulfamethoxazole)
UK	=	United Kingdom
UNDP	=	United Nations Development Programme
URI	=	upper respiratory infection
USA	=	United States of America
USDA	=	U.S. Department of Agriculture
USPHS	=	U.S. Public Health Service
UV	=	ultraviolet
v	=	versus
WBC	=	white blood cell
WHO	=	World Health Organization

DEFINITIONS
(Technical meaning of terms used in the text)

1. **Carrier**—A person or animal that harbors a specific infectious agent without discernible clinical disease and serves as a potential source of infection. The carrier state may exist in an individual with an infection that is inapparent throughout its course (commonly known as **healthy** or **asymptomatic carrier**), or during the incubation period, convalescence and postconvalescence of an individual with a clinically recognizable disease (commonly known as an **incubatory** or **convalescent carrier**). Under either circumstance the carrier state may be of short or long duration (**temporary** or **transient carrier**, or **chronic carrier**).

2. **Case-fatality rate**—Usually expressed as the percentage of persons diagnosed as having a specified disease who die as a result of that illness within a given period. This term is most frequently applied to a specific outbreak of acute disease in which all patients have been followed for an adequate period of time to include all attributable deaths. The **case-fatality rate** must be clearly differentiated from the **mortality rate** (q.v.). (Synonyms: fatality rate, fatality percentage, case-fatality ratio)

3. **Chemoprophylaxis**—The administration of a chemical, including antibiotics, to prevent the development of an infection or the progression of an infection to active manifest disease, or to eliminate the carriage of a specific infectious agent to prevent transmission and disease in others. **Chemotherapy**, on the other hand, refers to use of a chemical to treat a clinically manifest disease or to limit its further progress.

4. **Cleaning**—The removal by scrubbing and washing, as with hot water, soap or suitable detergent or by vacuum cleaning, of infectious agents and of organic matter from surfaces on which and in which infectious agents may find favorable conditions for surviving or multiplying.

5. **Communicable disease**—An illness due to a specific infectious agent or its toxic products that arises through transmission of that agent or its products from an infected person, animal or inanimate reservoir to a susceptible host; either directly or indirectly through an intermediate plant or animal host, vector or the inanimate environment. (Synonym: infectious disease)

6. **Communicable period**—The time during which an infectious agent may be transferred directly or indirectly from an infected

person to another person, from an infected animal to humans, or from an infected person to animals, including arthropods.

In diseases such as diphtheria and streptococcal infection, in which mucous membranes are involved from the initial entry of the infectious agent, the period of communicability is from the date of first exposure to a source of infection until the infecting microorganism is no longer disseminated from the involved mucous membranes, i.e., from the period before the prodromata until termination of a carrier state, if the latter develops. Some diseases are more communicable during the incubation period than during the actual illness (e.g., hepatitis A, measles).

In diseases such as tuberculosis, leprosy, syphilis, gonorrhea and some of the salmonelloses, the communicable state may exist over a long and sometimes intermittent period when active chronic lesions permit the discharge of infectious agents from the surface of the skin or through any of the body orifices.

In diseases transmitted by arthropods, such as malaria and yellow fever, the periods of communicability (or more properly **infectivity**) are those during which the infectious agent occurs in the blood or other tissues of the infected person in sufficient numbers to permit infection of the vector. A period of communicability (**transmissibility**) is also to be noted for the arthropod vector, namely, when the agent is present in the tissues of the arthropod in such form and locus (**infective state**) as to be transmissible.

7. **Contact**—A person or animal that has been in such association with an infected person or animal or a contaminated environment as to have had an opportunity to acquire the infection.

8. **Contamination**—The presence of an infectious agent on a body surface, in clothes, bedding, toys, surgical instruments or dressings, or other inanimate articles or substances including water and food. **Pollution** is distinct from contamination and implies the presence of offensive, but not necessarily infectious, matter in the environment. Contamination of a body surface does not imply a carrier state.

9. **Disinfection**—Killing of infectious agents outside the body by direct exposure to chemical or physical agents. **High-level disinfection** may kill all microorganisms with the exception of high numbers of bacterial spores; it requires extended exposure to ensure killing of most bacterial spores. It is achieved, after thorough detergent cleaning, by exposure to specific concentrations of certain disinfectants (e.g., 2% glutaraldehyde, 6% stabilized hydrogen peroxide and up to 1% peracetic acid) for at least 20 minutes. **Intermediate-level disinfection** does not kill spores; it can be achieved by **pasteurization** (75°C [167°F] for 30 minutes) or by appropriate treatment with EPA-approved disinfectants.

Concurrent disinfection is the application of disinfective measures as soon as possible after the discharge of infectious material from the body of an infected person, or after the soiling of articles with such infectious discharges; all personal contact with such discharges or articles should be minimized prior to such disinfection.

Terminal disinfection is the application of disinfective measures after the patient has been removed by death or to a hospital, or has ceased to be a source of infection, or after hospital isolation or other practices have been discontinued. Terminal disinfection is rarely practiced; terminal cleaning generally suffices (see Cleaning), along with airing and sunning of rooms, furniture and bedding. Disinfection is necessary only for diseases spread by indirect contact; steam sterilization or incineration of bedding and other items is recommended after a disease such as Lassa fever or other highly infectious diseases.

Sterilization involves destruction of all forms of life by heat, irradiation, gas (ethylene oxide or formaldehyde) or chemical treatment.

10. **Disinfestation**—Any physical or chemical process serving to destroy or remove undesired small animal forms, particularly arthropods or rodents, present upon the person, the clothing, or in the environment of an individual, or on domestic animals. (See Insecticide and Rodenticide.) Disinfestation includes delousing for infestation with *Pediculus humanus,* the human body louse. Synonyms include the terms **disinsection** and **disinsectization** when only insects are involved.

11. **Endemic**—The constant presence of a disease or infectious agent within a given geographic area; it may also refer to the usual prevalence of a given disease within such area. **Hyperendemic** expresses a constant presence at a high level of incidence, and **holoendemic** a high level of prevalence with infections beginning early in life and affecting most of the population, e.g., malaria in some places. (See Zoonosis.)

12. **Epidemic**—The occurrence in a community or region of cases of an illness (or an outbreak) with a frequency clearly in excess of normal expectancy. The number of cases indicating presence of an epidemic will vary according to the infectious agent, size and type of population exposed, previous experience or lack of exposure to the disease, and time and place of occurrence; epidemicity is thus relative to usual frequency of the disease in the same area, among the specified population, at the same season of the year. A single case of a communicable disease long absent from a population or the first invasion by a disease not previously recognized in that area requires immediate reporting and epidemiologic investigation; two

cases of such a disease associated in time and place are sufficient evidence of transmission to be considered an epidemic. (See Report of a Disease and Zoonosis.)

13. **Food irradiation**—A technology that provides a specific dose of ionizing radiation from a source such as a radioisotope (e.g., Cobalt 60), or from machines that produce accelerated electron beams or x-rays. Doses for irradiation of food and materiel are: **low**, 1 or less kiloGrays (kGy), used for disinfestation of insects from fruit, spices and grain; and parasite disinfection from fish and meat; **medium**, 1-10 kGy (commonly 1-4 kGy), used for pasteurization and the destruction of bacteria and fungi; and **high**, 10-50 kGy, used for sterilization of food as well as medical supplies (including IV fluids, implants, syringes, needles, thread, clips and gowns).

14. **Fumigation**—Any process by which the killing of animal forms, especially arthropods and rodents, is accomplished by the use of gaseous agents. (See Insecticide and Rodenticide.)

15. **Health education**—Health education is the process by which individuals and groups of people learn to behave in a manner conducive to the promotion, maintenance or restoration of health. Education for health begins with people as they are, with whatever interests they may have in improving their living conditions. Its aim is to develop in them a sense of responsibility for health conditions, as individuals and as members of families and communities. In communicable disease control, health education commonly includes an appraisal of what is known by a population about a disease, an assessment of habits and attitudes of the people as they relate to spread and frequency of the disease, and the presentation of specific means to remedy observed deficiencies. (Synonyms: patient education, education for health, education of the public, public health education)

16. **Herd immunity**—The immunity of a group or community. The resistance of a group to invasion and spread of an infectious agent, based on the resistance to infection of a high proportion of individual members of the group.

17. **Host**—A person or other living animal, including birds and arthropods, that affords subsistence or lodgment to an infectious agent under natural (as opposed to experimental) conditions. Some protozoa and helminths pass successive stages in alternate hosts of different species. Hosts in which the parasite attains maturity or passes its sexual stage are **primary** or **definitive hosts**; those in which the parasite is in a larval or asexual state are **secondary** or **intermediate hosts**. A **transport host** is a carrier in which the organism remains alive but does not undergo development.

18. **Immune individual**—A person or animal that has specific protective antibodies and/or cellular immunity as a result of previous infection or immunization, or is so conditioned by such previous specific experience as to respond in such a way that prevents the development of infection and/or clinical illness following reexposure to the specific infectious agent. Immunity is relative: a level of protection that could be adequate under ordinary conditions may be overwhelmed by an excessive dose of the infectious agent or by exposure through an unusual portal of entry; protection may also be impaired by immunosuppressive drug therapy, concurrent disease or the aging process. (See Resistance.)

19. **Immunity**—That resistance usually associated with the presence of antibodies or cells having a specific action on the microorganism concerned with a particular infectious disease or on its toxin. Effective immunity includes both **cellular immunity,** which is conferred by T-lymphocyte sensitization, and/or **humoral immunity,** which is based on B-lymphocyte response. **Passive immunity** is attained either naturally by transplacental transfer from the mother, or artificially by inoculation of specific protective antibodies (from immunized animals, or convalescent hyperimmune serum or immune serum globulin [human]); it is of short duration (days to months). **Active humoral immunity**, which usually lasts for years, is attained either naturally by infection with or without clinical manifestations, or artificially by inoculation of the agent itself in killed, modified or variant form, or of fractions or products of the agent.

20. **Inapparent infection**—The presence of infection in a host without recognizable clinical signs or symptoms. Inapparent infections are identifiable only by laboratory means such as a blood test or by the development of positive reactivity to specific skin tests. (Synonyms: asymptomatic, subclinical, occult infection)

21. **Incidence rate**—The number of new cases of a specified disease diagnosed or reported during a defined period of time, divided by the number of persons in a stated population in which the cases occurred. This is usually expressed as cases per 1,000 or 100,000 per annum. This rate may be expressed as age- or gender-specific or as specific for any other population characteristic or subdivision. (See Morbidity rate and Prevalence rate.)

    Attack rate, or **case rate**, is a proportion measuring cumulative incidence often used for particular groups, observed for limited periods and under special circumstances, as in an epidemic; it is usually expressed as percent (cases per 100 in the group). The **secondary attack rate** is the number of cases among familial or institutional contacts occurring within the accepted incubation period following exposure to a primary case, in relation to the total of exposed contacts; the denominator may be restricted to susceptible contacts when determinable. **Infection rate** is a proportion that expresses the incidence of all identified infections, manifest and inapparent.

22. **Incubation period**—The time interval between initial contact with an infectious agent and the first appearance of symptoms associated with the infection. In a vector, it is the time between entrance of an organism into the vector and the time when that vector can transmit the infection (**extrinsic incubation period**). The period in people between the time of exposure to a parasite and the time when the parasite can be detected in blood or stool is called the **prepatent period.**

23. **Infected individual**—A person or animal that harbors an infectious agent and who has either manifest disease (see Patient or sick person) or inapparent infection (see Carrier). An **infectious person** or animal is one from whom the infectious agent can be naturally acquired.

24. **Infection**—The entry and development (of many parasites) or multiplication of an infectious agent in the body of persons or animals. Infection is not synonymous with infectious disease; the result may be inapparent (see Inapparent infection) or manifest (see Infectious disease). The presence of living infectious agents on exterior surfaces of the body, or on articles of apparel or soiled articles, is not infection, but represents contamination of such surfaces and articles. (See Infestation and Contamination.)

25. **Infectious agent**—An organism (virus, rickettsia, bacteria, fungus, protozoan or helminth) that is capable of producing infection or infectious disease. **Infectivity** expresses the ability of the disease agent to enter, survive and multiply in the host; **infectiousness** indicates the relative ease with which a disease is transmitted to other hosts.

26. **Infectious disease**—A clinically manifest disease of humans or animals resulting from an infection. (See Infection.)

27. **Infestation**—For persons or animals, the lodgment, development and reproduction of arthropods on the surface of the body or in the clothing. Infested articles or premises are those that harbor or give shelter to animal forms, especially arthropods and rodents.

28. **Insecticide**—Any chemical substance used for the destruction of insects, whether applied as powder, liquid, atomized liquid, aerosol or "paint" spray; residual action is usual. The term **larvicide** is generally used to designate insecticides applied specifically for destruction of immature stages of arthropods; **adulticide** or **imago-**

cide, to designate those applied to destroy mature or adult forms. The term **insecticide** is often used broadly to encompass substances for the destruction of all arthropods, but **acaricide** is more properly used for agents against ticks and mites. More specific terms such as **lousicide** and **miticide** are sometimes used.

29. **Isolation**—As applied to patients, isolation represents separation, for the period of communicability, of infected persons or animals from others in such places and under such conditions as to prevent or limit the direct or indirect transmission of the infectious agent from those infected to those who are susceptible to infection or who may spread the agent to others. In contrast, quarantine (q.v.) applies to restrictions on the healthy contacts of an infectious case.

CDC has recommended that **Universal Precautions** be used consistently for all patients (in hospital settings as well as outpatient settings) regardless of their bloodborne infection status. This practice is based on the possibility that blood and certain body fluids (any body secretion that is obviously bloody, semen, vaginal secretions, tissue, CSF, and synovial, pleural, peritoneal, pericardial and amniotic fluids) of all patients are potentially infectious for HIV, HBV and other bloodborne pathogens. Universal precautions are intended to prevent parenteral, mucous membrane and nonintact skin exposures of healthcare workers to bloodborne pathogens. Protective barriers include gloves, gowns, masks and protective eyewear or face shields. A private room is indicated if patient hygiene is poor. Waste management is controlled by local and state authority.

There are two basic requirements that are common for care of all potentially infectious cases:

• *Hands must be washed after contact with the patient or potentially contaminated articles and before taking care of another patient;* and

• *Articles contaminated with infectious material should be appropriately discarded or bagged and labeled before being sent for decontamination and reprocessing.*

Recommendations made for isolation of cases in section 9B2 of each disease may allude to the methods that had been recommended by CDC (*CDC Guideline for Isolation Precautions in Hospitals*) as category-specific isolation precautions, in addition to universal precautions, based on the mode of transmission of the specific disease. These categories are as follows:

1) **Strict isolation**: This category is designed to prevent transmission of highly contagious or virulent infections that may be spread by both air and contact. The specifications, in addition to those above, include a private room and the use of masks, gowns and gloves for all persons entering the room. Special ventilation require-

ments with the room at negative pressure to surrounding areas are desirable.

2) **Contact isolation**: For less highly transmissible or serious infections, for diseases or conditions that are spread primarily by close or direct contact. In addition to the basic requirements, a private room is indicated, but patients infected with the same pathogen may share a room. Masks are indicated for those who come close to the patient, gowns are indicated if soiling is likely and gloves are indicated for touching infectious material.

3) **Respiratory isolation**: To prevent transmission of infectious diseases over short distances through the air, a private room is indicated, but patients infected with the same organism may share a room. In addition to the basic requirements, masks are indicated for those who come in close contact with the patient; gowns and gloves are not indicated.

4) **Tuberculosis isolation (AFB isolation)**: For patients with pulmonary tuberculosis who have a positive sputum smear or a chest x-ray that strongly suggests active tuberculosis. Specifications include use of a private room with special ventilation and closed door. In addition to the basic requirements, respirator-type masks are used by those entering the room. Gowns are used to prevent gross contamination of clothing. Gloves are not indicated.

5) **Enteric precautions**: For infections transmitted by direct or indirect contact with feces. In addition to the basic requirements, specifications include use of a private room if patient hygiene is poor. Masks are not indicated; gowns should be used if soiling is likely and gloves are to be used for touching contaminated materials.

6) **Drainage/secretion precautions**: To prevent infections transmitted by direct or indirect contact with purulent material or drainage from an infected body site. A private room and masking are not indicated; in addition to the basic requirements, gowns should be used if soiling is likely and gloves should be used for touching contaminated materials.

30. **Molluscicide**—A chemical substance used for the destruction of snails and other molluscs.

31. **Morbidity rate**—An incidence rate (q.v.) used to include all persons in the population under consideration who become clinically ill during the period of time stated. The population may be limited to a specific gender or age group, or to those with certain other characteristics.

32. **Mortality rate**—A rate calculated in the same way as an **incidence rate** (q.v.), by dividing the number of deaths occurring in the population during the stated period of time, usually a year, by the number of persons at risk of dying during the period. A **total** or

crude mortality rate utilizes deaths from all causes, usually expressed as deaths per 1,000. A **disease-specific** mortality rate covers deaths due to only one disease and is often reported on the basis of 100,000 persons. The population base may be defined by gender, age or other characteristics. The mortality rate must not be confused with case-fatality rate (q.v.). (Synonym: death rate)

33. **Nosocomial infection**—An infection occurring in a patient in a hospital or other healthcare facility in whom it was not present or incubating at the time of admission; or the residual of an infection acquired during a previous admission. Includes infections acquired in the hospital but appearing after discharge, and also such infections among the staff of the facility. (Synonym: hospital-acquired infection)

34. **Pathogenicity**—The property of an infectious agent that determines the extent to which overt disease is produced in an infected population, or the power of an organism to produce disease.

35. **Patient or sick person**—A person who is ill.

36. **Personal hygiene**—In the field of infectious disease control, those protective measures, primarily within the responsibility of the individual, that promote health and limit the spread of infectious diseases, chiefly those transmitted by direct contact. Such measures encompass (1) washing hands in soap and water immediately after evacuating bowel or bladder and always before handling food or eating; (2) keeping hands and unclean articles, or articles that have been used for toilet purposes by others, away from the mouth, nose, eyes, ears, genitalia and wounds; (3) avoiding the use of common or unclean eating utensils, drinking cups, towels, handkerchiefs, combs, hairbrushes and pipes; (4) avoiding exposure of other persons to spray from the nose and mouth as in coughing, sneezing, laughing or talking; (5) washing hands thoroughly after handling a patient or the patient's belongings; and (6) keeping the body clean by frequent soap and water baths.

37. **Prevalence rate**—The total number of persons sick or portraying a certain condition in a stated population at a particular time (**point prevalence**), or during a stated period of time (**period prevalence**), regardless of when that illness or condition began, divided by the population at risk of having the disease or condition at the point in time or midway through the period in which they occurred.

38. **Quarantine**—Restriction of the activities of well persons or animals who have been exposed to a case of communicable disease during its period of communicability (i.e., contacts) to prevent disease transmission during the incubation period if infection should occur.

1) **Absolute** or **complete quarantine**: The limitation of freedom of movement of those exposed to a communicable disease for a period of time not longer than the longest usual incubation period of that disease, in such manner as to prevent effective contact with those not so exposed. (See Isolation.)

2) **Modified quarantine**: A selective, partial limitation of freedom of movement of contacts, commonly on the basis of known or presumed differences in susceptibility and related to the danger of disease transmission. It may be designed to accommodate particular situations. Examples are exclusion of children from school, exemption of immune persons from provisions applicable to susceptible persons, or restriction of military populations to the post or to quarters. It includes: **Personal surveillance**, the practice of close medical or other supervision of contacts to permit prompt recognition of infection or illness but without restricting their movements; and **Segregation**, the separation of some part of a group of persons or domestic animals from the others for special consideration, control or observation; removal of susceptible children to homes of immune persons; or establishment of a sanitary boundary to protect uninfected from infected portions of a population.

39. **Repellent**—A chemical applied to the skin or clothing or other places to discourage (1) arthropods from alighting on and attacking an individual, or (2) other agents, such as helminth larvae, from penetrating the skin.

40. **Report of a disease**—An official report notifying an appropriate authority of the occurrence of a specified communicable or other disease in humans or in animals. Diseases in humans are reported to the local health authority; those in animals, to the livestock, sanitary, veterinary or agriculture authority. Some few diseases in animals, also transmissible to humans, are reportable to both authorities. Each health jurisdiction declares a list of reportable diseases appropriate to its particular needs (see Communicable Disease Reporting). Reports should also list suspected cases of diseases of particular public health importance, ordinarily those requiring epidemiologic investigation or initiation of special control measures.

When a person is infected in one health jurisdiction and the case is reported from another, the health authority receiving the report should notify the jurisdiction where infection presumably occurred, especially when the disease requires examination of contacts for infection, or if food, water or other common vehicles of infection may be involved.

In addition to routine report of cases of specified diseases, special notification is required of all epidemics or outbreaks of disease, including diseases not listed as reportable. (See Epidemic.) Special reporting requirements specified in International Health Regulations are presented in Communicable Disease Reporting.

41. **Reservoir** (of infectious agents)—Any person, animal, arthropod, plant, soil or substance (or combination of these) in which an infectious agent normally lives and multiplies, on which it depends primarily for survival, and where it reproduces itself in such manner that it can be transmitted to a susceptible host.

42. **Resistance**—The sum total of body mechanisms that interpose barriers to the invasion or multiplication of infectious agents, or to damage by their toxic products. **Inherent resistance**—an ability to resist disease independent of immunity or of specifically developed tissue responses; it commonly resides in anatomic or physiologic characteristics of the host and may be genetic or acquired, permanent or temporary. (See Immunity.) (Synonym: Nonspecific immunity)

43. **Rodenticide**—A chemical substance used for the destruction of rodents, generally through ingestion. (See Fumigation.)

44. **Source of infection**—The person, animal, object or substance from which an infectious agent passes to a host. Source of infection should be clearly distinguished from **source of contamination**, such as overflow of a septic tank contaminating a water supply, or an infected cook contaminating a salad. (See Reservoir.)

45. **Surveillance of disease**—As distinct from surveillance of persons (see Quarantine, 2), surveillance of disease is the continuing scrutiny of all aspects of occurrence and spread of a disease that are pertinent to effective control. Included are the systematic collection and evaluation of

    1) morbidity and mortality reports;
    2) special reports of field investigations of epidemics and of individual cases;
    3) isolation and identification of infectious agents by laboratories;
    4) data concerning the availability, use and untoward effects of vaccines and toxoids, immune globulins, insecticides and other substances used in control;
    5) information regarding immunity levels in segments of the population; and
    6) other relevant epidemiologic data. A report summarizing the above data should be prepared and distributed to all cooperating persons and others with a need to know the results of the surveillance activities.

    The procedure applies to all jurisdictional levels of public health from local to international. **Serologic surveillance** identifies patterns of current and past infection using serologic tests.

46. **Susceptible**—A person or animal not possessing sufficient resistance against a particular pathogenic agent to prevent contracting infection or disease when exposed to the agent.

47. **Suspect**—In infectious disease control, illness in a person whose history and symptoms suggest that he or she may have or be developing a communicable disease.

48. **Transmission of infectious agents**—Any mechanism by which an infectious agent is spread from a source or reservoir to a person. These mechanisms are as follows:
    1) **Direct transmission**: Direct and essentially immediate transfer of infectious agents to a receptive portal of entry through which human or animal infection may take place. This may be by direct contact such as touching, biting, kissing or sexual intercourse, or by the direct projection (droplet spread) of droplet spray onto the conjunctiva or onto the mucous membranes of the eye, nose or mouth during sneezing, coughing, spitting, singing or talking (usually limited to a distance of about 1 m or less).
    2) **Indirect transmission**:
        a) Vehicle-borne—Contaminated inanimate materials or objects (fomites) such as toys, handkerchiefs, soiled clothes, bedding, cooking or eating utensils, surgical instruments or dressings; water, food, milk, and biological products including blood, serum, plasma, tissues or organs; or any substance serving as an intermediate means by which an infectious agent is transported and introduced into a susceptible host through a suitable portal of entry. The agent may or may not have multiplied or developed in or on the vehicle before being transmitted.
        b) Vector-borne—(i) Mechanical: Includes simple mechanical carriage by a crawling or flying insect through soiling of its feet or proboscis, or by passage of organisms through its gastrointestinal tract. This does not require multiplication or development of the organism. (ii) Biological: Propagation (multiplication), cyclic development, or a combination of these (cyclopropagative) is required before the arthropod can transmit the infective form of the agent to humans. An incubation period (extrinsic) is required following infection before the arthropod becomes **infective**. The infectious agent may be passed vertically to succeeding generations (**transovarian transmission**); **transstadial transmission** indicates its passage from one stage of life cycle to another, as nymph to adult. Transmission may be by injection of salivary gland fluid during biting, or by

regurgitation or deposition on the skin of feces or other material capable of penetrating through the bite wound or through an area of trauma from scratching or rubbing. This transmission is by an infected nonvertebrate host and not simple mechanical carriage by a vector as a vehicle. However, an arthropod in either role is termed a **vector**.

3) **Airborne:** The dissemination of microbial aerosols to a suitable portal of entry, usually the respiratory tract. Microbial aerosols are suspensions of particles in the air consisting partially or wholly of microorganisms. They may remain suspended in the air for long periods of time, some retaining and others losing infectivity or virulence. Particles in the 1- to 5-μm range are easily drawn into the alveoli of the lungs and may be retained there. Not considered as airborne are droplets and other large particles that promptly settle out (see Direct transmission, above).

   a) Droplet nuclei—Usually the small residues that result from evaporation of fluid from droplets emitted by an infected host (see above). They may also be created purposely by a variety of atomizing devices, or accidentally as in microbiology laboratories or in abattoirs, rendering plants or autopsy rooms. They usually remain suspended in the air for long periods of time.

   b) Dust—The small particles of widely varying size that may arise from soil (as, e.g., fungus spores separated from dry soil by wind or mechanical agitation), clothes, bedding or contaminated floors.

49. **Universal precautions**—See under Isolation, Universal blood/body fluid precautions.

50. **Virulence**—The degree of pathogenicity of an infectious agent, indicated by case-fatality rates and/or the ability of the agent to invade and damage tissues of the host.

51. **Zoonosis**—An infection or infectious disease transmissible under natural conditions from vertebrate animals to humans. May be enzootic or epizootic. (See Endemic and Epidemic.)

INDEX

A

Abacterial meningitis, 338-340
Abattoir workers
  brucellosis hazard, 76-77
  leptospirosis risk, 294
  listeriosis hazard, 297
  orf virus disease hazard, 367
  Q fever risk, 409
Abortion
  risk of, 296-297, 353, 436, 482
ABPA. *See* Allergic
  bronchopulmonary aspergillosis
Abscesses
  breast, **464-467**
  liver, 11-12, 14
  staphylococcal, **461-464**
Absidia spp., 562
Abuse. *See* Drug abuse; Sexual
  abuse
Acanthamebiases, **359-362**
Acanthamoeba spp., 359-361
Acariasis, 445-447
Acinetobacter spp.
  animal bites and, 89
Acquired immunodeficiency
  syndrome, **1-9**. *See also* Human
  immunodeficiency virus
  antiretroviral therapy, 3, 7-8
  Burkitt lymphoma and, 325
  case definition for developing
    countries, 1
  CDC National AIDS
    Clearinghouse, 7
  control of patient, contacts and
    environment, 6-9
  deaths from, 3
  disaster implications, 9
  as disease risk, 134-136, 288
  EBV and, 327
  epidemic measures, 9
  fatality rate, 1
  identification, 1-2

incubation period, 4
infants and children, 1
infectious agent, 2
international measures, 9
Kaposi's sarcoma and, 328
methods of control, 5-9
mode of transmission, 3-4
non-Hodgkin's lymphomas and,
  327
occurrence, 2-3
period of communicability, 4
pneumocystis pneumonia risk,
  393
preventive measures, 5-6
reservoir, 3
risk behaviors, 3-4
susceptibility and resistance, 4-5
treatment, 7
Acremonium spp., 358
Actinobacillus mallei, 338
Actinomadura spp., 358
Actinomyces spp., 10
Actinomycetoma, 10, **357-359**
Actinomycosis, **9-11**
Acupuncturists
  hepatitis B risk, 245
Acute bacterial conjunctivitis,
  119-121
Acute febrile mucocutaneous
  lymph node syndrome, 276-278
Acute febrile respiratory disease,
  427-430
Acute flaccid paralysis, 398-399
Acute hemorrhagic conjunctivitis,
  124-126
Acute lymphonodular pharyngitis,
  129-131
Acute viral rhinitis, 424-430
Adenoviral hemorrhagic
  conjunctivitis, **124-126**
Adenoviral keratoconjunctivitis,
  122-124

Adenoviruses, 124-125, 398, 427-428
Adult T-cell leukemia, 329
Aedes aegypti, 38, 143-144, 146, 554
Aedes communis, 38
Aedes mcintoshi, 49
Aedes polynesiensis, 38, 199
Aedes scapularis, 199
Aedes spp., 40-41, 46, 49, 143, 198, 554
Aedes vigilax, 38
Afipia felis, 88
Aflatoxins, 61
African Burkitt lymphoma, 325
African hemorrhagic fever, 174-176
African histoplasmosis, 265
African tick bite fever, **433-434**
African trypanosomiasis, **514-518**
Agricultural workers
  anthrax risk, 20
  arenaviral hemorrhagic fever risk, 26-27
  brucellosis risk, 76
  chromomycosis risk, 113-114
  leptospirosis risk, 294
  melioidosis risk, 336
  paracoccidioidomycosis risk, 369
  sporotrichosis risk, 459
AHC. *See* Acute hemorrhagic conjunctivitis
AIDS. *See* Acquired immunodeficiency syndrome
Ajellomyces capsulatus, 263
Ajellomyces dermatitidis, 69
Alastrim variola, 456
Alcoholism
  as disease risk, 110-111
Alenquer virus, 34, 53
Aleppo evil, 284-287
Alexandrium, 210-211
Alfalfa sprouts
  contaminated, 156
Algae, 210

Allergic bronchopulmonary aspergillosis, 60-62
Alpha herpesvirus 3, 93
Alpha-fetoprotein, 324
Alphaherpesviral disease, 257-261
Alphaherpesvirinae, 259
Alphaviruses, 29, 37, 40, 46
Alveolar hydatid disease, 179-180
Alzheimer disease, 184
Amblyomma americanum, 182
Amblyomma spp., 431, 434
Amebiasis, 11-15
Amebic dysentery, 11, 14
Amebic meningoencephalitis, primary, 359-362
Ameboflagellates, 359
Ameboma, 11
American histoplasmosis, 262-265
American Red Cross
  Blood Service Regional Offices, 96
American trypanosomiasis, **518-520**
Amnesic shellfish poisoning, **212**
Amoebiasis, **11-15**
Ancylostoma braziliense, **500**
Ancylostoma caninum, **500**
Ancylostoma spp., 266
Ancylostomiasis, 265-268
Andes virus, 234
Anemia, 66, 189, 265
Angina
  monocytic, 350-352
  Vincent's, 166
Angiostrongyliasis, **15-17**
Angiostrongyliasis, abdominal, **17-18**
Angiostrongyliasis, intestinal, **17-18**
Angiostrongylus cantonensis, 15
Angiostrongylus costaricensis, 17
Animal bites
  herpes B-virus, 261-262
  infections associated with, **89-90**
  rabies, 412-419
  rat-bite fever, 420-421
  treatment of, 415, 417

Animal handlers
  disease risk, 20, 55, 76, 237,
    240–241, 261–262, 294
Animals. *See also* Milk and milk
  products; *specific animal by
  name*
  anthrax infection, 20–24
  as disease reservoir, 39–43,
    45–47, 79–80, 87, 115,
    134–135, 148, 150, 171, 183,
    206, 221, 263, 285, 294, 297,
    336, 408, 441, 492, 509, 558
  skin and hides as reservoir,
    20–24
  small mammals as disease
    reservoir, 51
Anisakiasis, **18–19**
Anisakinae, 18
Anisakis, 18
Anogenital herpesviral infections,
  257–261
Anopheles A group arboviruses, 32
Anopheles spp., 38, 46, 199, 312
Anthrax, **20–25**
  bioterrorism measures, 24–25
  control of patient, contacts and
    environment, 23–24
  disaster implications, 24
  epidemic measures, 24
  identification, 20
  incubation period, 21
  infectious agent, 20
  international measures, 24
  methods of control, 22–24
  mode of transmission, 21
  occurrence, 20–21
  period of communicability, 21
  preventive measures, 22–23
  reservoir, 21
  susceptibility and resistance, 22
Antiretroviral therapy
  for AIDS, 3, 7–8
Antitoxins
  botulism, 74
  diphteria, 169–170
Apeu virus, 32, 48
Aphthous pharyngitis, 129–131

Apodemus spp., 232
Apollo 11 disease, 124–126
Apophysomyces spp., 562
Appendicitis
  similarity to other diseases,
    17–18, 79
Apple cider
  contaminated, 135, 156
Aquatic plants
  disease transmission by,
    194–197
Arachnia propionica, 10
Arachnia viscosus, 10
Arboviral diseases, 28–36
Archeologists
  coccidioidomycosis risk, 118
Arenaviral hemorrhagic fevers
  South American, **26–28**
Arenaviruses, 279, 307
Argentinian hemorrhagic fever,
  26–28
Armadillos
  as disease reservoir, 290
Arthalgia
  arthropod-borne viral disease
    and, 37
Arthritic erythema, epidemic,
  420–421
Arthritis
  arthropod-borne viral disease
    and, 28, 37–39
  erythema infectiosum and, 189
  gonococcal infection, 223
  Lyme disease, 306
  streptococcal, **461–464**
Arthroconidia, 117–118
Arthropathy, reactive, 451
Arthropod-borne viral diseases
  arthritis and rash, **37–39**
  Culicoides-borne, **45–50**
  encephalitides, **39–45**
  Flaviviridae, 31–32
  hemorrhagic fevers, **54–58**
  location of, 30–36
  mosquito-borne, **45–50, 54–56**
  Orthomyxoviridae, 36
  overview, 28–29

phlebotomine-borne, **52–54**
Reoviridae, 35
Rhabdoviridae, 36
tickborne, **43–45, 50–52, 54–56**
Togaviridae, 30
vectors for, 30-36
Ascariasis, **58–60**
Ascarid worms, 60
Ascaridiasis, 58-60
Ascaris lumbricoides, 58
Ascaris suum, 58
Aseptic meningitis, 28, 39, 302, 338-340
Asian taeniasis, **491**
Aspergillosis, **60–62**
Aspergillus spp., 60-61
Ataxia, 183, 186
Athlete's foot, 151-152
ATL. *See* Adult T-cell leukemia
Atypical cutaneous leishmaniasis, 285
Australia antigen hepatitis, 243-251
Australia bat lyssavirus, 411
Australian encephalitis, 39-43
Avian chlamydiosis, 405-407
Azidothymidine
HIV treatment, 8
AZT. *See* Azidothymidine

B

Babanki virus, 30
Babesia divergens, 63
Babesia isolate type WA1, 63
Babesia microti, 63-64
Babesiosis, **62–64**
Bacillary dysentery, 451-455
Bacillus anthracis, 20-22
Bacillus Calmette-Guérin, 292
Bacillus cereus
food intoxication, **207–208**
Bacterial meningitis, **340**
Baghdad boil, 284-287
Balamuthia mandrillaris, 359-361
Balantidial dysentery, 65-66

Balantidiasis, **65–66**
Balantidiosis, 65-66
Balantidium coli, 65
Bancroftian filariasis, 197-201
Bandicota spp., 16
Bangui virus, 31, 35
Banzi virus, 48
Barmah Forest virus, 30, 37
Bartholinitis
gonococcal, 223-227
Bartonella bacilliformis, 67
Bartonella henselae, 88
Bartonella quintana, 507
Bartonella spp., 87-88
Bartonellosis, **66–68**
Basidiobolus spp., **563–564**
Batai virus, 33
Bats
as disease reservoir, 236, 411-413
disease transmission by droppings, 263
Bayou virus, 234
BCG. *See Bacillus Calmette-Guérin*
Beard
ringworm infection, 147-149
Bears
as disease reservoir, 171, 201
Beavers
as disease reservoir, 221
Beef tapeworm, 488-491
Behaviors, risk. *See* Risk behaviors
Bejel, 486-487
Belgrade virus, 232
Benign lymphocytic meningitis, 306-308
Benign lymphoreticulosis, 87-89
Benign tertian malaria, 310
Beta hemolytic streptococci, **470–476**
Beta herpesvirus 5, 139
Betaherpesvirus, 139, 192
Bhanja virus, 35, 51
BIG. *See* Botulinal immune globulin

Bile duct
  clonorchiasis, 114–116
Bilharziasis, 447–450
Bioport Corporation, 22
Bioterrorism
  anthrax, 21–22, 24–25
  botulinum toxins, 75
  CDC response coordination
    hotline, xxiii, 457
  plague, 383, 387
  variola virus, 455
Birds
  as disease reservoir, 38, 41, 49,
    55, 79, 84, 133, 204, 272,
    405–406, 408, 441, 558
  disease transmission by
    droppings, 133, 263
  importation regulation, 406
Bites, animal
  infections associated with,
    89–90
BL. *See* Burkitt lymphoma
Black Creek Canal virus, 234
Blacks. *See* Minorities
Blastomyces dermatitidis, 69
Blastomycosis, **68–70**
Blindness, river, 363–367
Blood and blood products. *See also*
    Transfusions
  donor restrictions, 185, 249,
    253, 314
  FDA regulations for prevention
    of HIV contamination, 6
  HIV transmission, 3, 9
Blood Service Regional Offices, 96
Body fluid precautions. *See*
    Universal precautions
Body lice, 372–374
Boils, staphylococcal, **461–464**
Bolivian hemorrhagic fever, 26–28
Bone marrow transplants
  CMV infections, 139
Boophilus spp., 55
Boosting, 522
Borderline leprosy, 289
Bornholm disease, 356–357
Borrelia burgdorferi, 62, 303–305

Borrelia parapertussis, 375–376
Borrelia pertussis, 375, 377
Borrelia recurrentis, 372, 422
Botryomyces caespitatus, 113
Botulinal immune globulin, 74
Botulism, **70–75**
  antitoxin, 74
  bioterrorism measures, 75
  CDC emergency telephone
    numbers, 74
  control of patient, contacts and
    environment, 73–74
  epidemic measures, 75
  foodborne, 70
  identification, 70
  incubation period, 72
  infectious agent, 71
  international measures, 75
  intestinal, 70–71
  methods of control, 73–74
  mode of transmission, 72
  occurrence, 71–72
  period of communicability, 73
  preventive measures, 73
  reservoir, 72
  susceptibility and resistance, 73
  wound, 70
Boutonneuse fever, **432–433**
Bovine papular stomatitis virus,
    367
Bovine spongiform
    encephalopathy, 183–184
Bovine tuberculosis, 523–524
BPF. *See* Brazilian purpuric fever
Branhamella spp., 120
Brazilian hemorrhagic fever, 26–28
Brazilian purpuric fever, 119–121
Breakbone fever, 142–144
Breast abscesses, staphylococcal,
    464–467
Breast feeding. *See also*
    Maternal–infant transmission
  AIDS transmission, 4
  ATL risk, 329
  CMV transmission, 140

disease protection and, 103, 162-163, 452
Brevetoxin, 211
Brill-Zinsser disease, 542
Broad tapeworm infection, 171-172
Bronchiectasis
aspergillosis and, 60
Bronchitis
aspergillosis and, 60
bacterial, 391
Brucella abortus, 76-77
Brucella canis, 76
Brucella melitensis, 76-77
Brucella suis, 76
Brucellosis, **75-78**
Brugia malayi, 197-201
Brugia timori, 197-201
Brugian filariasis, 197-201
BSE. *See* Bovine spongiform encephalopathy
Buboes
inguinal, 308
syphilis, 481
tularemia, 532
Bubonic plague, 381-385
Bunyamwera group arboviruses, 33
Bunyamwera viral fever, **48-50**
Bunyamwera virus, 33
Bunyaviridae, 29, 32-35, 40, 53, 55, 231
Bunyaviruses, 29, 32-35, 40, 48
Bureau of Infectious Diseases, 138
Burial practices, 186
Burkitt lymphoma, **325**
Burkitt tumor, **324-325**
Bush dogs
as disease reservoir, 180
Bussuquara virus, 31
B-virus, 261-262
infection from animal bites, 89
Bwamba group arboviruses, 33
Bwamba virus, 33
Bwamba virus disease, **48-50**

C

Calabar swelling, 299-301
Calcium oxide
for soil decontamination, 23
Caliciviridae, 255-256
California Department of Health Services, 74
California encephalitis, 39-43
California encephalitis virus, 33
California group arboviruses, 33-34
Calomys callosus, 27
Calomys musculinus, 27
Calymmatobacterium granulomatis, 229
Cambaroides spp., 371
Campylobacter coli, 79, 81
Campylobacter enteritis, **79-81**
Campylobacter jejuni, 79-81
Campylobacter spp., 79
Cancer
cervical, **329**
chickenpox risk, 94
liver, 251, **324-325**
Candida spp., 82
Candidemia, 81
Candidiasis, **81-83,** 166
Candidosis, 81-83
Candiru virus, 34, 53
Candling
fish, 19
Canicola fever, 293-296
Canidae, 180, 288
Canines. *See* Dogs
Cannibalism, 186
Capillaria aerophila, 87
Capillaria hepatica, 85-86
Capillaria philippinensis, 84-85
Capillariasis
due to *Capillaria hepatica,* **85-86**
due to *Capillaria philippinensis,* **84-85**
pulmonary capillariasis, **87**
Capnocytophaga canimorsus, 89
Capnocytophaga cynodegmi, 90

Caraparu virus, 32, 48
Carate, 379–380
Carbuncles, staphylococcal, **461–464**
Carcinomas. *See also* Cancer
  hepatocellular, 244, 252, **324–325**
  nasopharyngeal, **325–326**
  uterine cervix, 329
Cardiopulmonary diseases
  hantaviral, 234–236
Caries
  dental, streptococcal, **477–478**
Carrión disease, 66–68
Case-fatality rates
  AIDS, 1
  anthrax, 20
  arenaviral hemorrhagic fevers in South America, 26
  arthropod-borne viral diseases, 39, 43, 55, 57
  botulism, 70–71
  Boutonneuse fever, 433
  Brazilian purpuric fever, 120
  brucellosis, 76
  bubonic plague, 381
  capillariasis, 84
  Capnocytophaga canimorsus, 89
  chickenpox, 92
  cholera, 100, 102
  dengue hemorrhagic fever, 145
  diphtheria, 166
  Ebola disease, 175
  Ebola-Marburg viral diseases, 175
  group B streptococcal sepsis, 477
  hantaviral diseases, 231
  Hendra viral disease, 236
  hepatitis E, 255
  Kawasaki syndrome, 276
  Lassa fever, 279
  Legionnaires' disease, 281
  leptospirosis, 294
  listeriosis, 297
  malaria, 310
  measles, 330
  meningitis, 340
  monkeypox, 458
  Nipah viral disease, 236
  Oroya fever, 66
  pertussis, 375
  pneumonia, 387
  puffer fish poisoning, 212
  Q fever, 408
  relapsing fever, 422
  Rocky Mountain spotted fever, 431
  shigellosis, 451
  smallpox, 456
  spirillosis, 421
  tetanus, 491
  tularemia, 532
  typhus fever, 541, 544, 546
  yellow fever, 553
Catarrhal jaundice, 238–243
Catheters, intravascular
  disease transmission by, 81–83
Cats
  as disease reservoir, 148, 201, 263, 266, 371, 382–383, 408, 412, 441, 479, 497–501
  disease transmission by, 79–80, 87–90, 115–116, 199
Cat-scratch disease, **87–89**
Cattle. *See also* Meat and meat products; Milk and milk products
  bovine spongiform encephalopathy, 183–184
  as disease reservoir, 63, 79–80, 135, 148, 156, 193–194, 204, 263, 294, 303, 408, 441, 523–524
Catu virus, 34
Caves
  as disease reservoir, 264
CCDM website, 217
CD4 count
  HIV infection evaluation, 2

CDC. *See* Centers for Disease
  Control and Prevention
CDC group DF-2. *See*
  Capnocytophaga canimorsus
Cellulitis
  animal bites and, 89
  staphylococcal, **461–464**
  streptococcal, 471
  V. vulnificus and, 112
Centers for Disease Control and
  Prevention
  bioterrorism response
    coordination hotline, 457
  botulism emergency telephone
    numbers, 74
  Division of Parasitic Diseases,
    138
  Drug Service, 169, 457
  immunization website, 217
  Malaria Section, 311
  National AIDS Clearinghouse, 7
  travel web site, 311
Central Asian hemorrhagic fever,
  54–56
Central European tickborne
  encephalitis, 43–45
Centrifugal rash distribution, 456
Cercopithecine herpesvirus-1,
  261–262
  from animal bites, 89
Cercopithecus aethiops, 175
Cerebrospinal fever, 340–345
Cervical cancer, **329**
Cervicitis
  chlamydial, 97–98, 127
  gonococcal, 223–227
Cestodes, 171
Ceviche
  undertreated, 18
Chagas' disease, 518–520
Chagres virus, 34, 53
Chancre
  syphilis, 481
  trypanosomiasis, 514
Chancroid, **90–91**
  AIDS and, 4

Chandipura virus, 36, 53
Changuinola fever, 52–54
Changuinola group arboviruses, 35
Changuinola virus, 35, 53
Changuinola virus disease, **52–54**
Cheese. *See* Milk and milk
  products
Chicken. *See* Poultry
Chickenpox, **92–97**
  control of patient, contacts and
    environment, 95–96
  differentiated from smallpox,
    456
  disaster implications, 97
  epidemic measures, 96–97
  identification, 92–93
  incubation period, 93
  infectious agent, 93
  international measures, 97
  methods of control, 94–96
  mode of transmission, 93
  occurrence, 93
  period of communicability, 94
  preventive measures, 94–95
  reservoir, 93
  susceptibility and resistance, 94
Chickens
  disease transmission by
    droppings, 263
Chiclero ulcer, 284–287
Chikungunya virus, 30
Chikungunya virus disease, 37–39
Childbirth, disease transmission.
  See Maternal–infant transmission
Children. *See also* Infants
  chickenpox and, 92
  dental caries, streptococcal,
    477–478
  encephalitis risk, 40–41
  EPI vaccine for HIV-infected
    children, 6
  HIV infection, 1
  severe viral gastroenteritis,
    215–218
  sexual abuse, 90, 223–224, 259

Chimpanzees
  as disease reservoir, 245,
    252-256, 290
China paralytic syndrome, 399
Chinese liver fluke disease,
  114-116
Chlamydia pneumoniae, 97,
  396-398, 406
Chlamydia psittaci, 97, 127, 405
Chlamydia psittaci infection,
  405-407
Chlamydia trachomatis, 97-99,
  127, 227, 309, 394-396, 504
Chlamydial conjunctivitis, 97,
  126–129, 504-506
Chlamydial infections
  genital, **97–99,** 226
  lymphogranuloma venereum,
    308-310
  psittacosis, 405-407
  urethritis, **100**
Chlamydial pneumonias, 97, 126,
  394–398
Cholera
  control of patient, contacts and
    environment, 104-107
  disaster implications, 107
  epidemic measures, 107
  gravis, 100-101, 103
  identification, 100
  incubation period, 103
  infection with other *Vibrios,*
    113
  infectious agent, 100-101
  international measures, 107-108
  methods of control, 104-107
  mode of transmission, 103
  occurrence, 101-103
  period of communicability, 103
  preventive measures, 104
  reservoir, 103
  susceptibility and resistance,
    103-104
  traveler's, 102-103
  V. cholerae serogroups O1 and
    O139, **100–108**

V. cholerae serogroups other
    than O1 and O139, **108–110**
V. parahaemolyticus enteritis,
    110–111
V. vulnificus infection, **111–113**
Choriomeningitis
  lymphocytic, **306–308**
Chromoblastomycosis, 113-114
Chromomycosis, **113–114**
Chronic wasting disease, 183
Chrysops spp., 300
Ciguatera fish poisoning, **209–210**
Circumcision
  disease susceptibility and, 4, 91
Cirrhosis
  as disease risk, 112
  hepatitis A, 251
  hepatitis B, 244
  hepatitis C, 252
Civets
  disease transmission by, 199
CJD. *See* Creutzfeldt-Jakob disease
Cladosporium carrionii, 113
Clams
  amnesic shellfish poisoning, 212
  diarrhetic shellfish poisoning,
    211
"Clap," 223-227
Classic typhus fever, 541-544
Clethrionomys spp., 232
Climatic bubo, 308-310
Clonorchiasis, **114–116**
Clonorchis sinensis, 115
Clostridium baratii, 71
Clostridium botulinum, 70-73
Clostridium butyricum, 71
Clostridium difficile, 154
Clostridium perfringens
  food intoxication, **206–207**
Clostridium tetani, 491
Clostridium welchii food
  poisoning, 206-207
CMV. *See* Cytomegalovirus
  infections
CNS syphilis, 481-482
Coccidioidal granuloma, 117-119

Coccidioides immitis, 117–118
Coccidioidomycosis, **117–119**
Cockle agent, 219
Cohorting, 466
Cold, common, **425–427**
Colitis
amebic, 11–12
Colorado tick fever, 35, **50–52**
Colorado tick fever virus, 35, 51
Common cold, **425–427**
Common wart, 548–550
Compost piles
as disease reservoir, 61
Condoms
for disease prevention, 5, 99,
127, 225, 260
Condyloma acuminatum, 548–550
Congenital disease. *See also*
Maternal-infant transmission
cytomegalovirus infection,
138–141
rubella, **435–440**
syphilis, 482
toxoplasmosis, **500–503**
Conidia, 61, 69, 264, 358
Conidiobolus spp., **563–564**
Conjunctivitis
Acanthamoeba, 359
acute bacterial, **119–121**
adenoviral hemorrhagic,
124–126
chlamydial, 97, **126–129,**
504–506
enteroviral hemorrhagic,
124–126
gonococcal, 223, **227–228**
keratoconjunctivitis, adenoviral,
122–124
Construction sites
as disease reservoir, 264–265
Contact lens
as disease risk, 360
Contagious ecthyma parapoxvirus,
367
Contagious pustular dermatitis,
367–368

Contraceptive devices
growth of *A. israelii,* 10
salpingitis risk, 224
TSS risk, 469
Coquillettidia spp., 41
Corneal infections. *See*
Keratoconjunctivitis
Coronary artery disease
chlamydial, 97
Coronaviruses, 426–427
Correctional facilities
hepatitis B risk, 249
Corynebacterium diphtheriae,
120, 166
Coryza, acute, 425–427
Cough, whooping, 375–379
Council of State and Territorial
Epidemiologists, 138
Counseling programs
HIV/AIDS prevention, 5–6
Cows. *See* Cattle
Coxiella burnetti, 408
Coxsackievirus carditis, **131–132**
Coxsackievirus diseases, **129–132**
Coxsackieviruses
A24 variant, 125
Group A, 427
Group B, 339, 356, 427
Crab lice, 372–374
Crabs
amnesic shellfish poisoning, 212
disease transmission, 371
Cranial neuritis, 302
Creeping eruption, 500
Creutzfeldt-Jakob disease,
183–186
new variant, 183–184
Crimean-Congo hemorrhagic
fever, **54–56**
Crimean-Congo hemorrhagic fever
virus, 35, 55
Crohn disease, 531
Cryptococcosis, **132–134**
Cryptococcus neoformans,
132–133
Cryptosporidiosis, **134–138**

Cryptosporidium parvum, 135
CSD. *See* Cat-scratch disease
CTF. *See* Colorado tick fever
Culex annulirostris, 38
Culex modestus, 49
Culex morsitans, 38
Culex pipiens molestus, 49
Culex quinquefasciatus, 199
Culex spp., 41, 46
Culex univittatus, 38, 49
Culicoides paraensis, 49
Culicoides spp., 34, 202
Culicoides-borne viral fevers,
   45–50
Culiseta melanura, 41
Cunninghamella spp., 562
Cutaneous anthrax, 20–24
Cutaneous diphtheria, 166,
   168-169
Cutaneous larva migrans, **500**
Cutaneous leishmaniasis, **284–287**
Cutting boards
   disease transmission, 80
Cyclops spp., 173
Cyclospora cayetanensis, 137
Cyclospora diarrhea, **137–138**
Cystic echinococcosis, 177–179
Cystic hydatid disease, 177–179
Cysticerciasis, 488–491
Cysticercosis, **488–491**
Cytomegalovirus disease, **138–141**
Cytomegalovirus infections,
   138–141
   "mono syndrome," 351

D

Dacca solution, 106
DAEC. *See* Diffuse-adherence *E.
   coli*
Dairy products. *See* Milk and milk
   products
DAT. *See* Diphtheria antitoxin

Day care centers
   disease transmission, 80, 96,
      135, 141, 157, 190, 216, 221,
      239, 343,
452
Deafness, 436
Deer
   chronic wasting disease, 183
   as disease reservoir, 156, 294,
      303, 367
Deer flies
   disease transmission by, 300,
      533
Deer fly fever, 532-535
Deer mice
   as disease reservoir, 63, 235
Dehydration. *See* Rehydration
   therapy
Dehydroemetine
   amoebiasis treatment, 14-15
Deinocerites spp., 46
Delhi boil, 284-287
Delta hepatitis, **253–255**
Dementia, 183-184
Democratic Republic of the Congo
   Ebola, 175
Dendritic ulcers, 261
Dengue fever, 29, **142–147**
Dengue hemorrhagic fever,
   145–147
Dengue shock syndrome, **145–147**
Dengue viruses, 31
Dental caries
   streptococcal, **477–478**
Dental plaque
   growth of *A. israelii,* 10
Dermacentor andersoni, 51
Dermacentor marginatus, 57
Dermacentor reticulatus, 57
Dermacentor spp., 431, 434
Dermal eruptions, 66
Dermatitis
   contagious pustular, 367-368
Dermatitis verrucosa, 113-114
Dermatomycosis, 147-153

Dermatophytosis, **147–153**
Desert fever, 117-119
Desert rheumatism, 117-119
Developing countries
  acute hemorrhagic
    conjunctivitis, 125
  AIDS case definition, 1
  incidence of AIDS, 3
  maternal–infant transmission of
    AIDS, 8
Devil's grippe, 356-357
DHF. *See* Dengue hemorrhagic
  fever
Dhori virus, 36
Diabetes mellitus
  candidiasis and, 82
  as disease risk, 282
Dialysis centers
  hepatitis B risk, 245, 249
Diaphragm, contraceptive
  as disease risk, 469
Diarrhea
  acute, **154**
  amebic dysentery, 11
  balantidial, 65
  C. perfringens, 206-207
  Campylobacter and, 79
  cholera and, 100-113
  clonorchiasis, 114-115
  cryptosporidial, 134
  Cyclospora and, **137–138**
  E. coli and, **155–165**
  enteritis, *V. parahaemolyticus*,
    110-111
  epidemic, 218-220
  foodborne diseases and,
    203-211
  Giardia, 220-221
  Helicobacter, 213
  rotaviral, 215-217
  salmonellosis, 440
  schistosomiasis, 447
  shigellosis, 451-455
  travelers', 79, 109, 158-159, 216
  treatment solution, 106
  viral gastroenteritis, 218
  yersiniosis, 558-561

Diarrhetic shellfish poisoning, **211**
Dibothriocephaliasis, 171-172
Diffuse-adherence *E. coli*, **165**
Diloxanide furoate
  amoebiasis treatment, 14-15
Dinophysis acuminata, 211
Dinophysis fortii, 211
Dipetalonema spp., 300
Diphasic milk fever, 43-44
Diphteria, **165–170**
Diphteria antitoxin, 169-170
Diphyllobothriasis, **171–172**
Diphyllobothrium spp., 171
Dipylidiasis, **270**
Dipylidium caninum, 270
Dirofilaria spp., 201
Dirofilariasis, 201
Disinfection
  AIDS prevention, 7
Disseminated disease, 531
Ditchling agent, 219
Diural subperiodicity, 198-199
Division of Disease Surveillance,
  138
Dobrava virus, 231-232
Dogs
  as disease reservoir, 148, 171,
    177-180, 196, 201, 204, 266,
    285, 288, 294, 303, 371, 408,
    412-413, 433, 441, 479,
    497-500
  disease transmission by, 76,
    79-80, 87, 89-90, 115
Dog-tapeworm infection, 270
Domoic acid, 212
Donkeys
  as disease reservoir, 337-338
Donovania granulomatis, 229
Donovanosis, 229-230
Dorsal root ganglia, 92
"Dose," 223-227
Down syndrome
  as risk for disease, 247
Dracontiasis, 172-174
Dracunculiasis, **172–174**
Dracunculus medinensis, 172

Drug abuse
  AIDS and, 3, 5
  botulinum infection and, 72
  hepatitis A risk, 239-241
  hepatitis B risk, 245-246
  hepatitis D risk, 254
  tetanus and, 491-492
DSS. *See* Dengue shock syndrome
Ducrey bacillus. *See Haemophilus*
    ducreyi
Dugbe virus, 35, 51
Duodenal ulcer disease, 213
Dust. *See also* Soil
  control measures, 118-119
  disease transmission by, 118,
    187, 264, 336, 362
  preventive measures, 264
Dwarf tapeworm infection,
  268-269
Dysentery
  amebic, 11, 14
  bacillary, 451-455
  balantidial, 65-66

E

EAggEC. *See* Enteroaggregative *E.*
    coli
Eastern equine encephalitis, 39-43
Eastern equine encephalomyelitis
  virus, 30
Ebola virus hemorrhagic fever,
  174-176
Ebola-Marburg viral diseases,
  174-176
EBV. *See* Epstein-Barr virus
Echinococcosis, **176-180**
  cystic, 177-179
  multilocular, 179-180
  polycystic hydatid disease, 180
  unilocular, 177-179
Echinococcus granulosus,
  177-179

Echinococcus multilocularis,
  179-180
Echinococcus spp., 176
Echinococcus vogeli, 180
Echoviruses, 339, 356, 427
Ecthyma contagiosum, 367-368
Ectopic pregnancy, 98
Edema
  malignant, 20-25
  pulmonary, 235
Edge Hill virus, 31
Education
  amoebiasis prevention, 13
  anthrax transmission, 22
  brucellosis prevention, 77
  health education, 99
  HIV/AIDS prevention, 5
  home canning, 73
  oral hygiene, 11
  personal hygiene, 13, 59, 65
  sex education, 99, 484
Eggs and egg products
  disease transmission by,
    441-443, 474
EHEC. *See* Enterohemorrhagic *E.*
    coli
Ehrlichia chaffeensis, 181
Ehrlichia equi, 181
Ehrlichia ewingi, 181-182
Ehrlichia phagocytophila, 181
Ehrlichia sennetsu, 181
Ehrlichiosis, **181-183**
EIEC. *See* Enteroinvasive *E. coli*
EKC. *See* Epidemic
  keratoconjunctivitis
El Tor biotype *(V. cholerae),*
  100-104
Elderly persons
E. coli caused diarrhea and, 156
  encephalitis risk, 40-41
  herpes zoster, 92, 94
  postherpetic neuralgia, 92
Electrolyte solution, 106, 146, 158,
  218
Elephantiasis, 198-199, 308

Elk
  chronic wasting disease, 183
EM. *See* Erythema migrans
Encephalitides, arthropod-borne
  viral, **39–43**
Encephalitides, tickborne viral,
  43–45
Encephalitis
  arboviral, 28
  arthropod-borne viral diseases
    and, 28–29
  herpes simplex, 261
  mosquito-borne, 39–43
  tickborne, 43–45, 57
  viral, 236
Encephalopathy
  bovine spongiform, 183
  loa loa, 301
  mink, transmissible, 183
  subacute spongiform, **183–186**
Endemic Burkitt lymphoma, 325
Endemic fleaborne typhus fever,
  544–545
Endemic syphilis, nonvenereal,
  486–487
Endocarditis, 223, 408
  infective, 166
  staphylococcal, **461–464**
Entamoeba dispar, 12, 32
Entamoeba histolytica, 12, 14–15,
  360
Enteric fever, 535–541
Enterically transmitted non-A
  non-B hepatitis, 255–257
Enteritis
  enteropathogenic *E. coli*,
    161–164
  epidemic viral
    gastroenteropathy, **218–220**
  Giardia, 220–222
  necrotizing, 206
  rotaviral, **215–218**
  Vibrio parahaemolyticus,
    110–111
Enteritis necroticans, 206–207
Enteroaggregative *E. coli*, **164–165**
Enterobiasis, **186–188**

Enterobius vermicularis, 187
Enterocolitis
  salmonellosis and, 440, 444
Enterohemorrhagic *E. coli*,
  155–158
Enteroinvasive *E. coli*, **160–161**
Enteropathogenic *E. coli*, **161–164**
Enteropathogenic *E. coli* enteritis,
  161–164
Enterotoxigenic *E. coli*, **158–160**
Enteroviral carditis, 131–132
Enteroviral hemorrhagic
  conjunctivitis, **124–126**
Enteroviral lymphonodular
  pharyngitis, **129–131**
Enteroviral vesicular pharyngitis,
  129–131
Enteroviral vesicular stomatitis
  with exanthem, **129–131**
Enterovirus 70, 125
Enteroviruses, 339, 400
Entomophthoramycosis, **563–564**
Eosinophilia
  capillariasis, 85
  tropical pulmonary, 198
Eosinophilic meningitis, 15–17
Eosinophilic meningoencephalitis,
  15–17
EPEC. *See* Enteropathogenic *E. coli*
EPI. *See* Expanded Programme on
  Immunizations
Epidemic arthritic erythema,
  420–421
Epidemic hemorrhagic fever,
  231–234
Epidemic hepatitis, 238–243
Epidemic keratoconjunctivitis,
  122–124
Epidemic non-A non-B hepatitis,
  255–257
Epidemic pleurodynia, 356–357
Epidemic polyarthritis, 37–39
Epidemic viral gastroenteritis,
  218–220
Epidemic viral gastroenteropathy,
  218–220

Epidemics. *See also specific disease by name*
acute hemorrhagic conjunctivitis, 125
arthropod-borne viral hemorrhagic fevers, 57
balantidiasis, 65
capillariasis, 84
cholera, 101–103
conjunctivitis, 120
dengue hemorrhagic fever, 146
diphtheria, 166–167
enteropathogenic *E. coli* enteritis, 164
Hepatitis A, 239
HIV, 3
influenza, 270–272
meningitis, 341
pneumonia, 391
reporting, xxvii
rubella, 436–437
salmonellosis, 441–442
TB, 523
tinea capitis, 148–149
trench fever, 507
Epidermophyton floccosum, 150–151
Epidermophytosis, 147–153
Epididymitis, 97
Epilepsy
focal, 43
Epithelial keratitis, 124
EP-NANB. *See* Enterically transmitted non-A non-B hepatitis
Epstein-Barr virus
Burkitt lymphoma and, 325
Kaposi's sarcoma and, 327–329
malignancies related to, **326–329**
mononucleosis, 350–352
non-Hodgkin's lymphomas and, 327
NPC and, 326–327
Equine encephalitis, 39–43, 45–47
Eriocheir spp., 371
Erysipelas, 470–476

Erythema, epidemic arthritic, 420–421
Erythema infectiosum, **189–191**
Erythema migrans, 302–303, 305
Erythema nodosum leprosum, 289
Eschars, 432–433, 545
Escherichia coli, 348
diarrhea caused by, **155–165**
diffuse-adherence strains, **165**
E. coli O157:H7, 155–158
enteroaggregative strains, **164–165**
enterohemorrhagic strains, **155–158**
enteroinvasive strains, **160–161**
enteropathogenic strains, **161–164**
enterotoxigenic strains, **158–160**
Esophagus
candidiasis, 81–83
Espundia, 284–287
ETEC. *See* Enterotoxigenic *E. coli*
Eumycetoma, **357–359**
European encephalitis viruses, 31
Everglades virus, 30
Exanthem
enteroviral vesicular stomatitis and, 129–131
Exanthem subitum, **191–193**
Exanthematicus, typhus, 541–544
Exophiala spp., 113, 358
Expanded Programme on Immunizations
vaccines for HIV-infected children, 6
Extraintestinal yersiniosis, **558–561**
Eye infections. *See* Conjunctivitis
Eyeworm disease of Africa, 299–301

F

Falciparum malaria, 310–317, 321
Familial insomnia, fatal, 183
Far Eastern encephalitis/viruses, 31

Far Eastern tickborne encephalitis, 43-45

Farm workers. *See* Agricultural workers

Fasciola gigantica, 194

Fasciola hepatica, 194-195

Fascioliasis, **193-195**

Fasciolopsiasis, **195-197**

Fasciolopsis buski, 196

Fatal familial insomnia, 183

Fatality rates. *See* Case-fatality rates

Faucial diphtheria, 166

Favus, 147-149

FBI. *See* Federal Bureau of Investigation

FDA. *See* Food and Drug Administration

Febrile mucocutaneous lymph node syndrome, 276-278

Febrile respiratory disease, acute, **427-430**

Fecal contamination of food or water. *See* Food, fecal contamination; Water, fecal contamination

Fecal-oral disease transmission, 135, 213, 216, 219, 221, 239-241, 256, 268, 356, 401, 428, 441, 452, 489, 559

Fecal-oral non-A non-B hepatitis, 255-257

Feces
disease transmission by, 58-59, 65, 79-80, 82, 86, 130, 156, 221-222, 239-240, 497-499
preventing contamination of food and water, 13, 81, 222

Federal Bureau of Investigation bioterrorism investigation, 24-25

Feet
ringworm infection, 151-152

Felidae, 180

Fifth disease, 189-191

Filariasis, **197-202**
Bancroftian, 197-201
Brugian, 197-201
Malayan, 197-201
other nematode-produced microfilariae, 201-202
Timorean, 197-201
zoonotic, 201

Filarioidea, 197

Filiform warts, 548

Filobasidiella neoformans, 133

Filoviridae, 175

Fish
ciguatera fish poisoning, **209-210**
as disease reservoir, 18, 71, 72, 84-85
raw or undertreated, 18, 84-85, 103, 109-113, 115-116, 171-172, 219, 239, 371, 499
scombroid fish poisoning, **209**

Fish tapeworm infection, 171-172

Flat papillomas, 548

Flat warts, 548

Flaviviridae, 29, 31-32, 40, 252, 554

Flaviviruses, 29, 31-32, 40, 48, 57, 142, 554

Flea-borne diseases
control of, 383-385
plague, 381-387
transmission among cats, 88
typhus fever, 544-545

"Flesh-eating bacteria," 472

Flies
disease transmission by, 120, 364, 505, 514-516
preventive measures, 365

Floors
disease transmission by, 150-153

"Floppy baby," 70

Fluid replacement therapy, 105-106, 146-147, 158

Focal epilepsy, 43

Fonsecaea spp., 113

Food. *See also* Milk and milk
   products
   aflatoxins, 61
   bulging lids, 73
   eggs and egg products, 441–443
   fecal contamination, 13-14, 65,
      103, 159, 178, 206, 268,
      441-443, 537, 559
   fish, 18, 84–85, 115–116,
      171-172, 209–210, 499
   improper processing or storage,
      71
   irradiation, 19, 80, 157, 209
   meat pies, 206–207
   preventive measures, 16, 80,
      203
   raw meat, 489, 501, 509
   raw or undertreated fish and
      shellfish, 18, 84–85, 103,
      109-113, 115- 116, 171-172,
      219, 239, 371, 499
   rice, 208
   Safe Food Preparation Rules, 203
   seafood, 103, 109-113
   shellfish, 219, 239, 371
   unpasteurized milk, 44, 76–77,
      79, 156, 167
Food and Drug Administration
   Food Code, 157
   regulations for the prevention of
      HIV contamination of blood
      products, 6
   Treatment Investigational New
      Drug protocol, 74
Food handlers
   disease transmission by, 14, 80,
      157, 169, 204-205, 239, 442
   education and supervision, 65,
      110-111, 205, 442-443
Food poisoning. *See also*
   Food-borne diseases
   intestinal anthrax and, 20
Food Safety Inspection Service,
   157
Food-borne diseases, **202–212**
   amnesic shellfish poisoning, **212**
   Bacillus cereus, **207–208**

botulism, 70–75
   Campylobacter enteritis, 79
   ciguatera fish poisoning,
      209–210
   Clostridium perfringens,
      206–207
   diarrhetic shellfish poisoning,
      211
   listeriosis, 296-299
   neurotoxic shellfish poisoning,
      211
   paralytic shellfish poisoning,
      210–211
   puffer-fish poisoning, **212**
   salmonellosis, 440-444
   scombroid fish poisoning, **209**
   staphylococcal food
      intoxication, **203–206**
   streptococcal, 474
Fort Sherman virus, 33
Foxes
   as disease reservoir, 180, 263,
      294, 412
Frambesia tropica, 550-553
Francis disease, 532-535
Francisella tularensis, 533
Frozen fish
   undertreated, 18
Fruits
   disease transmission by, 239,
      441-442
Fugitive swelling, 300
Fungus balls, 60–61
Funisciurus spp., 458
Furuncles, staphylococcal,
   461–464

G

Gabon and Sudan Ebola, 175
Gambiense disease, 515
Gambierdiscus toxicus, 210
Gammaherpesviral mononucleosis,
   350-352
Gammaherpesvirus, 328
GanGan virus, 34

Gastritis
  caused by *H. pylori,* 212–215
Gastroenteritis
  acute infectious nonbacterial,
    218-220
  acute viral, **215–220**
  epidemic viral
    gastroenteropathy, **218–220**
  rotaviral, **215–218**
  V. cholerae, 108-110
Gastroenteropathy
  epidemic viral, **218–220**
GBS. *See* Guillain Barré syndrome
GC. *See* Gonococcal infections
Genital herpes, 258, 260-261
Genital infections
  chancroid, 90-91
  chlamydial, **97–99**
Gerbils
  as disease reservoir, 53, 84, 286
German measles, 435–440
Germiston virus, 33
Gerstmann-Sträussler-Scheinker
  syndrome, 183
Giardia enteritis, 220-222
Giardia lamblia, 220-221
Giardiasis, **220–222**
Gilchrist disease, 68-70
Glanders, **337–338**
Glandular fever, 350-352
"Gleet," 223-227
Global Polio Eradication
  Laboratory Network, 404
Glomerulonephritis, 445
Glossina spp., 515-516
Gnathostoma spinigerum, 499
Gnathostomiasis, **499**
Gnats
  disease transmission by, 46, 120
Goat hair
  anthrax hazard, 20-24
Goats. *See also* Milk and milk
  products
  as disease reservoir, 367, 408
  scrapie, 183
Gonococcal infections, **223–228**
  cervicitis, **223–227**

conjunctivitis, 120, **227–228**
  neonatorum, **227–228**
  urethritis, **223–227**
Gonorrhea, 98, **223–227**
Granulocytic ehrlichiosis, 181
Granuloma inguinale, **229–230**
Granulomatous amebic
  encephalitis, 359
Granulomatous lymphadenitis, 87
Gravlax
  undertreated, 18
Groin
  ringworm infection, 149-151
Ground meat. *See* Meat and meat
  products
Group A streptococci, **470–476**
Group B streptococci
  sepsis of the newborn, **477**
Group C arboviruses, 32
Group C virus disease, **48–50**
GSS. *See*
  Gerstmann-Sträussler-Scheinker
  syndrome
Guama group arboviruses, 34
Guama virus, 34
Guanarito hemorrhagic fever,
  26–28
Guanarito virus, 26-27
Guaroa virus, 33
Guillain Barré syndrome, 79, 273,
  399
Guinea-worm infection, 172-174
Gymnodinium breve, 211

H

HA. *See* Hepatitis A
Haemagogus spp., 38, 46
Haemaphysalis spinigera, 57
Haemaphysalis spp., 434
Haemophilus ducreyi, 90-91
Haemophilus influenzae,
  343-344
  biogroup *aegyptius,* 120
  meningitis, 345-347
  type b, 120, 167-168, 346
Haemophilus meningitis, **345–347**

Hair
  ringworm infection, 147–149
Hairy cell leukemia, 329
Hamburger. *See* Meat and meat
  products
Hamsters
  as disease reservoir, 307–308
Hand, foot and mouth disease,
  129–131
"Hanging groin," 363
Hansen's disease, 289–293
Hantaan virus, 231–232
Hantaviral diseases, **230–236**
  adult respiratory distress
    syndrome, 234–236
  cardiopulmonary syndrome,
    234–236
  hemorrhagic fever with renal
    syndrome, **231–234**
  pulmonary syndrome, **234–236**
Hard measles, 330–335
Hares
  as disease reservoir, 55
HAV. *See* Hepatitis A virus
Haverhill fever, 420–421
Hawaii agent, 219
HB. *See* Hepatitis B
HBIG. *See* Hepatitis B
  immunoglobulin
HBV. *See* Hepatitis B virus
HCC. *See* Hepatocellular
  carcinoma
HCV. *See* Hepatitis C virus
HCV infection, 251–253
HCWs. *See* Health care workers
HDV. *See* Hepatitis D virus
Head lice, 372–374
Health care workers
  AIDS protection, 6, 8–9
  AIDS transmission, 4
  CMV protection, 141
  diphtheria immunization, 168
  hepatitis B risk, 245, 249
  herpes simplex virus, 259
Health education, 99
Hearing loss, 353

Heart disease
  coxsackievirus carditis, 131–132
Heartworms, 201
Helicobacter pylori, 323
  gastritis, **212–215**
Helicobacter spp., 213
Heliosciurus spp., 458
Hemochromatosis, 111–112
Hemodialysis
  as disease risk, 247
Hemolysis, 322
Hemolytic uremic syndrome, 155,
  451
Hemophilia
  as disease risk, 254, 328
Hemorrhagic conjunctivitis,
  124–126
Hemorrhagic fevers
  arenaviral, South American, 26–28
  arthropod-borne viral, 28–29,
    54–58
  dengue, 145–147
  with renal syndrome, **231–234**
Hemorrhagic jaundice, 293–296
Hemorrhagic nephrosonephritis,
  231–234
Hemorrhagic sarcoma, **327–329**
Henderson–Paterson bodies, 349
Hendra viral disease, **236–238**
HEPA filters. *See* High–efficiency
  particle air filters
Hepacaviruses, 252
Hepadnaviruses, 244–246
Hepatic capillariasis, 85–86
Hepaticola hepatica, 85
Hepatitis
  delta, **253–255**
  epidemic, 238–243
  infectious, 238–243
  non-B transfusion associated,
    251–253
  parenterally transmitted non-A
    non-B, 251–253
  posttransfusion non-A non-B,
    251–253
  Type A, 238–243
  viral, **238–257**

Hepatitis A, **238–243**
Hepatitis A virus, 238–239
Hepatitis B, **243–251**
Hepatitis B immunoglobulin, 247–250, 325
Hepatitis B virus, 243–251, 324
Hepatitis C, **251–253**
Hepatitis C virus, 251–253, 324
Hepatitis D virus, 253–255
Hepatitis E, **255–257**
Hepatitis E virus, 255–257
Hepatocellular carcinoma, 244, 252, **324–325**. See also Cancer
Hepatoviruses, 239
Herpangina, 129–131
Herpes labialis, 258
Herpes simplex, **257–262**
  anogenital herpesviral infections, **257–261**
  meningoencephalitis due to cercopithecine herpes virus 1, **261–262**
Herpes simplex virus
  types 1 and 2, 257–258
Herpes zoster, **92–97**
Herpesviridae, 139, 259
Herpesvirus saimiri, 328
Herpesvirus simplex, 100
Herpesvirus type 6, 351
Herpesviruses, 93, 139
Herpetic keratitis, 261
Herpetic whitlow, 259, 261
Herring
  undertreated, 18
Heterophiles, 350–351
HEV. See Hepatitis E virus
HGE. See Human granulocytic ehrlichiosis
HHV-6B. See Human herpesvirus 6B
Hide processing
  anthrax hazard, 20–24
High-efficiency particle air filters, 25, 62

Hikojima serotype *(V. cholerae),* 101
Histamine poisoning
  from fish, 209
Histoplasma capsulatum
  infection, **262–265**
Histoplasmosis, **262–265**
  capsulati, 261–265
  duboisii, **265**
HIV. See Acquired immunodeficiency syndrome; Human immunodeficiency virus
HME. See Human monocytic ehrlichiosis
Hodgkin's disease, **326–327**
  as risk for disease, 133
Home-canned foods
  botulism transmission, 72–73, 75
Homologous serum jaundice, 243–251
Homosexuality
  amoebiasis and, 11–12
  chlamydial infections, 97
  CMV infections, 140
  cryptosporidiosis risk, 135
  gonococcal infection, 223
Helicobacter diarrhea, 213
  hepatitis A risk, 239–241
  hepatitis B risk, 245–246, 249
  hepatitis D risk, 254
  incidence of AIDS and, 3
  Kaposi's sarcoma risk, 328
  LGV risk, 308–309
  shigellosis risk, 451
  syphilis risk, 482
Honey
  as botulism reservoir, 72–73
Hookworm disease, 60, **265–268,** 500
Horses
  as disease reservoir, 236–237, 263, 303, 337–338, 492
  equine encephalitis, 39–43, 45–47

Hospitals
  cohorting, 466
  disease transmission, 80
  staphylococcal diseases in
      nurseries, 464–467
  staphylococcal diseases on
      medical and surgical wards,
      467–469
HPV. *See* Human papillomaviruses
HSV. *See* Herpes simplex virus
HTLV. *See* Human T-cell
  lymphotropic virus
Human ehrlichiosis, 181–183
Human granulocytic ehrlichiosis,
  181
Human herpesvirus 3, 93
Human herpesvirus 5, 139
Human herpesvirus 6, 192
Human herpesvirus 7, 192
Human herpesvirus 8, 324, 328
Human herpesvirus 6B, 191–192
Human herpesviruses 1 and 2,
  257–261
Human immunodeficiency virus
  (HIV). *See also* Acquired
  immunodeficiency syndrome
  chancroid ulcers and, 90
  counseling programs, 5–6
  HIV infection, 1
  human T-cell leukemia and, 324
  interaction with *Mycobacterium
      tuberculosis*, 4–5
  Kaposi's sarcoma and, 328
  mononucleosis-like illness, 351
  non-Hodgkin's lymphomas and,
      327
  oropharyngeal infection and, 82
  postexposure prophylaxis, 8–9
  proportion of untreated persons
      who develop AIDS, 1
  as risk for disease, 118, 133, 247
  serologic tests, 2
  TB and, 521, 527
  testing, 5
Human monocytic ehrlichiosis,
  181
Human orf, 367–368

Human papillomaviruses, 324, 329,
  548
Human parvovirus infection,
  189–191
Human T-cell lymphotropic virus,
  324
HUS. *See* Hemolytic uremic
  syndrome
Hyalomma spp., 55
Hydatid diseases, 177–180
Hydraxes
  as disease reservoir, 285
Hydrophobia, 411–419
Hygiene. *See* Oral hygiene;
  Personal hygiene
Hymenolepiasis, 268–270
Hymenolepis diminuta, 269–270
Hymenolepis nana, 268–269
Hypochlorhydria, 156
Hypovolemic shock, 106

I

Idiopathic multiple pigmented
  hemorrhagic sarcoma, 327–329
IG. *See* Immune globulin
Ilesha virus, 33
Ilheus virus, 31
Immune globulin, 241–243,
  277–278, 429
Immunization Practices Advisory
  Committee, 457
Immunizations. *See also* Vaccines
  pediatric schedule, 168, 217,
      248, 332, 354–355, 377, 402,
      438, 493
Immunosuppression
  as disease risk, 110, 112, 118,
      244, 282, 298, 327, 350
Impetigo
  staphylococcal, 461–464
  streptococcal, 470–476
Impetigo neonatorum, 464–467
Inaba serotype *(V. cholerae),*
  101–103
Inclusion conjunctivitis, 126–129

Incubation period. *See also specific disease by name*
Indeterminate leprosy, 289
India tick typhus, 432–433
Indiana vesicular stomatitis virus, 36
Indirect fluorescent antibody test for HIV antibodies, 2
Infant botulism. *See* Intestinal botulism
Infant diarrhea, 161–165
Infant formula, contaminated, 162–163
Infant pneumonia, 97
Infantile paralysis, 398–405
Infants. *See also* Breast feeding; Children; Maternal–infant transmission; Neonates
  botulism, 72–73
  CMV infections, 138–140
  conjunctivitis, 120
  encephalitis risk, 41
  enteroaggregative *E. coli* diarrhea, 164–165
  enteropathogenic *E. coli* enteritis, 161–164
  "floppy baby," 70
  HIV infection, 1, 2, 4
  severe viral gastroenteritis, 215–218
  thrush, 82–83
Infectious hepatitis, 238–243
Infectious parotitis, 353–355
Infertility, 97–98
Inflammatory bowel disease confusion with amebic colitis, 12
Influenza, **270–276**
Inhalation anthrax, 20–24
Inkoo virus, 33
Insomnia fatal familial, 183
International Certificate of Vaccination against Yellow Fever, 558

International Health Regulations, 104, 108, 384, 386, 557
International issues
  AIDS prevention and care program, 9
  cholera immunization, 108
  Global Polio Eradication Laboratory Network, 404
International Travel and Health, 315
Internet. *See* Web sites
Interstitial plasma–cell pneumonia, 392–394
Intertrigo, 81–82
Intestinal anthrax, 20–21
Intestinal botulism, **70–75**
Intestinal capillariasis, 84–85
Intestinal disease amoebiasis, 11
Intestinal yersiniosis, **558–561**
Intrauterine contraceptive devices
  growth of *A. israelii,* 10
  salpingitis risk, 224
Intravenous immune globulin, 277–278
Intussusception, 217
Iodine treatment of water, 13
Iodoquinol amoebiasis treatment, 14
Irradiation of food
  disease prevention, 80
  fish, 19
  meat, 157
Israeli tick typhus, 432–433
Issyk-Kul virus, 35
Itaqui virus, 32, 48
IVIG. *See* Intravenous immune globulin
Ivory Coast Ebola, 175
Ixodes cookei, 44
Ixodes pacificus, 303
Ixodes persulcatus, 44, 303
Ixodes ricinus, 44, 63, 303
Ixodes scapularis, 63, 182, 303
Ixodes spp., 434
Izumi fever, 558

J

Jakob-Creutzfeldt disease, 183-186
Jamestown Canyon encephalitis, 39-43
Jamestown Canyon virus, 33
Japanese encephalitis, 39-43
Japanese encephalitis virus, 31
Jaundice. *See also* Hepatitis
    arthropod-borne viral diseases and, 28
    epidemic, 238-243
    homologous serum, 243-251
    mononucleosis and, 350
Jellison organisms, 532
Junín hemorrhagic fever, 26-28
Junin virus, 26-27
Juquitiba virus, 234
Jurona virus, 36

K

Kala-azar, 287-289
Kaposi's sarcoma, **327–329**
Kaposi's sarcoma associated herpesvirus, 324, 328
Karelian fever, 37-39
Karshi virus, 31
Kasokero virus, 35
Katayama fever, 449
Kawasaki syndrome, **276–278**
Keloidal blastomycosis, 369
Kemerovo group arboviruses, 35
Kemerovo virus, 35, 51
Kenya tick typhus, 432-433
Keratitis. *See also* Conjunctivitis
    epithelial, 124
    herpetic, 261
    keratoconjunctivitis, adenoviral, **122–124**
Keratoconjunctivitis
    Acanthamoeba, 359
    adenoviral, **122–124**
Kerion, 147-149
Keterah virus, 35
Kittens. *See* Cats

Klebsiella-Enterobacter-Serratia group, 348
Koch-Weeks bacillus, 120
Kokobera virus, 31
Korean hemorrhagic fever, 231-234
Koutango virus, 31
KSHV. *See* Kaposi's sarcoma associated herpesvirus
Kunjin virus, 48
Kuru, 183, 186
Kwashiorkor, 330
Kyasanur Forest disease, **56–58**
Kyasanur Forest disease virus, 31

L

Laboratory Center for Disease Control, 138
Laboratory workers
    anthrax hazard, 21-22
    arthropod-borne viral diseases and, 29
    listeriosis hazard, 297
LaCrosse encephalitis, 39-43
LaCrosse virus, 33
Laguna Negra virus, 234
Larva migrans cutaneous, 500
Larva migrans visceralis, 497-499
Laryngeal papillomas, 548
Laryngitis
    viral, 424-430
Lassa fever, **278–281**
    relation to arenaviral hemorrhagic fever, 26
LCM. *See* Lymphocytic choriomeningitis
LeDantec group arboviruses, 36
LeDantec virus, 36
Legionella spp., 281-282
Legionellosis, **281–283**
Legionnaires' disease, 281-283
Legionnaires' pneumonia, 281-283
Leishman-Donovan bodies, 287
Leishmania spp., 284-285, 287
Leishmaniasis
    cutaneous, **284–287**

mucosal, **284–287**
visceral, **287–289**
Leishmaniasis recidivans, 284
"Leopard skin," 363
Lepromatous leprosy, 289–292
Lepromin test, 291
Leprosy, **289–293**
Leptosphaeria spp., 358
Leptospira spp., 294, 339
Leptospires, 294
Leptospirosis, **293–296**
Leptotrombidium spp., 546
Leukemia
  adult T-cell, 329
  chickenpox risk, 92, 94
  hairy cell, 329
  lymphatic tissue, malignancy,
    329
Leukocytosis, 391
Leukopenia, 330, 435
LGV. *See* Lymphogranuloma
  venereum
Lice, 372–374. *See also*
  Louseborne diseases
  preventive measures, 507–508
Liponyssoides sanguineus, 435
Lipovnik virus, 51
Listeria monocytogenes, 297–298,
  348
Listeriosis, **296–299**
Liver abscesses
  amoebiasis and, 11–12, 14
Liver cancer, 251, **324–325**
Liver cysts
  echinococcosis and, 176–180
Liver disease
  as disease risk, 110–113, 238
  hepatitis B, 244
Loa loa, 201
Loa loa infection, 299–301
Lobo disease, 369
Loboa loboi, 369
Lockjaw, 491–495
Loiasis, **299–301**
Louping ill, 43–45, 57
Louping ill virus, 31
Louseborne diseases

relapsing fever, 421–424
trench fever, 506–508
typhus fever, **541–544**
Lues, 481–486
Lung disease. *See also* Respiratory
  disease
  aspergillosis and, 60–61
  as disease risk, 282
Lung fluke disease, 370–372
Lutzomyia spp., 53, 67
Lutzomyia verrucarum, 67
Lyme borreliosis, 302–306
Lyme disease, **302–306**
Lymnaeidae, 194
Lymphadenitis, 531
Lymphadenitis, granulomatous, 87
Lymphatic tissue
  malignancy, **329**
Lymphocytic choriomeningitis,
  306–308
  relation to arenaviral
    hemorrhagic fever, 26
Lymphocytosis, 351
Lymphogranuloma inguinale,
  308–310
Lymphogranuloma venereum, 97,
  308–310
Lymphomas
  Burkitt, **325**
  lymphatic tissue, malignancy,
    329
  non-Hodgkin's, **327**
  peripheral T-cell, 329
Lymphonodular pharyngitis,
  129–131
Lymphoproliferative
  as risk for disease, 247
Lymphosarcoma, T-cell, 329
Lyssa, 411–419
Lyssavirus, 411

M

Macacca fascicularis, 176
Macaques
  as disease reservoir, 256,
    261–262

Machupo hemorrhagic fever, 26–28
Machupo virus, 26–27
Mad cow disease, 183
Madrid virus, 32, 48
Madura foot, 357–359
Madurella spp., 358
Maduromycosis, 357–359
Malaria, **310–323**
  community based preventive measures, 313–315
  control of patient, contacts and environment, 320–322
  disaster implications, 322–323
  epidemic measures, 322
  identification, 310–311
  incubation periods, 313
  infectious agents, 311
  methods of control, 313–322
  mode of transmission, 312–313
  occurrence, 311
  period of communicability, 313
  personal protective measures, 315–320
  preventive measures, 313–320
  reservoir, 312
  susceptibility and resistance, 313
Malariae malaria, 310–314
Malayan filariasis, 197–201
Malignant edema, 20–25
Malignant neoplasms, **323–329**
  Burkitt lymphoma, **324–325**
  cervical cancer, **329**
  hepatocellular carcinoma, **324–325**
  Hodgkin's disease, **326–327**
  Kaposi's sarcoma, **327–329**
  lymphatic tissue, malignancy, **329**
  nasopharyngeal carcinoma, **325–326**
  non–Hodgkin's lymphomas, **327**
Malignant pustule, 20–25
Malignant tertian malaria, 310
Malnutrition
  as contributor to disease, 16

Malta fever, 75–78
Mammals. *See also* Animals
  as disease reservoir, 87
Mansonella spp., 202, 300
Mansonia spp., 38, 46, 199–200
Mantoux method, 527
Mapputta group arboviruses, 34
Marburg virus disease, 174–176
Marinated fish
  undertreated, 18
Marine mammals
  as disease reservoir, 71
Marituba virus, 32, 48
Marseilles fever, 432–433
Mastitis, 353
Mastomys spp., 279, 281
Maternal–infant transmission. *See also* Breast feeding
  AIDS, 4, 8
  babcsiosis, 63
  candidiasis, 82
  chickenpox, 96
  chlamydia, 97–98, 126–129
  chlamydial pneumonia, 394–396
  CMV infections, 138–140
  conjunctivitis, 126–129, 227–228
  dental caries, 478
  erythema infectiosum, 189–190
  gonococcal conjunctivitis, 227–228
  HBV, 325
  hepatitis B, 244, 246
  herpes simplex virus, 258–260
  listeriosis, 296–298
  lymphocytic choriomeningitis, 307
  malaria, 313
  rubella, 436
  syphilis, 482–483
  tetanus, neonatal, 495–496
  warts, 549
Mayaro virus, 30
Mayaro virus disease, 37–39
Mazzotti reaction, 364
Measles, **330–335**
"Measly pork," 489

Meat and meat products
  contaminated, 204, 206-207,
    441-443
  as disease reservoir, 71, 298
  irradiation of, 157
  meat pies, 206-207
  undercooked, 21, 79, 156, 489,
    501, 509
Medical workers
  arthropod-borne hemorrhagic
    fever risk, 55
  disease transmission by,
    122-123
Mediterranean fever, 75-78
Mediterranean spotted fever,
  432-433
Mediterranean tick fever, 432-433
Melanoconion spp., 46, 49
Melioidosis, **335-337**
Meningitis, **338-348**
  arthropod-borne viral diseases
    and, 28
  aseptic, 28, 39, 302
  bacterial, **340**
Campylobacter enteritis and, 79
  coccidioidal, 117
  cryptococcal, 132
  eosinophilic, 15-17
Haemophilus, **345-347**
  lymphocytic, 306-308
  meningococcal, **340-345**
  neonatal, **348**
  pneumococcal, **348**
  syphilic, 481
  viral, **338-340**
Meningococcal meningitis,
  340-345
Meningococcemia, 340
Meningoencephalitis
  cercopithecine herpes virus-1,
    261-262
  diphasic, 43
  eosinophilic, 15-17
  listeriosis, 296
  loiasis and, 301

lymphocytic choriomeningitis,
    307
  primary amebic, 359-362
Menstrual TSS, 469-470
Metronidazole
  amoebiasis treatment, 14-15
Microfilariae, 197-202, 299-301,
    363-366
Micropannus, 126
Microsporosis, 147-153
Microsporum audouinii, 148
Microsporum canis, 148
Microsporum spp., 150
Microtus pennsylvanicus, 63
Midges
  arthropod-borne viral disease
    vectors, 29, 53
Midwives, 496
Migrant workers. *See* Occupational
  risk of disease
Military personnel
  acute viral respiratory disease,
    428
  anthrax vaccination, 22
  coccidioidomycosis risk, 118
  leptospirosis risk, 294
  meningitis risk, 341-342
  pneumonia risk, 391
  trench fever risk, 507
Milk and milk products
  contaminated, 204, 474, 501
  disease transmission by,
    297-298
  unpasteurized, 44, 76-77, 79,
    156, 167, 409, 441
Milk fever, diphasic, 43-44
Milker's nodule virus, 367
Mink encephalopathy, 183
Minorities
  disease risk of, 118
  incidence of AIDS, 3
  resistance to *P. vivax* infection,
    313
Miteborne diseases
  rickettsialpox, 435
  scabies, 445-447
  typhus fever, 545-548

Mitsuda reaction, 291
Molluscipoxvirus, 349
Molluscs
  as disease reservoir, 15–17,
    210–211, 239
Molluscum contagiosum, **348–350**
Moniliasis, 81–83
Monkeypox, **458–459**
Monkeys
  as disease reservoir, 57, 84, 89,
    142, 175–176, 261–262, 290
"Mono syndrome," 351
Monocytic angina, 350–352
Monocytic ehrlichiosis, 181
Monongahela virus, 234
Mononucleosis
  CMV, 139
  diphtheria and, 166
  infectious, **350–352**
Monosporium apiospermum, 358
Moraxella spp., 120
Morbidity rates
  ciguatera fish poisoning, 210
Morbilli, 330–335
Morbillivirus, 330
Mortality rates. *See also*
  Case–fatality rates
  cholera, 112
  Creutzfeldt-Jakob disease, 184
  hantaviral diseases, 234
  hepatitis, viral, 238
  measles, 330
Morumbi virus, 34
Mosquito–borne diseases
  hemorrhagic fevers, **54–56**
  yellow fever, 553–558
Mosquito–borne viral
  encephalitides, 39–43
Mosquito–borne viral fevers,
  45–50
Mosquitoes
  as arthropod-borne viral disease
    vectors, 29–36
  as disease reservoir, 46, 143,
    145–146, 198–201
  disease transmission by,
    312–315

epidemic measures, 42–43
preventive measures, 41–42, 47,
  143–144, 199–200, 313–314
as reservoir of arthropod-borne
  viral arthritis and rash, 38
MOTT. *See* Mycobacteria other
  than tuberculosis
Mouth
  candidiasis, 81–83
MPC. *See* Mucopurulent cervicitis
Mtbc. *See Mycobacterium
  tuberculosis*
Mucambo virus, 30
Mucocutaneous lymph node
  syndrome, 276–278
Mucopurulent cervicitis, 223–224
Mucor spp., 562
Mucorales, 562–563
Mucormycosis, **562–563**
Mucosal leishmaniasis, **284–287**
Mud fever, 293–296
Mules
  as disease reservoir, 337–338
Multibacillary leprosy, 291–293
Multilocular echinococcosis,
  179–180
Mumps, **353–355**
  meningitis and, 339
Murine typhus, 544–545
Murray Valley encephalitis, 39–43
Murray Valley encephalitis virus,
  31
Murutucu virus, 32
Mus musculus, 307, 435
Muskrats
  as disease reservoir, 57
Mussels
  amnesic shellfish poisoning, 212
  diarrhetic shellfish poisoning,
    211
Myalgia, epidemic, **356–357**
Mycetoma, **357–359**
Mycobacteria other than
  tuberculosis, 530–532
Mycobacterium avium complex,
  531–532
Mycobacterium bovis, 523

Mycobacterium leprae, 290–292
Mycobacterium spp., 530–532
Mycobacterium tuberculosis,
    522–523
    interaction with HIV infection,
    4–5
Mycoplasma pneumoniae,
    391–392
Mycoplasmal pneumonia, **391–392**
Mycoses, 369–370
    candidiasis, 81
    cryptococcosis, 132
Mycotoxins, 61
Myocarditis
    coxsackievirus carditis, 131–132
Myositis
    V. vulnificus and, 112

N

Naegleria fowler, 360–361
Naegleriasis, **359–362**
NAGs. *See* Nonagglutinable vibrios
NAG-ST, 108–109
Nails
    ringworm infection, 153
Nairobi sheep disease virus, 35, 51
Nairovirus arboviruses, 35
Nairoviruses, 55
Naples virus, 53
Nasal diphtheria, 166
Nasopharyngeal carcinoma,
    325–326
National AIDS Clearinghouse, 7
National Immunization Day, 331,
    333
National Immunization Program,
    169
National Response Center, 25
Nausea
    epidemic, 218–220
NCVs. *See* Noncholera vibrios
Necator spp., 266
Necatoriasis, 265–268
Necrotizing enteritis, 206
Needles, contaminated
    AIDS transmission, 3–4

    education and exchange
        programs, 5
    hepatitis B transmission, 245
    Lassa fever transmission, 279
    malaria risk, 313
    treatment for needle stick, 250
Negishi virus, 31
Neisseria gonorrhoeae, 98, 224,
    227
Neisseria meningitidis, 120,
    340–341
Nematode diseases
    angiostrongyliasis, 15–17
    anisakiasis, 18–19
    dracunculiasis, 172–174
    enterobiasis, 186–188
    filariasis, 197–202
    gnathostomiasis, 499
    loiasis, 299–301
    pulmonary capillariasis, 87
    trichuriasis, 513–514
Neonatal inclusion blennorrhea,
    126–129
Neonatal meningitis, **348**
Neonates
    chickenpox and, 92, 94, 96
    chlamydial infections, 99,
        126–129
    conjunctivitis, 126–129, 223,
        227–228
    coxsackievirus carditis, 132
    gonococcal conjunctivitis, 223
    Group B streptococcal sepsis,
        477
    herpes simplex virus, 258–259
    staphylococcal disease in
        hospital nurseries, **464–467**
Neonatorum
    gonococcal, **227–228**
    impetigo, **464–467**
Neonatorum, tetanus, **495–496**
Neotestudina spp., 358
Neotoma spp., 303
Nephropathia epidemica, 231–234
Nepuyo virus, 32, 48
Neuralgia, postherpetic, 92

Neuritis
  cranial, 302
Neurotoxic shellfish poisoning,
  211
Nevirapine
  HIV treatment, 8
New Jersey vesicular stomatitis
  virus, 36
New World spotted fever, 430–432
New York-1 virus, 234
Newborns. *See* Neonates
NGU. *See* Nongonococcal
  urethritis
NIP. *See* National Immunization
  Program
Nipah viral disease, **236–238**
Nits, 372–373
Njovera, 486–487
Nocardia spp., 358, 362–363
Nocardiopsis spp., 358
Nocardiosis, **362–363**
Nocturnal periodicity, 197–199
Nonagglutinable vibrios, 101
Nonbacterial meningitis, 338–340
Noncholera vibrios, 101
Nongonococcal urethritis, 98, **100**,
  224
Non-Hodgkin's lymphomas, **327**
Nonpneumonic legionellosis,
  281–283
Nonpyogenic meningitis, 338–340
Nonspecific urethritis, **100**
Nonvenereal endemic syphilis,
  486–487
North American blastomycosis,
  68–70
North Asian tick fever, **434–435**
North Asian tick typhus, 430–432
Norwalk agent disease, 218–220
Norwalk-like disease, 218–220
Norwegian scabies, 445
Nosocomial disease, 531
Nosocomial transmission, 280, 297
Novartis Pharmaceuticals AG, 195
NPC. *See* Nasopharyngeal
  carcinoma

NSU. *See* Nonspecific urethritis
Nyando virus, 35

O

Obstetrical tetanus, 491–495
Occult filariasis, 198
Occupational risk of disease. *See
  also* Health care workers
  anthrax, 20–24
  arenaviral hemorrhagic fever,
    26–27
  arthropod-borne viral diseases,
    49, 55, 57
  brucellosis, 76
  cholera, 112
  chromomycosis, 113–114
  coccidioidomycosis, 118
  cryptosporidiosis, 135
  glanders, 338
  Hendra viral disease, 237
  hepatitis A, 240–241
  hepatitis B, 245, 249
  leishmaniasis, 285
  leptospirosis, 294
  listeriosis, 297
  melioidosis, 336
  Nipah viral disease, 237
  orf virus disease, 367
  paracoccicioidomycosis, 369
  plague, 383
  psittacosis, 406
  Q fever, 408–409
  rabies, 414
  sporotrichosis, 459
  yellow fever, 554
Ockelbo virus, 30
Ockelbo virus disease, 37–39
Octopus
  undertreated, 18
Ocular larva migrans, 497–499
Ogawa serotype *(V. cholerae)*, 101
Ohara disease, 532–535
Oklahoma agent, 219
Omsk hemorrhagic fever, **56–58**
Omsk hemorrhagic fever virus, 31

Onchocerca volvulus, 201, 300, 364

Onchocerciasis, **363–367**

Onchocerciasis Control Programme, 364, 366

Onchocerciasis Elimination Programme for the Americas, 367

Onychomycosis, 81, 153

O'nyong–nyong fever, 37–39

O'nyong–nyong virus, 30

Opisthorchiasis, **116**

Opisthorchis felineus, 116

Opossums
as disease reservoir, 263, 294

Oral cavity
growth of *A. israelii,* 10

Oral hygiene
actinomycosis prevention, 11
dental caries reduction, 478

Oral thrush, 81–82

Orbiviruses, 35, 53

Orchitis, 353

Ordinary variola, 456

Orf virus disease, **367–368**
anthrax and, 20

Organ transplants. *See* Transplants, organ

Oriboca virus, 32, 48

Oriental liver fluke disease, 114–116

Oriental sore, 284–287

Orientia tsutsugamushi, 546

Ornithodoros spp., 422

Ornithosis, 405–407

Oropharyngeal anthrax, 20–21

Oropouche virus, 34, 48

Oropouche virus disease, **48–50**

Oroya fever, 66–68

Orthomyxoviridae, 36

Orthopoxviruses, 456, 458

Orungo virus, 36

Ossa virus, 32, 48

Osteomyelitis
streptococcal, **461–464**

Otomycosis, 61

Ovale malaria, 310–311, 320

Oxygen therapy, 146

Oxyuriasis, 186–188

Oysters
as disease reservoir, 112–113

P

Pacas
as disease reservoir, 180

Pan American Health Organization (PAHO), 404–405

Papatasi fever, 52–54

Papilloma venereum, 548–550

Paracoccidioidal granuloma, 369–370

Paracoccidioides brasiliensis, 369

Paracoccidioidomycosis, **369–370**

Paragonimiasis, **370–372**

Paragonimus spp., 370

Parainfluenza viruses, 398, 427–428

Paralysis, acute flaccid, 398–399

Paralytic shellfish poisoning, **210–211**

Paramyxoviridae, 236, 330, 353

Parapertussis, **375–379**

Parapoxvirus, 367

Parasitemia, 311–313, 321

Parastrongylus cantonensis, 15

Parastrongylus costaricensis, 17

Paratrachoma, 126–129

Paratyphoid fever, **535–541**

Parenterally transmitted non-A non-B hepatitis, 251–253

Parinaud oculoglandular syndrome, 87

Paromomycin
amoebiasis treatment, 14

Paronychia, 81–82

Parotitis, infectious, 353–355

Parramatta agent, 219

Parrot fever, 405–407

Parvoviridae, 189

Parvovirus B19, 189–190

Parvovirus infection, human, 189–191

Pasteurella haemolytica, 89

Pasteurella multocida, 89
Pasteurella tularensis, 533
Pasteurellosis
    from animal bites, 89
Pasteurization
    disease prevention, 80
    radiation, 16
Paucibacillary leprosy, 293
PCF. *See* Pharyngoconjunctival
    fever
PCP. *See* Plasma-cell pneumonia
Pediculosis, **372–374**
Pediculus spp., 372, 422, 507, 542
Penicillinase producing *N.
    gonorrhoeae,* 224, 226
PEP. *See* Postexposure prophylaxis
Perianal region
    ringworm infection, 149-151
Pericarditis
    coxsackievirus carditis, 131-132
Peripheral T-cell lymphoma, 329
Peromyscus leucopus, 63
Peromyscus spp., 51, 235, 303
Personal hygiene
    amoebiasis prevention, 13
    ascariasis prevention, 59
    balantidiasis prevention, 65
    dermatophytosis prevention,
        150, 152
    enterobiasis prevention,
        187-188
    staphylococcal diseases and, 462
Pertussis, **375–379**
    immunization, 167-168
Pestis, 381-387
Petechial rash, 340
Pets. *See* Animals
Peyer patches, 535
Pharyngeal diphtheria, 168-169
Pharyngitis
    bacterial, 391
    enteroviral lymphonodular,
        129-131
    enteroviral vesicular, 129-131
    gonococcal, 223, 226
    viral, 166, 424-430

Pharyngoconjunctival fever,
    124-126
Pharyngotonsillar diphtheria, 166
Pharyngotonsillitis, 258
Phialophora spp., 358
Phialophora verrucosa, 113
Phlebotomine-borne arboviruses,
    34-36
Phlebotomine-borne viral fevers,
    52–54
Phlebotomines
    preventive measures, 286
Phlebotomus fever, 52-54
Phlebotomus papatasi, 53
Phleboviruses, 29, 34, 48, 53
Phthiriasis, **371–374**
Phycomycosis, 561-564
Pica, 498
Picornaviridae, 129, 239
Picornaviruses, 124-125
Piedraia hortai, 148
Pigbel, 206-207
Pigeons
    droppings as disease reservoir,
        133
Pigs
    adequate cooking for pork,
        509-510
    as disease reservoir, 65-66, 79,
        115, 196, 236-237, 256, 272,
        294, 371,
441, 558
    roundworm infection, 58
Pinkeye, 119-121
Pinta, **379–380**
Pinworm infection, 186-188
Piry virus, 36
Pistia, 200
Plague, **381–387**
    from animal bites, 89
Plantar warts, 548
Plasma-cell pneumonia, 392-394
Plasmodium falciparum, 63,
    311-319
Plasmodium spp., 311-314
Pleurodynia, epidemic, 356-357
Pneumococcal meningitis, **348**

Pneumococcal pneumonia, **387–390**

Pneumocystis carinii, 393
AIDS and, 1, 7
Pneumocystis pneumonia, **392–394**
Pneumonia
bacterial, 375
chlamydial, 97, 126, **394–398**
infant, 97
Legionnaires' disease, 281–282
melioidosis, 335
mycoplasmal, **391–392**
plague, 381–387
pneumococcal, **387–390**
pneumocystis, **392–394**
staphylococcal, **461–464**
Pneumonitis, 236
Pogosta disease, 37–39
Poliomyelitis, acute, **398–405**
Polioviral fever, 398–405
Polyarthritis
arthropod-borne viral disease and, 28, 37–39
Polycystic hydatid disease, 180
Pongola virus, 33
Pontiac fever, 281–283
Pork. *See* Pigs
Pork tapeworm, 488–491
Postexposure prophylaxis
anthrax, 24–25
HIV, 8
rabies, 419
Postherpetic neuralgia, 92
Postpolio syndrome, 399
Post-traumatic wound infections, 531
Potamon spp., 371
Poultry. *See also* Meat and meat products
as disease reservoir, 79–80, 441–442, 499
Powassan virus, 31
Powassan virus encephalitis, 43–45
Poxviridae, 349
Poxviruses, 367

PPNG. *See* Penicillinase producing *N. gonorrhoeae*
Pregnancy. *See also* Maternal–infant transmission
chickenpox and, 96
chlamydial infection and, 98
disease risk, 118
ectopic, 98
fetal anemia, 189
hepatitis E and, 255
HIV counseling programs, 5–6
HIV transmission to infants, 4
listeriosis and, 296–297
malaria and, 316–318
tetanus immunization, 495–496
toxoplasmosis risk, 500–501
vulvovaginal candidiasis, 82
Prepatent period, 312
Prevalence rates
leprosy, 290
Primary amebic meningoencephalitis, 359–362
Primary atypical pneumonia, 391–392
Primary liver cancer, **324–325**
Prion, 183–185
Proctitis
chlamydial, 97, 308
Propionibacterium propionicus, 10
Prostitutes
chancroid transmission, 90–91
Pruritis, 300
Pseudallescheria spp, 358
Pseudomonas aeruginosa, 120
Pseudomonas mallei, 338
Pseudomonas pseudomallei, 336
Pseudonitzschia pungens, 212
Pseudoterranova, 18
Psittacosis, 97, **405–407**
Psorophora spp., 46
PSP. *See* Paralytic shellfish poisoning
PT-NANB. *See* Parenterally transmitted non-A non-B hepatitis

Public safety workers
hepatitis B risk, 245, 249
Puerperal fever, 470–476
Puffer-fish poisoning, **212**
Pulex irritans, 383
Pulmonary disease resembling
tuberculosis, 531
Pulmonary diseases
blastomycosis, 68–69
capillariasis, 87
hantaviral, 234–236
histoplasmosis, 262–265
mucormycosis, 562–563
pneumocystis pneumonia,
392–394
sporotrichosis, 459–460
TB, 521–532
Pulmonary distomiasis, 370–372
Pulmonary edema, 235
Punta Toro virus, 34, 53
Puppies. *See* Dogs
Pustule, malignant, 20–25
Puumala virus, 231–232
Pyrenochaeta spp., 358

Q

Q fever, **407–411**
Quaranfil virus, 36, 51
Quartan malaria, 310
Queensland tick typhus, **434**
Query fever, 407–411
Quicklime
for soil decontamination, 23
Quintana fever, 506–508

R

Rabbit fever, 532–535
Rabbits
as disease reservoir, 55,
382–383, 533
Rabies, **411–419**
from animal bites, 89
Raccoons
as disease reservoir, 201, 294,
412

Radiation pasteurization, 16
Ragpicker disease, 20–25
Rash
arthropod-borne viral disease,
28, 37–39
Boutonneuse fever, 433
centrifugal distribution, 456
erythema infectiosum, 189–190
exanthem subitum, 191–193
Kawasaki syndrome, 276–277
meningitis, 338, 340
rickettsialpox, 435
Rocky Mountain spotted fever,
430–431
rubella, 435
scarlet fever, 471
smallpox, 455–456
streptobacillosis, 420
toxic shock syndrome, 469
Raspberries
disease transmission by,
137–138
Rat tapeworm infection, 269–270
Rat-bite fever, 89, **420–421**
Rats. *See* Rodents
Rattus spp., 16, 232, 544
Reactive arthropathy, 451
Red measles, 330–335
"Red tides," 210–211
Reed Sternberg cell, 326
Rehydration therapy, 105–106,
146–147, 158, 218
Reiter syndrome, 97, 451
Relapsing fever, 372, **421–424**
Renal disease
as disease risk, 282
Renal syndrome
hemorrhagic fever, **231–234**
Reoviridae
arboviruses, 35
rotaviruses, 216
Reservoir of infectious agents. *See
specific disease by name*
Respiratory disease. *See also* Lung
disease
acute febrile, **427–430**
acute viral, **424–430**

acute viral rhinitis, **425–427**
adenoviruses and, 125
animal bites and, 89
chlamydial, 97
coccidioidomycosis, 117
Hantavirus pulmonary
  syndrome, 234–236
influenza, 270–276
pharyngoconjunctival fever and,
  124
Respiratory syncytial virus, 398,
  427–429
Restan virus, 32, 48
Reston Ebola, 175
Retroviruses, 324
Reye syndrome
  chickenpox and, 92
  influenza and, 271, 273
Rhabdoviridae, 36
Rhabdoviruses, 53, 411
Rhesus–based rotavirus vaccine,
  tetravalent, 217
Rheumatic fever, 470–476
Rhinitis
  acute viral, 424–430
Rhinocladiella aquaspersa, 113
Rhinoviruses, 425–427
Rhipicephalus sanguineus, 433
Rhizomucor spp. 562
Rhizopus spp., 562
Rice
  as disease reservoir, 208
*Rickettsia. See also Ehrlichia
  sennetsu*
Rickettsia africae, 433
Rickettsia akari, 435
Rickettsia australis, 434
Rickettsia conorii, 433
Rickettsia felis, 544
Rickettsia prowazekii, 372, 542
Rickettsia quintana, 372
Rickettsia rickettsii, 431
Rickettsia sibirica, 434
Rickettsia typhi, 544
Rickettsialpox, **435**
Rickettsioses, tickborne, **430–435**
Rift Valley fever, **48–50**

Rift Valley fever virus, 34, 48
Ringer's solution, 106, 146
Ringworm
  of the beard and scalp, 147–149
  of the body, 149–151
  of the foot, 151–152
  of the groin and perianal region,
    149–151
  of the nails, 153
Risk behaviors
  for AIDS, 3–4
  blood donations and, 6
  prevention programs, 5–6
Risus sardonicus, 491
Ritter's disease, 464–467
River blindness, 363–367
RMSF. *See* Rocky Mountain spotted
  fever
*Rochalimaea quintana. See
  Bartonella quintana*
Rochalimaea spp. *See Bartonella*
  spp.
Rocio encephalitis, 39–43
Rocio virus, 31
Rocky Mountain spotted fever,
  181, **430–432**
Rodents
  bites, 89
  disease in, 86
  as disease reservoir, 15–17, 27,
    46, 49, 53, 57, 63, 79, 89, 115,
    180, 230–236, 263, 269–270,
    279, 285, 294, 303, 307,
    381–383, 420–421, 435, 441,
    544
  preventive measures, 233,
    307–308, 383–386
Romaña sign, 518
Roseola infantum, 191–193
Roseolovirus, 192
Ross River virus, 30, 37–39
Rotaviral enteritis, 154, **215–218**
Roundworm infection, 58–60,
  508–511
RRV-TV. *See* Rhesus–based
  rotavirus vaccine, tetravalent
RSV. *See* Respiratory syncytial virus

Rubella, **435–440**
Rubella virus, 436
Rubeola, 330–335
Rubivirus, 436
Russian spring-summer
   encephalitis, 43–45

S

Sabethes spp., 46
Sabiá hemorrhagic fever, 26–28
Sabiá virus, 26–27
Saccharomyces cerevisiae, 247
Saksenaea spp., 562
Saliva
   disease transmission by, 140,
      351, 412, 420–421
   growth of *A. israelii,* 10
Salmonella spp., 440–444,
   536–537
Salmonellosis, **440–444**
Salpingitis, 98, 224
Salted fish
   undertreated, 18
San Joaquin fever, 117–119
Sand flies
   disease transmission, 29, 67–68,
      285–286, 288
   preventive measures, 53
Sand fly fever, **52–54**
Sand fly fever arboviruses, 34
Sand fly Napels type virus, 34
Sand fly Sicilian type virus, 34
Sanitation
   amoebiasis and, 12
   hepatitis A and, 239, 243
   hookworm disease and, 266
Sao Paulo fever, 430–432
Sarcoidosis
   as risk for disease, 133
Sarcoma, Kaposi's, **327–329**
Sarcoptes scabiei, 445
Sarcoptic itch, 445–447
Sashimi
   undertreated, 18
Saxitoxins, 210–211
Scabies, **445–447**

Scalded skin syndrome,
   staphylococcal, 461, **464–467**
Scallops
   diarrhetic shellfish poisoning,
      211
Scalp
   ringworm infection, 147–149
Scarlet fever, 470–476
SCBA. *See* Self-contained
   breathing apparatus
Scedosporium spp., 358
Schistosoma spp., 447–449
Schistosomiasis, **447–450**
Schizotrypanum cruzi, 518–519
Scombroid fish poisoning, **209**
Scrapie, 183
Scrub typhus, **545–548**
Scytalidium dimidiatum, 150
Scytalidium hyalinum, 150
Seabather's eruption, 448
Seafood
   as disease reservoir, 71
   disease transmission by, 103,
      109–113
Self-contained breathing
   apparatus, 25
Semliki Forest virus, 30
Sennetsu fever, 181–183
Seoul virus, 231–232
Sepik virus, 31
Sepsis
   staphylococcal, **461–464**
   streptococcal, **477**
Septicemia
   cholera, 109, 111–113
   GC, 223
   listeriosis, 296–297
   melioidosis, 335
   meningitis, 348
   plague, 381
   salmonellosis, 440
Septicemic disease
   V. cholerae, 108–110
Sergentomyia spp., 53
Serous lymphocytic meningitis,
   306–308
Serous meningitis, 338–340

Serra Norte, 34
Serum hepatitis, 243–251
Severe viral gastroenteritis,
    215–218
Sex education, 99, 484
Sexual abuse
    chancroid and, 90
    chlamydial conjunctivitis and,
        127
    gonococcal infection, 223–224
    herpes simplex virus, 259
Sexual transmission of diseases
    AIDS, 3–5
    AIDS and, 3–4
    amoebiasis, 11, 13
    chancroid, 90
    chlamydia, 97, 127
    CMV, 140
    conjunctivitis, 127
    crab lice, 372–374
    cryptosporidiosis, 135
    Ebola-Marburg disease, 176
    genital herpes, 258
    giardiasis, 221
    gonococcal infections, 223–228
    granuloma inguinale, 229–230
    hepatitis B, 245–246
    hepatitis D, 353–355
    HSV, 258, 260–261
    Lassa fever, 279
    lymphogranuloma venereum,
        308–310
    multiple sex partners as risk,
        245, 249, 329
    scabies, 445
    syphilis, 482–483
    trichomoniasis, 511–512
    warts, 549
Sézary disease, 329
Sheep. See also Milk and milk
    products
    as disease reservoir, 49, 79,
        177–179, 193–194, 367,
        408–410
    scrapie, 183
Shellfish
    amnesic shellfish poisoning, **212**

diarrhetic shellfish poisoning,
    211
disease transmission by, 103,
    109, 371
neurotoxic shellfish poisoning,
    211
paralytic shellfish poisoning,
    210–211
viral gastroenteritis, 219
Shiga toxin producing *E. coli,*
    155–158
Shigella dysenteriae, 155, 451
Shigella spp., 451–454
Shigellosis, **451–455**
Shingles, 92–97
Shipyard conjunctivitis, 122–124
Shipyard eye, 122–124
Shokwe virus, 33
Shop typhus, 544–545
Shower stalls
    disease transmission by,
        150–153
Shrews
    as disease reservoir, 57
Shuni virus, 34
Siberian tick typhus, 434–435
Sicilian virus, 53
Sickle cell trait, 313
SIDS. *See* Sudden infant death
    syndrome
Sigmodon hispidus, 17
Silage
    as disease reservoir, 297
Simbu group arboviruses, 34, 48
Simian B disease, 261–262
Simulium spp., 364–365
Sin Nombre virus, 234
Sindbis virus, 30
Sindbis virus disease, 37–39
Sixth disease, 191–193
Skin infections
    disease transmission by,
        204–206
    streptococcal, 470–471
Skin tests
    TB, 521–522, 527
Skin ulcers, 531, 545

Skunks
  as disease reservoir, 263, 413
"Slapped face," 189
Sleeping sickness, 514–518
Sloths
  as disease reservoir, 285
Slow virus infections, CNS,
    183–186
Slugs
  angiostrongyliasis transmission,
    17
Smallpox, **455–457**
Smoked fish
  undertreated, 18
Smoking
  as disease risk, 282
Snail fever, 447–450
Snails
  disease transmission by, 15–17,
    115, 194
Snow Mountain agent, 219
Snowshoe hare encephalitis, 39–43
Snowshoe hare virus, 33
Sodoku, 421
Soft chancre, 90–91
Soil. *See also* Vegetation, decaying
  anthrax contamination, 21–23
  decontamination of, 23
  as disease reservoir, 58–59, 69,
    71–72, 86–87, 114, 118, 133,
    150, 206, 208, 263, 297, 336,
    358, 369, 459, 492, 497–499,
    501–502
  fecal contamination, 178, 206,
    263, 266–267
Sore throats
  streptococcal, 470–476
South America
  arenaviral hemorrhagic fevers,
    26–28
South American blastomycosis,
    369–370
Spirillary fever, 421
Spirillosis, **421**
Spirillum minus, 421
Spirochaetales, 294
Spondweni virus, 31, 48

Sponges, contraceptive
  as disease risk, 469
Sporadic viral gastroenteritis,
    215–218
Sporothrix schenckii, 459
Sporotrichosis, **459–460**
Spotted fever group, 430–435
Squid
  undertreated, 18
Squirrels
  as disease reservoir, 382–383,
    458
SSSS. *See* Scalded skin syndrome,
  Staphylococcal
St. Louis encephalitis, 39–43
St. Louis encephalitis virus, 31
Standby treatment
  malaria, 316–317
Staphylococcal diseases, **460–470**
  animal bites and, 89
  in the community, **461–464**
  food intoxication, **203–206**
  on hospital medical and surgical
    wards, **467–469**
  in hospital nurseries, **464–467**
  toxic shock syndrome, **469–470**
Staphylococcal sepsis, **461–464**
Staphylococcus aureus, 204, 277,
    460–470
STD check, 511
STDs. *See* Sexual transmission of
  diseases
STEC. *See* Shiga toxin producing *E.
  coli*
Stevens–Johnson syndrome, 391
"Sticky eye," 119–121, 126–129
Stomatitis
  enteroviral vesicular with
    exanthem, 129–131
"Strain," 223–227
"Strawberry" spots, 511
"Strawberry" tongue, 276–277
Streptobacillary fever, 420–421
Streptobacillosis, **420–421**
Streptobacillus moniliformis, 89,
    420

Streptococcal diseases, 470–478
  animal bites and, 89
  dental caries, 477–478
  Group A, 470–476
  Group B, 477
Streptococcal infection, 470–476
Streptococcal sepsis, Group B, 477
Streptococcal skin infections,
  470–471
Streptococcal sore throat, 470–476
Streptococcus agalactiae, 477
Streptococcus mutans, 478
Streptococcus pneumoniae, 120,
  344, 388
Streptococcus pyogenes, 472
Streptococcus spp., 348
Streptococcus viridans, 120
Streptomyces somaliensis, 358
Strongloides spp., 479
Strongyloidiasis, 478–481
Subacute sclerosing
  panencephalitis, 330
Sudden infant death syndrome, 71
"Sulfur granules," 9
Surgical instruments
  disease transmission by,
    185–186
Surveillance, xxv
Sushi
  undertreated, 18
"Swimmer's itch," 448
Swimming pools
  conjunctivitis, 124–125, 127
  as disease reservoir, 124–125,
    127, 135, 221, 296, 360–361,
    428
Swine. *See* Pigs
Swineherd disease, 293–296
Syphilis, 226, 481–487
  diphtheria and, 166
  nonvenereal endemic, 486–487

T

TAC. *See* Transient aplastic crisis
Tacaiuma virus, 32

Tacaribe arenaviruses, 26
Tâche noire, 432
Taenia saginata taeniasis
  intestinal form, 488–491
Taenia solium taeniasis, 488–491
Taeniasis, 488–491
  Asian, 491
Tahyna virus, 33
Tamarins
  as disease reservoir, 256
Tamdy virus, 35
Tapeworms
  beef, 488–491
  broad, 171–172
  dog, 270
  dwarf, 268–269
  Echinococcus granulosus,
    177–179
  Echinococcus multilocularis,
    179–180
  Echinococcus vogeli, 180
  fish, 171–172
  pork, 488–491
  rat, 269–270
Tataguine virus, 35
Tattoo parlors
  hepatitis B risk, 245, 249
Taunton agent, 219
TB. *See* Tuberculosis
T-cell lymphosarcoma, 329
Teeth, carious
  growth of *A. israelii,* 10
  streptococcal, 477–478
Tensaw virus, 33
Testing programs
  HIV/AIDS prevention, 5
Tetanus, 491–496
  from animal bites, 89
  immunization, 167–168
  neonatorum, 495–496
Tetracycline resistant *N.*
  gonorrhoeae, 226
Tetrodotoxin, 212
T-helper cell count
  HIV infection evaluation, 2

Thermonuclease, 204
Thimerosal, 248
Thogoto virus, 36, 51
Thominx aerophila, 87
Thrombotic thrombocytopenic
  purpura, 155
Thrush, 81–83
Tickborne diseases
  African tick bite fever, **433–434**
  babesiosis, 62–64
  Boutonneuse fever, **432–433**
  ehrlichiosis, 182
  encephalitis viruses, 31
  encephalitis-louping ill
    complex, 57
  hemorrhagic fevers, **54–56**
  Lyme disease, **302–306**
  meningopolyneuritis, 302–306
  North Asian tick fever, **434–435**
  Queensland tick typhus, **434**
  relapsing fever, 421–424
  rickettsioses, **430–435**
  Rocky Mountain spotted fever,
    430–432
  typhus fever, 430–432
  viral encephalitides, **43–45**
  viral fevers, **50–52**
Ticks
  as arthropod-borne viral disease
    vectors, 29, 31, 35–36
  as disease reservoir, 44, 408, 533
  preventive measures, 52
Timorean filariasis, 197–201
Tinea barbae, **147–149**
Tinea capitis, **147–149**
Tinea corporis, **149–151**
Tinea cruris, **149–151**
Tinea pedis, **151–153**
Tinea unguium, **153**
TLCL. *See* T-cell lymphosarcoma
Togaviridae, 29–30, 40, 46, 436
Tonate virus, 30
Tonsils
  vesicular pharyngitis, 129
Torula, 132–134

Toscana virus, 34, 53
Toxic shock syndrome
  staphylococcal, **469–470**
  streptococcal, 471–472
Toxocara canis infection, 497–499
Toxocara cati infection, 497–499
Toxocariasis, **497–500**
Toxoplasma gondii, 501
Toxoplasma spp., 500
Toxoplasmosis, 351, **500–503**
Trachoma, 97, **504–506**
Transfusion associated hepatitis,
  251–253
Transfusions. *See also* Blood and
  blood products
  arthropod-borne viral fever
    transmission, 51
  babesiosis transmission, 63–64
  bartonellosis transmission, 67
  CMV mononucleosis, 139–140
  Creutzfeldt-Jakob disease risk,
    185
  erythema infectiosum risk, 189
  hepatitis A risk, 239
  hepatitis B risk, 249
  HIV risk, 6, 9
  Kaposi's sarcoma risk, 328
  Lassa fever risk, 279
  malaria risk, 312–314
  mononucleosis, 351
  Q fever risk, 409
  trypanosomiasis transmission,
    519
Transient aplastic crisis, 189
Transmissible mink
  encephalopathy, 183
Transmission of infectious agents.
  See specific disease by name
Transplants, organ
  AIDS transmission, 3
  CMV infection, 139–141
  Creutzfeldt-Jakob disease risk,
    185
  disease transmission by, 185
  exanthem subitum transmission,
    192

Kaposi's sarcoma and, 328
rabies transmission, 412
Traveler's cholera, 102–103
Travelers' diarrhea, 79, 109,
158–159, 216
Trees. *See also* Wood
as disease reservoir, 133
Trematode diseases
clonorchiasis, 114–116
fascioliasis, 193–195
fasciolopsiasis, 195–197
paragonimiasis, 370–372
schistosomiasis, 447–450
Trench fever, 372, **506–508**
Treponema carateum, 380
Treponema pallidum, 482, 487,
551
Trichinella spp., 509
Trichinellosis, **508–511**
Trichiniasis, 508–511
Trichinosis, 508–511
Trichocephaliasis, 513–514
Trichomonas vaginalis, 100, 512
Trichomoniasis, **511–513**
Trichophyton mentagrophytes,
148, 151
Trichophyton rubrum, 151
Trichophyton schoenleinii,
147–148
Trichophyton spp., 150, 153
Trichophyton tonsurans, 148
Trichophyton verrucosum, 148
Trichophytosis, 147–153
Trichosporon beigelii, 148
Trichosporon inkin, 148
Trichosporon ovoides, 148
Trichuriasis, 60, **513–514**
Trichuris trichiura, 60, 513
Trivittatus virus, 34
Tropical bubo, 308–310
Tropical pulmonary eosinophilia,
198
Tropical spastic paraparesis, 329
Trubanaman virus, 34
Trypanosoma brucei gambiense,
515

Trypanosoma brucei rhodesiense,
515
Trypanosoma cruzi, 518–519
Trypanosoma rangeli, 518
Trypanosomiasis
African, **514–518**
American, **518–520**
Tsetse fly
disease transmission by,
514–516
TSS. *See* Toxic shock syndrome
Tsutsugamushi disease, 545–548
TTP. *See* Thrombotic
thrombocytopenic purpura
Tuberculoid leprosy, 289, 291–293
Tuberculosis, **521–532**
HIV and, 5, 7
Tucunduba virus, 33
Tularemia, **532–535**
from animal bites, 89
Type A Hepatitis, 238–243
Type B Hepatitis, 243–251
Typhoid fever, **535–541**
Typhus
abdominalis, 535–541
endemic fleaborne, **544–545**
epidemic, 372
epidemic louseborne, **541–544**
exanthematicus, 541–544
scrub, **545–548**
Typhus fever, **541–548**
''Typhus islands,'' 546

U

Ulcerative colitis
confusion with amebic colitis,
12
Ulcers
candidiasis and, 81
chancroid, 90–91
leishmaniasis, 284
skin, 531, 545
Ulcus molle, 90–91

UNAIDS
  AIDS prevention and care
    program, 9
Uncinariasis, 265–268
Undulant fever, 75–78
Ungulates
  as disease reservoir, 367
Unilocular echinococcosis,
  177–179
Universal precautions, 141
  AIDS prevention, 6, 7, 9
Ureaplasma urealyticum, 100
Urethritis
  chlamydial, 97, 127
  gonococcal, 223–227
  nongonococcal and nonspecific,
    100
Urinary tract
  candidiasis, 81–83
Urine
  disease transmission by,
    294–295, 537
Uruma virus, 30
Uruma virus disease, 37–39
U.S. Army Medical Research and
  Materiel Command, 42, 47, 410
U.S. Department of Agriculture
  (USDA)
  Food Safety Inspection Service,
    157
Usutu virus, 32
Uta, 284–287

V

Vaccine Adverse Events Reporting
  System, 217
Vaccine associated paralytic polio,
  402–403
Vaccines. *See also* Immunizations
  adenoviruses, 427
  anthrax, 22, 24–25
  arenaviral hemorrhagic fever, 27
  arthropod-borne viral diseases,
    45, 47, 49, 55, 57–58
BCG, 527–528
brucellosis, 77
cholera, 104, 108
diphtheria, 167
encephalitis, 42
EPI vaccine for HIV-infected
  children, 6
hepatitis A, 240–243
hepatitis B, 247–250, 325
influenza, 273
Lyme disease, 304–305
measles, 331–334
meningitis, 342–343, 346–347
MMR, 332–333
mumps, 354
pertussis, 377
pneumonia, 389
poliomyelitis, 400–403
Q fever, 409
rabies, 413–416
rotavirus, 217
rubella, 437–438
tetanus, 493–494, 496
tuberculosis, 527–528
typhoid, 539
vaccinia, 457
varicella virus, 94–95
yellow fever, 555–556
Vaccinia, **457**
VAERS. *See* Vaccine Adverse
  Events Reporting System
Vaginal transmission. *See also*
  Sexual transmission of diseases
  candidiasis, 82–83
Vaginitis, 511
Valley fever, 117–119
Varicella, 92–97
Varicella–zoster immune globulin,
  95–96
Varicella–zoster virus, 93
Variola virus, 455
Varivax Coordinating Center, 94
vCJD, 183–184
Vegetables
  disease transmission by, 72,
    137–138, 239, 441

Vegetation, decaying. *See also* Soil
    as disease reservoir, 61, 114,
    358, 459
Venereal warts, 548
Venezuelan equine encephalitis,
    45–47
Venezuelan equine
    encephalomyelitis virus, 30
Venezuelan equine
    encephalomyelitis virus disease,
    45–47
Venezuelan equine fever, 45–47
Venezuelan hemorrhagic fever,
    26–28
Verotoxin producing *E. coli,*
    155–158
Verruca vulgaris, 548–550
Verruga peruana, 66–68
Vesicular pharyngitis, 129–131
Vesicular rickettsiosis, 435
Vesicular stomatitis fever, 52–54
Vesicular stomatitis group
    arboviruses, 36
Vesicular stomatitis virus, 36
Vesicular stomatitis virus disease,
    52–54
Vesicular stomatitis with
    exanthem, **129–131**
Veterinarians
    anthrax hazard, 20
    arthropod-borne hemorrhagic
        fever risk, 55
    brucellosis hazard, 76
    herpes B-virus, 261–262
    leptospirosis risk, 294
    orf virus disease hazard, 367
    plague hazard, 383
    Q fever risk, 408
    rabies hazard, 414
Vibrio cholerae
    Campylobacter enteritis and, 79
    classical biotype, 100, 104
    El Tor biotype, 100–104
    epidemic O139 strain, 101
    serogroup O139 Bengal, 102
    serogroups O1 and O139,
        100–108

serogroups other than O1 and
    O139, **108–110**
Vibrio parahaemolyticus enteritis,
    110–111
Vibrio spp.
    infections, **113**
Vibrio vulnificus infection,
    111–113
Vibrionic enteritis, 79–81
Vincent's angina, 166
Viral carditis, 131–132
Viral diarrhea, 218–220
Viral gastroenteritis
    in adults, 218–220
    severe, 215–218
    sporadic, 215–218
Viral gastroenteropathy, epidemic,
    218–220
Viral hepatitis, **238–257**
Viral meningitis, **338–340**
Viral rhinitis, acute, 424–430
Viral warts, **548–550**
Visceral larva migrans, 497–499
Visceral leishmaniasis, **287–289**
Vitamin A deficiency, 330
Vivax malaria, 310–311, 313, 319
Viverra tangalunga, 199
Voles
    as disease reservoir, 63
Vomiting
    epidemic, 218–220
VTEC. *See* Verotoxin producing *E.
    coli*
Vulvovaginitis, 81–82, 223–227
VZIG. *See* Varicella-zoster immune
    globulin
VZV. *See* Varicella-zoster virus

W

W agent, 219
Wanowrie virus, 35
Warts, viral, **548–550**
Wasting disease, chronic, 183

Water
  chlorination, 107, 157, 283
  contaminated, 173, 256,
    294–295, 449–450
  as disease reservoir, 103, 109,
    111, 135, 221, 256, 282–283,
    297, 336, 360–361
  disease transmission by,
    137–138, 156, 239
  fecal contamination, 13, 65, 103,
    268, 537, 559
  iodine treatment, 13
  nonchlorinated, 79, 124–125,
    156, 441
  superheating, 283
  swimming pools, 124–125, 127,
    135, 221, 296, 360–361, 428
  treatment of, 13, 65
  unfiltered drinking water, 221
Water-borne epidemics, 65
Web sites
  CCDM site, 217
  CDC immunization site, 217
  CDC National AIDS
    Clearinghouse, 7
  CDC travel site, 311
Weil disease, 293–296
Wesselsbron virus, 32
West Nile fever, **48–50**
West Nile virus, 32, 48
Western blot test
  for HIV antibodies, 2
Western equine encephalitis, 39–43
Western equine encephalomyelitis
  virus, 30
Whipworm disease, 513–514
Whitlow, herpetic, 259, 261
Whitmore disease, 335–337
WHO. *See* World Health
  Organization
Whooping cough, 375–379
Wild animals
  as disease reservoir, 180, 408,
    412, 441, 509, 533, 559
Wildlife workers
  anthrax hazard, 20
Winter vomiting disease, 218–220

Women. *See also* Pregnancy
  incidence of AIDS, 3
Wood. *See also* Trees; Vegetation,
  decaying
  as disease reservoir, 114, 459
Woodchucks
  as disease reservoir, 254
Woolsorter disease, 20–25
World Health Assembly, 174, 455
World Health Organization
  AIDS prevention and care
    program, 9
  diarrhea treatment solution, 106
  Expert Committee on Leprosy,
    291–292
  International Travel and Health,
    315
  Safe Food Preparation Rules, 203
World Wide Web. *See* Web sites
Wound infections
  chromomycosis, 113–114
  mycetoma, 358
  post-traumatic, 531
  tetanus, 492, 496
  V. cholerae, 109
  V. vulnificus, 112
  Vibrio spp., 113
  wound botulism, 70–75
Wuchereria bancrofti, 197–201,
  300
Wyeomyia virus, 33

X

Xenopsylla cheopis, 383, 544
Xingu virus, 33

Y

Yaws, **550–553**
Yellow fever, **553–558**
  dengue fever and, 144
  hepatic damage, 28
  humans as vectors, 29
Yellow fever virus, 32
Yersinia enterocolitica, 558–561
Yersinia pestis, 382, 387

Yersinia pseudotuberculosis,
558–561
Yersinia spp., 558–559
Yersiniosis, **558–561**

Z

Zaire Ebola. *See* Democratic
Republic of the Congo Ebola

ZDV. *See* Zidovudine
Zidovudine
HIV treatment, 4, 6, 8
Zika virus, 32, 48
Zoonotic filariasis, 201
Zoster, 92–94
Zygodontomys brevicauda, 27
Zygomycosis, **561–564**

NOTE: Page references in **bold** indicate main reference

Recommended Childhood Immunization Schedule[1] United States, January–December 1999

Vaccines are listed under routinely recommended ages. Bars indicate range of recommended ages for immunization. Any dose not given at the recommended age should be given as a "catch-up" immunization at any subsequent visit when indicated and feasible. Ovals indicate vaccines to be given if previously recommended doses were missed or given earlier than the recommended minimum age.

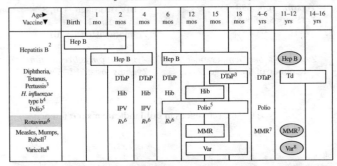

Age ▶ Vaccine ▼	Birth	1 mo	2 mos	4 mos	6 mos	12 mos	15 mos	18 mos	4–6 yrs	11–12 yrs	14–16 yrs
Hepatitis B[2]	Hep B									Hep B	
		Hep B			Hep B						
Diphtheria, Tetanus, Pertussis[3]			DTaP	DTaP	DTaP		DTaP[3]		DTaP	Td	
H. influenzae type b[4]			Hib	Hib	Hib	Hib					
Polio[5]			IPV	IPV	Polio[5]				Polio		
Rotavirus[6]			Rv[6]	Rv[6]	Rv[6]						
Measles, Mumps, Rubell[7]						MMR			MMR[7]	MMR[7]	
Varicella[8]						Var				Vav[8]	

Approved by the Advisory Committee on Immunization Practices (ACIP), the American Academy of Pediatrics (AAP), and the American Academy of Family Physicians (AAFP).

[1]This schedule indicates the recommended ages for routine administration of currently licensed childhood vaccines. Combination vaccines may be used whenever any components of the combination are indicated and its other components are not contraindicated. Providers should consult the manufacturers' package inserts for detailed recommendations.

[2]*Infants born to HBsAg-negative mothers* should receive the 2nd dose of hepatitis B (Hep B) vaccine at least one month after the 1st dose. The 3rd dose should be administered at least 4 months after the 1st dose and at least 2 months after the 2nd dose, but not before 6 months of age for infants.
Infants born to HBsAg-positive mothers should receive hepatitis B vaccine and 0.5 mL hepatitis B immune globulin (HBIG) within 12 hours of birth at separate sites. The 2nd dose is recommended at 1–2 months of age and the 3rd dose at 6 months of age.
Infants born to mothers whose HBsAg status is unknown should receive hepatitis B vaccine within 12 hours of birth. Maternal blood should be drawn at the time of delivery to determine the mother's HBsAg status; if the HBsAg test is positive, the infant should receive HBIG as soon as possible (no later than 1 week of age).
All children and adolescents (through 18 years of age) who have not been immunized against hepatitis B may begin the series during any visit. Special efforts should be made to immunize children who were born in or whose parents were born in areas of the world with moderate or high endemicity of hepatitis B virus infection.

[3]DTaP (diphtheria and tetanus toxoids and acellular pertussis vaccine) is the preferred vaccine for all doses in the immunization series, including completion of the series in children who have received 1 or more doses of whole-cell DTP vaccine. Whole-cell DTP is an acceptable alternative to DTaP. The 4th dose (DTP or DTaP) may be administered as early as 12 months of age, provided 6 months have elapsed since the 3rd dose and if the child is unlikely to return at age 15–18 months. Td (tetanus and diphtheria toxoids) is recommended at 11–12 years of age if at least 5 years have elapsed since the last dose of DTP, DTaP or DT. Subsequent routine Td boosters are recommended every 10 years.

[4]Three *Haemophilus influenzae* type b (Hib) conjugate vaccines are licensed for infant use. If PRP-OMP (PedvaxHIB® or ComVax® [Merck]) is administered at 2 and 4 months of age, a dose at 6 months is not required. Because clinical studies in infants have demonstrated that using some combination products may induce a lower immune response to the Hib vaccine component, DTaP/Hib combination products should not be used for primary immunization in infants at 2, 4 or 6 months of age, unless FDA-approved for these ages.

[5]Two poliovirus vaccines currently are licensed in the United States: inactivated poliovirus (IPV) vaccine and oral poliovirus (OPV) vaccine. The ACIP, AAP and AAFP now recommend that the first two doses of poliovirus vaccine should be IPV. The ACIP continues to recommend a sequential schedule of two doses of IPV administered at ages 2 and 4 months, followed by two doses of OPV at 12–18 months and 4–6 years. Use of IPV for all doses also is acceptable and is recommended for immunocompromised persons and their household contacts.
OPV is no longer recommended for the first two doses of the schedule and is acceptable only for special circumstances such as: children of parents who do not accept the recommended number of injections, late initiation of immunization which would require an unacceptable number of injections, and imminent travel to polio-endemic areas. OPV remains the vaccine of choice for mass immunization campaigns to control outbreaks due to wild poliovirus.

[6]Rotavirus (Rv) vaccine is shaded and italicized to indicate: 1) health-care providers may require time and resources to incorporate this new vaccine into practice; and 2) the AAFP feels that the decision to use rotavirus vaccine should be made by the parent or guardian in consultation with their physician or other health care provider. The first dose of Rv vaccine should not be administered before 6 weeks of age, and the minimum interval between doses is 3 weeks. The Rv vaccine series should not be initiated at 7 months of age or older, and all doses should be completed by the first birthday.
Use of this vaccine was suspended on July 16, 1999 and in October, 1999 when this Manual went to press, no decision had been made about resumption of its use. The most current vaccine recommendations will be posted on the CDC immunization website: (http://www.cdc.gov/nip)

[7]The 2nd dose of measles, mumps, and rubella (MMR) vaccine is recommended routinely at 4–6 years of age but may be administered during any visit, provided at least 4 weeks have elapsed since receipt of the 1st dose and that both doses are administered beginning at or after 12 months of age. Those who have not previously received the second dose should complete the schedule by the 11–12 year old visit.

[8]Varicella (Var) vaccine is recommended at any visit on or after the first birthday for susceptible children, i.e. those who lack a reliable history of chickenpox (as judged by a health care provider) and who have not been immunized. Susceptible persons 13 years of age or older should receive 2 doses, given a least 4 weeks apart.